"The *Mad Studies Reader* brings the world of mental health together with the world of critical intellectual scholarship and activism. It is invaluable reading that works out the central problem of sanism in the way we treat mental differences. I have no doubt it will be an instant classic and a 'go to' resource for people in the mad pride movement, disability studies, health humanities, narrative medicine, arts for health, critical mental health, and anyone interested in the complexities of today's mental health concerns."

Danielle Spencer, PhD, *Program in Narrative Medicine, Columbia University and author of* Metagnosis: Revelatory Narratives of Health and Identity

"In the relentless quest for liberation, echoes have resonated through time— voices of scholars, storytellers, and activists narrating the tale of defiance. The *Mad Studies Reader* stands as a testament within the tapestry of social justice movements embroiled in this struggle for emancipation. For me, its arrival marks a critical juncture, a turning tide where the silenced voices of society's marginalized find amplification. Mad people being recognized as bearers of transformative wisdom capable of reshaping our world."

Vesper Moore, *Activist and host of* GET MAD! *podcast devoted to transformative mental health, mad pride, and disability justice*

"So many questions: Do medical models want to eradicate mental illness? What is anti-psychiatry? Could depression be poetry? What does epistemic justice look like for mental health? Does capitalism fuel mental illness? In response to these questions and many more, The *Mad Studies Reader* is what our futuristic-politociz ed-neurodivergent-justice-fueled-(re)educational process needs to look like."

Jennifer Mullan, PhD, *Psychotherapist and author of* Decolonizing Therapy: Oppression, Historical Trauma, and Politicizing your Practice

"A groundbreaking cornucopia of art, activism, and critical thought. Required reading for artists, students, scholars and anyone interested in mental health."

Jussi Valtonen, PhD, *Novelist and psychologist,* They Know Not What They Do

Mad Studies Reader

THE LAST FEW YEARS HAVE BROUGHT increased writings from activists, artists, scholars, and concerned clinicians that cast a critical and constructive eye on psychiatry, mental health care, and the cultural relations of mental difference. With particular focus on accounts of lived experience and readings that cover issues of epistemic and social injustice in mental health discourse, the *Mad Studies Reader* brings together voices that advance anti-sanist approaches to scholarship, practice, art, and activism in this realm.

Beyond offering a theoretical and historical overview of mad studies, this Reader draws on the perspectives, voices, and experiences of artists, mad pride activists, humanities and social science scholars, and critical clinicians to explore the complexity of mental life and mental difference. Voices from these groups confront and challenge standard approaches to mental difference. They advance new structures of meaning and practice that are inclusive of those who have been systematically subjugated and promote anti-sanist approaches to counter inequalities, prejudices, and discrimination. Confronting modes of psychological oppression and the power of a few to interpret and define difference for so many, the *Mad Studies Reader* asks the critical question of how these approaches may be reconsidered, resisted, and reclaimed.

This collection will be of interest to mental health clinicians; students and scholars of the arts, humanities and social sciences; and anyone who has been affected by mental difference, directly or indirectly, who is curious to explore new perspectives.

Bradley Lewis is a psychiatrist and psychotherapist with a background in the arts and humanities. He is Associate Professor at New York University's Gallatin School of Individualized Study and he is on the editorial board of the *Journal of Medical Humanities*. His books include *Moving Beyond Prozac, DSM, and the New Psychiatry: The Birth of Postpsychiatry*; *Narrative Psychiatry: How Stories Can*

Shape Clinical Encounters; and *Experiencing Epiphanies in Literature, Cinema, and Everyday Life* (forthcoming).

Alisha Ali is Associate Professor in the Department of Applied Psychology at New York University. Her research focuses on the mental health effects of oppression, including violence, racism, discrimination, and trauma. She is the co-editor of the book *Silencing the Self Across Cultures* (Oxford University Press) as well as the co-editor of *The Crisis of Connection* (NYU Press).

Jazmine Russell is the co-founder of the Institute for the Development of Human Arts (IDHA), a transformative mental health training institute, and host of Depth Work: A Holistic Mental Health Podcast. She is an interdisciplinary scholar of mad studies, critical psychology, and neuroscience, with experience working both within and outside the mental health system.

Mad

Studies

Reader

Interdisciplinary

Innovations in

Mental Health

Edited by

Bradley Lewis, Alisha Ali and Jazmine Russell

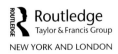
Routledge
Taylor & Francis Group

NEW YORK AND LONDON

Designed cover image: Jacks McNamara (www.jacksmcnamara.net)

First published 2025
by Routledge
605 Third Avenue, New York, NY 10158

and by Routledge
4 Park Square, Milton Park, Abingdon, Oxon, OX14 4RN

Routledge is an imprint of the Taylor & Francis Group, an informa business

Library of Congress Cataloging-in-Publication Data
Names: Lewis, Bradley, editor. | Ali, Alisha, editor. | Russell, Jazmine, editor.
Title: Mad studies reader : interdisciplinary innovations in mental health / edited by Bradley Lewis, Alisha Ali, and Jazmine Russell.
Description: New York, NY : Routledge, 2025. | Includes bibliographical references and index.
Identifiers: LCCN 2024020537 (print) | LCCN 2024020538 (ebook) | ISBN 9780367709099 (hardback) | ISBN 9780367709082 (paperback) | ISBN 9781003148456 (ebook)
Subjects: LCSH: Mental illness. | Mental health.
Classification: LCC RC454.4 .M26 2024 (print) | LCC RC454.4 (ebook) | DDC 616.89--dc23/eng/20240509
LC record available at https://lccn.loc.gov/2024020537
LC ebook record available at https://lccn.loc.gov/2024020538

ISBN: 9780367709099 (hbk)
ISBN: 9780367709082 (pbk)
ISBN: 9781003148456 (ebk)

DOI: 10.4324/9781003148456

Typeset in Perpetua
by Deanta Global Publishing Services, Chennai, India

Celia Brown – A relentless advocate, a fierce activist, and an inspiring embodiment of the mad pride movement. Celia died during the time we were developing this reader, but her legacy of resilience, compassion, and boundless love shine on as a beacon of hope for those who follow in her footsteps.

Messages in her memory from family, dearest friends, and colleagues are included in Chapter 37.

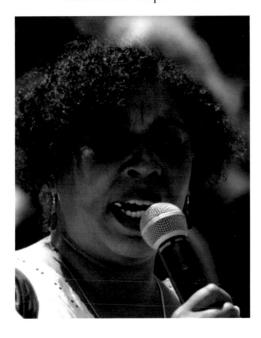

Contents

"Are You Conrad?" is a graphic narrative based on the 1980 Academy Award-winning film Ordinary People. *It investigates some of the many "juicy empowering choices" possible when one is going through times of psychic difference or trouble.*

The time of mad studies scholarship has arrived. The result is a flowering of mad studies work from a range of theoretical perspectives and positions. Mad studies scholar Erica Fletcher surveys this emerging scholarship and articulates some of its key themes, concerns, and tensions.

The rise of mad studies scholarship is fueled in no small part by the efforts of disability studies scholars. In this chapter, influential disability studies scholar Lennard Davis uses a biocultural and disability studies perspective to consider some of the many slips and slides from "obsession" in popular culture to "obsessive compulsive disorder" in manuals of psychopathology.

Hayley Stefan's chapter shows the value of mad studies for literary studies and humanities through a reading of Toni Morrison's Sula. At the same time, she shows the value of literary studies and humanities for mad studies.

La Marr Jurelle Bruce's chapter provides a poignant example of the way that scholarship at the intersection of mad studies, disability studies, and Black studies is flourishing in the humanities. Bruce uses this chapter to tease out overlapping meanings of "madness" needed to understand the power and provocation of Black radical art.

How does capitalism drive the mental health industry? What can be learned by exposing the inner workings of commercialism that shape psychiatric science? Using as their impetus philosopher Ian Hacking's guidance that "lively scholars do not stay still," Justin Karter, Lisa Cosgrove, and Farahdeba Herrawi argue that we can no longer afford to look the other way in the face of evidence of the profit-driven models that are rampant in the mental health field.

Many practitioners and consumers view spirituality as the core of their experience. Yet the mental health field has minimized the importance of individuals' spiritual lives. In this chapter, author and clinician Katrina Michelle guides the reader through an exploration of the spiritual as a ground for healing, growth, and self-understanding.

Marilyn Charles provides a psychoanalytic perspective that goes beyond Freud's early scientific and secular prejudice and dogmatism. She shows how innovative psychoanalytic approaches can be attuned to and supportive of experiences that can otherwise be personally overwhelming and socially ostracizing.

Bradley Lewis uses his chapter to rethink contemporary US psychiatry through a mad studies perspective. He provides an invitation to clinicians, even those working within dominant models, to move toward mad studies perspectives in their work.

Judi Chamberlin was a civil rights heroine who devoted her immense talent and passion to the cause of a more just world for mental difference. She took inspiration from other civil rights movements to help start something she liked to call mad pride—a movement for the rights and dignity of people diagnosable with mental illness.

The Icarus project was an activist and mutual-aid collective devoted to creating new languages and new communities around mental difference and diversity. Sascha DuBrul, one of the Icarus Project's cofounders, provides a window into its work and history.

In this chapter, Alberto Vásquez Encalada shares his experience as a former Peruvian congress member and researcher for the Office of the United Nations Special Rapporteur on the rights of persons with disabilities, fighting against coercion and navigating his own identity as a mad activist.

Introducing Mad Studies

OPHELIA: [sings]

And will he not come again?
And will he not come again?
No, no, he is dead.
Go to thy deathbed.
He never will come again.
His beard was as white as snow,
(All) flaxen was his pole.
He is gone, he is gone.
And we cast away moan.
God 'a mercy on his soul.
And of all Christians' souls, (I pray God.) God be wi' you. (*She exits.*)

Hamlet (4.5.212–24)

Mad studies scholarship, creative work, activism, and clinical reform are devoted to democratizing our understandings and practices surrounding mental difference and mental suffering.[1] Mad studies works against the grain of common approaches to mental life that organize these differences around a hierarchical binary of normal and pathological and that designate mental difference as "mental illness." The notion that mental difference is an "illness" or a "pathology" may at times be valuable, but it should not be the only option for considering mental difference. Many other options are possible, and the questions of mad studies are questions of playing fair with these options, opening up space for alternatives and diversity, and shifting the focus from "Who is right?" to "Who should decide?" which meaning-making options to choose.

To see the complexity and multiplicity of meaning-making in this domain consider the character of Ophelia in Shakespeare's *Hamlet* (Shakespeare, 1992). The song above contains the young Ophelia's last words. She is at the height of her troubles and recent losses, just before she dies in what seems like a passive suicide. She has come to the court, distraught and disheveled, to say goodbye to her family. She has not slept or been consoled, and she is wracked with despair. Laertes, her brother, stands aghast, calling her song a kind of "madness" (4.5.180). He laments the fragility of human lives and even our very minds, our "wits" (4.5.183). The king, a family

DOI: 10.4324/9781003148456-1

acquaintance, looks on with pity. He expounds that the "poison of deep grief" has caused her to become "divided from herself and her fair judgment" (4.5.80, 92).

After her song is complete, Ophelia goes outside by the willow tree and the brook to be alone, collect flowers, and chant old songs. She falls into the stream, but she does not try to save herself. She floats magically on the water at first, as though she and the water were a single unit. Tragically, as an eyewitness explains, it cannot last: "Her garments, heavy with their drink, pulled the poor wretch from her melodious lay to muddy death" (4.7.205–207). The church doctor diagnoses suicide and judges Ophelia harshly. But Laertes tells the doctor in no uncertain terms he is wrong to judge her so: "A minist'ring angel shall my sister be when thou liest howling [in hell]" (5.1.251–2).

If we consider the similarities between Ophelia's story and the ones we bring to mental health care today, how might we make sense of Ophelia's story? What variables could we use to begin the process? And how might Ophelia use these understandings to help take care of herself? Should our focus be on her grief and trauma as the king would recommend? And, if so, how far back should we go? Should we give attention to the immediate death of her father or the recent breakup with her boyfriend, or should we go back to her childhood and the loss of her mother? Perhaps, instead, we should look at Ophelia's story from an existential perspective. Perhaps her losses have put her in tune with the tragic edge of human existence. Perhaps she is reeling from having broken through our common denials of death.

Or perhaps we should not think in terms of grief or existentialism, which normalize her situation, but see Ophelia as suffering from an illness and a pathology. Perhaps we should argue that everyone suffers loss, so that alone cannot explain Ophelia's difference. Perhaps Ophelia harbors cognitive distortions that interfere with her ability to function in the world. Or maybe we should consider her song a symptom of biological abnormality. Perhaps we should dissect Ophelia's cadaver, open her brain, tease apart her neuronal circuits, and quantify her neurotransmitters? Perhaps Ophelia needed medication, neurosurgery, or electrical brain stimulation to treat her broken brain and chemical imbalances.

Or maybe we should go the other direction; perhaps we should see Ophelia as having a gift rather than a pathology. Perhaps, compared with others, she is more sensitive to the world and yearns more deeply than most for the world that could be. If so, perhaps we should not consider Ophelia in isolation but should consider her relationships and the familial and social world in which she lives. Perhaps we should see Ophelia's personal response as deeply connected to the political world in which she lives. Certainly, we know from the other characters that there is something rotten in Denmark—injustice, inequality, corruption, vice, toxic sexism. Perhaps these social problems will best help us understand Ophelia and perhaps, in the right circumstances, with support and community, Ophelia could be a social activist for a better world.

Or what about Ophelia's prayer at the end of her song? Perhaps the best variables for understanding Ophelia are in her religious and spiritual life. Perhaps Ophelia tunes in to the possibility of a higher spiritual consciousness and in other circumstances might be a spiritual teacher or a spiritual leader. Or, lastly, perhaps we should look to Ophelia's song itself to best understand. Perhaps Ophelia is best understood as an artist, someone who is in touch with the power of creativity. Perhaps, in different circumstances, she might be a kind of Shakespeare's sister and even write a drama as influential as *Hamlet* has become.

As if this array of questions were not daunting enough, we also must grapple with the question of which disciplines and interpretive communities we should work from in approaching this problem. Should it be a clinical discipline like psychology, psychiatry, psychoanalysis, or social work? Or should we think more in terms of culture or society and look to anthropology or sociology? Or maybe we should choose neuroscience or political science instead. Or perhaps we should avoid the "sciences" and look to the humanities or the arts. Maybe we should turn to history, philosophy, literature, or religious studies? Or perhaps music, or fiction, or drama, or painting? Or perhaps "disciplinary" thinking is more of a hindrance than a help. Perhaps the very structures that organize academic disciplines keep out or silence people who can really understand mental difference. Perhaps we must turn to interdisciplinary domains like gender studies, race studies, or disability studies. Or perhaps even these approaches to meaning-making are still too restrictive. Perhaps we must look to disability activists, mutual-aid groups, and mad pride communities who have organized around the common ground of lived-experience and the rallying cry of "Nothing about us without us!"

These questions take us into the complexity of mental life and mental difference and the need for a new kind of work in this domain. We, the editors of this volume, join with others to call this new kind of work "mad studies," and the *Mad Studies Reader* is about taking these kinds of questions seriously. Rather than close down uncertainty around mental difference, the *Mad Studies Reader* goes in the other direction. It opens up to the humility and the diversity of possibilities that so many questions can create.

From a mad studies perspective, what is even more striking than the complexity of meaning-making surrounding Ophelia is the anticomplexity—the narrowness and dogmatism—of cosmopolitan culture's standard approaches to mental difference. If Ophelia were to see a contemporary clinician, her experience would be quickly interpreted as a "mental illness." She would be diagnosed as having "Major depression with psychotic features" (*DSM-V* code 296.24, *ICD-10* code F32.3). She would likely be hospitalized and treated with a combination of antipsychotic and antidepressant medications, possibly electroconvulsive therapy. All this would be done against her will if necessary, using the courts to gain authorization to treat her over her protest if she was considered a danger to herself. Ophelia would most likely be told that she had a mental illness, a kind of medical condition, not unlike diabetes or high blood pressure, and that she would need to be treated for the rest of her life to avoid relapses.

For some of us, this response would be helpful, perhaps even deeply appreciated. Particularly so if Ophelia were able to use this kind of "treatment" to turn a corner beyond a suffering and tragic outcome. But, for many of us, this approach would be deeply off-putting and alienating. And, for a few, it would feel wrong, oppressive, and self-serving. For those of us in these last groups, this kind of treatment might not help at all. Indeed, if we are treated like the church "doctor" treated Ophelia, this kind of pathologizing, blame-the-victim response might generate outrage, trauma, add to Ophelia's problems, and even hasten tragic outcomes. Mad studies holds that this kind of narrowness and single-mindedness of interpretation of who we are in our difference and our suffering should be a source of deep critical concern. Human mental variance is too important to be left to a small group of authorities and experts who claim to tell us who we are in our difference.

Terminology

Before turning to a history of mad studies, let us say a word about terminology. As the above discussion implies, finding terms to talk about Ophelia's situation is difficult. If we use "mental illness," we assume from the beginning that Ophelia is medically ill. This overdetermines how we perceive Ophelia and leaves us unable to consider other possibilities. If we use "mental distress" or "mental suffering," we make it seem that she suffers all of the time or that her difference necessitates her suffering. Ophelia is clearly suffering in this scene, but it would not necessarily be so for Ophelia. If things had turned out differently, if the people around her had been more responsive to her concerns, or if she had found a way to navigate her difference in another way, she would not have suffered, or at least not in the same way and with the same consequences.

For these reasons, this reader tends to use the terms "mental difference" or "mental diversity." We also use "neurodiversity" and "cognitive diversity." And, of course, we use "mad," as in the term "mad studies." All these terms are more open-ended compared with "mental illness" or "brain disorders." The term "mad," although it takes a little getting used to, is particularly helpful because it facilitates a connection with the mad pride movement of activists, artists, and intellectuals who have followed in the footsteps of Black pride and gay pride to destabilize and reverse the binaries and hierarchies associated with mainstream psychiatry. In addition, "mad" is helpful because it evokes Foucault's work in *History of Madness* (2006), which tracks historical shifts in the terms used to understand psychic differences and the dividing practices associated with the language of mental difference. For Foucault, "mad" speaks to the variability of what we now call psychiatric knowledge and practice over time, and to the possibility that we might do things otherwise in the future. Finally, "mad" is often used by memoir writers to evoke aspects of psychic difference, suffering, and unusual states of consciousness that cannot be reached through a more sanitized and scientific language.[2]

A History of Critique

The history of deep concern and critical response to modern clinical disciplines is not new and goes back to the entire history of these fields. To highlight some examples from the United States alone, in 1886, Mrs. Elizabeth Ware Packard, a former mental hospital patient and the founder of the Anti-Insane Asylum Society, began publishing a series of books and pamphlets critical of psychiatry. Packard's writings challenged the subordination of women to their husbands and the remarkable complicity of the political and psychiatric establishment in this subordination (Packard, 1868, 1874). Historian Gerald Grob explains that "when Packard refused to play the role of obedient [minister's] wife and expressed religious ideas bordering on mysticism, her husband had her committed in 1860 to the Illinois State Hospital for the Insane" (Grob, 1994, p. 84). Packard remained incarcerated for three years and won her freedom only by going to court to challenge her confinement. She spent the next 20 years campaigning for personal liberty laws that would protect individuals from wrongful commitment and retention in asylums.

In the 1970s, reactions like Packard's began to coalesce in an activist movement that we think of today as "the mad pride movement." Mad pride activists during these years gained momentum from the civil rights movement, the women's movement, and the early stages of the gay and lesbian movement and the disability movement. Like Elizabeth Packard almost a century before, mad pride activists were motivated primarily by their negative treatment within the psychiatric system. Early founders of the movement shared common experiences of being treated with disrespect, disregard, and discrimination at the hands of psychiatry. Many also suffered from unjustified confinement, verbal and physical abuse, and exclusion from treatment decisions.

Leonard Roy Frank, cofounder of the Network Against Psychiatric Assault in 1972, provides insight into the experiences of many. After graduating from Wharton, Frank moved to San Francisco to sell commercial real estate. He was, in his own words, "an extraordinarily conventional person" (Farber, 1993, p. 191). Gradually he started discovering a new world within himself and began going through a "clash between … my emerging self and … my old self" (p. 191). He went through what he thought of as a "spiritual transformation." He lost his job, grew a beard, became a vegetarian, and devoted himself to full-time spiritual exploration. Frank was exhilarated by the process, but his parents thought he was having a "breakdown." They arranged an involuntary hospital commitment and Frank's psychiatrists documented symptoms of "not working, withdrawal, growing a beard, becoming a vegetarian, bizarre behavior, negativism, strong beliefs, piercing eyes, and religious preoccupations" (p. 193). They diagnosed him as having "paranoid schizophrenia" and started a sustained course of court-authorized insulin-electroshock treatments that lasted nine months and included 50 insulin comas and 35 electroshocks.

Frank came to realize that hospital resistance was futile, and, with the ever-increasing numbers of shock treatments, he also came to fear he was in a "life or death" situation: "These so-called [shock] treatments literally wiped out all my memory for the [previous] two-year period. … I realized that my high-school and college were all but gone; educationally, I was at about the eighth-grade level." Rather than risk more "treatments," Frank surrendered. He played the psychiatrists' game and did what they wanted: "I shaved voluntarily, ate some non-vegetarian foods like clam chowder and eggs, was somewhat sociable, and smiled 'appropriately' at my jailers" (p. 196). After his release, it took him six years to recover from his treatment. But he never gave up on his beliefs and he never saw another psychiatrist for treatment. He went on to become a major figure in early mad pride activism.

During the early 1970s, people like Frank began to recognize they were not alone and started organizing local consciousness-raising groups. This included the Insane Liberation Front in Portland, Oregon (1970), the Mental Patients' Liberation Project in New York City (1971), and the Mental Patients' Liberation Front in Boston (1971). These groups built support programs, advocated for hospitalized patients, lobbied for changes in the laws, and educated the public through guest lectures and newsletters. In addition, they began the process of developing alternative, creative, and artistic ways of dealing with emotional suffering and psychological difference outside the medical models of psychiatry. The publication of mad pride activist Judi Chamberlin's book *On Our Own* (1977) in the mainstream press was a milestone in the development of peer-run alternatives (Van Tosh & del Vecchio, 2000, p. 9). Chamberlin used the book to expose her own abuse at the hands of psychiatry and to give a detailed account of burgeoning consumer-run alternatives. The eloquence, optimism, and timing of the book were critical catalysts for many in the movement. As ex-patient Mary O'Hagan puts it:

> When my mood swings died away I was angry and amazed at how the mental health system could be so ineffective. There had to be a better way. I searched the library not quite knowing what I was looking for. And there it was, a book called *On Our Own* by Judi Chamberlin. It was all about ex-patients who set up their own alternatives to the mental health system and it set me on my journey into the psychiatric survivor movement.

> (Quoted in Chamberlin, 1977, back cover)

The newly formed local mad pride groups also organized the then annual Conference on Human Rights and Psychiatric Oppression to help connect local members with the wider movement. At these meetings, activists from across the country gathered to socialize, strategize, and share experiences. They gained solidarity and increasing momentum from being with like-minded activists. Between meetings, local groups communicated through a newspaper forum. The San Francisco local newsletter, *Madness Network News*, evolved into a newspaper format that covered ex-patient activities across North America and around the world. This publication became the major voice of the movement, each issue containing a rich selection of personal memoirs, creative writing, cartoons, humor, art, political commentary, and factual reporting—all from the ex-patient's point of view (Chamberlin, 1990, p. 327; Hirsch, 1974; see also Chamberlin's article in the Daring Activists section).

This early period of the mad pride movement was also the most radical in its epistemological critique. Leaders drew philosophical support from high-profile critical writers who, as a group, came to be known as "antipsychiatry." Writers such as Erving Goffman (1961), R. Laing (1967), Thomas Scheff (1966), and Thomas Szasz (1961) may have differed widely in their philosophies, but collectively their main tenets were clear: mental illness is not an objective medical reality but rather a strategy for coping in a mad world. As Laing (1968) put it, and one can see an obviously viable way of understanding Ophelia here, "the apparent irrationality of the single 'psychotic' individual" may often be understood "within the context of the family." And, in turn, the irrationality of the family can be understood if it is placed "within the context of yet larger organizations and institutions." Put in context in this way, madness has a legitimacy of its own, which is erased by medical-model approaches that can only pathologize it (Lewis, 2017). For many antipsychiatry writers, mental suffering can be the beginning of a healing process and should not be suppressed through aggressive behavioral or biological interventions.

The most epistemologically radical of the antipsychiatry writers, Thomas Szasz, had the strongest influence on US activists (see the Critical Scholars section for a sample of Szasz's writings). Szasz, a dissident psychiatrist, was shunned within his own field, but his prolific writings (over 25 books) and forceful prose gave him tremendous influence outside psychiatry (Leifer, 1997). Throughout his work, Szasz's argument was always twofold: (1) mental illness is a myth and (2) there should be a complete separation between psychiatry and the state. As Szasz (1998) put it in a summary statement:

> Involuntary mental hospitalization is imprisonment under the guise of treatment; it is a covert form of social control that subverts the rule of law. No one ought to be deprived of liberty except for a criminal offense, after a trial by jury guided by legal rules of evidence. No one ought to be detained against their will in a building called "hospital," or any other medical institution, on the basis of expert opinion.

Szasz based his criticism on a strong positivist philosophy of science that emphasized a sharp demarcation between observation and conjecture. For Szasz, *physical illness* was real because it was based on actual observation, but *mental illness* was at best a metaphor. A broken leg is real because you can see the X-ray, but a "broken brain" is a myth because there is no X-ray that will show it. Szasz argued that to see mental illness as "real" rather than as a metaphorical myth is to make a serious category error that opens the door to authoritarian control.

From Antipsychiatry to Mad Studies

Antipsychiatry's critique has been deeply influential for the mad pride movement and for popular culture and mainstream mental health care as well. The blockbuster film *One Flew Over the Cuckoo's Nest*, which won five Oscars in 1975, is a good marker of antipsychiatry's popular influence. Randle McMurphy, played by Jack Nicholson, arranges to have himself transferred from prison to a psychiatric ward in the belief that he will be better treated. But, rather than being treated better, by the end of the film, McMurphy is brutally lobotomized. The antipsychiatry perspective is powerfully portrayed in the film and the message resonates across popular culture: mental illness is not real but a label used to coerce nonconformists. As sociologists Mayes and Horowitz (2005) put it, "The antipsychiatry critics were not marginal eccentrics but major figures in an intellectually prominent counterculture. They found a receptive audience with many college students, intellectuals, and the anti-authority ethos of the time" (p. 252).

Inside mental health care, the influence of antipsychiatry contributed to a growing crisis of legitimization that by 1980 resulted in a major response. The American Psychiatric Association, attempting to be as rigorous as possible, published the *Diagnostic and Statistical Manual (DSM-III)*, which went on to have a major impact on the field. Leading psychiatrists at the time hailed the *DSM-III* as a revolutionary book that would lead "to a massive reorganization and modernization of psychiatric diagnosis" (Andreason, 1984, p. 155). Historian Edwin Shorter (1997) confirmed this theme years later when he argued that the *DSM-III* signaled "a redirection of the discipline toward a scientific course" (p. 302). This redirection brought a heightened emphasis on biomedical models and pharmacological interventions. It shifted the psychiatric gaze, particularly in outpatient settings, from psychoanalytically framed unconscious conflicts, unresolved griefs, and childhood traumas to biomedically framed broken brains and chemical imbalances.

Interestingly, 1980 also heralded the decline of antipsychiatry as the leading edge of mad pride movement criticism because of the way the *DSM-III* crafted an influential counterresponse. Antipsychiatrists had argued that psychiatry was problematic because it represented a false consciousness (a socially constructed myth that distorted the truth of psychic life) and because it was an illegitimate form of social control and coercion. *DSM-III* authors pulled the sting out of both of these criticisms by co-opting antipsychiatry concerns and providing a seemingly scientific solution. *DSM-III* authors agreed in principle, if not in manifest approval, that the psychiatric diagnoses of old were unreliable and intertwined with false (mostly psychoanalytic, from their point of view) theories that did not hold up to scrutiny. As a result, diagnosis *could* function as an illegitimate form of social control. These two problems became the grounds on which that group offered the new *DSM-III*, which, they claimed, would fix these problems by creating an operational and scientific classification system that assured both truth and value neutrality, and therefore legitimacy. Through this tactic, *DSM-III* authors successfully diverted antipsychiatry arguments, and the energy of this wave of psychiatric critique began to dissipate.

It is important to add that the pharmaceutical industry played a pivotal role in this story and 1980 marks a watershed moment for the pharmaceutical industry as well. That was the year Ronald Reagan was elected and it signifies a time of increasing neoliberal deregulation and the unleashing of corporate profiteering. That year also initiated the "decade of greed," and the pharmaceutical industry exploded during that time. Marcia Angell (2004), former editor of the *New England Journal of Medicine*, points out that 1980 was the year the pharmaceutical industry transitioned from a good business to the colossus we know today. "From 1960 to 1980, prescription drug sales were fairly static ... but from 1980 to 2000, they tripled," hitting over 200 billion dollars by 2002 (p. 3). The primary strategy of pharmaceutical growth during these latter decades has been the aggressive promotion of "lifestyle" drugs for chronic conditions (arthritis, hypertension, cholesterol, diabetes, allergies, heartburn, and psychiatric conditions) (Dumit, 2012). The new scientific psychiatry fit perfectly into this business plan and psychiatry's shift toward a biomedical model and was invaluable to big pharma's fortunes. The pharmaceutical industry used a version of the *DSM-III* message to promote drug research and medical interventions into psychic life, which effectively remade psychiatric training and practice. Without a pharmaceutical push, it is unlikely that the *DSM-III* would have transformed the field as dramatically as it did.[3]

But the mad pride movement and the corresponding critique of mental health care does not end with the *DSM-III*. Instead, we see a shift in the underlying philosophical perspectives away from antipsychiatry and toward mad studies during this time. Indeed, it is possible to see mad studies as critical work on psychiatry and mainstream mental health practices that emerged after *DSM-III* and after antipsychiatry. What is perhaps most important to understand about the shift to mad studies compared with antipsychiatry is the move away from binary models of epistemology and human values. Mad studies does not rest on the binaries of propsychiatry versus antipsychiatry nor on the related binaries of truth versus myth, right versus wrong, or good versus bad. Instead, mad studies rests on questions of democracy and interpretive choice. Who is included in the creation of psychiatric knowledge(s) and practices? Who is excluded? Why are these inclusions and exclusions created? How can we open up our knowledges and practices surrounding mental difference to a greater diversity of perspectives? How can we include more disciplines, more methods of knowing, more points of view, and more approach alternatives? And, most importantly, how can we include the perspectives of the key stakeholders, those of us who are impacted by these knowledges, and those of us who are most unhappy and aggrieved with how the knowledges and practices have emerged?

Sanism

These democracy-driven questions are organized, at their heart, around the logics of sanism. Mad studies is antisanist in the way that gender studies is antisexist, race studies is antiracist, and disability studies is anti-ableist. In that way, mad studies is antidiscriminatory more than it is "antipsychiatry." Mad studies, like gender studies, race studies, and disability studies, is a form of engaged scholarship and engaged meaning-making. Its goal is to make the world a better place for those of us who have been, or could be, labeled mentally ill. The target of mad studies criticism is therefore not psychiatry, science, pharmaceuticals, hospitals, particular mental health models, or the mental health system per se. The targets are oppression, subordination, and discrimination. The target is injustice. None of this means that mad studies never uses binaries or that it never has a place for antipsychiatry perspectives or propsychiatry perspectives. It means only that mad studies does not rest on these either/or logics as the sole foundation of its approach. It rests on democracy and justice.

The failure of democracy and the emergence of discrimination run deep in mainstream mental health approaches. These domains, sometimes called the "psy" domains, harbor exclusive knowledge-making practices that lead to epistemic injustice and reinforce sanist oppression. As the philosopher Miranda Fricker (2007) articulates, epistemic injustice is a form of injustice that affects us in "our most basic everyday practices: conveying knowledge to others by telling them, and making sense of our own social experiences" (p. 1). LeBlanc and Kinsella (2016) bring this perspective to the mad movement, pointing out that epistemic injustice is an insult and a wrong performed against people in their very capacity as knowers. As they explain, "If it is our ability to *know* that makes us distinctly human, as has been suggested, it is no wonder that the 'powerful' have historically undermined, insulted, or otherwise wronged the 'powerless' in this capacity, as a means for denouncing their humanity" (p. 61).

LeBlanc and Kinsella go on to argue that "epistemic injustice is inextricably linked with social and political injustice" (p. 61). This resonates with Judi Chamberlin's (2002) mad pride perspective:

> A basic premise of the disability rights movement is simply this: Nothing About Us Without Us. ... Just as women would not accept the legitimacy of a commission of "expert" men to define women's needs, or ethnic and racial minorities would not accept a panel of "expert" white people to define their needs, we similarly see [exclusive, expert-driven approaches to mental health] as basically irrelevant to our struggle to define our own needs.

Chamberlin was an early advocate of the use of terms that go beyond "stigma" to characterize this kind of oppression. She used the term "mentalism," disability activists use the term "ableism," and more recently there has been increasing use of the term "sanism" (Perlin, 1992; Poole et al., 2012). All of these terms do something that the term "stigma" tends not to do. They bring out critical anti-oppression perspectives that go beyond individual cognitive labeling to focus on larger power dynamics at the institutional and social/cultural levels (Holley et al., 2012). Holley et al. provide examples of focus at these larger levels, including language, representation, norms, rituals, traditions, practices, institutions (schools, businesses, workplaces, religion, housing, research, media, the arts), and systems/structures (legal, medical, mental health, political, economic).

Fricker (2007) points out two levels of epistemic injustice—testimonial injustice (where people's perspectives are discredited because of identity prejudice) and hermeneutical injustice (where larger structures of knowledge, practice, and institutional organization prejudice ways of knowing and being). This distinction is important because, although there has been some movement in mental health systems to reduce prejudice at the testimonial level—through emerging clinical models such as "open dialogue" or "narrative psychiatry"—these approaches have limited reach beyond individual encounters (Lewis, 2011; Seikkula, 2005). They are largely applicable to what Katheryn Pauly Morgan (1998) has called "micro-institutionalization" of oppressive frames through clinician-patient relations (see Figure 0.1). They do not effectively address larger, hermeneutic-level injustice, which Morgan calls "conceptualization" and "macro-institutionalization."

To reach these larger structures of meaning and practice around mental difference, we need larger-level responses. That is where mad studies comes in. Mad studies is an interdisciplinary approach to mental difference that is deeply conscious of

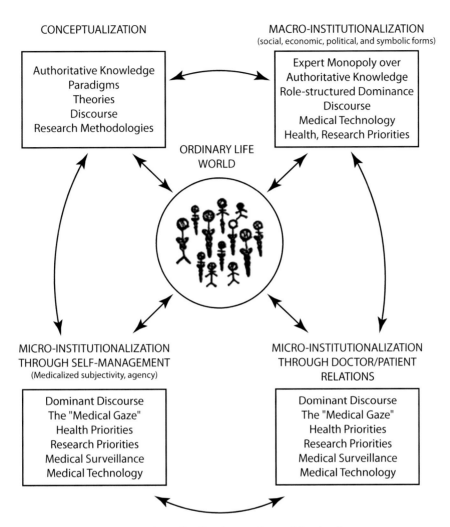

CONCEPTUALIZATION

Authoritative Knowledge
Paradigms
Theories
Discourse
Research Methodologies

MACRO-INSTITUTIONALIZATION
(social, economic, political, and symbolic forms)

Expert Monopoly over
Authoritative Knowledge
Role-structured Dominance
Discourse
Medical Technology
Health, Research Priorities

ORDINARY LIFE
WORLD

MICRO-INSTITUTIONALIZATION
THROUGH SELF-MANAGEMENT
(Medicalized subjectivity, agency)

Dominant Discourse
The "Medical Gaze"
Health Priorities
Research Priorities
Medical Surveillance
Medical Technology

MICRO-INSTITUTIONALIZATION
THROUGH DOCTOR/PATIENT
RELATIONS

Dominant Discourse
The "Medical Gaze"
Health Priorities
Research Priorities
Medical Surveillance
Medical Technology

Figure 0.1   Structures of medicalization and psychiatrization.
Source: Morgan, K. P. 1998, Contested bodies, contested knowledges: Women, health, and the politics of medicalization. In *The politics of women's health: Exploring agency and autonomy,* ed. S. Sherwin 83–122. Philadelphia: Temple Univ. Press. Reprinted with permission.

the problems of sanism and that works to combat social oppression through the creation of new structures of meaning and practice. These structures are inclusive of perspectives that have been systematically subjugated, and they engage with power dynamics, structural levels of analysis, and the promotion of social justice that have been invisible in most structures of knowledge production around mental difference.

Our goal with this edited volume is to bring together voices that advance antisanist approaches to scholarship, practice, art, and activism in the mental health realm. We aim to reach participants in the mad movement and mental health clinicians, but also community organizers, policymakers, researchers, and others who are invested in integrating neurodiversity and perspectives of mental difference into psychiatric discourse and practice. We also hope to reach those who have not before considered the ways that mainstream mental health care is too often predicated on discriminatory—and even abusive—theories, practices, and assumptions.

Overview of Sections and Conclusion

The best way to understand mad studies and its move toward democracy is through immersion in the world of mad studies. This means sitting down at the table of this emerging conversation and hearing the language being spoken. In the service of that goal, we have divided the reader into four sections that reflect four areas where this work has emerged. From our perspective, mad studies contributions often come from the work of

- Innovative Artists
- Critical Scholars
- Concerned Clinicians
- Daring Activists

These four subcultures of mad studies are often fragmented from one another, and the people involved are often separated from one another. The *Mad Studies Reader* works against this fragmentation to build a larger coalition of voices devoted to mad studies. At the same time, these four domains have to be held lightly, since many of our contributors identify across domains and create hybrid identities not captured by these categories. In that way, we offer these groupings for heuristic purposes only. The reader can easily be approached in any order. We start with the arts since, as we saw with Shakespeare's Ophelia, the arts can provide an invaluable opening to alternative perspectives and possibilities.

Collectively, mad studies advocates are fighting, often against tremendous odds, to reduce individualization, psychiatrization, and sanist approaches to psychic life. The work is arduous and at times a little "mad," but the stakes are high, and the struggle must continue. With the increasing coalition with the broader disability movement, the fight is becoming more and more mainstream. Soon the battle will be one about which we all know and in which we can all participate.

The editors of *Adbusters* summed up their early work on mad pride (20 years ago), with a call for a big-tent approach to a sanist world. As we see it, their conclusion is as accurate now as it was then. In a "normal" world of hardening inequality, greed, status, materialism, conflict, war, pandemic, and environmental degradation, a world not unlike Ophelia's:

> Mad Pride can be a broad embrace. It is a signal that we will allow ourselves our deep sorrow, our manic hope, or fierce anxiety, our imperfect rage. These will be our feedback into the system. We reserve the right to seek relief from both our most troubling symptoms and from society's most punitive norms. The sickness runs deep; without madness, there is no hope of cure.
>
> ("Deep sadness, manic hope," 2002)

Notes

1 For key mad studies references, see the following: Andersen et al., "Mad Resistance/Mad Alternatives"; Beresford and Russo, *The Routledge International Handbook of Mad Studies*; Burstow, LeFrançois, & Diamond, *Psychiatry Disrupted;* Davis, *Disability Studies Reader*; DuBrul, "The Icarus Project"; Green & Ubozoh, *We've Been Patient Too Long;* Hall, *Outside Mental Health: Voices and Visions of Madness*; LeFrancois, Menzies, & Reaume, *Mad Matters*; Lewis, "A Mad Fight"; Mad in America website; Ostrander & Henderson, *Disability and Madness*; Price, *"Defining Mental Disability";* Russo and Sweeney, *Searching for a Rose Garden;* and Spandler, Anderson, & Sapey, *Madness, Distress, and the Politics of Disablement*.

2 See Perring, "'Madness' and 'Brain Disorders': Stigma and Language," for a helpful review of the term "madness" and its use in memoir writing. Sample memoirs Perring considers include *The Loony-Bin Trip; Madness: A Bipolar Life; An Unquiet Mind: A Memoir of Moods and Madness; Brilliant Madness: Living with Manic Depressive Illness; The Quiet Room: A Journey Out of the Torment of Madness; Mad House: Growing Up in the Shadow of Mentally Ill Siblings; Beyond Crazy: Journeys Through Mental Illness; Out of Her Mind: Women Writing on Madness;* and *Crazy: A Father's Search Through America's Mental Health Madness*.

3 For the role of the pharmaceutical industry, see Dumit, *Drugs for Life*; Healy, *Pharmageddon*; Matheson, "Corporate Science and the Husbandry of Scientific and Medical Knowledge by the Pharmaceutical Industry"; Rose, "Neurochemical Selves"; and Sismondo & Green, *Pharmaceutical Studies Reader*. Also, another important player in the transition to biopsychiatry is the insurance industry's use of managed care to control costs (which often ended up in synergistic biopsychiatric models). For a discussion see Luhrmann, *Of Two Minds*, particularly her chapter "The Crisis of Managed Care."

References

Andersen, J., Altwise, E., Bossewitch, J., Brown, C., Cole, K., & Weber, C. L. (2017). Mad resistance/mad alternatives: Democratizing mental health care. In S. Rosenberg & J. Rosenberg (Eds.), *Community mental health: Challenges for the 21st century* (pp. 19–36). Routledge.

Andreason, N. (1984). *The broken brain: The biological revolution in psychiatry*. Harper and Row.

Angell, M. (2004). *The truth about drug companies: How they deceive us and what to do about it*. Random House.

Beresford, P., & Russo, J. (Eds.). (2022). *The Routledge international handbook of mad studies*. Routledge.

Burstow, B., LeFrançois, B. A., & Diamond, S. (Eds.). (2014). *Psychiatry disrupted: Theorizing resistance and crafting the (r)evolution*. McGill-Queen's University Press.

Chamberlin, J. (1977). *On our own: Patient-controlled alternatives to the mental health system*. National Empowerment Center.

Chamberlin, J. (1990). The ex-patients' movement: Where we've been and where we are going. *Journal of Mind and Behavior 11* (3 & 4), 323–336.

Chamberlin, J. (2002). *Testimony of Judi Chamberlin*. American Association of People with Disabilities Online. Retrieved June 17, 2005, from http://www.aapd-dc.org/News/disability/testjudichamberlin.html

Davis, L. (2016). *Disability studies reader*. Routledge.

Deep sadness, manic hope: A movement for liberty, and the pursuit of madness. (2002). *Adbusters* (10), 3.

DuBrul, S. (2014). The Icarus project: A counter narrative for psychic diversity. *Journal of Medical Humanities, 35*, 257–271.

Dumit, J. (2012). *Drugs for life: How the pharmaceutical industry defines our health*. Duke University Press.

Farber, S. (1993). From victim to revolutionary: An interview with Lennard Frank. In *Madness, heresy, and the rumor of angels: The revolt against the mental health system* (pp. 90-240). Open Court.

Foucault, M. (2006). *History of madness*. Routledge.

Fricker, M. (2007). *Epistemic injustice: Power and the ethics of knowing*. Oxford University Press.

Goffman, E. (1961). *Asylums: Essays on the social situation of mental patients and other inmates*. Doubleday.

Gorman, R. & LeFrancois, B. A. (2017). Mad studies. In B. Cohen (Ed.), *Routledge international handbook of critical mental health* (pp. 108–114). Routledge.

Green, L. D., & Ubozoh, K. (2019). *We've been patient too long: Voices from radical mental health*. North Atlantic Books.

Grob, G. (1994). *The mad among us: A history of the care of America's mentally ill*. Harvard University Press.

Hall, W. (2016). *Outside mental health: Voices and visions of madness*. Madness Radio.

Healy, D. (2012). *Pharmageddon*. University of California Press.

Hirsch, S. (Ed.). (1974). *Madness network news reader*. Glide Publications.

Holley, L., Stromwall, L., & Bashor, K. (2012). Reconceptualizing stigma: Toward a critical anti-oppression paradigm. *Stigma Research and Action, 2*(2), 51–61.

Laing, R. D. (1967). *The politics of experience*. Ballantine.

Laing, R. D. (1968). The obvious. In D. Cooper (Ed.), *The dialectics of liberation*. Penguin.

Leblanc, S., & Kinsella, E. (2016). Toward epistemic justice: A critically reflexive examination of "sanism" and implications for knowledge generation. *Studies in Social Justice, 10*(1), 59–78.

LeFrancois, B. A, Menzies, R., & Reaume, G. (Eds.). (2013). *Mad matters: A critical reader in Canadian mad studies*. Canadian Scholars Press.

Leifer, R. (1997). The psychiatric repression of Dr. Thomas Szasz: Its social and political significance. *Review of Existential Psychology and Psychiatry, XXIII*(1, 2 & 3), 85–107.

Lewis, B. (2011). *Narrative psychiatry: How stories can shape clinical practice*. John's Hopkins Press.

Lewis, B. (2013). A mad fight: Psychiatry and disability activism. In L. Davis (Ed.), *The disability studies reader* (4th ed.). Routledge.

Lewis, B. (2017). A deep ethics for mental difference and disability: The case of Vincent van Gogh. *Medical Humanities, 43*, 172–176.

Luhrmann, T. M. (2000). *Of two minds: An anthropologist looks at American psychiatry*. Vintage Books.

Mad in America. (2019). https://www.madinamerica.com/

Matheson, A. (2008). Corporate science and the husbandry of scientific and medical knowledge by the pharmaceutical industry. *BioSocieties, 3*, 355–382.

Mayes, R., & Horowitz, A. (2005). *DSM-III* and the revolution in the classification of mental illness. *Journal of the History of the Behavioral Sciences, 41*(3), 249–267.

Morgan, K. P. (1998). Contested bodies, contested knowledges: Women, health, and the politics of medicalization. In S. Sherwin (Ed.), *The politics of women's health: Exploring agency and autonomy* (pp. 83–122). Temple University Press.

Ostrander, N., & Henderson, B. (Eds.). (2013). Special issue: Disability and madness. *Disability Studies Quarterly, 33*(1).

Packard, E. (1868). *The prisoner's hidden life, or insane asylums unveiled: As demonstrated by the report of the investigating committee of the legislature of Illinois.* Published by the Author, A. B. Case.

Packard, E. (1874). *Modern persecutions, or married woman's liabilities.* Case, Lockwood, & Brainard.

Perlin, M. L. 1992. On "sanism." *Southern Methodist University Law Review, 46,* 373–407.

Perring, C. (2009). "Madness" and "brain disorders": Stigma and Language. In Kimberly White (Ed.), *Configuring madness: Representation, context and meaning.* Rodopi Press.

Poole, J. M., Jivraj, T., Arslanian, A., Bellows, K., Chiasson, S., Hakimy, H., & Reid, J. (2012). Sanism, 'mental health,' and social work/education: A review and call to action. *Intersectionalities: A Global Journal of Social Work Analysis, Research, Polity, and Practice, 1,* 20–36.

Price, M. (2013). Defining mental disability. In L. Davis (Ed.), *Disability studies reader.* Routledge.

Rose, N. (2003, November/December). Neuorchemical selves. *Society,* pp. 46–59.

Russo, J., & Sweeney, A. (2016). *Searching for a rose garden: Challenging psychiatry, fostering mad studies.* PCCS Books.

Scheff, T. (1966). *Being mentally ill.* Aldine.

Seikkula, J. (2005). Open dialogue integrates individual and systemic approaches in serious psychiatric cases. In Anita Lightburn & Phebe Sessions (Eds.), *Handbook of community based clinical practices* (pp. 502–529). Oxford University Press.

Shakespeare, W. (1992). *The tragedy of Hamlet Prince of Denmark.* Folger Shakespeare Library. Simon and Shuster.

Shorter, E. (1997). *A history of psychiatry: From the era of the asylum to the age of Prozac.* John Wiley and Sons.

Sismondo, S., & Green, J. (2015). *Pharmaceutical studies reader.* John Wiley and Sons.

Spandler, H., Anderson, J, & Sapey, B. (2015). *Madness, distress, and the politics of disablement.* Bristol University Press.

Szasz, T. (1961). *The myth of mental illness: Foundations of a theory of personal conduct.* Hoeber-Harper.

Szasz, T. (1998). *Thomas Szasz's summary statement and manifesto.* Retrieved July 20, 2005, from http://www.szasz.com/manifesto.html

Van Tosh, L., & del Vecchio, P. (2000). *Consumer-operated and self-help programs: A technical report.* U.S. Center for Mental Health Services.

Part I. Innovative Artists

DOI: 10.4324/9781003148456-2

WE COULD BEGIN THE *MAD STUDIES READER* with any of the four subgroups: innovative artists, critical scholars, concerned clinicians, or daring activists. We chose to start with art because it provides an ideal opportunity to see the world aslant. The arts can open new perspectives and new possibilities. They can help us step out of our usual frames so we can imagine, practice, embody, study, support, and lobby for new alternatives. Achieving this kind of opening-out of our usual ways of approaching mental difference is absolutely necessary for mad studies, because to understand mad studies is to understand the world afresh. Immersion in the *Mad Studies Reader* artwork unleashes our minds and provides nuance, complexity, and richness to our usual world views. Spending time with this work liberates us from the boxinations of our normative thinking and feeling around mental life. This is possible because many of the artists in this section self-identify with "lived experiences" that can be, or have been, labeled "mental illness." But they are living and expressing these experiences anew.

We could call this section "mad art" except that *all art is mad art*. All art, in other words, works with the full range of human experience. It is only through the lens of social structures—like the mental health system and the way the system bleeds into culture—that we label and separate some human experiences as normal and others as pathological. Artists bring their reactions to the mental health system into their art, but as artists, they are not mad or sane. They are simply artists working to bring into artistic configuration their experience and imagination. To be an artist, or to enter into an artistic world as an audience, is to have the potential to leave behind a world where hegemonic and sanist tags of "normal" and "abnormal" rule the roost. It is to enter a world that can equally value the dynamic flux and flow of the many experiences of life, beyond clunky binaries and hierarchies. It is to enter a world that Jacks McNamara (one of the contributing artists in this section and the cover artist for the *Mad Studies Reader*) calls the world of "lilies and urine" (Rosenthal, 2010). Bringing "lilies and urine" together allows an embrace of the world in all its complexity—without expectation of pure or impure, beautiful or spoiled, cleanliness or clarity, normality or pathology, sweet or stench.

That said, the arts are invaluable not only to introduce mad studies, but also because of the transformative cultural work they can do. The world we experience of mental difference and mental diversity does not come with pre-labeled tags and categories. It is through our personal, cultural, and political choices that we label and we organize the grids and hierarchies of meaning through which we understand ourselves and one another. This hierarchical grid helps create and reinforce sanist norms, expectations, and structures of inclusion and exclusion. These labels and hierarchies become the background assumptions of our everyday experiences and practices. They structure and constrain our self-and-other identifications. Mad studies, as a field, critiques problematic aspects of these background assumptions and affirms additional possibilities and options. The arts join in this cultural work in multiple ways.

To appreciate the cultural work of the arts in mad studies, it helps to have an aesthetic theory that combines philosophical hermeneutics and cultural studies. *Philosophical hermeneutics* tells us that artists create from their embedded and prefigured understandings of the world (Ricoeur, 1998; Sirowy, 2015). Artists create a configured work of art by combining their craft with their prefigured understandings. This configured artwork contains meanings, affects, percepts, and worldviews with which the audience engages and interacts. Through the aesthetic encounter, the audience can use the artwork to refigure their meanings, affects, percepts, and worldviews. The audience, in other words, can emerge from the artistic encounter with new understandings and new ways to experience the world. *Cultural studies* adds the understanding that aesthetic encounters are not just individual phenomena—they are also part of the larger circuits of culture (Fornas, 2017; Johnson et al., 2004). The arts not only help shape personal identifications, but they also feed into the cultural formations in which new art is made and released. The arts, as a result, become an invaluable source of both personal and cultural understanding and transformation (see Figure P.1 for a simplified illustration).

This model helps us understand how the arts have entered into therapeutic practice as well as how the arts have a role in personal and social transformation beyond therapeutic practice. Starting with therapeutic practice, the expressive arts therapies and creative arts therapies (such as art therapy, music therapy, dance therapy, drama therapy, and poetry therapy) combine the therapeutic process with the creative process (National Organization for Arts in Health, 2017, Malchiodi, 2006). For the expressive arts therapist, both the person in therapy and the artist have a common desire to explore their experience and their relations to the surrounding world. Both the person in therapy and the artist use this awareness to transform their experiences. Expressive arts therapists often understand this overlap between the therapeutic and the artistic through a continuum that places more or less emphasis on the therapy side or on the art side. One side of the continuum may be called "art *in* therapy" and the other side may be called "art *as*

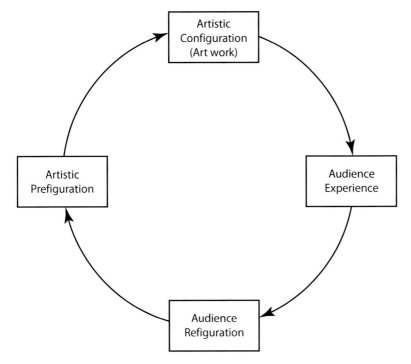

Figure P.1   Cultural circuit of the arts.

therapy" (Edwards, 2004, p. 1). The distinction sounds subtle, but the difference in lived experience between these two approaches can be tremendous.

The expressive therapist working from the art *in* therapy side of the continuum uses artistic expression to help the person access psychic materials that can then be processed through a therapeutic relationship. Art *in* therapy therefore functions similar to the way Freud used free association and dream analysis. Artistic expression helps the person and the therapist tune in to aspects of the person's thoughts, feelings, and perceptions that are difficult for the person to reach through direct conversation alone. Once this material becomes available through art, expressive therapists help the person process the material and work through it in ways similar to the methods of other therapists.

At the other end of the continuum, when the focus is on art *as* therapy, the expressive therapist focuses less on standard therapeutic goals and more on helping people achieve creative expression. This side of the continuum makes sense because art alone, independent of traditionally defined therapeutic goals, can be tremendously healing for several reasons. First, many people find art to be deeply engaging. When a person is absorbed in the process of art, other aspects of life, even painful aspects, may drift into the background. In addition, art allows people to take hard-to-reach experiences and share them with an audience. These experiences, which might otherwise be toxic or alienating, find a voice through creative expression so that the artist is no longer isolated and alone with them. Moreover, art rewards people for their sensitivity. To be an artist, one must be able to pick up on aspects of inner life, imagination, and the world that often escape other people. This sensitivity, which is often coded negatively in the context of most therapies (most therapeutic approaches suggest that people "stop being so sensitive"), is coded positively in the context of creative expression. A highly sensitive "patient" is often considered a bad thing. But a highly sensitive "artist" is nearly always a good thing. This shift of the kaleidoscope can take a denigrated identity (a pathologized patient) and transform it into a celebrated identity (a valued artist). Finally, art takes experience that may otherwise be seen as ugly or inappropriate and turns it into something beautiful, sublime, aesthetically desirable, and politically or spiritually moving. Art therefore brings the artist outside the artist's own preoccupations and into the community. It gives people an invaluable role in making the world a better place.

Expressive arts therapists vary in how much they emphasize art *in* therapy compared with art *as* therapy. Some primarily focus on the former, some on the latter. Most focus on a combination. It is important to see, however, that the further we move toward the art *as* therapy side, the more therapeutic language recedes and creative language emerges. If one goes far enough down this continuum, artistic work easily escapes the context of expressive therapy and becomes simply art. In other words, one does not need to be in expressive therapy to do artistic work and engage in art *as* therapy. One may simply become an artist. The practical implications of becoming an artist will mean not going to a therapist at all but rather taking art classes, setting up a studio, joining an artistic community, and so on. The ideas and language of "therapy" may be the furthest thing from the artist's mind.

The arts, in both of these formations, are invaluable to the mad studies' goal of critiquing problematic aspects of our understanding of mental difference. At the same time, the arts can take us out of the clinical situation as usual and provide affirmative alternative community resources for processing, transforming, and healing personal and cultural differences, antagonisms, conflicts, and prejudices— including sanism. The arts can do this for us as individuals as we use the arts to develop practices of self-care and mutual aid through which we narrate and navigate our psychic differences. And the arts can do this at the larger social level as well. In this latter role, not only can the arts help reconfigure our ideas around mental health and mental difference, but they can also help us shrink the mental health system and expand additional cultural resources beyond mental health care as usual. When the arts become a practice and a community resource, they provide an alternative outlet and a resource for personal and cultural processing, healing, and well-being. This can take the form of increased expressive arts therapies and increased community access to the arts. In the latter version, no mental health labels are required. What is required is public support for artistic spaces and artistic practices.

This larger community understanding of the value of art for well-being has recently gained momentum under the banner of arts and health promotion. The fields of arts and health are diverse and have multiple iterations, such as arts for health, arts in health, arts-health, creative public health, and arts into health (Ali et al., in press; Crawford, Brown, and Charise, 2020; Clift & Camic, 2016; Davies et al., 2016; Fancourt, 2017). The US National Organization for Arts in Health articulates this domain as "a maturing field dedicated to using the power of the arts to enhance health and well-being in diverse institutional and community contexts" (NOAH, 2017, p. 5). To date, the fields of arts and health have not been familiar with mad studies, but there is an alliance waiting to happen, as both see the arts as an invaluable human and cultural resource that should be much more widely promoted and developed. This does not mean that there are no tensions between the two approaches. Mad studies would be critical and cautious around the very idea of needing "health" and "well-being" to promote the arts because of the many ableist and sanist prejudices that can come in the back door with these terms. But, at the same time, "health" and "well-being," when held lightly and critically and used in the service of a social movement toward justice and equality, can be powerful rallying cries for social change in times of multiple public health crises and increasing mental health diagnoses, pharmaceutical treatments, and suicide rates.

Arts for health as a social movement, in other words, connects the dots between the personal, the political, and the environmental. It foregrounds that flourishing people require a healthier society and a healthier planet. The Manchester Institute for Arts, Health, and Social Change (MIAHSC) put this well in their "Manchester Declaration" (Parkinson, 2019). MIAHSC describes itself as "a collective of people and organizations committed to improving the health of communities and addressing inequalities and their causes across Greater Manchester, nationally and globally." They bring together citizens, artists, curators, educators, health and care professionals, and activists alongside academics and researchers to frame their social movement approach. Like all good social movements, the Manchester Declaration has a series of rallying cries at the center of their efforts:

WE ARE A COLLECTIVE of people driven by our experience, knowledge and commitment to promote health, wellbeing and social change through culture, creativity and the arts in all their forms.

WE ACKNOWLEDGE the role that participation in culture and the arts can play in the lives of all members of society, regardless of the factors that may create barriers to that participation.

WE BELIEVE that the arts enrich all our lives from the cradle to the grave and we are committed to everyone having access to culture and freedom of expression as a fundamental human right.

WE WILL PURSUE a rich and nuanced agenda for social change where the most exciting, profound and challenging cultural opportunities are available to everyone.

WE WILL CELEBRATE neurodiversity, nurturing and embracing difference in all its forms, supporting people to realize their potential through the arts.

WE ARE COMMITTED to creating the means to make culture and the arts accessible to the many.

WE WILL ENRICH our understanding of the potency of culture through ground-breaking and innovative research to better inform our shared approach to addressing inequalities.

WE WILL HARNESS stories and data to create new ways of understanding the reach and impact of our work.

WE CONSIDER that environmental public health and the wellbeing of communities and individuals are inseparable.

WE WILL EXPLORE practice, exchange and research between artists, carers and health professionals to learn from each other and develop a supportive culture of empathy and care.

WE WILL ENCOURAGE culture and the arts in our towns and cities to arouse people to be curious, inspired and critical of the status quo.

WE ACKNOWLEDGE that the arts are not a panacea for all life's ills, but we assert that they provide opportunities to give voice to multiple perspectives of lived experience. (Parkinson, 2019)

As we dive into the work of innovative artists in this section, it helps to keep these rallying cries close at hand. They allow us to see why this work matters for individuals, communities, and ecosystems.

References

Ali, A., Wolfert, S., Lam, I., Fahmy, P., Chaudry, A., & Healy, J. (in press). Treating the effects of military sexual trauma through a theatre-based program for veterans. *Women and Therapy*.

Clift, S., & Camic, P. (Eds.). (2016). *Oxford textbook of creative arts, health, and wellbeing: International perspectives on practice, policy, and research*. Oxford University Press.

Crawford, P., Brown, B., & Charise, A. (Eds.). (2020). *The Routledge companion to health humanities*. Routledge.

Davies, C., Pescud, M., Anwar-McHenry, J., & Wright, P. (2016). Arts, public health and the National Arts and Health Framework: A lexicon for health professionals. *Australian and New Zealand Journal of Public Health 40*(4), 304–306.

Edwards, D. (2004). *Art therapy*. Sage Publications.

Fancourt, D. (2017). *Arts in health: Designing and researching interventions*. Oxford University Press.

Fornas, J. (2017). *Defending culture: Conceptual foundations and contemporary debate*. Palgrave Macmillan.

Johnson, R., Chambers, D., Raghuram, P., & Tinknell, E. (2004). *The practice of cultural studies*. Sage Publications.

Malchiodi, C. A. (Ed.). (2006). *Expressive arts therapies*. Guildford Press.

Parkinson, C. (2019). *Manchester declaration*. Manchester Institute for Arts, Health, and Social Change

National Organization for Arts in Health (NOAH). (2017). *Arts, health, and wellbeing in America*. National Organization for Arts in Health.

Ricoeur, P. (1998). *Critique and conviction: Conversations with Francois Azouvi and Marc de Launay*. Polity Press.

Rosenthal, K. P. (Director). (2010). *Crooked Beauty* [Film].

Sirowy, B. (2015). Hermeneutics, aesthetics and the arts. In J. Malpas & H. Gander (Eds.), *The Routledge companion to hermeneutics* (pp. 519–540). Routledge.

Chapter 1

"Icarus Wing," "Taking Care of the Basics," and "National Association for the Eradication of Mental Illness"

Icarus Project

Summary

The Icarus Project (2002–2020) was started by artists and activists devoted to creating resources beyond the dominant models of mental illness. The project was kicked off by Sascha DuBrul and Jacks McNamara after they had deeply problematic experiences with the mental health system as usual. Here is how the Icarus Project articulated their initial mission and vision:

> The Icarus Project was created in the beginning of the 21st century by a group of people diagnosed in the contemporary language as Bipolar or Manic-Depressive. Defining ourselves outside convention we see our condition as a dangerous gift to be cultivated and taken care of rather than as a disease or disorder needing to be "cured." With this double edged blessing we have the ability to fly to places of great vision and creativity, but like the boy Icarus, we also have the potential to fly dangerously close to the sun—into realms of delusion and psychosis—and crash in a blaze of fire and confusion... Despite these risks, we recognize the intertwined threads of madness and creativity as tools of inspiration and hope in this repressed and damaged society. We understand that we are members of a group that has been misunderstood and persecuted throughout history, but has also been responsible for some of its most brilliant creations. And we are proud ...

> We hope to learn from each others' mistakes and victories, stories and art, and create a new culture and language that resonates with our actual experiences of this "disorder" rather than trying to fit our lives into the reductionist framework offered by the current mental health establishment. We would like this site to become a place that helps

DOI: 10.4324/9781003148456-3

people like us feel less alienated, and allows us, both as individuals and as a community, to tap into the true potential that lies between brilliance and madness. (Quoted in Chapter 34)

The images printed here, created by Icarus members Sarah Quinter ("Icarus Wing"; Figures 1.1), Sophie Crumb ("Taking Care of the Basics"; Figures 1.2), and Becky Cloonan ("National Association for the Eradication of Mental Illness"; Figures 1.3), showcase the "inspiration and hope" of TIP and their many participants.

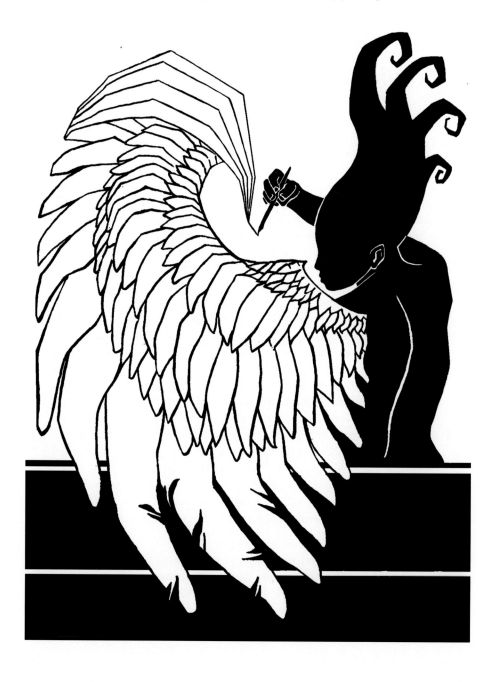

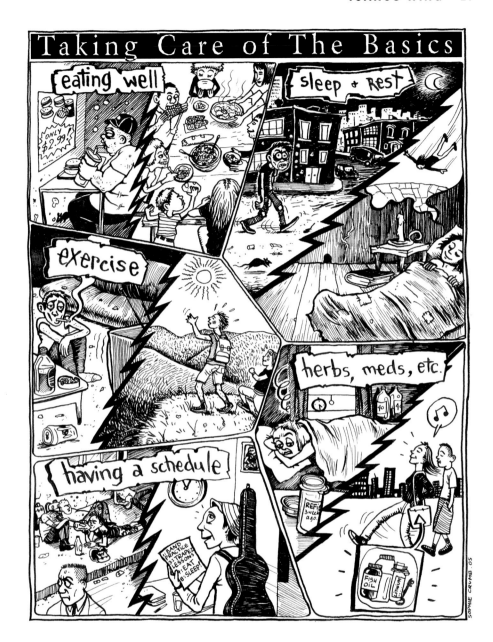

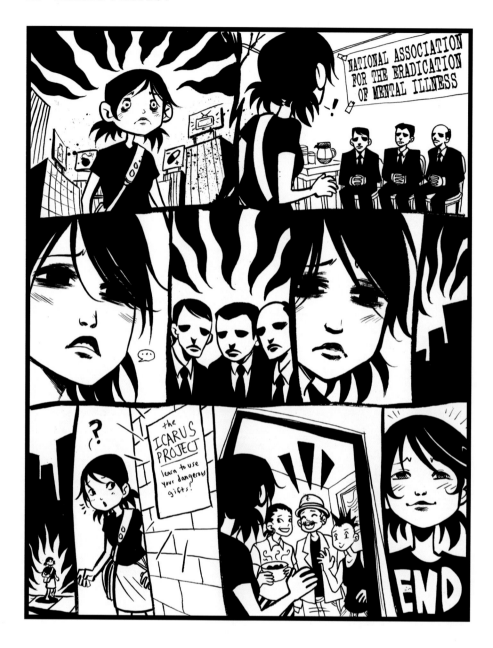

Chapter 2

Mad Studies and Mad-Positive Music[1]

Mark A. Castrodale

Summary

This chapter unpacks how mad-positive music may disrupt pathologizing mental health discourses and affirm mad subjectivities. Castrodale draws on the field of Mad Studies to discuss how mad-positive music recognizes the subjugated knowledge(s) of self-identifying mad persons, troubles the dominance of psy-disciplinary knowledge(s), and opens complex mad-positive spaces. He draws on Mad musicians' lyrical work to demonstrate how Mad music may be epistemologically dissonant with dominant mental health biomedical paradigms that pathologically root mental illness in individuals. Lastly, Castrodale suggests that mad-positive music inserts mad counterknowledge(s) and complex radical narratives that draw from mad persons' lived experiences. As such, mad-positive music offers new pedagogical insights into contemporary mental health systemic practices.

*

> Songs were sung, speeches were made and a moment of silence was held
> for those who were remembered at the end of that first [Mad] Pride Day.
> Geoffrey Reaume (2008, p. 3)

Madness or what we understand to be madness is learned. Mad identities are also lived and crafted. Music represents a pedagogical site where Mad musicians teach others about their lived experiences, and through self-expression carve their own identities. In this paper [chapter], I argue that the discursive meanings of Mad-positive music provide pedagogical insights into mental health systems, psychiatric violence, Mad experiences, Mad pride, and consumers/survivors/ex-patients (c/s/x) subjectivities.

As an amateur musician, I experienced music as a form of self-expression. I come from a musical family where music binds us. My musical history is also a family history. My grandfather Settimio Castrodale was a conductor and professional musician; he played for the local philharmonic orchestra, wrote and transposed music, founded and was the conductor of a local Italian-Canadian community band.

DOI: 10.4324/9781003148456-4

When my mother died from breast cancer I was fifteen years old (See also Castrodale & Zingaro, 2015) and I turned to my vinyl collection listening to the Beatles—"While My Guitar Gently Weeps", and Beach Boys' *Pet Sounds* entire album on repeat. My grandfather continued to give me extensive piano lessons. I also found ways to socialize by playing drums, which I learned from my father. Practicing in the basement, playing along with album tapes of Nirvana, Foo Fighters, Pixies, Sloan, [and] Weezer got me through my tough teenage years. I joined a band and practiced and played live often hiding behind my deliberately angled cymbals. I still write music and play from time to time. For me music represents a means of expression and was personally instrumental in times of grief. My history of loss and connections to Mad-identifying individuals and communities has led me to take up this trajectory of inquiry.

In my work, I view my research, teaching, and writing as interconnected praxis aimed at promoting peace, empathy, and social justice. I draw on Disability Studies, Mad Studies (See LeFrançois et al., 2013), and Geographies of Disability (Castrodale & Crooks, 2010). My positionality (Castrodale & Zingaro, 2015), lived experiences, and previous research with self-identifying Mad student activists (See also Castrodale, 2015) have motivated me to examine Mad-positive music.

Mental health language and imagery often represent mentally ill subjects as out of control, immoral, and violent individuals (LeFrançois et al., 2013). There is a paucity of critical perspectives unpacking sanism in music. Arts-based practices, such as survivor engagement in music may facilitate compassion, care, trust, and recovery (Crawford et al., 2013). I outline the field of Mad Studies and discuss how Mad-positive music may represent a site of pedagogy. I argue that more research is needed that draws directly on psychiatric survivors', consumers', ex-patients' (c/s/x) knowledge(s), and perspectives on music. How do c/s/x understand the role of music in their lives? How do c/s/x use music to actively challenge sanism and psy-violence? How is music linked to Mad pride?

I write this paper as an engaged academic (Castrodale, 2017a; Cresswell & Spandler, 2012) drawing on Mad Studies and survivors' narratives, and hoping for a more loving world. I discuss music therapy to unpack how music has been linked to discourses of wellness and the mediation of persons' conduct. Music therapy may thus represent a tool aimed at producing normal, subjects complacent with the status quo, who are certainly not Mad. Critical orientations toward understanding music as an anti-oppressive practice are needed to address power inequalities, social injustices (See Baines, 2000, 2013, 2014), and counter sanism. Subsequently, I introduce themes and avenues serving as platforms from which one may critique dominant mental-health-related discourses in mainstream music. Lastly, I draw on Daniel Mackler, Blue Panthers Party, and Evan Greer & Friends lyrics, who as psych-survivors trouble pathologizing psy-approaches, psy-violence, and psy-expertise. Through their song lyrics they introduce ideas of mental-health distress and recovery, and demonstrate music as a transformative radical site linked to their own subjectivity and self-care.

A deeper sustained analysis of Mad-positive music and lyrics is needed along with an examination of the pedagogical value of Mad music drawing on c/s/x knowledge(s).

Mad pedagogies have been absent from adult education, critical pedagogy (McLaren & Kincheloe, 2007), and teacher education (Castrodale, 2017a). This paper represents my attempt to catalogue the works of Mad-musical artists and ponder the pedagogical-value of such music. Mad Studies represents a site of education offering pedagogical insights drawing on c/s/x knowledge(s) to countering sanist oppression (Costa, 2014) and psychiatric violence (Brustow, 2013). Mad-positive music holds pedagogical value informing new Mad-subjectivities and countering sanism. Such music allows Mad and non-Mad adult learners to make sense of subjectivities in relation to mental-health oriented discourses, as well as constituting Mad-positive identities. Music can be instrumentally educative in countering sanism and crafting Mad-positive ways of being.

Music and the Psy-sciences

The therapeutic value of music has been well noted (Clarke, 2016). The (a/e)ffects of music are of keen interest to psy-investigation. Psy-informed mental-health-related music literature predominantly discusses the potential of music as therapy to restore normative positive emotional states of unwell subjects (Legge, 2015; Lin et al., 2011; Patterson et al., 2015). Music has been linked to discourses of health and well-being, alleviation of stress, and the overall promotion of positive mental health (Ansdell & Meehan, 2010; Lee & Thyer, 2013; Västfjäll et al., 2012). Performing music and singing can foster a sense of community and promote overall well-being (Dingle et al., 2013). Involvement of clients in music therapy is also viewed as beneficial in shaping the quality of music therapy (Rolvsjord, 2014). There is a need for more research on music drawing directly on the perspectives and experiences of service users (Baines, 2000, 2013, 2014; McCaffrey, 2014). The link between music and mental health represents an important area of investigation and scholarship.

When an individual or group of people do something nonconformist, distasteful, criminal, delinquent, [or] immoral, the question posed "what music were they listening too?" becomes part of the psy-investigation peering into the depths of human subjectivities. Music is broadly linked to the moral hygiene of the population (Baker & Bor, 2008). Music may alleviate individuals' distress, anxiety, and depression (Chen, 2014; Chen et al., 2015; Choi et al., 2008), and severe mental illness (Grocke et al., 2014). Yet, there is little critical examination of music as [a] disciplinary and regulatory tool aimed at conditioning behavior in relation to discourses of relaxation, therapy, and resilience (Spelman, 2012). In this way, music may be used as a way to normatively (re)align 'mentally ill' subjects' thoughts and conduct. As Baker and Bor (2008) attest music genres are often seen to play a role in shaping the attitudes, emotions, and conduct of individuals. Musical taste is thus conceptualized in some speculative psy-literature as having profound impacts on a person's (anti)social thoughts, behavior(s), conduct, and actions (Suetani & Batterham, 2015). The music to which one listens and the mental health of individuals are thus discursively connected. Music is implicitly said to play a role in shaping individuals' mental health, shaping their mood and mind in some way. This has implications for people's health and well-being.

If music is conceived to have therapeutic potential, I would also suggest that some music therapy might also represent a tool aimed at disciplinary regulation of subjects' conduct (Foucault, 1999, 2003, 2007). Music as therapy seeks to calm, render complacent, [and] encourage coping with the present world injustices. In much music therapy, the radical potential, rebellious, angry, loud, punk, and alternative is vacated. Music that screams, bashes, grapples with dissonance, cacophonies of sound, [and] unintelligible noises is thus not of therapeutic value.

Mad Studies

Mad Studies represents a growing field of inquiry and activism opening new ways of examining mental health discourses (Beresford & Russo, 2016). The term Mad stems from madness where Mad is reclaimed from its pejorative roots by self-identifying Mad persons as a source of pride and resistance. Mad Studies as a field draws on the knowledge(s) and perspectives of consumers, survivors, ex-patients (c/s/x), and people who have direct experiences with psy-oppression (Beresford & Russo, 2016; Burstow, 2013; Castrodale, 2015; Liegghio, 2013; LeFrançois et al., 2013; LeFrançois & Diamond, 2014; McWade et al., 2015; Procknow, 2017; Price, 2011; Reville & Church, 2012; Russo & Beresford, 2015). Mad Studies rips madness out of the biomedical clinical psy-expertise discursive grip that speaks with authority on all matters relating to 'mental illnesses' where Mad Studies offers counternarratives of madness and Mad knowledge(s) (Costa et al., 2012).

Mad Studies as a field represents:

> An area of education, scholarship, and analysis about the experiences, history, culture, political organising, narratives, writings and most importantly, the PEOPLE who identify as Mad; psychiatric survivors; consumers; service users; mentally ill; patients; neuro-diverse; inmates; disabled -to name a few of the 'identity labels' our community may choose to use.
>
> (Costa, 2014, What is Mad studies?, para.l)

Mad Studies as a field has been greatly informed by the Mad movement that has been instrumental in exposing the systemic oppression, violence, and power of the mental health system (Everett, 2000). As an area of education, Mad Studies offers pedagogical value. Mad Studies draws on Mad knowledge(s) to teach others about Mad experiences, counter-sanism, and proudly acknowledge Mad identities.

Mad positive politics values the subjectivities and knowledges of Mad persons and respects their human dignity. Mad-positive politics is intersectional, often seeking social justice and equality. Within this politics, Mad histories are valued and Mad pride is celebrated. Importantly, Mad positive politics carves out a place for madness in society (Adame, 2014). Allies may also take up Mad positive positions by supporting Mad persons' rights and agency (Church, 2018).

Mad Studies makes central psychiatric survivors' narratives whose direct experiences with psy-regimes of knowledge, expertise, practices, therapies, cures, onto-epistemological violence, and torture are brought to the fore.

Mad-positive activism has been instrumental in protesting the dominance of biomedical individualizing pathologizing psy-based interventions and treatments and in advocating for the human rights of c/s/x populations (Everett, 2000). Mad persons may celebrate madness, trouble distress (Rimke, 2016), value c/s/x histories and narratives, and seek to forge new compassionate networks of support, respect, mutual aid, and care.

Some Mad persons also align with anti-psychiatry as a means to contest and refute psy-authority and the real violence and harms done by psychiatry. Not all Mad persons share this political positioning. Nevertheless, "Mad studies is not colluding with Big Pharma, piss poor fabricated research on the 'mentally ill,' vapid ne-oliberal imperatives, and the morally bankrupt psy enterprise" (Castrodale, 2017a, p. 52).

As a field of activism and inquiry Mad Studies appreciates a polyphony of Mad voices (Clarke, 2016), experiences, and perspectives that are in some ways commonly tied to the pursuit of countering sanism and the dominant ways Mad persons are often subjugated, alienated, pathologized, and treated violently. Thereby recognizing a multitude of Mad identities, alterity, and various consciousnesses validating different experiences (Burstow, 2003), Mad Studies holds important lessons for adult education in teaching about sanism and rejecting deficit models of madness (Burstow, 2003). This also teaches about the oppression encountered by Mad persons, ways to understand trauma, and the need to understand and value alternate experiences (2003). Adult education can apprehend discourses on mental health through applying Mad Studies informed theories and onto-epistemological perspectives. Adult educators may incorporate teaching and learning that draws directly on c/s/x and Mad-positive knowledge(s) in ways that challenge labeling practices and deficit understandings of Mad identities in education.

Conceptual Framework

Music represents a site of resistance to psy-oppression and also a site for celebrating Mad pride identities. Madness has been a subject of popular music (Spelman, 2012). Yet, as Spelman (2012) attests: "to date, very little research has been conducted with respect to representations of madness in popular music … this paucity is quite surprising" (p. 9).

I draw on Spelman (2012) as a useful conceptual analytic framework. Spelman (2012) offers relevant thematic avenues to critique mental health discourses prevalent in music:

1. Characterizations, depictions, and representations of mad subjects
2. Madness and familial units and relations
3. "Criticism of psychiatric treatments" (p. 146)
4. "Criticism of involuntary psychiatric confinement" (p. 150)
5. Anti-psychiatric stances and sentiments

Spelman (2012) demonstrates Mad subjects as delinquent, deficient, abnormal, violent criminal and in need of intervention, treatment, [and] cure. Madness is represented as lacking and lesser than purportedly sane/normal individuals. The family is evoked as a center of relationships with familial bonds relating to mental health and well-being. Family relations play a role in shaping one's mental-subjectivity. Psychiatric treatments and violence such as confinement have a punitive torturously violent history. Psychiatric science when subject to scrutiny can be revealed as imperfect/flawed. Regimes of cure may also discipline individuals to shape their conduct (Spelman, 2012). Last, anti-psychiatric stances share a deep history of skepticism and rejection of the authority and expert status (Rose, 1998; Spelman, 2012). Such themes inform the basis of my discussions of Mad-positive music and represent conceptual threads for a deeper critical analysis of the political terrain of mental health discourses in music. Spelman's (2012) approach is commensurable with Mad-positive politics in offering a critique of the ways madness is understood and represented while advocating for the inclusion of c/s/x perspectives to transform existing understandings and practices.

I also draw theoretically on Foucault (1995, 1999, 2003) to examine psychiatric knowledge(s) and highlight the ways Mad subjects discursively understand themselves in relation to psy-knowledges to affirm Mad-positive subjectivities. Mad-positive music characteristically questions biomedical disciplinary knowledge(s) that constitute mental normality (Foucault, 1999; Frances, 2014) and conversely mental abnormality advocating for alternative understandings (Spelman, 2012). As with any movement, the Mad movement has tensions where some Mad persons may have more favorable relationships with psy-sciences, pharmacological interventions, psy-professionals, and psychiatric practitioners while others may not.

Methodology

*I adopted a qualitative exploratory case study approach (Denzin & Lincoln, 2010; Stake, 2000). In order to select Mad music I engaged in an extensive search. I connected with people in the Mad community and through social media to compile lists. Songs and artists were selected that addressed the considerations advanced by Spelman (2012) and [the] Foucault (1995, 1999, 2003) discursive analytic approach. Songs from self-identifying c/s/x individuals, Mad persons, and Mad allies were examined. Songs that demonstrated lyrics that most readily resonated with emergent analytic themes (Patton, 1990) were subjected to greater analysis.

Noteworthy musicians were compiled and songs were examined for their lyrical content where I drew on Spelman (1995, 1999, 2003) and Foucault (2003) analytically. Artists included: The Avalanches, "Frontier Psychiatrist" [song]; Michael Adams, SSRIs SSRLies [anti-psychiatry song]; Blue Panthers Party, "Murda Murda" [song]; Eels (band), "Electro-Shock Blues" [song]; Bonfire Madigan Shive [musician]; Wombats, Anti-D; Wendell Woody Cormier [psychiatric survivor musician]; Defiance, Ohio [band]; Johnny Matteson, "Rave" "Mad Musician" "Crazy People" [songs]; Sills and Smith (band), "Etched" [Album] and "Would it all be different" [song about Mad experience]; The Mad Pride (band), "Fade Away" [song]; Evan Greer & Friends, "Adderall song" [song]; Howie the Harp, "Crazy and Proud" [song]; and Vara Adams, No means yes [album], This list is partial, it is my own effort to catalogue, organize, and compile. I had help from peers and friends to which I am grateful. I encourage other Mad-positive advocates to share these songs, build this list, proliferate and disseminate, support Mad artists, and create more music. Key illustrative songs were selected from this list for deeper analysis and discussion. These selections represent an exploratory case (Stake, 2000) intended to encourage other researchers to expand this tangent of research examining the pedagogical value of Mad music.

Mad-Positive Music

Mad-positive music often refutes psy-authority, affirms Mad identities, counters sanism, and draws directly on c/s/x knowledges. Mad-positive musicians trouble psy-expertise, Big Pharma, psych-violent regimes of cure and treatment, and the pathologization of distress. Through tone, imagery, and lyrics, Mad-positive music plays in the face of psychiatric oppression and sanism. Raw, powerful, vulnerable, angry, eloquent, and beautiful, Mad music seeks to authentically tell powerful counter-narratives about mental health without normalizing experience or flattening emotion(s).

Mad music may also reflect Mad pride, the Mad persons' movement, Mad-positive identity politics, and celebrate Mad-subjectivities. Mad identities may thus be recognized and acknowledged as sites of difference, joy, and pride.

Lyrically, music may represent and shape human subjectivities constituting forms of mental subjects. Mental health imagery and language figure prominently in the contemporary music industry (Spelman, 2012). Music may reinforce systems of dominance such as patriarchy, racism, classism, sexism, sanism, and ableism, or may be a tool to unpack and speak back to such intersectionally contextual layers of privilege, access, and/or oppression (Spelman, 2012). There is a need to examine intersections of race, gender, sex, dis/ability, class, and in/sanity as these identity vectors are lyrically inscribed in popular mainstream music. A focus on complex identity markers and music as constitutive necessarily troubles dominant representations of mental health and the imagery, language, and associations attributed to 'mentally ill' subjects.

Self-identifying Mad persons' and psychiatric survivors' perspectives are largely absent from existing mental health music-therapy research (Rykov, 2006). Mad persons' knowledges may illuminate how music, situated in particular sonorous mental health-oriented terrains, composed music, and music as political art may shape our mental lives. Self-identifying Mad musicians are radically using musical forms of expression in ways that critique psychiatric violence, oppression, and pathologizing biomedical discourses.

Representing Madness

Mad and non-Mad musicians through mental-health-related lyrics represent madness. Madness may be represented in familiar tropes such as the imagery of being out of control, in need of a straightjacket, and medicated. However, Mad-allies or Mad-musicians may take Mad stances that challenge conventional discourses on mentally ill subjects. Some artists' music lyrically takes an openly Mad activist tone. Eels' album *Electroshock Blues* deals with [the] electroconvulsive shock his mother underwent. In this way, Mad-positive accounts can document the hardships encountered by others, speak against torturous treatments, and reflect upon Mad lives. Electric-convulsive therapy (ECT) has been viewed as a torturous treatment lacking beneficial efficacy (Breggin, 1994; Spelman, 2012). Mad Studies has troubled this practice particularly when lacking consent and forced (Breggin, 1994; Burstow, 2013, 2015).

Non-Mad identified popular artists play with mental-illness-related imagery. As an example, Rapper Marshall Mathers (aka Slim Shady or Eminem) has played extensively with Mad imagery and lyrics. He appears in straightjackets and sings lyrics about taking pride in being out of one's mind and out of control. Such imagery depicts delinquency and madness as linked to violent dangerous unruly conduct (Burstow, 2015). Devices such as straightjackets and ECT represent devices and mechanisms that are part of a historic trajectory that seeks to discipline and control the conduct of Mad individuals (LeFrançois et al., 2013). Mad Studies as a field has refuted the notion that Mad individuals are violent and instead posits and provides support to the contrary, where Mad persons are far more likely to be victims of violence than perpetrators (Burstow, 2015; LeFrançois et al., 2013).

Lyrically, he evokes madness-oriented discourses. In his song "I'm Friends with the Monster" he sings:

> Maybe I need a straightjacket, face facts. I'm nuts for real, but I'm okay with that… I'm friends with the monster that's under my bed. Get along with the voices inside of my head. You're trying to save me, stop holding your breath. And you think I'm crazy, yeah, you think I'm crazy.
>
> (Eminem et al., 2013)

This rejects a desire for cure regimes and instead posits that he is comfortable with who he is despite others' opinions. In the song "Monster" he also states: "I think I'm getting so huge I need a shrink. I'm beginning to lose sleep: one sheep, two sheep. Going cuckoo and cooky as Kool Keith. But I'm actually weirder than you think" (Eminem et al., 2013).

In this passage, Mathers lyrically makes reference to rapper Keith Thorton who was reportedly/disputably institutionalized to a mental hospital thereby interjecting his name into mainstream music. In my belief Mathers uses the term "shrink" a term that strips psy-expertise of authority and power and devalues the professional status and nature of psy-disciplinary knowledges to shrinkery. However problematic and imbued with stigmatizing imagery, Mathers draws on mental health language and imagery in his music lyrics and videos.

Popular Non-Mad identified artists such as Queen with "I'm going slightly mad" and David Bowie "Aladdin Insane" and Ozzy Osborne among others have also delved into topics of madness (Spelman, 2012). Madness has been a popularized music-lyrical topic explored by mainstream musicians. It matters who creates music and how such music needs to affirm and represent the experiential accounts of c/s/x persons without reducing, stigmatizing, or othering Mad lived narratives. Non-Mad identified performers may reflect accounts that do not resonate with the experiences of self-identifying Mad folk. Such accounts could reaffirm stigma. However, it is possible for Non-Mad musicians to create positive accounts of madness particularly when adopting allied stances and drawing on Mad-persons' lived experiences.

Mad Music Lyrics

Daniel Mackler, Howie the Harp, Blue Panthers Party, and Evan Greer offer lyrical insights into Mad lives. Artist Daniel Mackler (2016) whose examples of Mad Music include anti-psychiatry perspectives including "Bullshit-antipsychiatry and anti-medication song" and "The psych-med song" off the album "Songs from the locked ward." His music provides insights into his experiences with the psychiatric system and the violence and harm caused therein. In his "Bullshit—antipsychiatry and anti-medication song" (sung to the tune of "Bring back my Bonnie to me") Daniel Mackler (2016) sings:

> They tell me my problems genetic, I'm bom with a flaw in my brain, they tell me I need medication, and force me to bury my pain.
> [Bullshit Chorus]
> Bullshit, Bullshit, I've learned to smell bullshit from miles and miles [Repeat] I've learned to smell bullshit from miles.
> Their pills make me shaky and sweaty. I fear they're breaking my will.
> They told me that this is quite normal, and added another new pill.
> [Bullshit Chorus].
> They put me inside a straight jacket. They locked me inside of a cage.
> They inject me with Haldol to calm me, yet wonder why I'm full of rage.
> [Bullshit Chorus].
> They give me a shrink I can talk to, but she is just spiritually dead, she only repeats the same question, "are you still taking your meds"?
> [Bullshit Chorus].
> They force fed me E-fuller Torrey [American psychiatrist Edwin Fuller Torrey], but he is sadistic and gross. I asked them about Peter Breggin [American psychiatrist critical of psychiatry and medication] they replied by increasing my dose.
> [Bullshit Chorus]
> Their studies are so scientific, and based on assiduous work, but they don't share their affiliations, with Lilly and Janssen, and Merck. [Bullshit].
> They absolve all of my traumatizers, the horrors that they did to me, they tell me to put it behind me, and say that I need ECT [Electroconvulsive Therapy - 'electric shock therapy']
> [Bullshit Chorus].
> I said I think I can recover, and taper off all these meds, they tell me that's just my delusion, an illness that lives in my head [Bullshit].

Mad-positive survivor anthems such as these speak to theory and practice in Mad Studies relating to Mad activism and the desire for transformative Mad politics to make our lives better. Mackler rejects his subjectivity as someone flawed with genetic brain defects. Through Mackler's anti-psychiatry lyrics there are critiques launched against forcible confinement, criticisms of harsh violent treatments of electric shock therapy (ECT) (See Breggin, 1994), and the devaluation of psy-expertise and research coopted with Big Pharma interests. A substantial body of critical mental-health-related literature discusses how psy-based biomedical understandings of mental illness are often unreliable and of untrustworthy scientific validity (Rimke, 2016). Survivors' insights can inform mental health research and regimes of care in meaningful ways (Sweeney, 2016). Trauma inflicted is the fault of traumatizers and the consequent suffering is rejected as illness or delusion but as [a] consequence from [the] violence experienced. And, recovery is possible.

Mackler's lyrics speak of the side-effects experiences from pills, confinement, and control, [and] anger in the face of oppression. He attests to how his desire for freedom from psychiatric violence itself becomes pathologized. The psychiatric system insights he garnished from personal experience lead him to critique the ways medical practitioners and the politics of research production are influenced by Big Pharma-funding and affiliations (See also Whitaker, 2010).

Mad music holds important value in documenting the lived-realities of Mad persons and Mad survivors. Survivors use art to tell their own Mad histories. The Survivors History Group (2010) attests:

> [W]e seek to record, preserve, collate, and make widely available the diversity and creativity of [survivors] through personal accounts, writings, poetry, art, music, drama, photography, campaigning, speaking, influencing and all other expressions. Our basic founding principle is that [survivors] own their history.

Archival records of Mad survivor art share stories that may otherwise remain untold. In this way, music as a form of artistic expression tells rich Mad survivor's narratives.

Music also is a way for Mad-persons to engage in positive expressions of Mad identities and Mad pride. The late Howie the Harp (2018) sang lyrics to express Mad pride in the Mad pride movement. In "Crazy and Proud," Howie proclaims:

Well, they're always calling me crazy
And they're always putting me down
They always say they'll be my friend
But they never come around.
'Cause I'm not like normal people
I won't fit in their mold.
And for that crime
they either lock me up
or put me out in the cold.
'Cause I'm Crazeeeee, and I'm Proud!
Well 1 won't be a 9 to 5 robot

Well-oiled and made of chrome
I'll never have your ulcers
or your split-level home.
You tried so hard to change me
You bullied and you sneered
But I'll always remain just like I am
Loony, Crazy and Weird!
'Cause I'm Crazy… And I'm Proud
Well, you say I'll always be locked up
Unless I stop being me
But I'm not like that so stay off my back
I just wanna be free
'Cause I'm telling all you people
Don't give me those funny looks
You think you're great but you're the
Kind I hate
American Psychiatry Crooks
'Cause I'm Crazy… And I'm Proud

Beyond critiquing psychiatry, Howie affirms Mad identity and being loony, crazy, and weird. Howie troubles the stresses of everyday work/life, troubles normalcy, and proudly identifies as crazy. He desires Mad subjectivity and freedom. As a Mad musician, Howie uses music to resist the tyranny of sane-life. Resoundingly, Mad advocacy and use of musical lyrics demonstrate madness as a source of pride, and point to social factors in society as problematic places of stress and turmoil. Mad advocate musicians can teach able-bodied/sane persons ways to critique the current state of affairs, how so many normates (Thomson, 2017) live - the mold.

Among forms of art and expression, music is a means to document survivors' narratives, and unpack existing power-knowledge relations. Music holds rich value as a historic record of survivors' voices and knowledges. Psy-discourses of progress, innovation, rehabilitation, and cure no longer seem progressive when psy-histories are critically examined though [sic] a Mad-history lens. Yet, such lyrics may be seen as alienating for consumers who may find psy-interventions therapeutic and manage their well being through medications or other psy-informed practices.

Music holds educational value in shifting conversations around mental-health systems. Artists take political stances against diagnostic labeling practices and harms done by the collusions between medical authority, academia, neoliberalism, and the psy-enterprise.

Mad music may be used to resist psy-expertise. Psy-expertise represents the unquestioned authoritative status of psy-based practitioners to make judgments, observations, and pronouncements on all matters relating to mental-illness (Rose, 1998). Mad music may challenge such authority by lyrically denouncing psy-sciences informed discourses, pathologizing gaze, and regimes of truths (Foucault, 1999, 2003, 2007). As an example of music lyrics content as pedagogical discursive refutation of psy-authority, Blue Panthers Party directly implicates the violent death dealing psy-Big Pharma-enterprise loudly singing in "Murda Murda":

Its funny how they don't give out degrees in fantasy.
Oh wait I forgot about psychiatry
Silly me how could I forget they don't cure things
But they're good at naming things they call a disease
We all get sad but they're 'callin' that depression
We all get mad but they say that's aggressive
The DSM five knows a lot about problems
But they haven't published one book to get close to solve em
Correct me if I'm wrong, tell me if they made a difference
By altering the lives of family, wives, and their children
Let's get to work I'm fired up like a pistol
And if you feel the same way - it's time to get em
They think we suckas and can tell us whatever works
For their pockets but they never tell you bout the perks
Ask the doctor if he shares his kickbacks with the nurse
Its okay they still get paid while you up in a hurse
Lets gettem no longer can we hide
Lets show them that we have more than a pride
Murda Murda here comes the docta
We can't sit around we gotta get up and stop em
They've killed millions so we gonna give em problems
They tellin people they sick but nobody cured once
It's murda murda murda
To the first degree lets not let it go any further

Songs such as these draw on lyrics and imagery to trouble psy-discourses and a corrupt system that may harm persons while deriving massive profits. A system rife with kickbacks and perks is problematic and does not seek to be curative but to capture and expand mental-health clients and customers (See also Burstow et al., 2014). This is particularly insidious when children and vulnerable populations are targeted. As a pedagogical intervention, Mad musicians point to collusions between psy-sciences and Big Pharma as undermining the integrity of psy-diagnostic practices and curative interventions.

In this vein of thought Greer (2017) demonstrates intersections of pathologization of childhood, class issues, gender inequality, militarism, and his lived experiences as a former pill-taker who recovered and rejects pharmacological interventions:

> mrs greer your son acts up in class, he asks the questions that you're not supposed to ask, mr. greer, it's pretty plain to see, your son has got adhd and the doctors say he needs, 30 milligrams of amphetamines, (go!) when I turned eight years old, they put me on the pills, one to focus me at school, help me follow all the rules, and one to keep my tears away, cuz little boys should never cry, one to help me through my day, one to help, me sleep at night, and i had so few memories, of what it was like before that i took those damn pills everyday, since 1994, now i recognize the, system, i see what they're really for, i'm not giving you my money, i

won't take them anymore, i was in the dead center of the country, when i popped my final pill, i sold the rest of the bottle, to some kids from Chicago, then turned toward something new, and for the first time in my life, i felt at peace with who i was, i couldn't wait to share the new world out there, with all the people that i loved, and i had so few memories of what it was like before, the first week i went without them felt like i had been reborn, now i recognize the system i see what they're really for, i'm not giving you my money i won't take them anymore, that's when i got to thinking, about this society, and how there's something wrong, when a kid, so young's put on amphetamines, at first i blamed my parents, then the, doctors then the schools, but if you wanna fight back, look higher than that at the filthy frat cat with the big contract, at those puppy killing labs the results come back, taking science fiction and calling it fact, and if it screws you up they don't give a crap, cuz they can still drive home in their Cadillacs, making money off a game where the decks are stacked, and if that's not enough it's bigger than that, that's just one of this system's many attacks on you, so what are we gonna do? and do i have so few memories of what it was like before, that i can write this song with smoke in my lungs, and a bottle on the floor? now i recognize those systems, i see what they're really for, i'm not giving you my money, i won't buy it anymore!

Greer unpacks woven systems of education and health. He examines childhood experience, familial relations, and psy-interventions encountered as a child with limited agency. Lyrics demonstrate introspection in regards to being diagnosed and labeled with ADHD and subsequent psy-science interventions for not following rules. As a boy he was pathologized and relates this to gendered norms that boys are not supposed to cry. He acknowledges that his memory was negatively impacted due to [the] prescribed pills he took. No longer taking pills for Greer felt akin to being reborn. Mad politics and disability politics converge in understanding the implications of psychiatric diagnostic labeling practices (Beresford, 2000). Greer lyrically notes his distrust in profit motivated mental health systems for being uncaring and damaging lives.

Mad-Positive Music as Pedagogy

Mad music represents a pedagogical site. A pedagogy of madness seeks to unpack sanist oppression, and appreciate the gap in Mad-knowledge non-mad folks may miss. Mad musicians teach others about their lives and in so doing promote learning about mental health systems and Mad-positive subjectivities. Although there is no consensus or formal definition of what constitutes being Mad-positive, I would point to some anchor points to enacting and operationalizing Mad-positivity. Mad-positive stances counter pathologizing discourses surrounding mental illness and seek to transform understandings of madness. A mad-positive ethic seeks empathy, care, community, and compassion. This entails recognizing Mad histories and celebrating Mad pride.

A deficit model of Mad identities is refuted, and self-identifying Mad people often reclaim pejorative terms such as crazy and Mad. Sanism is recognized along with oppression encountered by Mad-persons. Mad-positive is also an identificatory label. Identifying as Mad-positive could indicate a person who may be Mad/ non-Mad however aligns themselves with the Mad peoples' movement and Mad political imperatives. Mad-positive, thus could mean one who aspires to be a Mad-ally. Hence, such a commitment expresses a desire to engage with Mad politics, and to learn from self-identifying Mad-persons' knowledge(s). It acknowledges the right of individuals to be Mad.

In relation to psy-sciences and mental health systems, C/S/X may have differing perspectives toward the psy-sciences and psychiatric systems. Some Mad persons, particularly consumers, may currently view psy-based interventions as beneficial and thus may not share anti-psychiatric viewpoints.

Mad pedagogy offers insights to examine sanism in Adult Education and celebrate Mad identities. Furthermore:

> Mad pedagogies may resist the influence of Big Pharma, unchecked diagnostic inflation, and the pathologization of normal, through the manufacturing of dis/ability and new disorders. Such a pedagogy can critique existing psy dominance of ways of knowing and being in the world.
>
> (Castrodale, 2017a, p. 58)

Mad music represents a form of expression permitting nuanced critiques of dominant mental health discourses permeating much of our contemporary daily lives. It may create communities of Mad pride, care, empathy, support, and shared experiences. Alternative non-pathologizng paths to recovery from distress might be realized. Mad musicians may reclaim normal (See Frances, 2014) and reject being pathologized or labeled as mentally ill. Mad music may teach non-Mad persons about sanism and oppression encountered by Mad persons. In this way, Mad persons' voices and histories may gain prominence in adult education curriculum. Moreover, in educational settings de-pathologizing/non-clinical peer-inspired approaches to support may be offered for students experiencing distress.

Music serves a pedagogical function, disseminating counter-knowledges and discourses warning others about the potential risks of flirting with psychiatry. Such Mad survivor narratives may refute psy-authority and offer pedagogical value (Burstow, 2003; Castrodale, 2017a) teaching others about psychiatric systemic violence through the sharing of lived experiences. Song singing is connected with recognition and remembrance, preserving those histories of Mad persons who did not survive psychiatric violence and connecting Mad pride community members (Reaume, 2008). Critical pedagogy is concerned with revealing and understanding the workings of unequal power-relations, contesting psy-authority (Rose, 1998), and hopes to generate emancipation from oppression (See Freire, 2009). Such a pedagogy values voice and agency of knowledges that are often subjugated (Castrodale, 2017b) drawing directly on Mad perspectives to transgress psychiatric systemic oppression.

Mad-positive musicians are not anti-science, anti-intellectualism, or anti-evidence. Rather, they often seek greater transparency and advocate for inclusion of Mad knowledge(s) to inform mental health systems. They are actively challenging the unquestioned power-authority vested in psychiatry (See Foucault, 2003). Unchallenged psy-expertise disempowers c/s/x populations, leaves societal inequalities and psycniatric violence unquestioned, and perpetuates harms through collusions with Big Pharma (Rimke, 2016) including confinement, forced treatments, and other damaging biomedical interventions.

Through their lyrics Mad musicians may challenge the reported efficacy of psy-interventions, lack of reliability, under-reporting of Pharma side-effects, psy-authority, and rampant collusion of psy-sciences with systems of regulation [and] control. This represents a refusal to be docile (Foucault, 2003) and comply unquestionably with psy-expert orders. Mounting lawsuits against the Pharma drug cartels have exposed unethical research practices (See Burstow, 2015). Music represents an artful form of resistance, a way of speaking truth to power (Foucault, 1995, 2007) and revealing injustices. People are churned through the academia-psy-pharma research pipeline. These musicians often regard psychiatry with deep and well-founded skepticism (Rimke, 2016). Where psy-sciences are to be distrusted given its history and contemporary apparent corrupt collusions running through research networks, psy-workers, and biomedical enterprising health systems (Rimke, 2016). The psy-web infiltrates educational systems, health, military, and human resources among other domains touching human life.

Conclusion: Fin

Music represents a political pedagogical site of learning for self-identifying mad and non-mad persons alike. Music holds rich pedagogical potential to educate and caution members of society of the potential risks/ benefits associated with particular psy-informed interventions. Mad-positive music dynamically embraces a wide range of emotions, ways of being, [and] relating to oneself and others while de-pathologizing madness. Mad music may reveal contemporary orientations to madness and dominant mental-health-related discourses. Music may also be a site of resistance where pathologizing individualizing ways of being made "mental," constituted as a subject in relation to mental health discourses, in this world may be challenged and troubled.

Mad experiences may teach us about our humanity and our world. For Mad listeners there may be commonalities, shared narrative experiences, and activist stances voiced for collective change. For Mad artists Mad music is a place of expression and self-constitutive work, a place of learning and identity carving. Non-mad persons may someday also consider themselves to be Mad and thereby encounter psychiatric systems more intimately. Both Mad and non-Mad persons may learn about psy-authority, psychiatric discourses, psy-systems, and regimes of treatment as well as Mad-positive identities through Mad-positive music. Non-mad persons may also engage in crafting Mad-positive music through ethical collaborations with Mad-persons.

Music may also entail exploration, imagination, and improvisation opening safe democratic spaces of resistance (Clarke, 2016). For Clarke (2016), music expands notions of identity appreciating a multitude of voices and diverse identity constitutions. Music represents a site implicated in Self-crafting and is thereby useful for Mad persons in challenging normalcy.

Mad music seeks to disrupt normal sane complacency. Mad music is not necessarily angry, although at times anger may be evoked in the face of unrelenting oppression. In contrast to music that seeks to inspire individual resilience, [and the] ability to cope with an oppressive world, Mad music is revolutionary, inspires counter-dialogue, and seeks to critique existing forms of sanist violence and marginalization.

Mad music, including anti-psychiatry inspired songs and lyrics are often integral pieces of the Mad pride movement. As part of Mad organizing and events, music and poetry are often components of anti-oppressive activism, education, and mental health advocacy for transformative social justice (See Icarus, 2017). For some members, music expression is part of the artistic tapestry involved in being Mad. It is a way to express one's identity, to heal from trauma, to speak against psy-based oppression, and to connect with others.

Anti-psychiatry inspired music thus represents a means to question the authority psychiatry bestows upon itself, to question the legitimacy of claims to scientific neutrality that often underpin psy-science, and [to] realize the real harms inflicted by psy-endorsed interventions. Lived environments and social relationships with others impact our mental health and interventions need to fix our social world rather than encouraging resiliency, normalcy, and complacency. Music thus represents a mode of expression and means to speak with agency about trauma, alienation, psy-violence, forced confinement, and harsh treatments Mackler experienced in the name of cure. Survivors' accounts and expression through music may shape better regimes of care and understanding, advocacy, and peer support that take positions against sanism and the oppression of Mad persons toward an inclusive transformative Mad-positive politics.

Mad-positive music rearticulates a different therapeutic value recasting music as anti-oppressive, a means to constitute oneself through affirming positive identities and countering sanism. Mad music is a radical and transgressive reimagining of the relationship between music and mental well-being. Mad-positive music offers de-pathologizing arts-based survivor-initiated approaches to overall health promotion. There is much that can be learned about mental health experiences and systems through survivor lyrics and narrative accounts musically expressed. More work is needed to draw on consumer offerings of mad positive lyrics who identify as Mad, relay bouts with madness, and may not identify as psychiatrically oppressed. This would provide a deeper and more nuanced sample of Mad musicians' perspectives.

There are now growing international hubs of self-identifying Mad and Mad-positive musicians. As an example Toronto Mad Pride (2018) website features a Mad music performer directory. Similarly, Mindfreedom (2017) has linked Mad politics and activism to Mad music artists. Music and song-writing is [sic] used to celebrate "free minds, and challeng[e] psychiatric human rights violations" (Mindfreedom, 2017).

Vara Adams, a psychiatric survivor musician describes her motivations for engaging in the process of songwriting for her album as follows:

I decided that it was time to tell the world how I feel about the system that labelled, drugged and shocked me. I know the songs are raw, but they very clearly express the way I view psychiatric treatment as a whole. It makes me angry that people labeled as mentally ill immediately become nameless and are subjected to coercion and abuse. I have survived that label, and I won't be nameless anymore.

(Mindfreedom, 2017)

As Vara attests, music represents a means to contest coercion, violence, and a psychiatric system that shocks and harms often in the name of cure. The impetus of writing is to educate others, to inform others about labeling practices and psychiatric systemic violence.

Mad-positive music articulates a polyphony of Mad persons' voices and perspectives that may be working harmoniously and in dissonant ways. Survivors unpack ways medical systems and society may oppress, alienate, and do real harm to certain individuals. Such individuals are often understood and named as non-conforming, irrational, unintelligible, dangerous, and difficult to control subjects. Subsequently such subjects are pathologized, labeled in ways to subjugate and nullify, normalize these odd subjects (Foucault, 1999; Frances, 2014).

Mad positive music may take many forms, and be expressed through diverse musical genres and by a range of different artists. Mad music represents a site of contestation and activism, to counter the psy-dominance of everything that is mental in this world. As a mode of expression, music delivers complex messages, conveys emotions, and is a language in and of itself. Lyrically music may convey meanings about mental discourses, making sense of the world, and fitting in with or contesting and complicating broader systems of thoughts and actions. As a pedagogical tool, music can be a mode to unpack the complex ways mad subjects are constituted through lyrics.

Music is also a means and mechanism for Mad subjects to construct their identities and dynamic subjectivities. There is a need for researchers to examine mental health-related discourses inscribed in mainstream music, and also how Mad persons may use music as a tool to express their own knowledge(s) through music. Arts informed methods may enrich our understandings of mental health, and mental health systems (Johnson, 2010). Self-identifying Mad persons onto-epistemologically unpack the links between music and medicine. Mad positive music embraces that complex, nuanced, dynamic, dissonant potential in music to shape new and radical subjectivities.

Why not be profoundly Mad in the face of violence, inequality, and oppression? The question should not be about restoring positive mental health at the level of individuals but instead, in a world so violent, with strife, war, inequality, discrimination, suffering, and hardships why are not more people positively Mad? Why are there so many seemingly fine able-bodied sane normates and neuro-typicals? Mad-positive music may provide insights into the mental health system, the distress encountered by people in their daily lives, and ways Mad people are understood and treated in society while providing new avenues for thought and action. Mad-persons may also adopt different stances towards psychiatry, psy-discourses, psy-interventions, and psychprofessionals. However, a common thread is the unpacking of power-knowledge relations, a desire to affirm positive identities, to create means for care and empathy and reject individual pathologizing models often in favour [sic] of social determinants of mental health and well-being. Mental health is political, socio-cultural, and complex and needs to be understood as such beyond simplistic narrow biomedical discourses.

Pedagogically, adult learners both Mad and non-Mad alike may learn about Mad identities, Mad pride, psychiatric systems, sanism, and psy-oppression. Mad music shares narrative insights that educate listeners about their lives and Mad knowledge(s). It is far from a simple binary Mad/non-Mad but non-Mad persons may become Mad, and Mad persons may at times no longer identity [sic] as Mad individuals. Nevertheless, Mad music offers something different, a new way of unpacking mental-health discourses and rethinking psy-authority and pathologizing labeling practices. Mad musical lyrics teaches [sic] new ways of understanding how mental illness is treated in society. Mad music also provides insights to ponder who is deemed to be mentally ill, when, where, how, and why, and what this means in how they become subsequently treated. Music represents a site for Mad musicians to create songs with agency, to resist being pathologized, and to share their complex nuanced mental-health lived narratives.

Mad positive music could be used in medical student training to education students on Mad persons' experiences with psychiatric systems and teach about Mad Pride. This would promote de-pathologizing approaches to Madness, discourses of recovery, problematizing the influence of Big Pharma, and rethinking sanism in mental health. Such lyrics could also be shared and circulated with Mad activists, scholars, [and] c/s/x populations encouraging community building. Adult educators can learn new ways of understanding and speaking about mental health.

In this paper [chapter], I have drawn on self-identifying survivors' music, highlighting songs and lyrics. Mad music may illustrate psychiatric violence, psychiatric systems, and Mad positive subjectivities. An essential extension of this work would be to directly discuss the significance, meanings, and implications of these songs with self-identifying c/s/x individual music writers, listening audiences, and Mad-positive communities. Additional research is needed on the educational implications of sanism, and how Mad persons may transform educational pedagogical possibilities (Castrodale, 2017a; Procknow, 2017). Research that connects with Mad musicians and asks them to share their insights about their lyrics is greatly needed to better understand how they understand their music in relation to c/s/x knowledges(s). Mad Studies and Mad-positive music inserts [sic] Mad positive knowledge(s) in curriculum, unpacks sanism, and de-pathologizes the subjects of education.

Note

1 Originally printed in *New Horizons in Adult Education & Human Resource Development 31*(1), 40–58. Reprinted with permission.

References

Adame, A. (2014). "There needs to be a place in society for madness": The psychiatric survivor movement and new directions in mental health care. *Journal of Humanistic Psychology, 54*(4), 456–475.

Ansdell, G., & Meehan, J. (2010). "Some light at the end of the tunnel" exploring users' evidence for the effectiveness of music therapy in adult mental health settings. *Music and Medicine, 2*(1), 29–40.

Baines, S. (2000). A consumer-directed and partnered community mental health music therapy program. *Canadian Journal of Music Therapy, 7*(1).

Baines, S. (2013). Music therapy as an anti-oppressive practice. *Arts in Psychotherapy, 40*(1), 1–5.

Baines, S. (2014). *Giving voice to service-user choice: Music therapy as an anti-oppressive practice* [Doctoral Thesis]. University of Limerick, Ireland.

Baker, F., & Bor, W. (2008). Can music preference indicate mental health status in young people? *Australasian Psychiatry, 16*(4), 284–288.

Beresford, P. (2000). What have madness and psychiatric system survivors got to do with disability and Disability Studies? *Disability and Society, 15*(1), 167–172.

Beresford, P., & Russo, J. (2016). Supporting the sustainability of Mad Studies and preventing its co-option. *Disability and Society, 31*(2), 1–5.

Breggin, P. R. (1994). *Toxic psychiatry: Why therapy, empathy, and love must replace the drugs, electroshock, and biochemical theories of the "new psychiatry."* New York: Macmillan.

Burstow, B. (2003). From pills to praxis: Psychiatric survivors and adult education. *Canadian Journal for the Study of Adult Education, 17*(1), 1–18.

Burstow, B. (2013). A rose by any other name: Naming and the battle against psychiatry. In B. A., Lefrançois, R. Menzies, & G. Reaume's (Eds.), *Mad Matters: A critical reader in Canadian Mad Studies* (pp. 79–90). Toronto, Ontario: Canadian Scholar's Press Inc.

Burstow, B. (2015). *Psychiatry and the business of madness: An epistemological accounting.* New York: Palgrave MacMillan.

Burstow, B., Lefrancois, B., & Diamond, S. (Eds.) (2014). *Psychiatry disrupted: Theorizing resistance and crafting the (Revolution).* Montreal: McGill-Queen's University Press.

Castrodale, M. A. (2014). Mad matters: A critical reader in Canadian mad studies. *Scandinavian Journal of Disability Research.* https://doi.org/10.1080/15017419.2014.895415.

Castrodale, M. A. (2015). *Examining the socio-spatial knowledge(s) of disabled and mad students in higher education* [Electronic Thesis and Dissertation Repository], p. 3229. https://ir.lib.uwo.ca/etd/3229

Castrodale, M. A. (2017a). Critical disability studies and mad studies: Enabling new pedagogies in practice. *Canadian Journal for the Study of Adult Education, 29*(1), 49–66.

Castrodale, M. A. (2017b). Mobilizing dis/ability research: A critical discussion of qualitative go-along interviews in practice. *Qualitative Inquriy, 24*(1), 45–55.

Castrodale, M. A., & Crooks, V. A. (2010). The production of disability research in human geography: An introspective examination. *Disability and Society, 25*(1), 89–102.

Castrodale, M. A., & Zingaro, D. (2015). "You're such a good friend": A woven autoethnographic narrative discussion of disability and friendship in higher education. *Disability Studies Quarterly, 35*(1).

Chen, X. J. (2014). *Music therapy for improving mental health problems of offenders in correctional settings* [PhD Thesis]. Doctoral Programme in Music Therapy. Department of Communication and Psychology, Aalborg University.

Chen, X. J., Hannibal, N., & Gold, C. (2015). Randomized trial of group music therapy with Chinese prisoners impact on anxiety, depression, and self-esteem. *International Journal of Offender Therapy and Comparative Criminology.* https://doi.org/10.1177/0306624X15572795.

Choi, A. N., Lee, M. S., & Lim, H. J. (2008). Effects of group music intervention on depression, anxiety, and relationships in psychiatric patients: A pilot study. *The Journal of Alternative and Complementary Medicine, 14*(5), 567–570.

Church, K. (2018). *Mad positive in the academy: From conference to curriculum.* Ryerson University. Retrieved January 5, 2018, from https://www.ryerson.ca/ds/madpositive/

Clarke, L. F. (2016). Embracing polyphony: Voices, improvisation, and the hearing voices network. *Intersec-tionalities: A Global Journal of Social Work Analysis, Research, Polity, and Practice, 5*(2), 1–11.

Costa, L. (2014). *Mad studies - What is it and why should you care?* Retrieved April 1, 2016, from https://madstudies2014. wordpress.com

Costa, L., Voronka, J., Landry, D., Reid, J., Mcfarlane, B., Reville, D., & Church, K. (2012). "Recovering our stories": A small act of resistance. *Studies in Social Justice, 6*(1), 85–101.

Crawford, P., Lewis, L., Brown, B., & Manning, N. (2013). Creative practice as mutual recovery in mental health. *Mental Health Review Journal, 18*(2), 44–64.

Cresswell, M., & Spandler, H. (2012). The engaged academic: Academic intellectuals and the psychiatric survivor movement. Social movement Studies. *Journal of Social, Cultural and Political Protest, 11*(4), 138–154. ISSN 1474-2837

Denzin, N. K., & Lincoln, Y. S. (Eds.). (2010). *The handbook of qualitative research.* Thousand Oaks, CA: Sage Publications, Ltd.

Dingle, G. A., Brander, C., Ballantyne, J., & Baker, F. A. (2013). 'To be heard': The social and mental health benefits of choir singing for disadvantaged adults. *Psychology of Music, 41*(4), 405–421.

Eminem, Rihanna, Bellion, J., & Rexha, B. (2013). The monster. On *The Marshall Mathers LP 2*, CD. Recorded by Frequency. New York: Aftermath.

Everett, B. (2000). *A fragile revolution: Consumers and psychiatric survivors confront the oppression of the mental health system.* Waterloo, ON: Wilfred Laurier University Press.

Foucault, M. (1995). *Discipline and punish: The birth of the prison* (2nd ed.). New York: Vintage Books.

Foucault, M. (1999). *Abnormal: Lectures at the college de France 1974–1975.* New York: Picador.

Foucault, M. (2003). *Psychiatric power: Lectures at the college de France 1973–1974.* New York: Picador.

Foucault, M. (2007). *The politics of truth.* Los Angeles: Semiotext(e).

Frances, A. (2014). *Saving normal: An insider's revolt against out of control psychiatric diagnosis, DSM5, big pharma, and the medicalization of ordinary life.* New York: William Morrow.

Freire, P. (2009). *Pedagogy of the oppressed.* New York: Continuum.

Greer, E. (2017). *Evan Greer bandcamp.* https://evangreer.bandcamp.com/album/evan-greer-friends-never-surrender

Grocke, D., Bloch, S., Castle, D., Thompson, G., Newton, R., Stewart, S., & Gold, C. (2014). Group music therapy for severe mental illness: A randomized embedded-experimental mixed methods study. *Acta Psy-Chiatrica Scandinavica, 130*(2), 144–153.

Howie the Harp. (2018). *Crazy and proud.* Retrieved June 24, 2018, from http://www.mindfreedom.org

Icarus Project. (2017). Retrieved May 30, 2017, from http://legacy.theicarusproject.net/

Johnston, K. (2010). Performing depression: The workman theatre project and the making of Joy. A musical. About depression. In B. Henderson & N. Ostrander (Eds.), *Understanding disability studies and performance studies* (pp. 206–224). New York, NY: Routledge.

Lee, J., & Thyer, B. A. (2013). Does music therapy improve mental health in adults? A review. *Journal of Human Behavior in the Social Environment, 23*(5), 591–603.

LeFrançois, B. A., & Diamond, S. (2014). *Psychiatry disrupted: Theorizing resistance and crafting the (r)evolution.* McGill-Queen's University Press.

LeFrançois, B. A., Menzies, R., & Reaume, G. (Eds.) (2013). *Mad matters: A critical reader in Canadian mad studies.* Canadian Scholars' Press.

Legge, A. W. (2015). *On the neural mechanisms of music therapy in mental health care: Literature review and clinical implications.* Music Therapy Perspectives, miv025.

Liegghio, M. (2013). A denial of being: Psychiatrization as epistemic violence. In B. A. LeFrançois, R. Menzies, & G. Reaume (Eds.), *Mad matters: A critical reader in Canadian Mad studies* (pp. 122–129). Toronto, ON: Canadian Scholars' Press.

Lin, S. T., Yang, P., Lai, C. Y., Su, Y. Y., Yeh, Y. C., Huang, M. F., & Chen, C. C. (2011). Mental health implications of music: Insight from neuroscientific and clinical studies. *Harvard Review of Psychiatry, 19*(1), 34–46.

Mackler, D. (2016). *Songs from the locked ward: Bullshit-anti-psychiatry and anti-medication song.* http://wildtruth.net

McCaffrey, T. M. (2014). *Experts' by experience perspectives of music therapy in mental health care: A multimodal evaluation through art, song and words.* Ireland: University of Limerick.

McLaren, P., & Kincheloe, J. L. (Eds.) (2007). *Critical pedagogy: Where are we now?, 299.* Peter Lang.

McWade, B., Milton, D., & Beresford, P. (2015). Mad Studies and neurodiversity: A dialogue. *Disability and Society, 30*(2), 305–309.

Patterson, S., Duhig, M., Darbyshire, C., Counsel, R., Higgins, N., & Williams, I. (2015). Implementing music therapy on an adolescent inpatient unit: A mixed-methods evaluation of acceptability, experience of participation and perceived impact. *Australasian Psychiatry.* https://doi.org/10.1177/1039856215592320

Patton, M. Q. (1990). *Qualitative research and evaluation methods* (2nd ed.). Newbury Park, CA: Sage.

Price, M. (2011). *Mad at school: Rhetorics of mental disability and academic life.* University of Michigan Press.

Procknow, G. (2017). Silence or sanism: A review of the dearth of discussions on mental illness in adult education. *New Horizons in Adult Education and Human Resource Development, 29*(2), 4–24.

Reaume, G. (2008). A history of psychiatric survivor pride day during the 1990s. [Bulletin 374, 1-10, Mad Pride Issue July 14, 2008]. Toronto, ON: The Consumer/Survivor Information Resource Centre. http://csinfo.ca/bulletin/Bulletin_374.pdf

Reville, D., & Church, K. (2012). Mad activism enters its fifth decade: Psychiatric survivor organizing in Toronto. *Organize*, 189–201.

Rimke, H. (2016). Mental and emotional distress as a social justice issue: Beyond psychocentrism. *Studies in Social Justice, 10*(1), 4–7.

Rolvsjord, R. (2014). What clients do to make music therapy work: A qualitative multiple case study in adult mental health care. *Nordic Journal of Music Therapy*, 1–26.

Rose, N. (1998). *Inventing our selves: Psychology, power, and personhood.* Cambridge, UK: Cambridge University Press.

Russo, J., & Beresford, P. (2015). Between exclusion and colonization: Seeking a place for mad people's knowledge in academia. *Disability and Society, 30*(1), 153–157.

Rykov, M. H. (2006). Voicing the song of music therapy cancer support. In *Proceedings of the 25th CASAE conference* (pp. 204–209). Toronto, Canada: York University.

Spelman, N. (2012). *Popular music and the myths of madness.* Surrey, England: Ashgate.

Stake, R. E. (2000). Case studies. In N. K. Denzin & Y. S. Lincoln (Eds.), *Handbook of qualitative research* (2nd ed., pp. 435–454). Thousand Oaks, CA: SAGE.

Suetani, S., & Batterham, M. (2015). Un-rapping teen spirit: Use of rap music as a treatment tool in adolescence psychiatry. *Australian and New Zealand Journal of Psychiatry.* https://doi.org/10.1177/0004867415576978.

Survivors' History Group. (2010) *'Survivors' history and the survivors history group' on the rethink mental illness.* Retrieved January, 5, 2018, from http://www.rethink.org/document.rm7id.6373

Sweeney, A. (2016). An introduction to survivor research. In J. Russo & A. Sweeney (Eds.), *Searching for a rose garden: Challenging psychiatry, fostering Mad Studies.* Ross-on-Wye, UK: PCCS Books.

Thomson, R. G. (2017). *Extraordinary bodies: Figuring physical disability in American culture and literature.* New York: Columbia University Press.

Toronto Mad Pride (2018). *Toronto Mad Pride: Culture, advocacy, history and fun with Mad, crazy, consumers / survivors and labelled folk - Mad Music and performer directory.* Retrieved January 1, 2018, from www.torontomadpride.com

Västfjäll, D., Juslin, P. N., & Hartig, T. (2012). Music, subjective wellbeing, and health: The role of everyday emotions. *Music, Health and Wellbeing*, 405–423.

Walker, W. (2011). Alterity: Learning polyvalent selves, resisting disabling notions of the self. *New Directions for Adult and Continuing Education, 132*, 43–52.

Whitaker, R. (2010). *Anatomy of an epidemic: Magic bullets, psychiatric drugs, and the astonishing rise of mental illness in America.* New York: Broadway Books.

Chapter 3

Woody Guthrie's Brain

Issa Ibrahim

Summary

Over 250 institutions for the "insane," first called "lunatic asylums," were built throughout the United States from the mid-nineteenth century to the early twentieth century. By 1948, they housed more than a half-million people. Michel Foucault's *History of Madness* (2006) tells the story of this process in Europe. Foucault makes the compelling argument that this physical exclusion and physical othering set the stage for medical, psychological, and social othering that followed. Indeed, this physical othering becomes the founding act of the sanism we must all cope with today. In the United States, the institutional aspects of this began to shift in the 1960s, as the process of deinstitutionalization nearly emptied the psychiatric wards. But the state continues various forms of involuntary treatment and confinement to this day.

Issa Ibrahim brings his experiences as a writer, artist, and former psychiatric "inmate" to counter the relentless othering of these institutional processes. In this chapter, Ibrahim uses creative nonfiction to take us into the world of one of these institutions: Creedmoor Psychiatric Center, as it is now called. Ibrahim tells the story of his life at Creedmoor, his interactions with hospital chaplain Father Chuck, and the legend of how Woody Guthrie's ghost came to haunt the grounds. For Father Chuck, if you listen closely, you can still here Guthrie singing "Worried Man Blues" in the halls and corridors of Creedmoor Psychiatric Institute:

I went across the river
I lay down to sleep
I went across the river
I lay down to sleep
When I woke up
Had shackles on my feet …

*

I was in the main yard on a scorching August afternoon when I saw him step out, slower than usual, his huge bear-like frame shuffling almost aimlessly when I waved him over. His bearded face was slackened, as if in shock. Even in the brilliant sun he

DOI: 10.4324/9781003148456-5

wasn't wearing his customary shades. His eyes were vacant, like a child who has lost his dog or his best friend, and I discovered that he had.

"Jerry has left us. Jerry has left us," he repeated softly, as if to convince himself that his spiritual mentor and idol Jerry Garcia has died and he will never again see God after one of Garcia's 14-minute solos and a hit of grass. Father Chuck was never the same after Jerry Garcia's death. His sermons lost their trippy, otherworldly leanings and slow-dived into more traditionally Catholic guilt-inspired cautions bereft of his humor and quirkiness.

Becoming more preoccupied with death and admittedly disappointed with how Creedmoor handled its patients, Father Chuck would often go on tangents about mistreatment, malpractice, and the hospital's history of quickly and quietly settling lawsuits to prevent the further soiling of its already shaky reputation. He was one of the rare few employees who spoke the truth to the patients about what went on, and what still goes on, here in Creedmoor. Perhaps the creepiest injustice in Father Chuck's recurring nuthouse nightmares is his understanding of the tragic story of Woody Guthrie, who reputedly walked through the gothic iron gates of Creedmoor Hospital and left a vital part of himself behind.

Father Chuck and I grew close by talking music. I'd often ask him if there was anything new or good he was listening to.

"Well, the new Tom Petty is pretty good. A lot like his other stuff but he's pretty reliable. And I heard the latest offering from The Stones, which wasn't too bad. I don't know why they still bother to make records; I guess they need the money. They've got an artistic and creative range that's an inch wide but a mile deep that they've been mining since 1963. There's an audience for them though. And I think they could possibly do it till they die."

I came to realize that if I wanted a review or commentary on any artist under the age of 30, I should probably look elsewhere, but I also recognized a lot of myself in him. Not terribly impressed with any of the Seattle grunge bands besides the first wave, suspicious of the annoying adenoidal White boy whine of the alternative pop-rockers popping up in the 1990s, and basically holding on for dear life to the new wave icons that moved me as a teenager some 20 years previous, I was slowly becoming an old rock and roll fart.

Still, I always enjoyed talking tunes with Father Chuck whenever he made his rounds of the wards, or if I happened to run into him while I was on my grounds privileges as he traveled to the increasingly few open buildings. He saw the deinstitutionalization of this hospital that started decades ago and was pleased that the wards and buildings were emptying out and shutting down. That I was committed in the early 1990s, when New York State realized that policy wasn't working and started locking us mental patients down harder, upset Father Chuck. He thought me and the other Insanity Plea patients deserved the shot at freedom that many other less politically uncomfortable patients received. I saw this compassion in him and it moved me. He was one of the few whom I could open up to, about my crime, my remorse, reveal my fear of not ever getting out, my anger at the system, my frustration at the everyday indignities, and my hopes for a better life, symptom-free, marijuana free.

"Well, I guess reefer isn't for everybody," he'd often say enigmatically.

Like a good chaplain and soul supporter Father Chuck remembered all the things I said to him. He got to know me, and he would comment on a new song or local concert appearance by an artist I might have mentioned liking. I delighted in his giving me a song by song account of the reunion concert he saw of Elvis Costello and the Attractions, saying "they played their hearts out but in the end the audience didn't seem to appreciate the specialness of it besides a few committed fans. I bet you would have loved it, though."

"Yeah, I probably would've," I sighed ruefully, but also grateful for his review.

Father Chuck was born Charles Edward Brodeur in Rural Valley, Pennsylvania, in 1937. Fifty miles northeast from American songwriting pioneer Stephen Foster's hometown of Pittsburgh. Charles grew up on a modest farm with his God-fearing parents and protective older sister. Charles and Emily would spend many evenings after their chores and homework were done listening intently to radio dramas, laughing at the various comedic programs, and dancing together to ballroom waltzes and the polite jazz sounds of the Paul Whiteman Orchestra when their parents had gone off to bed. Charles had an affinity for music. He was an avid listener though he never learned to play an instrument, his parents likening it to dereliction in deference to his studies and their hopes for him being the first in their family to go to college and possibly even pursue his talents in youth counseling into a life in the clergy.

Charles did indeed graduate with honors from Saint Joseph's University in Philadelphia with a degree in psychology and followed that up with a master's in divinity from The Lutheran Theological Seminary and fellowship in Saint John Lutheran Rectory. However, though his nose was in the good book his ears were always tuned to the radio, seeking out the best sounds broadcasting the Negro beat music for juvenile delinquents that was scaring the bejeezus out of America that was dubbed "rhythm and blues." While he would be flogged by his parents were he to be caught listening to the bebop and hard swing that he caught fleeting sonic glimpses of as his sister Emily whizzed the dial on the family RCA, searching for Jack Benny and Dinah Shore, he was happy to have studied away from home so he could have access to the driving drum thunder of Gene Krupa, the blistering blare of trumpeter Harry 'Sweets' Edison, and the confounding but still satisfying scat of Ella Fitzgerald.

We are talking music, as usual, when Father Chuck suggests as a topic "classic shows that blew your mind." I mention catching The Clash playing Bond's Casino on Broadway when I was 15.

"I cut school that day and got on line at 10 a.m. to ensure a good place for the General Admission show and after a lot of pushing and shouting and a near riot during the opening act I wound up stage center, looking up Joe Strummer's nostrils, impressed by the dental work done on his once-infamous atrocious teeth and baptized by his sweat, saliva, and soul. Absolutely life changing!"

Father Chuck nominates the Dead, of course, but on a double bill with Bob Dylan in the summer of 1987. "While the Dead were better than usual Dylan was transcendent," he says with awe and reverence.

"Yeah, I hear ya," I enthuse, "I saw him at Radio City in '88. He was amazing. What was really cool was he had grown tired of doing all his old stuff the same old way so by this time he was re-inventing the hits. Like, more than halfway through a song you'd find yourself saying, 'Oh, that's "Like a Rolling Stone," or 'Oh, that's "Just Like a Woman."' It was wild. I overheard some fans, or so-called fans, walking out complaining but Dylan's cool to do that, if for no one else than himself. He's gotta keep it fresh, you know?"

"Well, Dylan learned from the best. I give him credit for continuing to grow as an artist while still to a degree after all these years remaining true to the very root of where he came from musically. Blues, traditional folk and even the standards."

"Even though he freaked Pete Seeger and the die-hards out by going electric?"

"Especially! It's the message, what you're saying that's important, not so much the vehicle that you drive up in to deliver it. Woody Guthrie would've been proud. But only the two of them know how he really felt about that. Bob made the long trek to New York City to seek out his idol. Haunted Woody's old apartment on Mermaid Avenue in Coney Island in brutal winter weather with just the bare clothes on his back to catch a glimpse of the now infirm and reclusive troubadour. Bob eventually tracked Woody down with the help of Guthrie's protégé, Ramblin' Jack Elliott. With Woody sick with Huntington's disease at Greystone Psych Hospital in Trenton, New Jersey, Bob was taking notes. Not actually writing stuff down, although who knows, maybe he was, but that young kid was sitting with this living legend, this folk icon, the great Woody Guthrie, stricken with this progressive genetic neurological disorder inherited from his mother, Nora."

"Bob was soaking it all up. Like a 22-year-old baby-faced sponge, carting his cheap, battered acoustic guitar with him, him and Ramblin' Jack sitting at Guthrie's bedside, Elliott acting as a medium in a séance for someone not yet dead, schooling Bob on the ways of Woody. In his rare lucid moments Guthrie would proclaim, 'If you want to learn something just steal it—that's the way I learned from Lead Belly.' The three kindred spirits traded folk and roots music passed by the oral tradition, political songs, labor songs, and children's songs and ballads, most of which came from Stephen Foster's quill, even some of Woody's tunes, rare ones, some even Woody forgot and others that he would remember and tell Bob where he was when he wrote them, what they meant to him, what they really mean. And Woody, in the delicate state that he was in, befriended Bob Dylan, AKA Robert Allen Zimmerman, the wandering Jew from Hibbing, Minnesota."

"And Woody's wife and kids took Bob in when he visited, amused by this youthful pretender, who at that time was nakedly emulating Woody's style, while also appreciating Bob's open, childlike awe of this man who was just a husband and father and musician and loudmouth and was now bed-ridden, discombobulated with jerky body movements, and behavioral and psychiatric problems. Woody would have good days and bad days and eventually suffer worse days. Bob would sing to Woody for hours during some visits, challenging himself, trying to remember every song he knew. On others, Woody would berate Bob mercilessly. With increasing muscular distress, unable to control his movements, declining health, and erratic mood swings, Woody endured various misdiagnoses including alcoholism and schizophrenia. Woody got sicker and sicker, and his condition and illness weren't fully understood by most of the doctors he visited. Due to a lack of information about the disease at the time, his illness went essentially untreated. Had he more money or access to better medical care maybe he could've been more comfortable. Either way, he grew difficult to be around. He had a deficient memory, egocentrism, aggression, and compulsive behavior and eventually he was committed to Creedmoor."

"Get out!"

"Yep."

"Seriously?"

"Yep."

"Woody Guthrie was here? In *this* dump?!"

Come his senior year of high school, Father Chuck first heard what was salaciously called "rock and roll" in the form of Bill Haley and the Comets' "Rock Around the Clock" via the film "The Blackboard Jungle" and his mind, his *soul* was rocked. Though he was changed forever, in another profound way he was bound, professing a lifelong love of rock and rhythm and blues yet chastened by his familial obligation and commitment to the church. Like rock architect Richard Penniman, Charles adored the beat and the attitude of the new form yet was torn by the perception that it was "the devil's music." While Little Richard wrestled with his demons, dropping out and then returning repeatedly to his obvious calling as a musical visionary, Charles spent the 1960s hiding his Beatles and Stones LPs beneath the quaint efforts of Mantovani and Englebert Humperdinck. He attended landmark concerts from Café Wha? to the Fillmore East, making the scene, blowing his mind, and covering his tracks with invented tales of bible studies and peaceful retreats.

In the late 1960s, Charles discovered The Grateful Dead and marijuana, two potent mind-altering forces that continue to influence his sermons to this very day. Through bleary eyes and a bemused smile, Father Chuck would quote an eerily appropriate line from The Dead and weave a dizzying 45-minute tapestry infusing the lyrical relevance of "Death Don't Have No Mercy" or "Attics of My Life" with the wisdom of Solomon or the compassion of Christ himself. Sometimes he would nail it and other times he would meander to a mumble, lidded eyes indicating a carelessness, and blissed out dry mouthed smacks suggesting his high had long since peaked, the sermon was over, and he was now eager to dig into the Hostess cupcakes waiting for him in his desk drawer.

This is not to suggest Father Chuck was a habitual stoner, however, during the 1970s and 1980s the laissez-faire Creedmoor hospital administration didn't notice or care if one of their more popular chaplains rambled occasionally during services or wore sunglasses indoors. He had excellent time and attendance, performed compelling and inspired memorial services including a taped rendition of The Dead's "Ripple" whenever an inpatient passed away, and was exceptionally good relating to the current crop of MICA patients, mentally ill chemical abusers, like me.

"Believe it," [Father Chuck says to me]. "One time bound for glory, Woody Guthrie ended up one of the many institutionalized mentally ill. He was pretty bad off by the time he got here. His muscular coordination was shot, he'd suffered significant cognitive decline and had developed dementia. I heard stories of a paranoid/post-motorcycle accident Dylan coming down from his reclusive retreat up in Woodstock to visit Woody here in Creedmoor, but some people who were there say he showed up in disguise and was acting really strange and stayed only five or ten minutes, saw the state Woody was in, and started freaking out because Woody didn't recognize him. Bob caused a ruckus and was practically thrown out of the place. I don't know if *that's* true but it could've happened. I wouldn't dismiss it out of hand. So, Woody finally passed away. I think it was in the fall of '67. He was 55."

"Damn, that's young. My dad died of cancer at the same age."

"And apparently the hospital got him or his family to sign away his brain. For study."

"What?"

"Yeah, Creedmoor took Woody Guthrie's brain. Though I don't think it was legal, or let's just say someone may have signed the paperwork but it's morally questionable. When his son Arlo became somewhat famous in the late 60s for that silly song,"

"'Alice's Restaurant?'"

"Ugh, yes. Well there was talk of having him come out here and sing and play in a concert, to honor his father, raise a little money for research, maybe help improve the hospital's image but he wasn't interested. He was fairly disgusted by the whole thing. Marjorie, Woody's wife, did a lot to raise awareness of the disease which led to the founding of the Huntington's Disease Society of America, although there's still no cure. When I came here in '73 and heard the story I started to look into it and discovered the usual sloppy record keeping and convenient amnesia which suggested to me that the Guthrie family may have been coerced or Woody might not have even been competent enough to sign that waiver."

"So what happened to it?"

"Woody's brain sat in a jar of muddy formaldehyde in the basement of Building 40 in a storage room down the hall from the hospital morgue where they kept excised organs and body parts from patients who died of unnatural causes. There were other brains in jars down there, stacked on dusty metal shelves, with index cards strung to the lids all with no names and only patient identification numbers and the disorder that the particular brain suffered from. It was a shame and seemed a crime that the body and soul of the writer of "This Land Is Your Land" wandered this lunatic's landscape toward the great beyond like a zombie with empty eyes and a concave skull while his brain sat unsung amidst the remnants of the homeless and the hopelessly mentally infirm. But perhaps Woody would see the beauty in that, champion of the downtrodden, friend of the forgotten, up-lifter of the underdog that he was. Perhaps the most important part of him, the part besides his heart that conjured up those haunting melodies and stirring lyrics, perhaps his nameless, fameless brain wading in those staid chemicals would find a sense of peace and contentment. Not getting any special treatment in death, no amenities or privileges of the pampered pop culture put-on artists, of which his acolyte Bob Zimmerman has struggled successfully against, would make Woody proud."

"Wow. But there's no more morgue here, is there? I mean, when I first came here in '92 I saw the sign in the back of the building but since the renovation…"

"You're right. After the renovation in the 90s where they updated the medical records office, restructured the clinic, and gutted the basement to put the Rec center down there, basically changing their identity from 'Creedmoor Hospital' to a 'psychiatric center' all of the old equipment was modified and whatever didn't adhere to the new mode of treatment and protocols was eliminated. Nobody I know is aware of what happened to the bodies, body parts, and brains that were housed down there, and the few who were around in the 30 or so years it took to phase out the old system and implement the current way of doing things aren't talking."

"Man, that's wild."

"Yes, but that's not all. Here's something you as an artist will find interesting. While most of the remains went missing, probably rudely and disrespectfully disposed of, I'd been hearing talk of the former director's interest in collecting what now goes by the name of Outsider Art, most of the "found objects" variety, are you familiar with that?"

"Definitely. I've done some pieces, artwork, sculptures comprised of found objects."

"Hmmm. Well it seems our former CEO may have had a morbid fascination with the macabre, and though I've never been in her office, Rabbi Rosenberg has told me that he's seen, sitting deep in her mahogany bookshelf among Haitian fetish objects, a large, filmy, glass jar with a brain in it and propped up next to it is a framed photograph of Woody Guthrie famously strumming his guitar emblazoned with the slogan 'This Machine Kills Fascists.'"

"Aw, now that's just sick!"

"No, it gets better. I've been working here a long time and I've made a lot of friends, some in medical records. And I'm not ashamed to say that as a music lover and fan of Woody's, I went down there to see if I could look up his records and do my own little investigations."

"Really? Whadya find?"

"Not much. There was little on him years ago when I went down to check his file and in recent years, due again to the renovation and overhaul and consolidation of the records, there's virtually nothing. Except, Rabbi Rosenberg would swear that he saw what looked like an old yellowed death certificate framed and sitting next to the photo and the brain."

"Well, I dunno, Father Chuck. Rabbi Rosenberg is also said to frequent prostitutes and carry a loaded gun in his briefcase."

"Ah yes, I've heard that too."

We sit in silence for a little while, Father Chuck resting his thick arms over his prosperous belly as if just finishing a filling meal, my face screwed up into a knotted mask of stupefaction. I look into his eyes, stoic yet sad. I can see that he will mourn Jerry Garcia for the rest of his days, as he's mourned John Lennon, and Phil Ochs, and Jimi Hendrix, and Janis Joplin and Brian Jones, and Otis Redding…and Woody Guthrie.

"So…"

"So what?"

"So did she take it? Did she take it with her when she left?"

"Well, you may remember she was let go. Asked to retire so as to avoid the ugliness of a forcible removal of a state figurehead, and under those circumstances she was not allowed to return to even clean out her desk…or her bookshelf."

"So, where is it?"

"Like I said, nobody's telling. But I stay late on some nights, preparing the next day's sacrament and though I'd like to think it's the wind rushing up and down and through this tall drafty building, sometimes, just as I'm leaving, I have heard what sounds like a low mournful whistling coming from the director's office. And I'll be damned if that whistling, like the chilling gust rattling through the bones in a graveyard, doesn't veer into a spectral wail of one of Woody's songs. That folk tune telling the story of a man imprisoned for unknown reasons...the song 'Worried Man Blues.'"

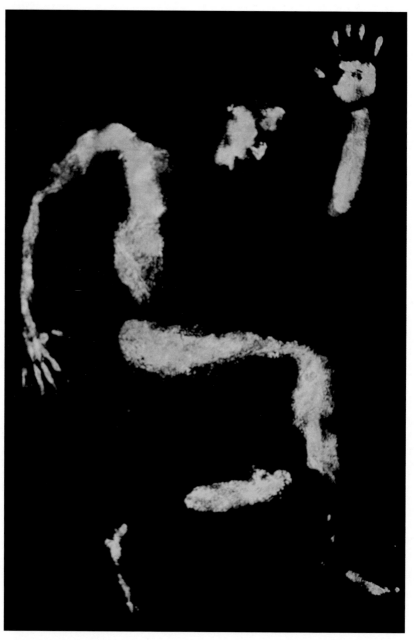

Man in a Box (body print) acrylic, enamel on unstretched canvas. 62×49 (1997). Artist: Issa Ibrahim.

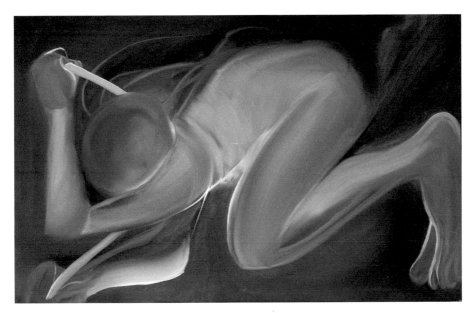

Turmoil, oil on canvas, 24×48 (1995). Artist: Issa Ibrahim.

Editor's Reference

Foucault, M. (2006). *History of madness.* Routledge.

Chapter 4

The Invisible Line of Madness

Sabrina Chap

Summary

Sabrina Chap is a Brooklyn-based songwriter, composer, and performer noted for her live shows, where she mixes high theatricality with gut punches of truth. She has performed both on large stages and in small barrooms across the country. Chap is also the editor of the Lambda-nominated anthology *Live Through This: On Creativity and Self-Destruction*. The collection explores the frequent entanglement of seemingly contradictive destructive and creative forces, not simply one or the other, but the often invaluable yet volatile ways they mix together.

In this chapter, Chap explores another contradiction that often goes together: the experiences that are pathologized in the clinician's office and in normal society can also be experiences that are most appreciated and valued onstage and in the arts. Chap does not romanticize these experiences, but at the same time, her perspective opens up a point of view rarely understood in mainstream approaches to mental difference.

*

The invisible line that divides an audience from the stage is a powerful one. Sometimes, it's a raised platform. Sometimes, it's a spotlight. And sometimes, it's simply one person facing a hundred others; just one person with a mic, peering into hundreds of judging eyes and delivering whatever cockamamie thoughts they've developed in the privacy of their bedroom. Of course, if someone saw us in our bedroom, talking to ourselves, muttering the lyrics to songs, or practicing poses in the mirror, they'd call us crazy. But when we're on stage, they applaud.

Years ago, in college, a doctor listened to me for less than five minutes and said, 'You're manic bipolar,' and then looked down at her clipboard, checking off a box. She said it like it was a bad thing. Like something was wrong with me. Sure, I had had a hard time sleeping and was writing deep into the morning hours. And, sure, I'd realized that the line between me and the other 'normal' students was tenuous at best. But when I asked her how she could tell, she said, 'You speak too fast.'

I always speak too fast.

I speak too fast, I think too fast, I judge too fast, and my feelings may go deeper and higher than most people with basic nine-to-five jobs. But is that a bad thing? Well, it depends on where you're standing.

DOI: 10.4324/9781003148456-6

I'm often standing on a stage. In fact, I grew up on stages. As a pianist, I began competing at five years old, quickly memorizing the crystallized tension in the air as a room stares at you as you express yourself. I've stood on several stages through the years – as an actress, a spoken word performer, a folk singer, a public speaker, an avant-garde composer, and most recently, a cabaret performer.

Each time I step on a stage, it's after a period of intense creation. I mutter to myself, memorizing lines. As a songwriter, I follow the tunes in my head, looking for the words to anchor them as I wander the streets of Brooklyn. As a writer, I plunge into the depths of my sorrow and joy, hoping to scavenge a few glistening words or truths that might help me process my emotions and calm my spinning head. The act of creation, if done right, would be seen as madness to anyone who doesn't understand the process. Perhaps it's the physical elevation of 'the stage' that allows audiences to accept me in my elevated states.

Case in point – one of my early gigs as a cabaret performer was at a show called, 'Book Club Burlesque,' where all the performers would read the same book and then create a piece inspired by it. For one performance, we were all supposed to read 'Geek Love' by Katherine Dunn and write a piece from it. I wrote a song called, 'Freaks,' which was about the power of being an outsider. The song was one built on rage, devotion, and the sly smile of the wicked. I was excited to share it, but since it was a wordy song, I needed to focus the audience to hear it properly.

There was a group of men seated towards the front, who'd been heckling acts throughout the show. They were mostly entertaining themselves, not being funny at all, and pulling focus from the performers. At one point, they started heckling me. Not in an evil-spirited way, but in a drunk, 'We think we're *hilarious!*' sort of way…

Time froze. I wanted to shut them down in flames but was afraid to do it in front of everyone. Two selves battled internally as I continued playing, the Devil me saying, 'Burn them, shut them down!' the Angel me saying, 'Oh, let it go – they're just having fun. Who cares if they ruin your song with their incessant chatting?' As someone who rarely thinks before she speaks, this struggle seemed to last forever in my mind, until part of me thought, 'Oh well, it's too late to say something now.' Finally, I couldn't help myself, and without thinking, shut them down in front of everyone with a few words and continued with my song.

In my head, it felt like at least a minute had passed between them speaking and me responding – an eternity. However, I had taped this performance, and looking back at the tape, I realized that I responded so fast, I almost cut them off. They had hardly finished their sentences.

It was the first time I realized how fast I really was, and the difference between what the audience saw versus what I experienced. I was shocked. The measure of time in my mind didn't match 'real-time.' In fact, I soon became known for how much I loved responding to hecklers. It felt like a kind of superpower, to be able to shut down assholes yelling at the stage without even blinking. I yearned for people to just even fucking try me, marveling at how my sarcastic wit was met with applause while on stage when it usually was met with silence in the real world.

In the 'normal' world, this quick, honest reaction is something that wouldn't go over very well. Many's the time I've gotten in trouble for blurting out what I was thinking. However, once I began performing on stage, it was interesting: my quick responses, my hyper-sensitivity, and my awareness *were* superpowers. People often respond with joy and laughter when I use these powers on stage. Offstage, these non-polite responses would never be accepted. In fact, they would be diagnosed.

Listening to my song, 'The Denial Rag,' most people laugh. It's a patter song, a brisk tempo song crammed with a ton of words. In it, I'm a woman who's pretending she's not sleeping with some man's sister. It's an anxious denial of queerness, all the while alluding to the fact that she is, indeed, bedding the sis. When I perform it, people laugh at the anxiety and fast-paced denial, because it's something they've felt themselves. We've all experienced that heart-pounding, 'not wanting to be found out'-ness, and know that it makes words inexplicably tumble out of our mouths in verbal diarrhea.

However, my mind works in a way that I could recreate that emotional anxiety, put words to it, and deliver the lightning-fast song easily. Because I do, indeed, talk and think that fast. On stage, what others may deem as signs of a 'mental illness' are often seen as 'talent.'

So what is the magic of this invisible line that divides our society into audience and performer? And more importantly, how are we – as artists – able to exist on the other side of the line? Can we? Or are we doomed to madness? Doomed to suicide and institutions, pills, and patient in-takes? Doomed to diagnoses or self-destruction?

These questions were the ones I reckoned with back in college after that first doctor bluntly said, 'You're manic bipolar.' Her diagnosis seemed like a death sentence at a time where I finally had discovered living. At the time, I had finally begun writing my own texts and experimenting on the stage. I staged a piano duet accompanying an artist painting on stage. I wrote a duet for a psychiatrist locked in a battle against her own intellect, represented by a typewriter gone mad. It was in the exuberance of my art-making that my emotional peaks and valleys emerged. As I began to contend with my desire to be an artist, I looked for a roadmap left by other artists whose work I admired and was sobered by what I'd found.

All of my art heroes had killed themselves: Sarah Kane, Virginia Woolf, Sylvia Plath. In fact, all the women artists that I'd resonated with had committed suicide. As someone who often felt her creative output was often twinned with self-destructive behaviors, I wondered if I was doomed to do the same.

For the rest of college, I danced between manic artistic expression and terrifying highs. It was exhilarating until it wasn't. Until I realized I had terrified everyone that ever loved me, alienated friends, and had painted a path towards my own eventual self-destruction. After my senior thesis, the president of our college took me aside, amazed at what I'd produced, and eagerly asked me my plans after school. Flatly, I responded, 'I'm going to work at a bookstore and get a boyfriend.' He looked at me, aghast, 'Sabrina! You can't just go work at a bookstore. What you just produced was incredible.' I returned his gaze and said, 'I'm going to go work at a bookstore because if I don't, I'm going to kill myself.'

I knew I had two paths – one as the brilliant artist who produces a few works of genius and then burns out, and another. I didn't know what that other path looked like, other than it was 'stable' and 'normal.' But since I knew how the first path ended, I decided to simply find out. I resigned myself to stop making art for a year and learn how to be normal.

After a time of healing, I couldn't help but start creating again. But always, was the fear that each time I created, I would be creeping towards a manic spiral. I kept on looking for examples of people who had lived close to the edge of art and sanity and survived, and time and time again, all I found were suicides, alcoholics, and masters of self-destruction.

Finally, I decided to see if I could find some artists who'd admit that they'd dealt with self-destruction, but not let it define them. I needed a badass group of artists to assure me that I could both be a creative artist and also a happy and healthy person. I approached over 60 living artists, asking if they had ever dealt with self-destructive tendencies and if so, if they'd be willing to write about how they balanced that with their art-making. In the end, I had essays from about 20 of them, which made up my book, *Live Through This: On Creativity and Self-Destruction*.

The book was an anthology where I asked a wide array of women and trans artists (dancers, composers, writers, cartoonists, and more) about the relationship between their self-destructive and creative impulses. I approached artists who'd dealt with a variety of self-destructive impulses, from eating disorders and alcoholism to drug abuse and suicidal ideations so I could focus on the common act of self-destruction. In editing the book, and working intensely with most of the artists to tell their stories, I began unraveling themes that coincided with both creative and destructive acts.

At the guidance of one of the book's contributors, revolutionary gender theorist and author, Kate Bornstein, I began lecturing on the book at colleges. I lectured on several themes that occur in both creative and destructive impulses: ritual, control, power, shame, and how it coincides with gender. The ritual of an artist is much like the ritual of someone on the path towards self-destruction. An artist sets up their easel, their keyboard, plays jazz in the background to settle their mind, and makes a cup of coffee to accompany them as they write. As the ritual is completed, the act of art begins, where they can safely allow their mind and craft to explore their emotions. For a cutter, they might have their own ritual – turning off all the bathroom lights, making sure their roommate is asleep, and looking at their face in the bathroom mirror before they open the drawer quietly to retrieve their razors. For alcoholics, they might know, 'If I drive down that street, I'll take a right, and if I take a right, I'll end up at that bar, and if I end up at that bar, I'll get wasted.' Rituals can act as a clearing of space for either self-destructive or creative action.

Control plays a big part in both actions as well. As an artist, when we face our demons, we're able to manipulate their claws outwardly, to make something beautiful, instead of turning them in on ourselves. As self-destructive people, we often unconsciously use our self-destruction as an act of controlling our own pain, i.e., if we damage ourselves, then we are laying claim to our pain as opposed to allowing ourselves to be hurt by others. The topic of control shifts greatly when talking about gender, as it is often conversely reflected by the amount of control each individual has in their place in society.

Shame is vital to self-destructive behaviors, but once tackled, often unlocks the key to an artist's work. In her essay for the book, groundbreaking author and social activist bell hooks mentions how as a child she cried endlessly, 'a survival strategy that aided me in my distress was the intense expression of grief, a conscious sorrow' (hooks, 2012, p. 195). She goes on to reveal the depth of her tears as a young, black girl, and how her tears were shamed by her mother as a sign of not only weakness but of whiteness. Only after delving into fictional narratives where she saw that 'children were often the unjust targets for adult rage,' hooks realized that she needn't accept responsibility for her trauma, that the trauma may have been born of a situation she was placed in (p. 195). This allowed her to stop crying and delve further into what these systems may be, where she then cried out for the rest of her life, now in a highly literate and crafted manner, against injustices across the board.

I lectured and developed workshops where I explored all these themes, suddenly being booked by the budding mental health advocacy groups that slowly began flowering across the nation: The National Alliance on Mental Illness, Active Minds, Icarus Collective, Psychology classes, and Centers for Gender and Sexuality. Soon, my audiences were filled with others who were just like me. Suddenly, there was no line between me and the audience, so there didn't need to be a stage. I didn't need to be elevated. My audience was elevated with me.

We all understood how our minds worked and how it stigmatizes us in the real world. We all understood we had to keep our superpowers secret, although they are the only currency we have in a very blah world. We knew that admitting we weren't exactly 'sane' meant that others would try and categorize us or shame us. When I spoke to artists, we knew that being open about these issues would then allow others to classify our work, especially as women. Sylvia Plath is still seen as a tragic figure, while Hemingway is still seen as the 'manliest of men,' although both of them killed themselves.

As I finally stepped into my own strength as a songwriter and performer, I was very private about my own struggles and that single diagnosis received years ago. I didn't want to be known as 'crazy,' I wanted to be known on the merit of my artistic talents. Privately, I tested the waters, finally telling my best friend of ten years in Brooklyn that I'd been 'diagnosed' as a 'manic bipolar' in college. I said this casually, anecdotally, while talking about another friend I suspected might have an undiagnosed condition.

Suddenly, his tone changed and he began interrogating me: Was I on meds? Was I still crazy? Question after question, every stereotypical fear I had about admitting my diagnosis was confirmed. That night, we texted casually and spoke briefly in the evening. The next morning, his tone had changed completely, and he said to me, 'Last night you were acting crazy.' An accusation I was shocked to hear after ten years of friendship. When I asked in what way I was acting crazy, he replied, 'You were speaking too fast.'

There it was, again. Twenty years later. Simply telling someone I'd dealt with mania allowed them to dismiss me as a crazy person. I told him I thought it was suspicious that the day I had told him of my diagnosis ten years previous, he had suddenly labeled me as crazy. The more I tried to make him understand he was being insensitive and reactionary, the crazier I seemed in his eyes. Our ten-year friendship stopped immediately. I haven't spoken to him since.

I know, firsthand, how my superpower can be used against me in the real world. However, it is the deepest part of me, and the part that I'm most proud of. I'm glad I'm able to dive into my deepest emotions. I'm proud of being able to empathize with people so deeply I'm spurred into action. I love that my mind is so fast and quick that I often see things and patterns before others, but it's been a balancing act of knowing when to pull out my cape, and when to put on my Clark Kent glasses of normalcy to blend in with the blah-ness of the masses to simply survive.

And as an artist, I've learned how to balance my mania for work or float on the sorrows of my depressive episodes when they come. I do think I have a lighter time of it than most, and in ten years of speaking to students and exploring the themes of self-destruction, I understand that the same tools we use to destruct can be turned towards creation. I'm mindful of my patterns, and more importantly, love speaking to others about how to wield these sharpened tools of our minds.

It gives me great joy to attack the stigmas surrounding mental health. Because there is so much shame around mental illness and self-destructive behaviors. It is deemed bad. Shameful. Weak. Like something is wrong with you. Like you're a box to be checked on a clipboard.

But sometimes, when I speak, I see hope in some of the students' eyes. Because, for once, someone isn't telling them that something is wrong with them. Or that they're weak. Or they're small enough to fit in a box. Someone is saying, 'You're more powerful than you know. And, once you learn how to wield your powers, trust me. They'll applaud.'

Reference

hooks, b. (2012). No more crying. In S. Chapadjiev (Ed.), *Live through this: On creativity and self-destruction* (pp. 193–198). Seven Stories Press.

Chapter 5

Cry Havoc

THE MADNESS OF RETURNING HOME FROM WAR

Stephan Wolfert

Summary

In this excerpt from his award-winning one-man play, Stephan Wolfert recounts a moment in his transition from military life to civilian life that left him on the edge of suicide. Wolfert's play uses characters, verses, and themes from Shakespeare's plays to portray the struggle of this transition. He shows the many ways that veterans are left isolated and alone in trying to deal with both the aftermath of time in combat and the realities of a world that does not understand or address their need for compassion, community, and connection. We see in Wolfert's story the roots of experience that led him to found the DE-CRUIT program, which uses structured, routinized practices from classical actor training—along with an experiential analysis of the many veteran and soldier characters in Shakespeare's plays—to help veterans heal and move forward with their lives in meaningful ways.[1]

*

I left a successful career in the US military after seeing Shakespeare's "Richard III" for the first time during a moment of crisis precipitated by the death of my best friend during a routine military training mission. I went on to become a classically trained Shakespearean actor and to found the DE-CRUIT Veterans Trauma Program. I tell my story in my one-man autobiographical play "Cry Havoc" which I have performed to audiences around the world. This is an excerpt from that play.

Los Angeles. Nine years ago. I am catering a tea party. Not the political tea party, but a Disney princess tea party. These gorgeous little four, five, and six year old girls are dressed in their Disney princess gowns and they're running by these gigantic tables piled high with frosted sugary goodness disguised as cake. They grab fistfuls of it and jam it somewhere near their mouths, and they throw the rest on the ground. And my job as a caterer is to bend over and pick up these saliva-strewn balls.

DOI: 10.4324/9781003148456-7

As I bent over to pick one up, I saw my hand as it was when I served in the military. I saw the dirt and gun oil actually in the cracks of my hands. Then I blinked and it was gone, and I saw what I was actually doing… It was a kick in the groin. These hands that served this country. These hands that held my best friend's head together before he died, and handed several folded flags to weeping family members. Called in airstrikes, medevacs, saluted people that were calling me sir and looking me in the eyes and now I'm picking up… blehhh.

And as I knelt there for, I don't know how long—I might have been kneeling three tenths of a second, three minutes, I have no idea. A little girl walked up. She looked me right in the eyes—the first one all day to look me in the eyes—and she threw her cake at me. And my body's reaction—not my thought, but my body's impulse—was to crush her skull. I lurched at her. I caught myself. I didn't hit her. We locked eyes. Horrified, she turned, ran screaming to her mother. More horrified, I pulled myself up, I ran to my jeep in the parking ramp, drove home to my apartment in Venice, locked the door, pulled out my sawed-off shotgun, opened up the breech, jammed a shell in, closed the breech, locked back the hammer…

> *To be, or not to be: that is the question:*
> *Whether 'tis nobler in the mind to suffer*
> *The slings and arrows of outrageous fortune,*
> *Or to take arms against a sea of troubles,*
> *And by opposing end them? To die: to sleep;*
> *No more; and by a sleep to say we end*
> *The heart-ache and the thousand natural shocks*
> *That flesh is heir to, 'tis a consummation*
> *Devoutly to be wish'd. To die, to sleep;*
> *To sleep: perchance to dream: ay, there's the rub;*
> *For in that sleep of death what dreams may come*
> *When we have shuffled off this mortal coil,*
> *Must give us pause: there's the respect*
> *That makes calamity of so long life;*
> *For who would bear the whips and scorns of time,*
> *To grunt and sweat under a weary life,*
> *But that the dread of something after death,*
> *The undiscover'd country from whose bourn*
> *No traveller returns, puzzles the will*
> *And makes us rather bear those ills we have*
> *Than fly to others that we know not of?*
> *Thus conscience does make cowards of us all;*

[Hamlet, *HAMLET*, ACT III, Scene 1]

As soldiers, we are wired for war through our military training, But, as veterans, we are never un-wired from war, never rewired for society. When I went into the military, I had a recruiter prepare me for life in the military. But when I got out, where was my de-cruiter to help prepare me for life after the military? And I know people say, "*Well the VA. Isn't that what it's for?*" Well, no. I want to say, honestly,

I am not here to tag on the VA. I know there's scandals, I know there's problems, but there's a great many veterans getting a great deal of good from the VA. There's more good than bad, and it's better than the alternatives, so let me just say that. But what most people don't know is we are not automatically signed up for the VA. It's a laborious process, as some of us have heard and know, and even for those of us who go through that process we are not automatically covered by the VA. And even for those who are, the VA does not de-cruit.

If I'm wrong about us needing de-cruiting, then why are twenty-two veterans killing themselves every single day? And if I'm wrong about us needing de-cruiting, then ask yourself: Who's catering your kid's party?

Note

1 The DE-CRUIT website can be found here: https://www.decruit.org/

Chapter 6

Betty and Veronica

Emily Allan and Leah Hennessey

Summary

Emily Allan and Leah Hennessey are playwrights, directors, and actors known for their web series *Zhe Zhe*, a camp satire of New York City's performance scene. They have also created and starred in work exploring "Slash fiction," a genre of fan fiction that focuses on homoerotic pairings of canonically straight characters from popular culture. This genre was developed primarily by women writers and uses the power of the erotic imagination to undermine patriarchal traditions of authorship and ownership. In their two-person show *Slash*, Allan and Hennessey bring to life favorite characters from film, TV, literature, and history—such as Sherlock Holmes, Harry Potter, and The Beatles.

The selection included here is an excerpt from *Slash*. Betty and Veronica, two teenage characters from the classic and long-running *Archie* comic-book series, begin to reflect on their lives, their roles, their ongoing conflicts, and the stories they inhabit. Living in the past, perhaps 1950s America, although with anachronistic elements—such as taking psychiatric medications from the present—Betty and Veronica start to wonder why they feel so alienated and disenchanted with their lives. At first, they blame themselves and try a range of mental health treatments to change who they are. But then, on second thought, maybe there is more to it than that.

*

ACT I

BLACKOUT. MUSIC PLAYS, "TRISTAN UND ISOLDE: PRELUDE"

Veronica's house.
Lights up and music cuts as Veronica appears alone onstage, *brushing her hair, looking into an invisible mirror.*

DOI: 10.4324/9781003148456-8

VERONICA

I am beautiful. I am rich. I am fashionable. I am sexy. I am brunette. I am beautiful. I am rich. I am fashionable. I am sexy. I am brunette. I am beautiful.

DING DONG

Veronica looks confused. Betty stands in the doorway.

VERONICA

Betty! I wasn't expecting you.

BETTY

Yeah I know, can I come in?

VERONICA

Of course! Hey it's almost six, shouldn't you be getting ready for the dance?

BETTY

I'm not. Going. To the dance.

VERONICA

(drops hairbrush)
What??

BETTY

That's what I wanted to talk to you about. That and…I don't know. A lot of things.

VERONICA

Sit down sit down. Are you sure you're not going to the dance? What about Archie?

BETTY

Look. I know I'm supposed to go to the dance with Archie, but we both know what's going to happen. You're gonna do something to get Archie's attention and then I'm going to freak out trying to win him back and then at the next dance you'll go with Archie and I'll do something to get his attention and you'll be the one freaking out and then at the next dance…

VERONICA

Okay okay I get it.

BETTY

I just wanted to say: you can have him. I can't do this anymore. I'm done.
SILENCE.

VERONICA

Oh Betty, I'm not falling for one of your tricks again.

BETTY

No this isn't a trick. This isn't even about Archie, or you, it's about me. I need to break—I need to at least try—to break out of this cycle.

VERONICA

Betty, you're scaring me. Are you sure you're feeling okay?

BETTY

I'm not feeling ok actually. I haven't felt okay in a really long time. I feel fucking trapped…in this…this…I don't know—

VERONICA

…role?

BETTY

Yeah. Exactly. It's like what is my life even? I'm the girl next door. I like Archie. I compete with you. I'm blond. I go to school—and then it's like, I go to school but I don't ever learn anything. I feel like I'm never even in class, I'm always in the hallway, or a dance or at a bake sale, or at the fucking diner. It's like, when am I going to graduate? I wanna go to college! I wanna get out of Riverdale! I feel like I've been in high school for decades, I feel so old! I know this sounds crazy—

VERONICA

It doesn't. It doesn't sound crazy.

BETTY

I just don't have anyone else to talk to…

VERONICA

Betty, I understand. I understand more than you know.

BETTY

What, what do you mean?

VERONICA

Betty, it sounds like you're suffering from depression.

BETTY

No, I'm not sad—I'm paralyzed—nothing seems real—I feel like a character, trapped in some—

VERONICA

Betty, there are a lot of popular misconceptions about depression. Depression isn't a feeling, it's not like sadness or anger—clinical depression is a disease caused by a neurochemical imbalance in the brain, and it can be life threatening. Have you ever thought about self harm?

BETTY

You mean like, suicide?

VERONICA

Yeah, but not just that.

BETTY

Well. Remember last year? When you went to the dance with Archie, and then we all went to Pops, and I was flirting with Archie and sharing a milkshake, but then I just left?

VERONICA

Yes.

BETTY

Well. That night I went home and I tried to kill myself.

VERONICA

Wait. Really?

BETTY

Yeah. I had to go to the hospital and get my stomach pumped.
Silence

VERONICA

Betty. That night, after you left the diner, I went home alone. And. I slit my wrists.

BETTY

What?? Why???

VERONICA

Because I wanted to feel something. Everything seemed so meaningless. I guess in my own way, I was trying to break the cycle.

BETTY

Ronnie, I had no idea.

VERONICA

Since then I've been taking pretty heavy-duty SSRIs. At first they really helped but now I just feel sluggish, and out of it. And I have no sex drive.

BETTY

Wait, that's so crazy. I've been doing cognitive behavioral therapy and going to this meditation workshop and like, I'm eating better and sleeping better and I haven't wanted to kill myself but I feel like we're never getting to the root of the problem—like maybe the problem isn't my personal trauma or existential despair, maybe there's something actually wrong, with my, my reality. Plus, all that shit is so expensive and I only have one more session of CBT covered by my insurance.

VERONICA

I think I know what you mean. It does go beyond depression.

BETTY

Right? Like there's something objectively wrong with the reality status of our lives, our lives in particular are particularly meaningless and you and I are unusually devoid of agency.

VERONICA

Yeah. I know.

BETTY

> You do?

VERONICA

> Yeah I've felt this way for a long time, and there is something.

BETTY

> What?

VERONICA

> There's something I've been wanting to try.

BETTY

> Yeah?

VERONICA

> It's a little unorthodox.

BETTY

> At this point I'm willing to try anything.

VERONICA

> Okay. Um. Well. So. When you were little. No. Okay. So. How do I start. Did you ever fantasize about homoerotic relationships between "straight: male fictional or historical characters"?

BETTY

> You mean like thinking about Captain Kirk and Mr. Spock having sex?

VERONICA

> Yes, but not just sex. Like, thinking about the depth of the connection between Kirk and Spock that is canon, but then also allowing yourself to expand upon that very real dynamic and to imagine their fully realized, sexual, erotic, relationship.

BETTY

> Yeah. I've done that.

VERONICA

> Me too. But have you ever acted out any of your fantasies with another person?

BETTY

> No, who would want to do that with me? Archie?
>> *They both laugh.*

VERONICA

> Awkward!
>> *They smile.*

VERONICA

> So. Do you want to try it with me?

BETTY
> Yeah.

VERONICA
> Cool.

BETTY
> But, don't you have to go to the dance?

VERONICA
> Fuck the dance. Let's do it.

Chapter 7

The Uses of Depression

THE WAY AROUND IS THROUGH[1]

David Budbill

Summary

David Budbill lyrically describes the way he used poetry and spirituality to develop a "give in" approach to depression. Rather than fight depression or try to consciously change it, he found that "the only way around my periods of depression is directly through them: in other words, the sooner I can resign myself to the Angel of Depression, the sooner she will be done with me and leave me alone." Surprisingly, when Budbill used his give-in approach, he found that there were aspects of depression, what he calls the "uses of depression," that were valuable to him both as a writer and as a person.

Depression slowed him down, heightened his sensitivity, opened him to humility, and helped him receive the world as a passive receptacle. This was not easy, of course. Giving in to depression, allowing himself to feel what he felt, put him outside the norm, particularly in the United States. Emptiness, sloth, slowing down seems un-American when one is surrounded by a culture that prizes speed and busyness. But these very non-normative dimensions also increased Budbill's imagination time, his compassion, and his contact with human suffering. And not only that, it helped him tap into a Zen Buddhist wisdom of fullness and wonder in the heart of the everyday and the ordinary. Budbill does not advocate this method for everyone; he describes himself as different from most—he even calls himself a "rebellious, contrary sort of person and writer, always going against the mainstream, no matter what the mainstream is." But, of course, that is the point in many ways. We need non-normative ways of approaching life, not for everyone, but for the people who tend to find themselves in non-normative positions. If most people want fast food, that does not mean that fast food is for everyone.

*

DOI: 10.4324/9781003148456-9

When I was a teenager, I was involved in music and theater. I played jazz trumpet pretty seriously and I was in a couple of high school plays. I didn't get interested in writing poetry until I was a senior. The deeper, the more intense my interest in writing poetry grew, the deeper and more intense my periods of depression became also. By the time I was half way through college I was writing a lot of poetry and spending a lot of time lying on a cot in a depressive and paralytic daze down in the dark of a basement furnace room. Clearly, or so it seemed to me, poetry and depression were lovers doing some kind of macabre dance in and with my life, and I was, it appeared, helpless, no matter how much I resisted, to do anything about it. This was in the late 1950s.

This pattern of bursts of creativity—making poems, stories, plays, essays—alternating with periods of paralytic depression was to be the way I lived my life for the next thirty years. I started calling "her" The Angel of Depression.

LETTER TO THE ANGEL OF DEPRESSION

O, Angel of depression, I give myself to you.
I give myself to you Angel of darkness, Angel
of quiet pain, Angel of numbness, Angel of a
stillness still as death, Angel of the eyes that stare,
Angel of the breath that barely moves, Angel of
dullness, I give myself to you. I give myself to you.
I praise you. I pay homage to you. I attend to you.
I do not turn my back on you. I make this prayer
for you. I speak it openly in front of everyone. O,
Angel of darkness, Angel of depression, dark Angel
of life, I do not forget you. Therefore, now,
I pray you, give me leave,
release me, let me go.

uncollected poem

But my ablutions didn't get me much absolution. For many years in my twenties, thirties, and forties, it sometimes seemed that I was going to lose this battle with depression. Sometimes I thought suicide was the only way out.

I HAVE ALWAYS BEEN and still am a rebellious, contrary sort of person and writer, always going against the mainstream, no matter what that mainstream is.

FLAWED VERSE: AFTER A POEM BY HAN SHAN

Vinegar Bob, The Academic, laughs at my flawed verse and says,
He writes short stories, then chops up the lines so he can pretend they're poems.
I say: What's wrong with short stories?

Vinegar Bob, The Academic, laughs at my flawed verse and says,
He has no command of prosody. He just throws words down anywhere on the page.
I say: Yeah, that's right. I'll throw 'em down anywhere I like.

from *Moment to Moment: Poems of a Mountain Recluse*

Thirty years alone at the foot of Judevine Mountain raising vegetables, cutting
firewood, talking to the birds and making poems, hasn't exactly
made Judevine Mountain a household word in the poetry academy.

Once a friend recommended him to the academy and they all cried,
Who's this Judevine Mountain guy? Another friend—who just
happened to be there—said, *Everybody in these parts knows who he is.*
Why, he's the most famous unknown poet for miles around. The only people
around here who don't know who he is, is you! Which, of course, proved
to the academy that he didn't exist at all. And therefore

Judevine Mountain was set free to continue on his mountainside
raising vegetables, cutting firewood, talking to the birds and making poems,
which he is doing to this very day, in his non-existent sort of way.

from While We've Still Got Feet

In 1981, at the age of forty-one, I received a Guggenheim Fellowship in Poetry. The
Establishment—with a capital T and a capital E—had opened its arms and welcomed
me in. It was more than I could stand. Almost immediately I fell into a depression
deeper and more profound than any I had ever experienced. I sat in a chair all day,
day after day, and cried.

for my daughter, Nadine

When you were four and I was forty-one
and sunk in my depression deeper than I'd ever been—
when all day each day all I could do was sit in a chair
and stare and weep at nothing in particular—
in the morning you'd come down the stairs still in
your pink sleeper and find me there already in my chair
or still there from the night before already staring
or weeping in that paralysis that was my life then,
you'd climb up into the chair and settle yourself,
fit yourself, curl yourself, into my lap so I could
hold you in my sadness while I wept and never,
not ever, not once, did you ask me why
I was crying, nor did you ever ask me to explain.

Now, twenty years later, now that you are twenty-four
and I am sixty-one I write this to say to you, Nadine,
you were such warmth, such sweet serenity,
such peace and comfort to me then. Thank You, Nadine,
My Daughter, for the chance to hold you when you were four
and I was forty-one.

uncollected poem

I was beginning to get an ulcer. My doctor put me on the Sippy Diet—only bland foods, no booze, no tomatoes, no spicy food of any kind. In other words, none of the foods I loved the most. No red wine, pasta, and red sauce. My god! forbidden to eat the most calming, relaxing, soporific meal known to humanity! I got worse—fast.

Next my doctor prescribed Ativan, but, because I'm hypersensitive to all drugs, my reaction to it was horrific. I felt so detached from myself I thought I had died. Over and over again, I had a vision of myself standing inside a telephone booth looking outside at myself while the self outside jumped up and down waving his arms and screaming at the top of his lungs, but the self inside the telephone booth just stood there motionless—and *emotion*less—staring at the self outside. All the self inside the booth could hear was a slight wind blowing. I was scared to death. It was as if the drug had split me in two: there was still a real self full of emotion out there jumping around waving his arms, but he was unapproachable, unreachable. The self I knew was a zombie. How was I going to create anything in this condition?

Then one night, while I was on the road for a reading in Buffalo, New York, I lay awake all night, my heart racing, beating maybe two hundred fifty beats a minute, maybe more. I don't know why. Perhaps it was a side effect of Ativan.

The next morning my heart rate had returned, somehow, to something like normal. I swore that morning never to take another tablet of Ativan or any other psychotropic drug again. I never have. It was clear to me that I'd have to deal with this problem without pharmaceuticals.

OVER THE ALMOST twenty-five years since then I've developed my own way of dealing with and using my depression. And as I've grown older, my periods of depression have lessened in both duration and intensity. I don't know why.

I've developed for myself what I call the "give in" method. I've discovered that the only way around my periods of depression is directly through them; in other words, the sooner I can resign myself to the Angel of Depression, the sooner she will be done with me and leave me alone. I should note here that I've been able to resign myself to her when necessary because I've been a freelance writer for the past more than thirty-five years and therefore I don't have a nine-to-five job. I do have to travel quite a bit, and the Angel seems to be kind enough to let me have those trips out and not bother me. This is an agreement we've come to later in my life. When I was younger she took me over whenever and wherever she wanted, with no consideration for what I had to do. In short, the quicker I can let the Angel of Depression take over my life completely and have her way with me for as long as she needs to, the sooner I can get back to my life.

WHEN I GET DEPRESSED

I get silent and I stare
at nothing all day long,
or I lie down and read
the ancient masters who
move me to even greater
depths of melancholy,

and then,
refreshed,
I get up
and
join the world
again.

from Moment to Moment: Poems of a Mountain Recluse

My depressions come most predictably near or just after the equinoxes.

THE END OF WINTER

The delicate and lovely emptiness of winter
gone now today, suddenly gone,
this last week
of May.
The glut of summer rushed in,
grass crowding everything,
trees thick again
with green.
The whole world full of life and noise
closing in, and nowhere for us
dark ones, depressed ones
to hide.

from Moment to Moment: Poems of a Mountain Recluse

NO POEMS

Yellow leaves
pile up
on the Scholar's
ink stone.
His brush
is dry.
He lies
still as death
on his cot
curled in
upon
himself.
Gone away
on his
autumnal
wander
through
Depression.

from While We've Still Got Feet

But, as I've said, as I've grown older both the duration and the intensity of these periods of depression have lessened. However, I want to try to explain why I think these periods of depression are actually good and useful and important to my writing life and to my life in general.

I WANT TO TALK about the Writer as Receptacle and then about Imagination Time in order to talk about Depression as Emptiness, all of which are a way of talking about The Uses of Depression.

THE WRITER AS RECEPTACLE

I have a little sign on my wall that says: "Don't think. Listen. Watch." When I apply my mind to the task at hand I can't hear what is there to be heard. In other words, if I think, I can't listen; when I use my head, my ears fall off.

I understand myself as a writer as someone who is a receiver, a receptacle. After I am filled up, or while I am being filled up, I can then attempt to become a transmitter of what I have received. I listen for the voices, and if I'm lucky I hear them and I write them down.

I'm a recordist, a stenographer, a secretary. If you want to get fancy about it, you could call me an intermediary, a priest. I don't invent what I write, I don't think it up, I record what I hear and see, both outside of me in the world and inside of me in my imagination, and most often in that combination of the two in which what is outside of me gets transformed into something new as it passes into the inside of me.

I do all this with language, which is not an end in itself, but a means to an end, the end of getting down on paper what I have received. My responsibility is to get down clearly and articulately what I have heard. Only as my capacity to be accepting and receiving comes together with my articulate use of the language is good work produced. If I haven't been articulate enough with the language, if my technique isn't good enough—well, too bad for me; I have failed. All of which is to say, I am responsible *only* for my mediocre and bad work. I can't take credit for my good work, since I am only the conduit for it. This notion has a pleasant sense of humility about it which appeals to me.

I want to dwell for a moment on the passive, accepting, receiving aspect of being a writer. This may be an issue particularly for men, since to be open, passive, receptive, and fecund is not the way most boys are raised; but increasingly it is an issue for women writers, too, inasmuch as we live in an age that gives so much credence and value to aggressiveness, assertiveness, and to the positive, optimistic, light, active, "male," Yang virtues. At the same time, our age denigrates the "female," Yin virtues of darkness, passivity, receptiveness, and so on. I understand that the idea of the Yielding Female—whether applied to men or women—is not currently a popular idea.

All that notwithstanding, here are a few excerpts pertaining to the idea of the Yielding Female, to the dark, passive, receptive, unknowing Yin virtues, from *The Tao Te Ching*. (These translations are my own compilations and inventions based on translations by Robert Payne, Witter Bynner, Gia-Fu Feng, and Jane English.)

Chapter 6 of *The Tao Te Ching* says:

The dark valley spring never dies.
It is called the Mysterious Female.
The entrance to the Mysterious Female
is the root of Heaven and Earth.
The entrance is quiet and hidden, seldom seen.
Touch it. Use it. It will never fail, never run dry.

Chapter 10 says:

At the entrance to the Mysterious Female
Can you take the part of the woman?
All seeing, all knowing, open to everything
Can you lie back and do nothing?

Chapter 20 says:

All men are beaming with pleasure
. . . .
I alone am silent. I am a simpleton,
a do-nothing. I am like an infant.
Abandoned, like someone homeless.
Men of the world are rich and successful,
They have position, power, prestige.
I alone seem to have nothing.
I am a man with the mind of an idiot.
A pure fool. I am dull and stupid.
Everywhere men are so clever and witty,
They are always so self-confident.
I never know what I'm doing.
I alone am dark and disquieted.
I am restless as a nervous sea,
All I ever do is drift. I never get anywhere.
Everywhere men are making their mark on the world
While I am depressed and sad,
aimless and full of regret.
I am different from all these others!
All I want to do is lie with the Mysterious Female.
All I want to do is suck at the mother's breast.

Chapter 28 says:

Know the male, but cleave to the female.
Know the light, but love the dark
Thus you will become the root of heaven and earth,
the womb of the world, and you will give birth
continuously, endlessly.

But how do you conceive? What is the proper atmosphere for fertile conception?

IMAGINATION TIME

I need—I think we all do—the one thing it seems is the most difficult to get in our lives: time. Very few of us can knock out poems in every little spare moment or two the way William Carlos Williams did between patients in his doctor's office. We need time to empty ourselves out so that we can be filled up again. We need time for emptiness, not for business, for busyness.

This kind of emptiness, sloth, laziness, is absolutely un-American. It runs contrary to the hurrying, consumptive, thingy, acquisitive, thoughtless American way. We are all busy, so busy busy busy, and we are proud of being busy. In fact, if you aren't so busy you are about to go nuts, you really aren't successful, and everybody knows it. Besides, being busy means you are the one in charge.

THE BUSY MAN SPEAKS

Appointments, schedules, deadlines.
Demands on my time from everywhere.
I've got to plan every minute.

I'm so busy and important I don't have time to
trust the current like an unmoored boat.

I wouldn't want to anyway.
I make the current go
where *I* want it to go.
I'm in charge here.

from *While We've Still Got Feet*

Trust the current like an unmoored boat—in other words, just drift along—is a quote from the ancient Chinese poet, Han Shan, one of the great do-nothing guys of all time, the exact opposite of an in-charge kind of guy. In fact, I'd say, bluntly, if you need to be in charge, you can't be a poet.

SUCH SELF-INDULGENCE AND SLOTH!

All morning I sit at my desk drinking tea,
reading ancient poets
and writing my own ridiculous poems.

In the afternoon I go wandering through the woods
to see wildflowers and listen to birds
and the wind singing through the trees.

Then I sit beside the brook down in the bottom
of the ravine where the rock outcroppings loom
over my head, and I listen to the waterfall.

Such self-indulgence and sloth makes me so happy!
I wonder who will pay me to be useless and in love?

from Moment to Moment: Poems of a Mountain Recluse

We have to be—I have to be, at least—empty, open, quiet, passive, receptive, dark. I have to do nothing in order to be filled.

This kind of emptiness is akin to the Zen Buddhist concept of Emptiness or what, in Zen art, would be called "negative space," all that blank paper surrounding the little ink painting of the bowl down in the lower right-hand corner, all that silence in and around much shakuhachi music, all that incredibly slow slow slow Butoh dancing.

WHERE I LIVE
Where I live is
emptiness.
Time to watch
and listen.
Space between
events and people.
Room for thoughts
to wander.
There they go—
drifting
wherever
they want to.
I've got no discipline at all!

from Moment to Moment: Poems of a Mountain Recluse

DEPRESSION AS EMPTINESS

In my life at least, depression is a kind of emptiness, a slothful, no-thing, withdrawal from the world. Although I've said that giving in to these periods of depression is the quickest way through them, I want to also say that over the years I've discovered that these periods of depression are not entirely negative. There is a positive aspect to depression.

I've come to understand my periods of depression not as useless periods in my life, periods that are to be fought against and resisted, but as dormancy periods, gestation periods, to be accepted, given in to, welcomed.

Over the years many very interesting and useful notes, images, situations, phrases, and so forth have appeared to me, have come to me—I've heard them—during these periods of depression. But more often I have no idea what is going on during the period of depression. Only much later do I realize that, because of that period of emptiness, I am now full of something new.

Botanists know that trees require their period of dormancy in the winter in order to grow during the summer. It appears that trees, while dormant, aren't really asleep, but rather are storing up energy for the coming burst of growth. No periods of growth without also periods of rest. Could this be one of the functions of depression?

Another great and useful use of depression is that it keeps you in touch with an acute sense of failure—not that most of us most of the time need any reminding of what it is like to fail. This contact with a sense of failure is especially necessary for anyone who is lucky enough to become even modestly successful. Not only does it keep you in touch with your real self, the self you know in the privacy of your own despair, but it also keeps you in touch with the depths of common humanity. This intense sense of failure, especially at the times of success, creates wholeness. It's a wholesome and honest blend of light and dark.

The Yin/Yang symbol is a circle evenly divided into half dark and half light, but the halves are not opposing; they are wrapped around each other. The line between them is not a straight line but a French curve; the dark and the light embrace each other; they are inseparably entwined, as in the number 69. Furthermore, within the dark space there is a nucleus of light, and within the light space a nucleus of dark.

The back and forth in my own life between periods of active writing and passive, do-nothing periods of depression seem to keep me going. I can't have one without the other. And now, as I grow older—I'm sixty-seven—my periods of depression are fewer and fewer and their intensity less and less. Maybe I'm not so compulsive or ambitious anymore. I don't worry so much about my periods of not writing. I actually enjoy them. I work in my gardens, cut wood, play my shakuhachi, do nothing. In other words, I wait.

A CAVE ON JUDEVINE MOUNTAIN

> There is a cave on Judevine Mountain, a secret place,
> way back in the woods, high up on a hidden slope,
> in a place no one ever goes. Only I know where it is.
> No one else has ever been there. I go up there a lot
> and sit around, make a little fire, boil some tea,
> sometimes cook a little meal, but mostly what I do is
> sit and wait, poke at the fire, add a twig or two
> and wait and wait and stare, until suddenly
> I know what to do.

> from *While We've Still Got Feet*

And sometimes what I suddenly know what to do is more of nothing.

Which brings me to wonder about the function of psychotropic drugs and whether in some cases they actually hinder a creative person from getting in touch with his or her dark, depressive side, actually get in the way of that dormancy some call depression, which may actually be a period of important creative gestation for what comes next.

Note

1 Berlin, Richard M., MD, ed. *Poets on Prozac: Mental Illness, Treatment, and the Creative Process.* pp. 80–91. © 2008 The Johns Hopkins University Press. Reprinted with permission of Johns Hopkins University Press.

Chapter 8

Inbetweenland

Jacks McNamara

Summary

Jacks McNamara's work at the intersection of politics, art, spirituality, and healing is a deep inspiration for many in the world of mad studies. They were a cofounder of the Icarus Project and they currently host a podcast, *So Many Wings*,[1] which is a series of conversations at the intersection of transformative mental health and social justice. In addition to their activist and artistic work, Jacks has developed their own healing arts practice.[2]

In the poems published here, Jacks puts into practice a poetic principle of "lilies and urine" they talked about in the experimental documentary *Crooked Beauty* – a film by Ken Rosenthal. The poetic principle of "lilies and urine" calls for an embrace of the world in all its complexity, without expectation of cleanliness or clarity. This approach to life and poetry goes against the grain of the sanitized normal/pathological binaries of mental health definitions, diagnoses, and treatment protocols. The phrase "lilies and urine," first articulated by Chilean poet Pablo Neruda (1994), calls for

> a poetry impure as the clothing we wear, or our bodies, soup-stained, soiled with our shameful behavior, our wrinkles and vigils and dreams, observations and prophecies, declarations of loathing and love, idylls and beasts, the shocks of encounter, political loyalties, denials and doubts, affirmations and taxes.
>
> (p. 39)

Or, as Jacks puts it, "You don't have to choose between sanity and the roofless night."

*

Inbetweenland

I wish someone had told me I would get out of the burning house –
or that I had already escaped
a long time ago – and it lived on
only in my muscles and my mind.
I wish someone had handed me the word

DOI: 10.4324/9781003148456-10

survivor
placed it in my palms
like a blossom or a drill
told me to build altars and hang
hinges. Carefully. I wish
they had told me
I could stand up any time
open the door
leave.

~

It is 1986. I am lying
on my back in a hot room.
My father blocks the door
tells me fairy tales with cruel endings
Goldilocks shut in a closet and forced
to eat beetles
by her parents
after she gets lost in the woods.

He leans over to kiss me
on the lips where I don't want
to be kissed. Wishes me
good night. Again.

~

It is 2006. I am lying
on my back in a room with red velvet
curtains, walls covered
in fairies and pelts. Lying on the table
of a psychic named Sue
whose hands know things
I can't explain.

She touches my shoulders and asks where I am.

In space.

Asteroids   comets   a large
silence of almost nothing.
That far away?
No wonder I can't find you.

My eyes are closed.
I cannot tell if I am sinking or floating.

You haven't chosen
to stay on this earth yet
have you? No.
26 years and counting.

~

I wish someone had told us that the years spent journeying back and forth across Inbetweenland would not be a waste. That the miles and blizzards could not be avoided. That we would find the necessary roads, the necessary words, the mystery between them both. I wish they had told us about earthquakes. That we were not crazy. That sometimes the unspeakable

    erupts out of the fault lines
    in your spine. That the body
    stops shaking the ground
    stops buckling despite
    aftershocks despite fire
    eventually
    something settles
    water turns clear
    birds come back in the morning
    you choose earth
    make breakfast
    go on.

~

    My best friend and I used to talk
    about choosing earth and sky
    we traveled between borders leading
    workshops for survivors
    who had known rocks that whisper
    billboards who shout conspiracies
    and cosmic truths, electric hearts
    impaled on apocalypse sunsets
    over ruined cities and paper mountains
    speaking myths that evaporate
    like water off hot pavement
    when you finally come down

    into the world of toothpaste and toilet paper
    fathers and sons
    appointments, diagnoses –
    mania, psychosis – but we knew
    we were caught trying to fly
    out of the mazes built by kings and corporations

where your wings melt
once you finally make it over the sea.

When we mentioned keeping one foot
in both worlds, everyone in the room
would exhale
eyes like fireflies
switching on at dusk.
Permission. This too is real.
Inbetweenland. Both. Our own maps.
You don't have to choose
between sanity and the roofless night.

~

It is 2012 and I am lying
on the floor of a small room
while a therapist in a black muscle tee
emblazoned with Hope in white letters
draws infinity symbols over my eyes.
I follow her fingers I freeze as usual
until the images come. The shadow shapes of men
my father leaning over thick
stories heat
suddenly
the impulse to roll onto my side
stand up
open the door
leave. For the first time

I do.

Outside the world is big as snow
bright as a waxing moon.
Full of people. My hands
are full of tools my eyes
full of horizon.
I am enormous.
A child landing in an adult's miraculous skin.

Why Bodhisattvas Stare at Walls

The old winter light like the desert.
The memory of war in green places. The dryness
in our mouths, the paralysis in our limbs, the way it feels
to let your skull be heavy against the floor, the rising

and falling, the walk we should be taking
to end the word *should*, the way it all wells up
between our ears; the songs, the grief, the attempts
to keep the sun on our skin for a thousand years,
to balance at the edge of a ruined hill,
to stand under the planets when the night is so cold
breathe through our bellies in the dark
and look up. To be full of horizon when the wind is gray
and there is no grave to visit, to yell at the rain, to wake up
anyway, be kissed anyway, chop onions
fold clothes, talk to angels, and sit still
even though he is leaving, even though she is gone, even though
we are coughing and parched and the ending
is unclear, even though the empty hours are coming –
the empty hours are here. Her hair is in a silver box.
The morning glory died. The cactus downstairs
has small pink flowers
that bloom like stars in November
on broken arms covered in spikes.

Towards Fire

1

I remember when I painted Grace as a place
with no people. Grace as a doorway
into the moon. Or hills rolling
out to horizon. Desert, sea,
a circle of perfect blue.

Grace the water
that held me aloft
under a sky with no skin
kind only in its emptiness
whispering, *Vast*.

2

I aspired to a slow heartbeat
in all situations.
Weightless bones
plenty of time.
I did not wear a watch or ride
in ambulances. I never burst
into tears and argued with cops.

Grace was a clean floor
before dawn, sitting in lotus
facing a wall. No late nights
nothing smoking. Just the murmur
of chants in a foreign language
I didn't even speak. 9 bows
3 bells. Grace
the space behind clouds.

3

One May I woke up red.

I was sure my soul had jumped
outside my skin, turned flat
as a shadow stitched on at the heels.

I set fires.

I flew 3000 miles
drank wine at lunch
sang ballads to weeds
seduced other people's trouble.

Eventually I wanted
messy things. A child
requiring haircuts. A lover
requiring meals. The other side
of a hard fight.

4

It took many years of dislocation
and weeping to shake the ribs,
many nights of scratching
scars, and startling
awake to remember
how women leave
and men violate
how women violate
and men leave
before I swallowed my soul back inside.

It grew like a child and made me nauseous
with truth. It got stuck
in my windpipe. The soul screamed.

I fought to swallow
the sound. Painkillers
did not work. The struggle
became louder. Finally
I looked for Grace to encourage
the soul's extension
into my hands, its descent
through my legs.

5

A canyon, a sister, a misfit monk
to cradle my ankles, a medicine woman
to press hard on my heart. Sandbags,
needles, pens. Queers
crips and beloved crazies
to listen and know. The experiments –
lovers reaching inside
and leaving, lovers holding
me down. Fists inside muscles, shaking
with what it might mean to stay.

One day a teacher to insist
I find the dignity in my spine
extend my quaking arms
toward something like a future
beside others extending theirs.
The soul filled out abandoned spaces.
The stories began burning
down into my feet, making light.
My steps began to hum.
Grace became a verb.

6

I carried my questions then
back to the sea and the patient desert. Still
they spoke of Grace. Grace, and storms.
Storms and justice.
Justice and the heartbeats
of our people. *Dreamers*
healers, rebels, you must walk
with your singing feet
toward the blood of sunrise
next to others grown full
from the walking.

Notes

1 So Many Wings website accessible here: https://www.somanywings.org/
2 Jacks McNamara's healing arts practice website accessible here: https://jacksmcnamara
   .net/

Editor's Reference

Neruda, P. (1994). Toward an impure poetry. In B. Belitt (Ed.), *Selected poems: Pablo Neruda* (pp. 39–41). Grove Press.

Chapter 9

Sometimes/I Slip

L. D. Green

Summary

L. D. Green is an artivist: a non-binary writer, performer, college professor, mad studies scholar, and mental health advocate. Among their many publications, they coedited and contributed to the anthology *We've Been Too Patient: Voices from Radical Mental Health*.[1] Green's poem "Sometimes/I Slip" joins the anthology to ask, "So what will you call me/[us]?" at times when life leaves us "howling at the sun and gathering fruit under the moon." One answer, which Green feels was inflicted on them by the "mental health industrial complex," was "bipolar disorder," implying chemical imbalances and broken brains. But Green came to see possibilities as much more complex and contradictory:

> While I chose to take medication as one tool to mitigate the intensity that characterizes my life, I have many other tools: mutual aid, therapy, creativity, spirituality. Those are the tools that save me. Personally I am suspicious of any narrative that says medication is *the* method of solving something so complex as mental and emotional distress. … [I] actively resist the mainstream pseudoscience of the biomedical model in favor of other alternative frameworks such as the recovery model, trauma-informed care, the mad pride movement, the consumer movement, the neurodiversity framework, and … radical acceptance that I will have hard days.
>
> (Green & Ubozoh, 2019, pp. 3–4).

Green's poem published here asserts that whatever the "ableist, capitalist power structure" may call us, we have the possibility to narrate alternative stories. We have the possibility of embracing the ideal of "nothing about us without us" even when others do not. It is in that spirit that the speaker of the poem chooses, out of the many possible options, to represent the complexities and contradictions of their life in perhaps the simplest terms: I am only/human.

*

DOI: 10.4324/9781003148456-11

Sometimes/I Slip

They say when you see a wild beast, the last thing
You should ever do is make yourself small.
Don't tremble.
Raise your arms like you're calling down lightning,
Scream.
Let your voice echo through the canyon

Forty five years ago, a man died here, trying to kill a grassfire.
He was the solitary doctor in a sanitarium.
These fields used to cradle a crazy house
When shipped to Wildcat Canyon,
You would be safely quarantined.
Miles from the disgrace of a loving family.
This was not vacation. This was a colony.
And the doctor ran it, for forty three years.
Until fire consumed him in his effort to beat it back.

I have vacationed in spots like this before.
Four times in my life, I have been too patient
with the good intentions of this secular priesthood.
I held my mouth open to commune with the corporate body
While my blood was measured to determine
The diagnosis of my curse.

But today I am only a spectator to these specters,
I do not believe the patterns in the grass to hold any more truth
Than a passing laugh, and mine is not maniacal.
But every day I live with the fear that the mirror will see
That the predator is me.

I can only hold myself back from the edge
of the canyon so long
until it's the effort itself, the awkward shaking,
the denial of my desire to jump
feet first into the unknown--
That makes me small.
Makes me tremble.
Makes me look like prey.

So today I choose to raise my hands high,
like I can call down rain.
Maybe some kind of lightning caused that grassfire,
but only water and time can make things right.

Lightning does strike in the same place twice,
But each time I was institutionalized
In a synthetic expansion of adolescent nights,
I howled at the sun and gathered fruit under the moon,
Grew fangs as a mouse and the wolf in me trembled.
Hunting my own flesh and gathering his
This distortion of civilization has rendered wrong
Every action along the both poles of my reason
Into dueling serpents of logic and feeling
I must be spreading some kind of treasonous disease,
Something to quarantine.
So what will you call me?
When the sky opens next time,
When everything I say becomes
Indecipherable rhyme.
Those adolescent nights did not
Shudder off into a dawn the color of Depakote.
I walk carefully around my edges to avoid this, but
Sometimes
I slip. I'm only
        Human.

Note

1 For more about LD and their writing, please see www.ldgreen.org.

Editor's Reference

Green, L. D., & Ubozoh, K. (Eds.). (2019). *We've been too patient: Voices from radical mental health*. North Atlantic Books.

Chapter 10

The Mystery of Madness through Art and Mad Studies[1]

Ekaterina Netchitailova

Summary

This chapter explores how the world of art can show a different view of "madness." Mad studies, as an emergent academic field, has the possibility to offer alternative and contrasting views on madness. Netchitailova argues that the current biomedical model where "madness" is reduced to "mental illness" denies us the possibility to hear different views and see a person behind a diagnosis. The art world, through visual representation, can present us with an "unknown" factor of "madness" in which madness remains a mystery that we will never truly grasp. Visual art can also depict the complexities and contradictions of human beings and the many stories behind the "diagnoses."

*

The current medical model of 'mental illness' tries to make out of madness an object of 'brain study', an object of purely medical enquiry which can be reduced to scientific explanations, denied of its mystery.

The current system of diagnoses tries to make out of madness a chemical chart, where we have 'bipolar disorder', 'schizophrenia', or 'schizoid disorder', hiding behind the classification many different lives, totally distinct from each other's stories, and various people with often fascinating narratives.

Mad Studies, by contrast, as an emergent academic field, challenges the predominant view of 'mental illness', where the purely medical model dominates the debate in most countries in the western hemisphere. Mad Studies proposes 'a critical discussion of mental health and madness in ways that demonstrate the struggles, oppression, resistance, agency and perspectives of Mad people to challenge dominant understanding of "mental illness"' (Castrodale 2015). Thus, it gives space for additional exploration of madness, from different views, which could challenge the status quo of the 'biochemical' model.

However, it becomes ever more difficult to offer alternatives where the purely medical model sees itself increasingly incorporated across society. Mad Studies, as Beresford and Russo (2016) argue, risks being assimilated into the status quo of

DOI: 10.4324/9781003148456-12

the main biochemical model, where stories of 'survivors' will be heard only if they reflect the predominant understanding of 'mental illness' like 'any other illness', where only those survivors who agree with 'mental illness' will be heard.

But madness should retain its aura of mystery, and it should always leave room for different views and stories, where some 'mad' people or 'survivors' want a place in the exploration of the unknown, where there is still room to laugh about one's madness, and where some 'patients' want to offer different stories, different perspectives, different views on 'madness', sometimes mysterious, but sometimes very mundane.

The art world is a world which still offers us these alternatives. It is also a world that shows the dilemma of 'madness'. The dilemma of doctors trying to put a definite label on something which cannot really be explained. Or when it explains something, we want to hear the 'other' side, the real, human story. We want to see what each 'diagnosis' hides. Behind each 'depression' is its own story of sadness, and behind each 'psychosis' there is a distinct and unusual journey, sometimes terrifying and, on occasions, very exciting.

The art world also demonstrates that we, as human beings, will always remain attracted to the mystery of madness. People are fascinated by madness, by what it hides. The art world is the world where madness belongs, where it should belong: in the narrative of the 'unknown', of the unexplored. 'Psychosis' might be defined as a loss of touch with reality by scientists, but for those who experience it, it is a reality which can be magical. It can also be trivial, but, as a human being, I am also interested in the 'small' details behind each 'madness'. I am interested in a 'patient', in his story, in his experience with madness.

The story of the current psychiatry and its reduction of the humankind to an object of scientific enquiry can be seen in the famous painting by Pierre Aristide André Brouillet (1887), *A Clinical Lesson at the Salpêtriére* (Image 10.1). It shows us a clinical demonstration given to postgraduate students by the famous neurologist Jean-Martin Charcot (Netchitailova 2019).

This painting was painted before the official history of psychiatry started, but it shows the state of psychiatry as it is now. There are several doctors who claim to understand madness through words, without clear medical tests confirming the 'diagnosis'.

But as a human being, when I look at this painting, I am not interested in what Charcot has to say. I can guess what he is trying to say.

I am interested in the patient. Her name is Blanche and I want to hear her story. I want to know what happened to her, and I want to know how she ended up where she is: in the middle of a clinical demonstration. I am also curious as to why no one tries to put a jacket on her, and why she seems like she is 'asleep'. From the rare mentions of Blanche, I learned that she worked as seamstress, and that she was affected by epilepsy. Charcot used her for his weekly demonstrations to show his 'skills' in hypnosis, during which Blanche would suffer from convulsions. They stopped after Charcot had died.

The art world is one world that still shows us the mystery of madness, and our fascination with it as human beings.

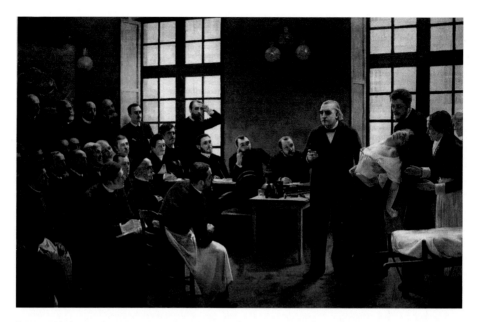

Image 10.1   *A Clinical Lesson at the Salpetriere*, by Pierre Aristide Andre Brouillet (1887). *Source*: Wikimedia Commons/Public Domain.

We are fascinated by Van Gogh not only because of his genius paintings but also due to his history of 'madness'. Modern doctors try to impose occasional diagnoses on Van Gogh, such as 'schizophrenia', 'bipolar disorder', or 'personality disorder'.

But as a sociologist and a fellow human being, I am interested in the story of Van Gogh, in the glimpses of his 'battle' with the unknown. I want to read that after his spell in an asylum, he painted 75 paintings in 70 days and completed more than 100 drawings and sketches. I read with deep curiosity about his life, that he was unlucky in love and was once rejected by Eugenie Loyer when he lived in London. I am less interested in what exactly happened with his ear, but more in the final moments of his life, when, before attempting to take his own life, he painted his *Tree Roots* (1890).[2]

On this painting we can see different leaves and roots giving way to trees, where the colourful 'palette' so unique to Van Gogh is very much present.

The painting, of course, created a lot of debates and controversies. Can we really see any moments of 'madness' in it? Can we witness the state of mind of the artist right when he was contemplating ending his own life?

Or we take another painting by Van Gogh as an example: *The Starry Night* (1889) that he painted while living in the asylum.[3]

What does it tell us, this painting? It is an amazing painting, one of the best, with stark colours and unusual sky. We can see a small village in it, and a church, and a beautiful sky, with yellow stars and moon. But I am also fascinated by the 'human story' of the painting. How was life in the mental asylums then? What were the patients eating? What kind of 'activities' did they have?

The biological model of 'mental illness', or its recent argument that 'mental illness is like any other illness', deprives us of these 'background' stories. It tries to create a narrative that something tragic, but sometimes beautiful, can be reduced to the notion of 'bipolar disorder'; that something which cannot be explained is defined as 'hallucinations'.

But as a human being I am curious about each particular 'hallucination'. Where do they come from? What do they hide? I refuse to believe that it is biologically based, and that they are not real. They are real for the person experiencing them, so why do we deny, then, the person the truth of his journey?

What if the hallucinations are actually real, and only few of us have the possibility to witness the parallel reality?

This fascination of what is behind 'madness' can be seen in a painting by Mathias Grunewald, *The Temptation of St. Anthony* (1512–1516).[4]

Saint Anthony was a Christian monk who was tempted by demons during his sojourn in the Egyptian desert. Today, his mystical experience would be called 'psychosis', with his temptation described as 'hallucinations'. But it is the numerous paintings depicting the mystical experience of Saint Anthony which present us with a different view, a different story, and a different view on madness.

On the painting by Grunewald we can see the real demons, and these demons were real for Saint Anthony too. Who should we believe: the psychiatrists or a person telling us his own story, his visions?

The view of madness as something that we can explain started, of course, during the enlightenment, the age of reason. It was Foucault, the French philosopher, who said that how we view madness, is defined by social constructs of any given time.

Thus, during the Renaissance period, mad people were looked upon with curiosity and sometimes even with admiration. They would also be put on the ships and sent into 'nowhere', but they were not locked up, and some artists asked the eternal question: but what is really madness? Should we look at some individuals as mad, or judge, rather, the society which is also mad?

Thus, the famous painting by Bosch, *The Ship of Fools*, or *The Satire of the Debauched Revelers*, presents us with a different view on madness (Image 10.2).

On this painting we can witness the debauchery caused by some highstanding members of society. The two figures in front are a Franciscan friar and a nun, which was quite unthinkable at the time of the painting (1490–1500) (Netchitailova 2019).

But this painting, in particular, has an additional meaning. The ship itself holds the biggest symbolism. Because it was on this kind of ship that the mad were put and sent into the fools' paradise (into nowhere) in the Middle Ages.

On this painting, however, there is only one fool, who is put there with a purpose: to remind the viewers that it is the ship of fools indeed which is depicted. But by placing other characters, so-called 'sane' members of the society on it, Bosh made his view on madness quite clear.

Who is really mad? An innocent fool, not harming anyone, or those who harm others in the name of God?

By looking at this painting, I also want to know the story of this 'fool'. Who was he? What happened to him? How was life on the ships for people who were put on them?

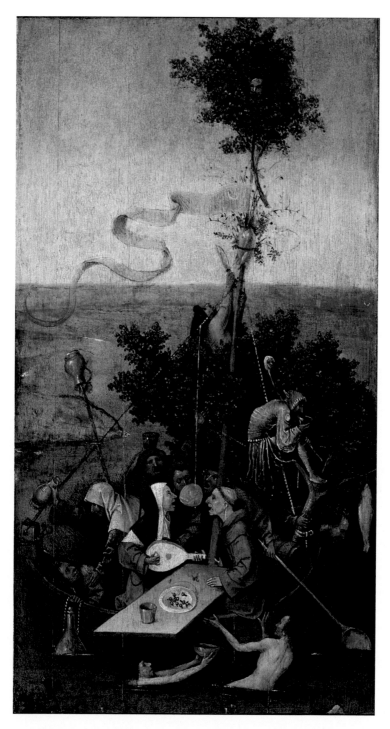

Image 10.2 *The Ship of Fools* by Hieronymous Bosch (1490–1500).
Source: Wikimedia Commons/Public Domain.

Another painting, The *Scream* painted by the Norwegian painter Edward Munch (1893), also poses the existential question of 'madness'. The *Scream* shows us a lonely figure of a man, who is obviously distressed, with two hands on his head, as if trying to shut oneself from the world.[5]

Is this how 'depression' looks or anxiety? Or is it the society itself which we can witness on this *oeuvre d'art*? Or was it indeed provoked by the fact that the sister of the painter happened to be in the mental asylum when Munch painted it? Does this painting express indeed the 'anxiety' of the modern man?

By looking at paintings we can ask these questions. Unlike the modern diagnoses, art gives us the possibility to explore, to venture into different views and interpretations. It gives us stories and a narrative behind. There is no real narrative anymore behind the classification of diagnoses and symptoms; it reduces different aspects of human life to 'mental illness', to 'mental illness like any other 'illness'.

The art and painters, however, always explored and continue to explore the remaining mystery of 'madness'. They paint us stories and possibilities of different interpretations. As human beings, we always want 'stories', we want more details of real human life, hiding behind the increasing number of diagnoses.

When I contemplate the paintings by Kim Noble,[6] a modern artist, who has 'dissociative identity disorder', I am interested in what is behind. I want to learn more about different personalities that make the paintings.

I am listening with great curiosity when Kim talks and gives interviews and I want to learn more about her as a person. Her art is a way for different personalities to express themselves, and her art is beautiful. When I look at her paintings, I do not think of 'mental illness', I think of an extremely interesting and vibrant person, who gives us a gift of her art.

I am glad that art still retains the mystery of 'madness'; that it removes the scientific explanation of all human misery, and presents questions rather than answers.

Doctors try to give us succinct, definite answers, but is there really an answer to the human psyche?

Should we not retain some mystery?

Should we not leave some space for the unknown, for something that we cannot really explain?

Notes

1 Ekaterina Netchitailova (2019). The mystery of madness through art and Mad Studies, Disability & Society, 34:9–10, 1509–1515, DOI: 10.1080/09687599.2019.1619236. Reprinted with Permission from Taylor and Francis.

2 *Tree Roots* by Van Gogh can be seen online: https://artsandculture.google.com/asset/tree-roots/WQGYd-7iPjW88g?hl=en-GB&ms=%7B%22x%22%3A0.5%2C%22y%22%3A0.5%2C%22z%22%3A9.295089552092103%2C%22size%22%3A%7B%22width%22%3A1. 2548849463499612%2C%22height%22%3A1.23749999999999 96%7D%7D. Accessed on 23.03.19.

3 *The Starry Night* by Van Gogh can be seen online: https://www.google.com/search?q =van+gogh+the+starry+night&source=lnms&tbm=isch&sa=X&ved=0ahUKEwjex_

PbvdzgAhUjonEKHTYED08Q_AUIDigB&biw=1366&bih=657#imgrc=qqSZWcd-voaRUNM. Accessed on 23.03.19.

4   *The Temptation of Saint Anthony* by Grunewald can be seen online: https://www. googl e.com/search?q=grunewald+The+Temptation+of+St.+Anthony%E2%80%99& sou rce=lnms&tbm=isch&sa=X&ved=0ahUKEwjhsqC5vtzgAhX_URUIHcDCBK8Q_ AUIDigB&biw=1366&bih=657#imgrc=-MgxfknQcPzxmM. Accessed on 23. 03.1 9.

5   *The Scream* by Munch can be seen online: https://www.google.com/search?q= the+s cream+munch&tbm=isch&source=iu&ictx=1&fir=-4j9OW6FXR40KM%253A%2 52CliewB9Kj8MJFQM%252C%252Fm%252F01f3_n&usg=AI4_-kT3BPhjBX8ABsHP wWL7PtDJB7QaPQ&sa=X&ved=2ahUKEwi4mIiOwNzgAhXOVBUIHc3_A3QQ_B0 wHHoECAMQEQ# imgrc=-4j9OW6FXR40KM. Accessed on 23.03.19.

6   See the website of Kim Noble: http://www.kimnobleartist.com/). Accessed on 23. 03.19.

References

Beresford, P., and J. Russo. 2016. "Supporting the Sustainability of Mad Studies and Preventing Its Co-Option." *Disability and Society* 31(2): 270–274. doi: 10.1080/09687599.2016.1145380.

Castrodale, M. A. 2015. "Book Review 'Mad Matters: A Critical Reader in Canadian Mad Studies'." *Scandinavian Journal of Disability Research* 17(3): 284–286. doi: 10.1080/15017419.2014.895415.

Netchitailova, E. 2019. "The Mystery of Madness Throughout the Ages." *Mad in America*. https://www.madinamerica.com/2019/01/mystery-madness/

Chapter 11

Mad Art Makes Sense

Lorna Collins[1]

Summary

Lorna Collins turned her personal experiences with hallucinations into a catalyst for academic study as well as the creation of alternative creative arts practices and workshops. Her book, *Making Sense: Art Practice and Transformative Therapeutics* (2014), utilizes art practice and aesthetic experience as a proactive way to make sense of the world. It develops a theoretical and applied understanding of how we can use art as a method of healing and as a critical method of research. Drawing from poststructuralist philosophy, psychoanalysis, arts therapies, and the creative processes of contemporary artists, the book combines art theory, arts therapies, aesthetics, and art practice. Art, for Collins, helps us to make sense of the world by activating, nourishing, and understanding a particular worldview or situation therein. This insight is an inspiration for her work to make the creative and healing properties of artistic expression widely accessible, practical, and useful.

Collins's chapter gives us a personal account of how she used her arts practice to work through a period of extraordinary, vehement, destructive images, which her clinicians called a "psychotic breakdown." Rather than simply taking more medications, as her clinicians recommended, Collins brought these experiences into her creative practice. Whatever one might decide to call what Collins went through, as she puts it, "these images are dark and absurd, but they [also] initiate and celebrate a way to continue as and with pure creativity. This is Mad Studies."

*

My Scenario

I use art (painting, drawing, collage, writing, film) to narrate my psychotic experiences. Making art helps me make sense of these experiences in a world where no one understands me or them. In this chapter, I am going to immerse the reader in a series of hallucinatory scenarios and show what I make with them. This sets up my journey, both inside the clinic and outside the clinic, where such creative exercise is discouraged. I find sense beyond the barrier lines the clinic advises me to raise: when nourishing and fostering my creativity is the only way to come to terms with these violent, disturbing hallucinatory experiences. Finally, I will describe my new practice,

DOI: 10.4324/9781003148456-13

which opens creative art groups for a number of communities in the UK. These are arts in health workshops, in which participants simply make art. Together, we create a "free" space, which proves to be revitalizing and liberal. Here mad art makes sense.

To elucidate these ideas and practice, I turn to Félix Guattari and Michel Foucault. When I express my hallucinations, and when I open a "Being Creative" workshop, we tread on the outside of thought and build a schizoanalytic practice. This is "chaosmosis" (Guattari, 1995).

First, I invite you to enter my scenario. It is early 2020, at the beginning of the pandemic, and I've just started working for the National Health Service as a peer support worker. In this role, I use my lived experience of having been diagnosed with an eating disorder and psychosis to support eating disorder patients in their recovery journeys. But, suddenly, my daily life is engulfed by constant visual and aural hallucinations and flashbacks from my own illness—seemingly out of nowhere. This sets me off on a journey of self-care and I will describe how it turns out in the postscript. For now, I will describe these experiences at length, so you can see what I'm going through.

These descriptions of my hallucinations are short, stark poems. They become pieces of "minor literature," which Deleuze and Guattari define as an "expression machine" that can, they argue, "break forms, encourage ruptures and new sproutings … [and] necessarily be part of a rupture in the order of things" (Deleuze & Guattari, 1986, p. 28). My words rupture and recreate sense and subjectivity. Take a look.

*

I am walking down the street, I see a dead man. Suddenly, I am dead.
Flashback: I am suddenly at "Sick Bay" in Jesus College, Cambridge University,
    unable to walk. They take me to hospital.
VERY LOUD NOISE—deafening, taking me.

I go to a yoga class. I see blood burning in the sky. My legs are open; they tear
    into pieces. Rape. I die.
Constant rattling noises, piercing my temples.

A man appears and shoots me. A white moth enters my mouth and chokes me.
I am in hospital in Cambridge, my key nurse asks me to "let him know" when
    I'm going to kill myself. I am desperate.
Piercing whistles through my temples. A lady screaming.

Ominous lights, they're about to shoot me.
I see shackles in the ground.
I'm tied to the bed (flashback, in France, 2012).
Deafening noises. Whispering.
A man grabs the rucksack on my back, pulls me back, down and away. [I'm not
    wearing a rucksack.]

Flashback: I am in hospital in London (2003–5), water-loading 5 kilograms, to
    falsify my weight. I am coerced to "agree" to have ECT on my damaged brain
    (the only way I agree is because they tell me ECT may kill me).

Horses gallop around my stomach (very loud noise and physical sensations), which then explodes.
Strange animals appear: a crocodile, a baboon.

Flashback: I run out of the ward [Haleacre, Amersham, 2001], to the bridge. I try to leap off; 2 men rush up and hold me down.
I am in a white cube, talking about my experiences. Double transposition: I am in France [2012]. The worst—reoccurs. I see myself dissociating. Weird disorientation. I hear horses galloping [no horses actually there].

LOUD NOISES pierce me. Hard to concentrate on anything else.
I see and feel a star inside my head explode.
I see my head is open. Torrents of flashbacks:
A patient sets fire to her hair.
I carve myself to pieces in the bathroom; I lose 2 litres of blood.
My roommate tells me about their conspiracy, in great detail. She or her illness grooms me; I am drawn into her battle.

I confess to the police officer my crime: existence. "Take me away, lock me up, I deserve to die," I say. But I'm already there, here. Taken.
At work: ongoing, piercing flashbacks (different hospital admissions: Addenbrooke's, Fulbourn, Whiteleaf).
Impaled by sound—humungous noise, all-encompassing—through my temples, invading my brain, my entire being.
On the ledge of a cliff. I leap off. Nothingness.

I am running. My body falls out of me, lying on the floor. There is a horse straddling me, rolling over me. Dead.
My head explodes.
Overwhelming noise.
A bird flies ahead in the sky, leaving a flood of green entrails in its wake.
The radio is on. A 3-part harmony is playing. [The radio is not on.]

A moon is divided into halves by a zip.
Flashing lights (peripheral vision).
A giant, shiny, purple beetle.
Piercing ringing bursts my temples.
My ears are going to explode.

There is a whole new world—elevated.
Incessant, intricate patterns.
Sounds become tactile, clasping me.
Flashback: acid rots my flesh.

The radio is on. [The radio is not on.]
Flashback: cutting "DIE" and "DNR" across my chest and arm, repeatedly.
Flashback: putting iron on my arms, to burn it. Irons saturate my vision—everywhere.

I see my body, being hacked into two by a rusty, corrugated iron saw.
The butterfly crashes into a black wall.

At the end of the path, a man rushes out and shoots me.
Flickering images.
Piercing sounds dissect my brain.

A car crashes into my car. [A car does not crash into my car.]
Dizzy rounds of noise sever through my temples.
A mosquito net sucks me up; I am a bat, enclosed and hiding in my own wings.

Flashback: I am at the Complex Cases ward in Cambridge. Everyone is obese
    and has scores of self-harm scars. A competition. Swapping tips on how to
    kill oneself.
My head is squashed down onto a ping-pong table. Someone thumps me with a
    black mallet. Smithereens.

Flashes of light in my peripheral vision.
A vision of my head in profile. It's very dark. Stars explode inside my head,
    destroy my brain . . . reeking outside and oozing into the darkness.

Flashback: I am running away from The Priory (Roehampton). I jump on a train.
    No one follows me. I escape; still trapped.
Disembodied, withered, grey torso. I am decapitated, my body is weightless and
    has no bones: a vast, opaque ghost.

Bleeding from down below—rush of blood. [This is not happening.]
Flashback: I see the patient who set fire to her hair, Adrian House Ward,
    Fulbourn Hospital. I let it go. The scene disappears, as quickly as it came.

A black gingerbread man crosses the road. A red car speeds by and tramples
    them. Dead.
A swarm of bees cluster around my head. They suffocate me.
Flashback: I am in my room at Cotswold House, Oxford, January 2018. My
    mother leaves a voicemail on my phone. She says: "I am sorry to hear you
    have relapsed." I have relapsed.
Flashback: bandaging swathes of ACID around my arm.

*

I make a note of all these experiences. Writing this down helps me, in a way, since it
makes what I am seeing (etc.) more tangible and real.

I am drawn to convey all this as images, using a pencil, pen, and paint. I develop a
ritual: every day, I create artworks of what I can see. I fill several books with them.
These images are incredibly disturbing, but I am captured, enraptured by them.

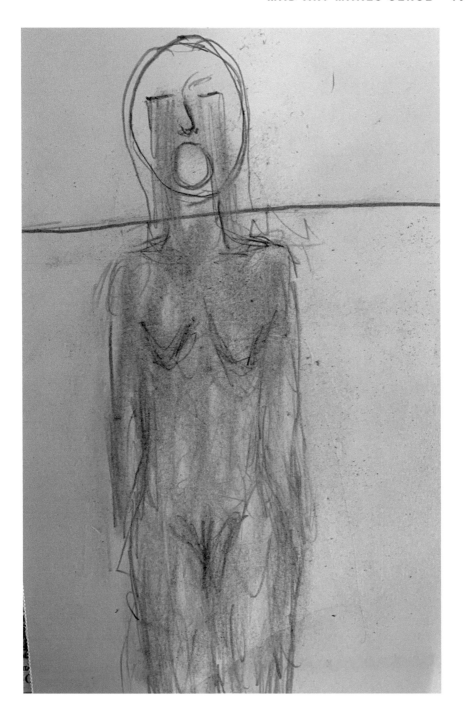

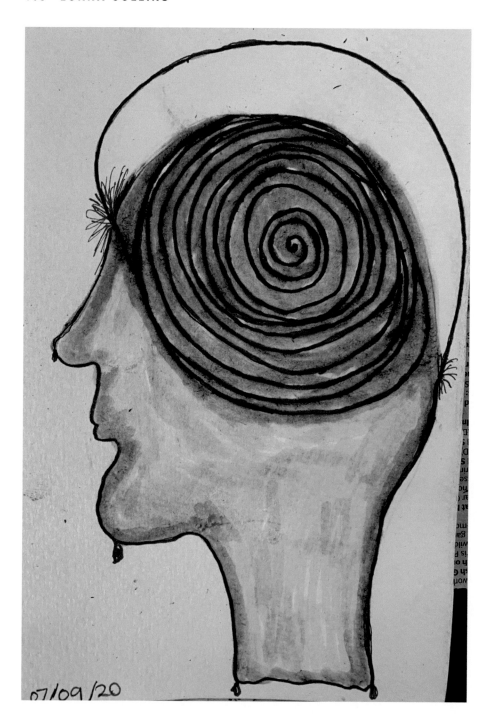

07/09/20

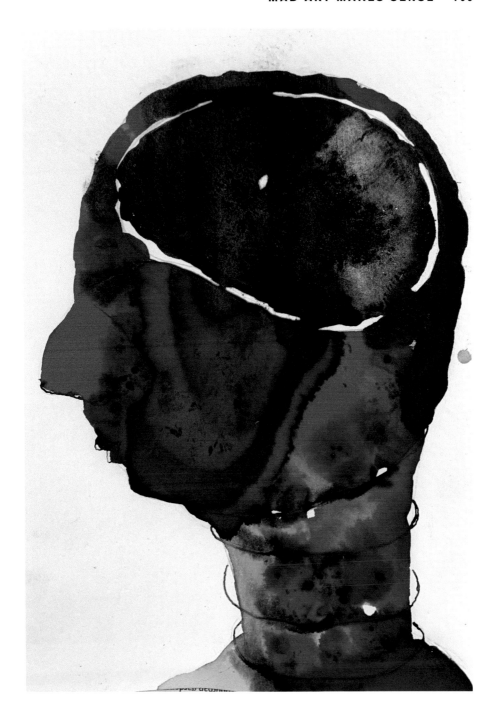

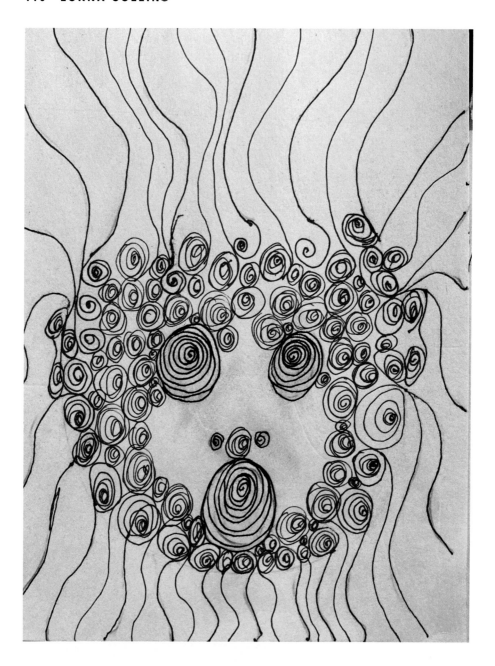

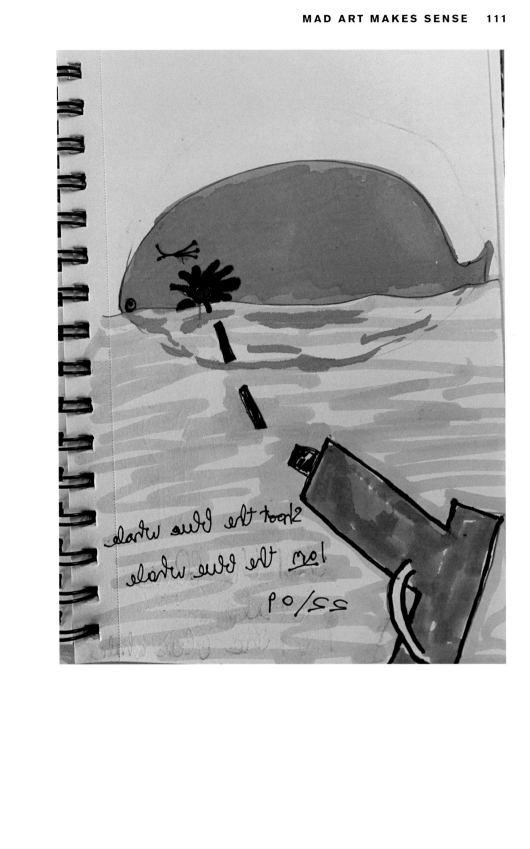

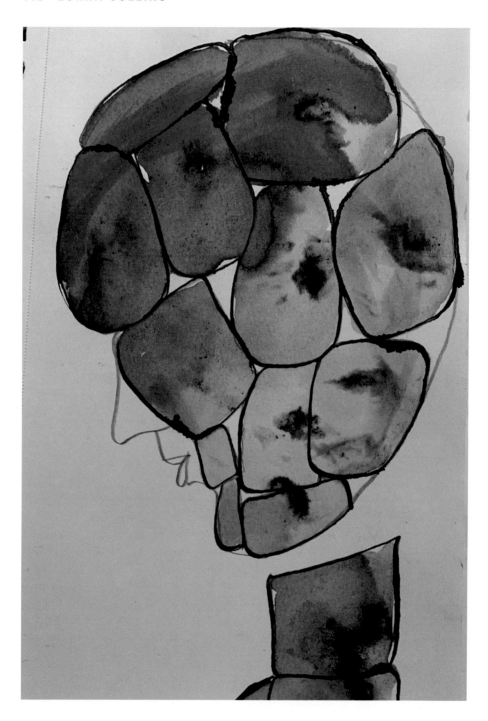

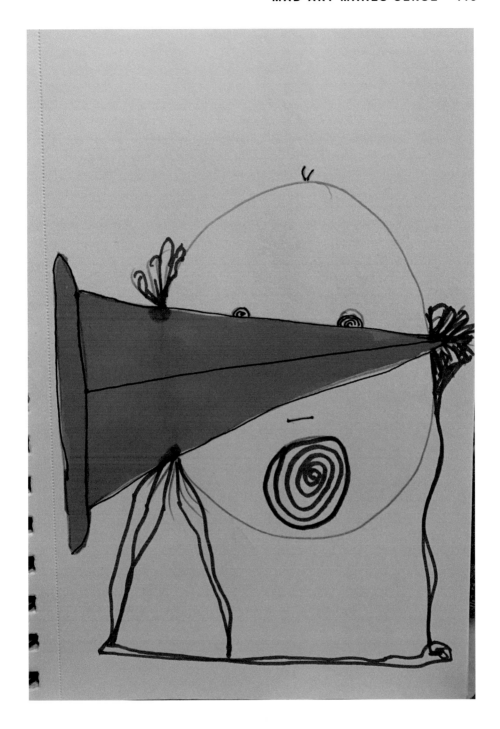

I wonder what to make of these images, which create a "cartography" of my "own universe" (Guattari & Rolnik, 2008, p. 359). I have always heard noises and sounds. But not as loud as they are now. I have always seen colors and shapes dissolve into fractal patterns, but not such extensive images and scenes. My hallucinations used to command me to die; now, I am already dead. My brain blows up, I am decapitated, my body withers—an opaque, weightless ghost. It's very, very dark.

As I write these things, I hear a constant, acute, pure, unfiltered daggers of sound shoot through my temples. This gives me the experience of having my skull broken, my brain dissected. All the gory flesh extrudes, escapes, out of the hole picked apart by the sound. I am trapped between the two holes, in my temples, whilst my brain and body evade me, escapes.

I hear, see, and fathom all this in the aural sensate. It is so loud I can't think.

I have previously been diagnosed with treatment-resistant schizophrenia. Clinicians disagree. Now they call my "illness" "Organic Psychotic Disorder (Undefined): F06.9," whatever that means.

There was a time when I could only hear this noise and the whispering voices when I attended to it. Most of the time, it left me alone. Or, rather, I did not concentrate on it, I was not entrapped by it. It was much quieter.

Now, I am drenched by the tsunami of sound. I also hear music. It sounds like the radio is on, when it isn't. I hear complex harmonies and orchestras.

But all of these things are not as alarming as what I can see. I am—at best—dead. My body is cut off from my head, it disappears. I am the grenade inside my head, which explodes.

What on earth am I supposed to do with any or all of this? Take even more olanzapine (antipsychotic medication)? Is it really a magic potion?

My medical team note my presentation and suggest I take more or less medication (different people disagree). When I say that I am drawing what I see, my care coordinator says this is "not a good idea," because it puts too much focus on the hallucinations. She says I should neither paint nor write about them.

What do I do, then?

I wonder about the hallucinations. They are constant, always fascinating, compelling. These transitory images are very interesting and I wonder where they come from. I draw everything. It is good to make art and express myself. It appears that I have infinite source material; my creativity is extraordinary, limitless.

Sometimes I think I am going to go POP.

And explode, beneath the weight and implications of my experiences.

Apparently, I am "in crisis" (says my care coordinator).

Hits me. Am I?

I have negated ideas.

I have *MANY* ideas. But I don't know what this is.

Too many things in my head. They excrete. Oozing shit. Baffling and absurd, weird.
It's odd.

For example, this morning: Head crammed full, about to go pop. A circus elephant, in fancy dress, is eating me. A traffic cone pierces through my temples, dissecting my brain. My body is a bomb made out of lead.

I don't understand it.

Suddenly, people (in the clinic) tell me I am "very, very ill at the moment," calling this a "psychotic breakdown." They say I should not work, I must not drive, and I must take more pills. I must stay at home and rest, get rid of the absurd. Before it gets rid of me.

Alarming.

All these medical people telling me to take chemicals, and what I can or cannot do.

My symptoms (and I) beguile explanation. There is no solution, other than being told to take more antipsychotic medication, over the maximum dose. Art becomes my sole means of coping with the extraordinary, vehement, destructive images that come to me, incessantly.

These images are dark and absurd, but they initiate and celebrate a way to continue as and with pure creativity. This is mad studies.

Chaosmosis

Spending time thinking about my madness, I realize that—with my painting and writing—I reenact the schizoanalytic cartographies seen in Guattari's philosophy (and new paradigm) about chaosmosis. My art shows that my madness is creative and chaosmotic, if not accurately defined by any clinical notion of "mad."

Art opens a level playing field on which I can "put" and situate my psychotic pathology. I have chaotic vertigo whilst experiencing these destructive images (etc.). It is disorientating; I wobble. When I enunciate and express how this makes me feel, my senses are liberated, orientated, grounded.

My creativity does not "cure" my psychosis. But it helps me understand and talk about these ravishing, disturbing experiences. When I respond to these by making an artwork, I am able to incorporate all the different voices and images (subjectivities) into a composed composition. I can continue.

The experiences open multiple subjectivities inside my identity. I see and connect lots of different beings (people, animals, objects); they lurch out of me, and I see them in the air around me. They are like partial objects (remnants of my psyche), in a primal sense (or Lacan's *objet petit a*).

I am curious to see the production of multiple elements in my subjectivity, by the means of my incessant creativity (and ontology). The people and objects (etc.) seem ruptured and autonomous; they flash by in an instant.

What remains? What Guattari (1995) calls "a more 'schizo' Unconscious, one liberated from familial shackles, turned more towards actual praxis than towards fixations on, and regressions to, the past" (p. 12). My own unconscious (if this is what causes these visions) breaks through my mind and body (rupturing their dichotomy) and ejects itself in front of me. I see and hear these visions: my inside is outside, dancing (or dying, or doing unmentionable things) in front of me. I reach out and try to grasp hold of what I can see; immediately, it eludes me, is gone. The rupturing or transcendence of dialectic logic is visible, is real, whilst also being intangible, ungraspable—beyond the human. I can sense it, but not know it, but it is real—for me, and my creativity.

When I write, or make art, to respond to my schizo selves, I create "existential refrains" (p. 15) and I build an "enunciative assemblage" (p. 29). My (plural) existence is enunciated; my artworks become assemblages of the different people (etc.) whom I proliferate.

At last, I can breathe. Making art helps me release the holds of the "crazy" visions, whilst retaining a sense of them.

The "chaotic vertigo" remains (p. 77). This is perhaps one of the most "privileged expressions in madness," when "psychosis starkly reveals an essential source of being-in-the-world" (p. 77).

In practical terms, what do I do? Get by, somehow. The clinical advice is to stop; take more pills. These experiences are proof that I have "broken" down; I am "very ill."

Guattari would say perhaps counter this, and applaud my "madness" as essential being, when he says that "delirious narrativity" is "a discursive power finalised by the crystallisation of a Universe of reference or a non-discursive substance, constitutes the paradigm for the construction and reconstruction of mythical, mystical, aesthetic, even scientific worlds" (p. 82).

My art is contaminated by my being(s) (and vice versa) reaching existence. I have the capacity to enunciate (to speak) through my art. The work of art then ruptures and unframes the "sense" dictated by the world (and the clinic). It enables me to recreate and reinvent subjectivity. In a way, I am subjected to the hallucinations; in another sense, they liberate my subjectivity because of the way I am able to express and enunciate them with my art. Art provides me with existential support.

Art and schizoanalysis

My interaction with the psychiatric clinic (the "Adult Mental Health Team") raises questions. I am influenced by reading of Deleuze and Guattari, who fire theoretical bullets, hell-for-leather, at all things Freudian, in all their works. I for one am very grateful for the outstanding care I have received during the past two decades of psychiatric illness, treatment, and recovery. But when the clinic says I am having a "psychotic breakdown," when they say I am "mad," I wonder what they mean.

My artworks recall one of Guattari's analysands, who had been diagnosed with schizophrenia and benefitted greatly from creative art: "In this new solitary assemblage, he began to create a mode of expression and develop it, creating a kind of cartography of his own universe" (Guattari & Rolnik, 2008, p. 360).

In the book Guattari wrote with Rolnik about schizoanalysis, he is not trying to eradicate the institution nor to destroy the clinic; he wants to change its logic and how it is run. Guattari wants to open a schizoanalytic practice that applies "a diversification of the means of semiotization" to build an understanding about subjectivity and subjectivization from a political, ethical, and psycho-clinical setting (p. 376).

Nor is Guattari trying to endorse psychiatric illnesses or problems such as addiction or schizophrenia ("that has *never* been among my intentions!") (p. 375). He says: "There is not the slightest doubt that it is absolutely necessary that asylums and refuges should exist" (p. 376). Rather, Guattari wants to expand and open the largely monadic, narrow, and punitive process of institutionalization so it can operate as a "polyphony" that can bring into play "anthropological, social, and ethical dimensions that concern the whole of society" (p. 376).

Guattari (with and after Deleuze) operates schizoanalysis first as a fervent critique of psychoanalysis and, as Guattari discusses in his own, later work, a "metamodeling" of its systematic malfunction in society (Guattari, 1995, pp. 58–76; 1996, p. 122).

This idea of "metamodeling" psychoanalysis, or modeling or creating or sculpting a practice *after* ("meta") psychoanalysis, brings to mind the dependence of *art* to realize schizoanalysis. Guattari metamodels to initiate his schizoanalytic practice. This means he remodels the model of psychoanalysis, reworking it, reforming it, so that it can address a new and updated clinical and political context. This process of remodeling ("metamodeling") is intrinsically artistic.

In *Anti-Oedipus* Deleuze and Guattari (2004) say that the psychiatric clinic actually *causes* rather than *cures* psychiatric illnesses. With their project of schizoanalysis they want to source an ethical "place of healing" that will build a new world—not just for those who have a psychiatric illness (although they base their argument around these cases) but for us all. They intend to do this by engaging with the schizophrenic *process* obtained and liberated from the schizophrenic *illness*. This is what I engage in my art.

Deleuze and Guattari imply an ethics to their schizoanalytic project. As Mark Seem argues, *Anti-Oedipus* "develops an approach that is decidedly *diagnostic* … and profoundly *healing* as well" (Deleuze & Guattari, 2004, p. xix). They are looking, not for a *cure* for the schizophrenic, but for a cure from the system that causes and detains this illness: "the schizophrenization that must cure us of the cure" (pp. 76, 80).

We begin to see how schizoanalysis can be carried out by practicing art. My own art provides me with relief and sense (making sense of my experiences). Deleuze and Guattari say that the *work* of art, art's work, art's job, is to change perception. That is, art must change how we see the world and make sense of it. Art has agency that disrupts and transforms the structure and authority of society. Because of this, art is intrinsically *political* as well as *aesthetic* (a Greek word meaning "of the senses"). From a schizoanalytic viewpoint, we are all artists. This means that we all have the capacity to challenge and change the world around us. Making and perceiving art gives us the opportunity to activate this motion, which is intrinsically schizoanalytic.

Guattari would call this application of schizoanalysis to generate therapy a process of "metamodeling." Guattari's practice of metamodeling helps us see how schizoanalysis is crucial for social therapy as art. Guattari was analyzed by Lacan and worked with him or from his ideas (in an unorthodox way) throughout his career as a psychiatrist, schizoanalyst, and militant.

Lacan used complex diagrams and "knots" to illustrate his theories (such as the "mathemes of the unconscious"). Although Guattari was critical of this, he also used diagrams and models throughout his writings. As Deleuze (2006) said: "His ideas are drawings, or even diagrams" (p. 238).

From this point of view, we can call Guattari an artist or designer. He sees his ideas in images. His drawing practice and the consequent diagrams he creates, which illustrate and explain his theories, are then forms of life drawing. They helped

Guattari to visualize what he was thinking about. Just so, looking at these diagrams can give us a different method of analyzing his thoughts and ideas.

Guattari's singular books contain diagrammatic material from a huge eclectic range of sources, such as linguistics, ethnology, anthropology, chaos theory, and thermodynamics. This process of diagramming can be called metamodeling being put into practice; that is, the construction of aesthetic models for his different theories in the drawing he composed on paper. Guattari and Deleuze's concept of the diagram is defined as a mode of thought that avoids language.

Guattari later defined schizoanalysis as "metamodeling" when he said that "schizoanalysis, I repeat, is not an alternative modeling. It is metamodeling" (Guattari, 1996, p. 122). It is "a discipline of reading other systems of modeling, not as a general model, but as instrument for deciphering modeling systems in various domains, or in other words, as a meta-model" (Guattari, 1989, p. 27).

For Guattari a "model" (or "pattern") is a taught pattern of behavior inherited from family, institutions, and society. This model consists of a preceding, prescribed norm that is imposed by the powers that be in society. A model is also, from another viewpoint, a way of mapping and organizing a process or a structure (of society, of the family, of the body, or of desire, for example).

Guattari says that we all feel alienated at some time in our lives. We react to this alienation by building our own "existential territories" out of whatever resources (social or semiotic) are available to us. We just about manage to hold everything together, despite our alienation from society. We do what we can to get by.

Guattari shows how schizophrenics, in particular, manage like this. They invent and build themselves a functional universe, even though they cannot by any means live by dominant social models. Guattari says: "Thus it's not simply a matter of remodelling a patient's subjectivity—as it existed before a psychotic crisis—but of a production *sui generis*" (Guattari, 1995, p. 6). That is, remodeling your existential territory means making up your own way of being that is unique, just for you.

Here we can see how Guattari puts forward schizoanalysis as a process of metamodeling, which then has a therapeutic function. Guattari's understanding and application of modeling is influenced by Lacan, who said: "Models are very important" even though "they mean nothing" (Lacan, 1988, p. 88). Humans respond to models because "that's the way we are—that's our animal weakness—we need images" (Lacan, 1988, p. 88).

We need images. Diagrams help us understand ideas where and when language cannot. This is why schizoanalysis (and metamodeling, its synonym) is so intrinsically linked to art. We have begun to see the therapeutic function and potential provided by Guattari's schizoanalytic practice, whilst (I am sure) we all recognize the therapeutic function and potential made possible through art.

"Being Creative"

I develop my efforts at metamodeling by inventing and opening "new assemblages of enunciation and analysis" (Guattari & Rolnik, 2008, p. 376), especially during the COVID-19 pandemic, by running a series of "Being Creative" art workshops remotely on Zoom. When these workshops began, they were attended by a small group of local friends' children. They soon expanded to include a larger number of different (random) people from across the UK.

"Being Creative" as a workshop model operates the "polyphony" that Guattari calls for in his schizoanalytic practice. It provides a "transformative therapeutics" for all participants, outside the clinic. The clinic does not even come into question: some participants are diagnosed with various disorders, some aren't. The point is to be creative and enjoy the manifest, potent benefits of doing so.

These workshops continue with a very simple premise: I presume that no one has any art materials and no one knows how to paint. But everyone has creativity (even if they don't know it yet). I provide the means by which participants can access, nourish, and enjoy being creative.

Participants enter as strangers, and then we make art together in a way that supplies synergy and replenishment from our mutually connecting imaginations.

I start the workshops by presenting a stimulus or idea (e.g., a mandala, a haiku poem, a potato print, or images from art history), then I guide participants through the practical process of accessing their imaginations and responding to the stimulus. Participants "go with it" and create. What results is a warm, nourishing fraternity, made from our reciprocal, interactive art-making. We learn, grow, and feed ourselves from what we create.

A variety of people now attend these virtual events: adults, kids, families, mental health service users. I also work with a charity for people who have eating disorders. The workshops provide connection, replenishment, and fun.

The sessions enable participants to create assemblages of enunciation and sense-making for people, accessing transformative therapeutics, outside the clinic. Pure creativity is utterly joyous.

The colorful consequences of these workshops contain pictures, writing, costumes, sculptures, dancing, collages, and happy faces. As one participant says: "This is the most motivated and happy that I've felt since the lockdown."

This practice (and model) recalls my work on "Making Sense," in which the artistic process creates objects (artworks), which have transformative effects (Collins, 2017). Being Creative situates these effects as specifically relating to but located outside the clinic. With participants who are themselves situated inside the clinic (in terms of their diagnosis or treatment) and those who have nothing to do with the clinic (random people), their mutual, powerful response to the art we create falls on the outside (of order, control, semiotics, representation). Here is, as one participant puts it, "a creative and therapeutic space to explore feelings through imagery, creativity, and imagination."

I have shown how looking at an artwork, engaging with art, and creating art are three processes that have extensive ontological, political, and social effects: they are transformative, transgressive, and therapeutic (Collins, 2017). These effects occur inside the artwork, inside us, and outside us, situated in the world. With my own art, and the Being Creative practice, I show how art's positive effects can be provoked, incurred, utilized.

As with my experiences, writing, and art shown earlier, here is "the outside of thought" (Foucault, 1987). The art we create is what Foucault refers to in his *Thought from Outside*. Our mutual creativity draws the threshold on the borders between the binary oppositions of reason and madness, with a new framework for language, logic, and thinking. The outside presents a rhizomatic plane of immanence and multiplicity—from the outside, where there need not be an outside, an inside, or a boundary line, but purely immanent from that chaotic "is," which discursive strategies seem to crush in their ordering. Here Foucault (1987) impels the need to leap, as he says,

> to the "outside": [where] language escapes the mode of being of discourse—in other words the dynasty of representation—and literary speech develops from itself, forming a network in which each point is distinct, distant from even its closest neighbours, and has a position in relation to every other point in a space that simultaneously holds and separates them all.
>
> (p. 12)

During our workshops, the most powerful moment is that elongated silence, broken only by the sound of pencils scribbling or paint swashing on paper. Here, we can breathe—separated but connected by our focus and eruption of pure creativity. Here is the "outside," which draws us in. It provides a "neutral" space, which has been lost from representational, discursive thinking; the incommensurable plain of immanence, which Foucault calls for in his *Thought from Outside*.

The Being Creative art workshops build what Guattari (1995) calls an "underground art" (pp. 90–91). Here is the opportunity to "find some of the most important cells of resistance against the steamroller of capitalist subjectivity" (p. 91). This happens when people are able to open barriers that have previously eluded them, by accessing their creativity and being surprised and delighted by the consequences. We open new communities and abilities with art, not as "established artists but [with] a whole subjective creativity which traverses the generations and oppressed peoples, ghettoes, minorities" (p. 91).

What is created, in response to the darkness and frustrations of COVID-19 lockdown, is a new aesthetic paradigm, when participants (say they) are "liberated" by this opening made by artistic endeavor and aesthetic composition: a new existence. We embody and realise Guattari's *Chaosmosis: An Ethico-Aesthetic Paradigm* (1995):

> The work of art, for those who use it, is an activity of unframing, of rupturing sense, of baroque proliferation of extreme impoverishment, which leads to a recreation and a reinvention of the subject itself. A new existential support will oscillate on the work of art.
>
> (p. 131)

In this way, mad art makes sense. It opens a practice (and a model of practice) that both ruptures and transcends the curtailing system we face in everyday life (inside or outside the clinic). My drawings, paintings, and writings build an assemblage from my experiences, from which I can enunciate and make sense of them. We all have different situations and perceptions; art provides a mirror and the means for each of us to express the unique version of reality we partake in. We can breathe through the chaos that besets us; our visions are elucidated, released. Here, the world makes sense.

I end this chapter with a poem I once wrote in response to my artistic practice and how mad art makes sense—healing, visionary sense.

Making Sense—a narrative

Here I am:

The Darkness Clings to my mind,
erupting through those barbed wire knots,
which itch beneath the pores of my skin,
burning and mutating me.

Sensations mix a melting pot of tension that must jump out. They exude pangs of masochistic violence. Mute here, there are no words (they only stilt what yearns to break free).

Cut it out.

Knashing thrash in this clash, I crash. I'm trash: crushed here.

Words frustrate; I ache.

What to do...

I sit down with a blank sheet of paper, some water and a pallet of watercolour paints:
I wet the page, soaking the sheet with a layer of water by stroking its upper sheath with my paintbrush. The horsehairs clasped on this brush come from a bay New Forest pony (caught from the time when I cantered across Exmoor, in search of wild ponies, two lives ago). I load these hairs with water and colour, and then let them drip together onto the paper.

The paper's thirst is quenched. Its edges creep in, curving upwards in a semi-circular hollow shape that lifts off the desk. Then the paint trickles down each side of the page in unpredictable dimensions. There it ferments and ripples in delicate, sensitive, tiny lines, and so the shadows quietly shake when you look at them.

Please look at them.

Here thoughts cease, my hand plays a game with chance, and the paper becomes a tool that dances through my fingers with the paint.

The colours I choose are often different shades of black, because of the Darkness Clinging. And yet, as they mingle with the water, run across the page, and there crystallise and dry, an infinite spectrum emerges.

The interacting colours and the water dry into creeping streaks or crackles, into dusky silhouettes and bounding lines of radiance, or sombre gestures from the deeply aching anguish, and the thirst for life (lynched by the Darkness) that feed and demand such expression.

Somehow, the finished product shows me what was in my mind whilst I was creating it. The painting speaks for me—*as me*. Its voice of colour *makes sense*.

And so the violence is redirected, and eased now. The painting captures something that is thwarted by words, but which can be softly held in this moment of expression that it shares with me.

Postscript

My hallucinations became less violent as soon as I stopped working in the clinic. Other factors were also evident—for instance, changing my medication also improved the contents and eruptions of my mind. But leaving my job as a peer support worker, and choosing a career away from being identified purely on my illness, made a significant difference.

I still hear and see things, and I am grateful for this presence, but the destructive circus no longer devastates me. I still use art to express my experiences. When I paint my visions, or write them down, or make a film, the violence recedes and what's left is pure, ravishing expression. Making art provides structure and boundaries, which give form to my ineffable experiences; they become more approachable, manageable, safe.

Note

1 Dr. Lorna Collins, FHEA, FRSPH, Independent scholar.

References

Collins, L. (2017). *Making sense: Art practice and transformative therapeutics*. Bloomsbury.

Deleuze, G. (2006). *Two regimes of madness: Text and interviews 1975–1995* (D. Lapoujade, Ed.; A. Hodges & M. Taormina, Trans.). Semiotext(e).

Deleuze, G., & Guattari, F. (1986). *Kafka: Toward a minor literature* (D. Polan, Trans.). Minnesota University Press (original work published 1975).

Deleuze, G., & Guattari, F. (2004). *Anti-Oedipus: Capitalism and schizophrenia* (R. Hurley, M. Seem, & H. R. Lane, Trans.). Continuum (original work published 1972).

Foucault, M. (1987). Maurice Blanchot: The thought from outside. In B. Massumi (Trans.), *Foucault: Blanchot*. Zone Books (original work published 1986).

Guattari, F. (1989). *Cartographies schizoanalytiques*. Galilée.

Guattari, F. (1995). *Chaosmosis: An ethico-aesthetic paradigm* (P. Bains & J. Pefanis, Trans.). Indiana University Press (original work published 1992).

Guattari, F. (1996). *The Guattari reader* (G. Genosko, Ed.). Blackwell.

Guattari, F., & Rolnik, S. (2008). *Molecular revolution in Brazil* (K. Clapshow & B. Holmes, Trans.). Semiotext(e) (original work published 2007).

Lacan, J. (1988). *The ego in Freud's theory and in the technique of psychoanalysis, 1954–55* (S. Tomaselli, Trans). W.W. Norton & Co.

Lacan, J. (2007). *Seminar, Book XVII, the other side of psychoanalysis* (R. Grigg, Trans.). W.W. Norton & Co. (original work published 1991).

Editor's Reference

Collins, L. (2014). *Making sense: Art practice and transformative therapeutics*. Bloomsbury.

Chapter 12

Are You Conrad?

Sophia Szamosi

Summary

Sofia Szamosi is an author and illustrator of graphic novels, zines, and artists' books. In this graphic narrative based on the film *Ordinary People* (1980), Szamosi reimagines the narrative framing of the story. When the film opens, Conrad, the main character, has been doing well, living a privileged, normative life in the suburban United States. But a tragic boating accident kills his brother, disrupting his life, throwing him into suicidal despair, and taking him out of the mainstream. The story is set just before the emergence of the *DSM-III* and the explosion of biopsychiatry. Consistent with that setting, Conrad seeks psychoanalysis to help make sense of his experiences. If it were today, he would likely seek biopsychiatry and medications.

Opening beyond either of those possibilities, Szamosi approaches and imagines Conrad's options from a mad studies perspective of multiple alternatives. She beautifully illustrates some of the many choices beyond psychoanalysis and medications that Conrad might utilize to make sense of and rework his situation. For Szamosi, "Choices open up space! Choices give us new possibilities we couldn't imagine before. Choices give us freedom and make things a lot more interesting!"

*

DOI: 10.4324/9781003148456-14

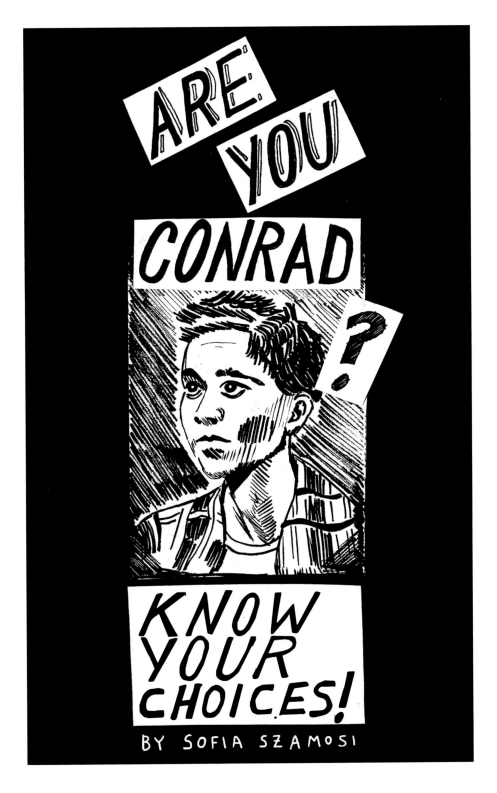

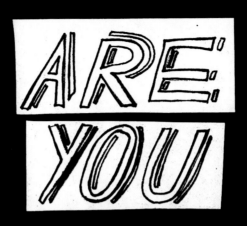

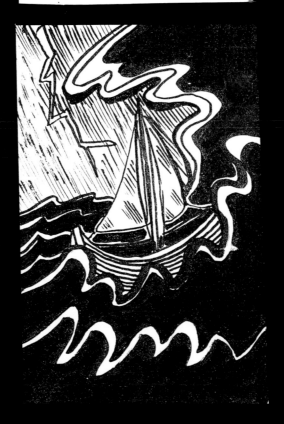

YOU COULD...
SEE A PSYCHOANALYST!

YOU COULD DIVE DEEP INTO UNCONSCIOUS PATTERNS OF FEELING THAT ORIGINATED IN CHILDHOOD AND HAVE BEEN TRANSFERED ON TO YOUR LIFE TODAY DO "THE WORK OF MOURNING" (FREUD)[2] AND FEEL ALL YOUR FEELINGS. IT WILL TAKE AS LONG AS IT TAKES.

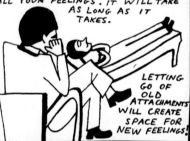

LETTING GO OF OLD ATTACHMENTS WILL CREATE SPACE FOR NEW FEELINGS!

YOU COULD...
SEE A COGNITIVE BEHAVIORAL THERAPIST!

YOU COULD UNDERSTAND YOUR SUFFERING AS BEING DUE TO FAULTY THINKING PATTERNS.[4] A THERAPIST COULD HELP YOU TO CONNECT YOUR THOUGHTS TO YOUR FEELINGS AND BEHAVIORS AND OVER A 12-WEEK PERIOD (OR LONGER) LEARN NEW TECHNIQUES AND WAYS OF THINKING AND BEHAVING SO THAT YOU COULD FEEL IN CONTROL OF YOUR MOODS AND THOUGHTS.

THOUGHTS

BEHAVIOR

FEELINGS

YOU COULD...
SEE A BIOPSYCHIATRIST!

YOU COULD UNDERSTAND YOURSELF AS HAVING A "BROKEN BRAIN",[3] A "MENTAL ILLNESS" OR A "DISEASE" THAT COULD BE LABELLED AND FIXED WITH MEDICATION. YOU COULD MEET WITH A PSYCHIATRIST AND DESCRIBE YOUR SYMPTOMS AND RECIEVE A DIAGNOSIS. YOU COULD UNDERSTAND THAT THIS IS NO ONES FAULT, YOU JUST HAVE A "CHEMICAL IMBALANCE" THAT CAN BE CORRECTED WITH MEDICINE.

RX LEXAPRO 2841937 BIG PHARMA

YOU COULD...
GO TO FAMILY THERAPY!

YOU COULD SEE YOURSELF AS ONE PART OF YOUR FAMILY UNIT AND FOCUS ON FINDING AND CHANGING UNHEALTHY OR DYSFUNCTIONAL PATTERNS IN THE FAMILY THROUGH FAMILY THERAPY SESSIONS FOCUSING ON THE PRESENT DYNAMICS YOU COULD DEVELOP NEW HEALTHY COPING AND COMMUNICATION SKILLS.[5]

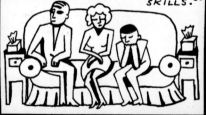

YOU COULD...
SEE AN INTERPERSONAL THERAPIST!

YOU COULD FOCUS ON YOUR INTERPERSONAL RELATIONSHIPS AS THE SOURCE OF YOUR EXPERIENCES AND FOCUS LESS ON WHAT IS GOING ON INSIDE YOUR HEAD. YOU COULD DO SHORT-TERM, STRUCTURED THERAPY WITH A GOAL OF ENRICHING YOUR RELATIONSHIPS AND REDUCING ISOLATION.[6]

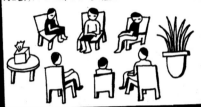

YOU COULD...
BECOME AN ACTIVIST!

YOU COULD UNDERSTAND YOUR EXPERIENCE AS BEING SHAPED BY YOUR SOCIAL, POLITICAL AND ECONOMIC CONTEXT. YOU COULD GET INVOLVED IN SOCIAL JUSTICE WORK, POLITICAL ORGANIZATIONS, OR COMMUNITY HEALING.

YOU COULD SEE A SOCIAL PSYCHIATRIST WHO COULD HELP YOU LINK THE PERSONAL TO THE POLITICAL AND SOCIOECONOMIC FACTORS AND FOCUS ON REHABILITATION.[8]

PERSONAL IS POLITICAL

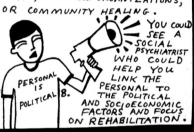

YOU COULD...
SEE A HUMANISTIC THERAPIST!

YOU COULD TAKE A PHENOMENOLOGICAL APPROACH AND SEE YOURSELF AS THE EXPERT OF YOUR OWN LIFE. YOU COULD READ SARTRE[7] AND GET INTO EXISTENTIALISM. YOU COULD BUILD A CLOSE RELATIONSHIP WITH YOUR THERAPIST WHO WOULD BE TOTALLY PRESENT WITH YOU, MIRRORING AND HEARING YOU, CREATING CONDITIONS WHERE YOU CAN FIX YOURSELF.

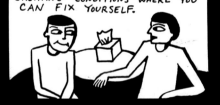

YOU COULD...
GET SPIRITUAL!

YOU COULD UNDERSTAND YOUR SUFFERING AS A "DARK NIGHT OF THE SOUL" THROUGH WHICH YOU MUST TRAVEL TO REACH ENLIGHTENMENT. YOU COULD HAVE A MYSTICAL EXPERIENCE, A SPIRITUAL AWAKENING, ADOPT A NEW RELIGION OR SPIRITUAL PRACTICE, OR SURRENDER YOUR WILL TO A POWER GREATER THAN YOUR SELF.[9]

YOU COULD...
JOIN A 12-STEP PROGRAM!

YOU COULD CHECK OUT [10.] ANY OF THE OVER 200 12-STEP MUTUAL AID FELLOWSHIPS DESIGNED TO HELP YOU RECOVER FROM BEHAVIORAL PROBLEMS BY SURRENDERING TO A HIGHER POWER OF YOUR UNDERSTANDING, TAKING A MORAL INVENTORY AND RIGHTING YOUR PAST WRONGS, AND HELPING OTHERS.

YOU COULD...
TRY EXPRESSIVE THERAPY!

YOU COULD USE ART IN A THERAPEUTIC SETTING TO ACCESS PSYCHIC MATERIALS TO THEN PROCESS IN THERAPY. OR, YOU COULD BECOME A PRACTICING ARTIST AND FIND HEALING THROUGH CREATIVE EXPRESSION.[12.]

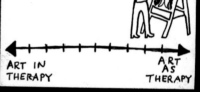

ART IN THERAPY   ART AS THERAPY

YOU COULD...
PRACTICE MINDFULNESS!

YOU COULD FOCUS ON HEALING YOUR MIND THROUGH MINDFULNESS-BASED THERAPY, AIMED AT REDUCING STRESS AND PREVENTING DEPRESSION THROUGH MINDFULNESS TECHNIQUES SUCH AS FOCUSING ON THE BREATH AND PRACTICING MEDITATION.[11.]

JUST SAY OM!

YOU COULD...
SEE A HOLISTIC HEALER!

YOU COULD SEE YOUR MIND, BODY, SPIRIT, EMOTIONS AND ENERGY AS ONE WHOLE ENTITY AND WORK WITH A HEALER WHO COULD OFFER NATURAL HEALING TREATMENTS SUCH AS HERBOLOGY, REIKI, ACUPRESSURE, ACUPUNCTURE, SOUND HEALING, TO NAME JUST A FEW.

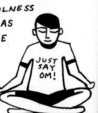

YOU COULD...
DO NOTHING!

YOU COULD DO ABSOLUTELY NOTHING. TIME COULD PASS AND HEAL ALL WOUNDS, OR MAYBE NOT. YOU COULD WAIT FOR CLARITY OR GUIDANCE, FOR SOMETHING TO SHIFT OR CHANGE, AND SEE WHAT HAPPENS.

YOU COULD...
BOTH/AND!

YOU COULD DO **BOTH** NOTHING **AND** EVERYTHING, AND THEN SOME! THERE ARE SO MANY MORE CHOICES THAN CAN EXIST IN A SINGLE PAMPHLET. THERE ARE INFINITE FRAMEWORKS AND METAPHORS FOR UNDERSTANDING YOUR HUMAN EXPERIENCE AND YOUR SUFFERING. YOU COULD GET CURIOUS ABOUT MULTIPLICITY AND FIND FREEDOM IN THE "POSSIBILITY OF POSSIBILITIES" [15.]

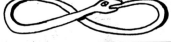

YOU COULD...
DO EVERYTHING!

YOU COULD TRY EVERYTHING UNDER THE SUN! EXPLORE ALL YOUR OPTIONS AND PICK AND CHOOSE PARTS YOU LIKE FROM EACH, "TAKE WHAT YOU LIKE AND LEAVE THE REST." [13.]

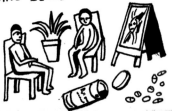

YOU COULD...
READ FICTION!

YOU COULD EXPAND YOUR MIND, UNFOLD THE WORLD AND UNFOLD NEW HORIZONS BY BRIDGING THE GAP BETWEEN LIVED LIFE AND TOLD STORIES. STORIES ARE LIVING PROCESSES, ONLY COMPLETED WHEN YOU THE READER INTERSECT YOUR WORLD WITH THE WORLD ON THE PAGE, MAKING READING ITSELF A WAY OF LIFE WITH INFINITE POSSIBILITIES. READING IS LIVING AND LIVING IS READING! LITERATURE CAN FREE US FROM OUR STINGY NARCISSISTIC EGOS BY OPENING OUR MINDS TO RADICALLY NEW PERSPECTIVES. [14.]

I KNOW WHAT YOU'RE THINKING...

WHY BOTHER?

WHY BOTHER WITH CHOICES?

WHAT'S SO BAD ABOUT DOMINANT STORIES?

KNOWLEDGE IS ALWAYS LINKED TO POWER.[15]

↓

THEREFORE QUESTS FOR UNIVERSAL TRUTHS WILL ALWAYS GET MESSY AND CORRUPTED.[16]

↓

HUMAN-MADE CATEGORIES, THEORIES AND DISTINCTIONS ARE DOOMED TO BE LIMITING AND CONSTRAINING.

↓

THEY CAN ALSO BE EXCITING AND ENABLING! [17]

↓

WHAT WORKS FOR ME MAY NOT WORK FOR YOU...

EXPAND YOUR TOOLKIT TODAY!

1. CONRAD JARRETT IS A FICTIONAL CHARACTER IN ROBERT REDFORD'S 1980 FILM *ORDINARY PEOPLE*. CONRAD IS THE TEENAGE SON OF THE JARRETT, AN UPPER-MIDDLE CLASS WHITE FAMILY LIVING IN THE CHICAGO SUBURBS. THE FILM FOLLOWS THE FAMILY AS THEY PROCESS CONRAD'S RECENT SUICIDE ATTEMPT AND HOSPITALIZATION AFTER THE ACCIDENTAL DEATH OF THE ELDEST SON, BUCK.

IT IS IMPORTANT TO CONSIDER HOW CONRAD'S RACE, GENDER, ORIENTATION, AGE AND CLASS ALL FACTOR IN TO THE AMOUNT AND QUALITY OF CARE AVAILABLE TO HIM, AND THAT NOT EVERYONE IS AFFORDED THE PRIVELEGE OF HAVING MANY CHOICES EASILY ACCESSIBLE.

2. AS DISCUSSED IN *MOURNING AND MELANCHOLIA* (1917) BY SIGMUND FREUD

3. AS DISCUSSED IN *THE BROKEN BRAIN* (1984) BY NANCY ANDREASEN

2.-13. ALL MODELS FEATURED IN THIS PAMPHLET DISCUSSED IN DEPTH IN *NARRATIVE PSYCHIATRY* (2011) BY BRADLEY LEWIS

7. AS DISCUSSED IN *EXISTENTIALISM IS A HUMANISM* BY JEAN-PAUL SARTRE (1946)

8. POLITICAL ARGUMENT MADE POPULAR IN SECOND-WAVE FEMINISM IN THE 1960'S BY CAROL HANISCH'S ESSAY *THE PERSONAL IS POLITICAL*

10. AS DISCUSSED IN *ALCOHOLICS ANONOMYS* (1939) BY BILL WILSON

11. AS DISCUSSED IN *MINDFULNESS, MYSTICISM AND NARRATIVE MEDICINE* (2016) BY BRADLEY LEWIS

13. A SLOGAN FROM TWELVE-STEP MEETINGS

14. AS DISCUSSED IN *LIFE IN THE QUEST OF NARRATIVE* BY PAUL RICOEUR

15. AS DISCUSSED BY MICHEL FOUCAULT IN *THE HISTORY OF SEXUALITY* (1981)

16.-17. AS DISCUSSED BY BRADLEY LEWIS IN *PSYCHIATRY AND POST-MODERN THEORY* (2000) AND JONATHAN CULLER IN *LITERARY THEORY: A VERY SHORT INTRODUCTION* (2011)

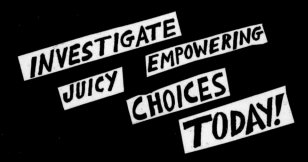

Part II. Critical Scholars

DOI: 10.4324/9781003148456-15

CRITICAL SCHOLARS OF MENTAL HEALTH HAVE been central in the conceptual shift from antipsychiatry to mad studies. This shift to mad studies involves a shift from antipsychiatry critiques of "myth of mental illness" to democracy-driven critiques of sanism and inclusion. Mad studies, from this perspective, is about the cultural work of increasing epistemic justice in the meaning-making practices around mental difference and mental suffering. To understand the role of critical scholars in this shift, it is useful to develop three background ideas and contexts: (1) Michel Foucault's theories of discursive practice and power; (2) the circuits of culture and medicalization; and (3) the role of affect, the body, materiality, and science in these circuits of culture. With this background, we can set up the kind of cultural work going on with critical scholars of mental health and mental difference.

The first background idea is Foucault's work on "discursive practice" and "power." For Foucault (1972), a *discursive practice* is a historically and culturally specific way of constructing meaning, experience, interpersonal relations, and lived practice (see also Ali, 2002; Lewis, 2006). Foucault's "discursive practice" is similar to Thomas Kuhn's concept of a "paradigm," and both a discursive practice and a paradigm can be helpfully compared to a game (Alcott, 2005). Games, like discursive practices more broadly, clearly involve the real world—with real equipment, costumes, practices, roles, rules, norms and rituals. But games, just as clearly, develop through social and cultural construction. As such, one does not usually ask if one game (e.g., chess) is more true to the real world than another game (e.g., basketball). One can certainly ask whether a particular move in chess or basketball is true to the rules and norms of chess or basketball. But it makes little sense to ask whether chess is more true than basketball. And if one prefers basketball to chess, one does not usually call chess is a myth. It is just a different way of being with the real. Similarly, in the world of mental health, when Western psychiatry transitioned from psychoanalysis to biopsychiatry in the 1970s and 1980s, this was not a shift in truth or "scientific progress" as much as a shift in discursive practice. From a discursive practice perspective, new capacities of knowledge and practice do emerge through the advent of biopsychiatry, but at the same time, many of the prior capacities of psychoanalysis were watered down or lost. Biopsychiatry as a discursive practice is not somehow more true than psychoanalysis, any more than chess is more true than basketball—although, as we saw, one can still ask local truth questions of biopsychiatry and psychoanalysis from within their respective discursive frames. And one can have preferences for biopsychiatry or psychoanalysis depending on how one wants to be with the real of mental life.

As a result, when Foucault (1972) compares discursive practices, he shifts the usual question, "Is it true?" to "Is it *in the true*?" in a particular time, place, culture, subculture, and so on. A discursive practice is "in the true" if it is legitimated as truth in a particular cultural formation (p. 224). This shift opens to questions of power. Foucault (1983) uses the term "power," or better yet, "power dynamics," to articulate a mode of "action upon action" (p. 222). Power is a "way in which certain actions modify other actions" (p. 219). In this definition, power is a force that, when exercised, structures the field such that particular actions are likely to follow. Power is the ability to make things happen in particular ways. It is here that Foucault parts company with Kuhn's idea of a paradigm. For Foucault (1980), a new discursive formation is not just a new "theoretical form, or something like a paradigm," it is a whole new "discursive regime" (p. 113). Knowledge and the power dynamics of knowledge creation must be thought of together. "Knowledge," which is shorthand for discursive practice, is not free from power. Knowledge is solidified through power, and power is solidified through knowledge. Power holds the elements of a discursive practice together, and power is a major determinant of why one discursive formation crystallizes rather than another.

This vision of power and knowledge, or power/knowledge, as co-constitutive shifts our usual concepts of power. For one, Foucault's power is not repressive but productive: it generates knowledge at the same time that knowledge generates power. Second, power always includes freedom and thus also always includes the seeds of resistance. For Foucault (1983), "The relationship between power and freedom's refusal to submit cannot therefore be separated" (p. 221). This approach to power is neither optimistic nor pessimistic. Power relations and power imbalances overdetermine discourse, but these power relations are not fixed, nor is their outcome always predictable. Power imbalances are unstable and often complex and contradictory. They are always in flux and always open to reversals. There is always room to shape, reshape, and resist knowledge/power claims within discursive formations, and there is always room to break out of hegemony to create and nurture counterhegemonic practices, approaches, communities, and mutual aid in which the power relations are more favorable. This empowered opening for change and alternative possibilities, though always available in theory, can be very limited on the ground of particular cultural circuits. But without seeing openings for change, and "wiggle room" for movement within current power relations, non-hegemonic possibilities and practices become even more difficult to access.

This brings us to our second background issue, the way interdisciplinary mad studies scholarship develops power/knowledge and related theories to understand the cultural circuits of mental difference. For example, feminist scholar Susan Bordo's work on eating disorder diagnoses, media studies scholars Toby Miller and Marie Clarie Leger's work on ADHD, sociologist Jackie Orr's work on panic disorder, anthropologist Joseph Dumit's work on brain images, American studies scholar Jonathan Metzl's work on pharmaceutic marketing and the racial dynamics of diagnosing psychosis, disability studies scholar Lennard Davis's work on obsession, psychologists Dana Jack's and Alisha Ali's work on gender and depression, comparative literature scholar Christopher Lane's work on the pathologization of shyness, sociologists Allan Horowitz's and Jerome Wakefield's work on sadness, feminist anthropologist Emily Martin's work on bipolar diagnoses, Bradley Lewis's work on the rise of biopsychiatry, Prozac, and the *Diagnostic and Statistical Manual III,* and sociologist Bruce Cohen's interdisciplinary work on critical mental health. These examples of mad studies scholarship only scratch the surface of the amount of work being done in this area, but they give a good feel for the way scholars are understanding the power dynamics around mental difference.

For a window into these power dynamics, it helps to return to Kathryn Pauly Morgan's (1998) work on the cultural circuits of medicalization, which we discussed in the "Introducing Mad Studies" section. Morgan draws on Foucault's ideas, but she also shows how Foucauldian-like concepts of power/knowledge are part of a much larger interdisciplinary lingua franca for scholarly critical cultural work. Morgan's interdisciplinary background includes philosophy of the body, feminist ethics and bioethics, critical disability studies, feminist bio-technoscience, medicalization theory, feminist pedagogy, and women and aging. When Morgan uses these resources to consider the legitimizing power dynamics of medicalization, she finds that the experiential life-world and pragmatic relations we have with our bodies and our minds are deeply influenced by the cultural circuits of medical-system discursive practice. As we saw in the introduction, she articulates these circuits into moments of conceptualization, macro-institutionalization, and micro-institutionalization (doctor/patient relations and internalized self-management) (see Figure 0.1 in "Introducing Mad Studies").

It is important to understand that the legitimizing medicalization circuits of Morgan's first figure are only the most proximal part of the story. In her next figure, she shows how the medicalization circuits are part of much larger cultural circuits (see Figure P.2). These larger circuits, which she calls "systemic hegemonic medicalization," include the forces and power dynamics of technocracy, patriarchy, structural alliances, and political economy. As a result, the legitimizing circuits of the first figure are reinforced and overdetermined by these larger cultural forces.

Morgan focuses on the medical system rather than the mental health system, but many of the issues overlap in four key ways. The first overlap is that mental health hegemony, like medical hegemony, overemphasizes and oversells a "biomedical

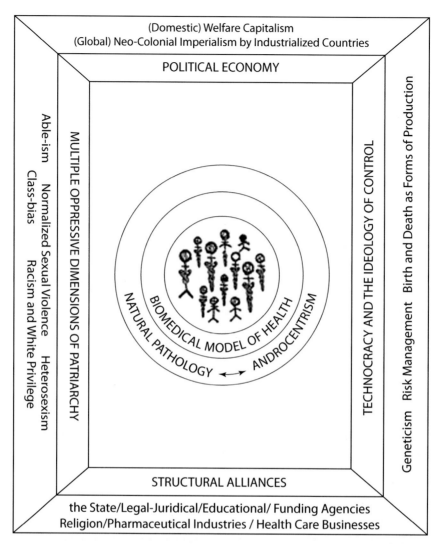

Figure P.2   Contextualized systemic hegemonic medicalization (Morgan, 1998, p. 106).

model" of mental difference. From a mad studies perspective, the biomedical model is not all bad, nor is it a "myth," but it does have limits and blind spots that often go unacknowledged in hegemonic mental health discourse. A key limitation is that when the biomedical model is applied to mental diversity it automatically pathologizes difference and turns mental difference into "mental illness." In addition, the biomedical model applied to mental difference reduces all relevant variables of mental difference to biological variables, genetic abnormalities, chemical "imbalances," and neuronal circuit "dysfunction." This narrow biomedical focus legitimates the overuse and overselling of biotechnological and pharmaceutical modes of assessment, diagnosis, treatment, and prevention. All of which feed in to biomedical and pharmaceutical profits and profiteering, which further feed back into the biomedical model, increasing its power relation over other possibilities. As a result, hegemonic mental health discourses overemphasize biological variables at the expense of personal, social/political, spiritual, aesthetic, and ecosystem variables.

The second overlap is that mental health system clinical models, including the biomedical model but also other mainstream models such as cognitive behavioral therapy, are reinforced, promoted, and propagated through systematic alliances with multiple other sectors of society—technocracy, patriarchy, structural alliances, and political economy. As Franz Fanon's (1986) work has so powerfully articulated, this means that shifting mainstream mental health models is not only about work in the mental health system; it is cultural work more broadly. The third overlap is the role of ableism—or in the case of mental health, sanism—in this hegemonic system: ableism/sanism is, on one hand, just a part of a larger context of hegemonic mental health and, on the other hand, the key value binary because the hierarchy of the normal and the abnormal creates structured pressure and internalized desire toward the norm. The fourth overlap is epistemic justice. As with Foucault's work, Morgan's interdisciplinary scholarship precedes Fricker's on epistemic injustice, but the power/knowledge perspective aligns nicely with it (Allen, 2017). Through Morgan's model of systemic hegemonic medicalization, we can see just how hard it is to actually get an epistemic voice around mental health knowledge formations. And yet, as with Foucault's notions of resistance and refusal, the balance between epistemic justice and injustice is not fixed, it involves a struggle.

The key reason epistemic injustice is so entrenched is that epistemic and social justice are linked across a range of intersectional differences. As social theorist Patricia Hill Collins (2017) puts it, "The term *intersectionality* references the critical insight that race, class, gender, sexuality, ethnicity, nation, ability and age operate not as unitary, mutually exclusive entities, but rather as reciprocally constructing phenomena that in turn shape complex social inequalities." Across all these differences "truth, ethics, and politics" are deeply linked, so that it would make little sense, for example, for "Black women to understand the truth of their lives without social justice as an ethical touchstone for action and political action to foster social justice in their lives" (p. 116). This link between epistemic agency and social justice is particularly important to see in the intersectional dimensions of sanism and mental difference. This is because the very same power dynamics of technocracy, patriarchy, structural alliances, and political economy that overmedicalize our mental lives also create the debilitating conditions of inequality that produce much of our distress and suffering in the first place.

Social and disability theorist Jasbir Puar's work (2017) on the "biopolitics of debilitation," which highlights the ways political economies of injustice mark out populations for "slow death" and "debility," is valuable here. Puar argues that we cannot understand individual mental distress without understanding the "knitting of finance capitalism and the medical industrial complex" (p. 1). These entrenched structures of "economic, racial, political, and social disenfranchisement" created an everyday world where "debility is endemic, perhaps even normative, to disenfranchised communities." Debility becomes the norm, "not exceptional, not that which is to come or can be avoided, but a banal feature of quotidian existence"

(p. 16). For certain neoliberal structures linked in tandem with medical industrial systems "debility pays, and pays well."

In the language of public health, when we look upstream from our individual lives, we find that structural inequality is causing much of our mental pain (McKinlay, 2019; Wilkinson & Pickett, 2020). As social epidemiologists Wilkinson and Pickett (2018) put it, inequality helps foster a social world of "dominance and subordination, superiority and inferiority. That affects how we treat each other and feel about ourselves. Inequality increases status competition and status insecurity. It increases anxieties about self-worth, and intensifies worries about how we are seen and judged." The amount of mental pain, much of it created through the stress of inequality, is staggering. The UK Mental Health Foundation Survey found that 74% of adults (83% of those 18–24 years old) were overwhelmed or unable to cope sometime in the past year; 32% of adults (39% of those 18–24 years old) had suicidal feelings as a result of stress. And 16% of adults (29% of those 18–24 years old) had self-harmed (referenced in Wilkinson and Pickett, 2018). Epistemic injustice forces us to pathologize our individual brains and cognitive processing as the only variables involved in this distress. Biomedical reductionism of social inequality creates a pernicious circle that psychologists Lisa Cosgrove and her colleagues link with Naomi Klein's concept of "disaster capitalism"–where an upstream political economy of inequality manufactures much of our distress and then offers us downstream reductive biotechnical solutions from which it can further profit (Cosgrove et al., 2020; Klein, 2007). This means that the struggle for epistemic agency around mental difference is inevitably also a struggle for larger social justice.

The third and last theoretical background issue for understanding mad studies scholarship involves topics that have often been underemphasized in mad studies but have emerged in recent years as important for cultural scholarship of all kinds. These topics all have to do with highlighting the importance of the material world, of bodies and affect, and of science for thinking about cultural circuits. In this vein, mad studies scholarship is increasingly careful to avoid reducing language and culture to nothing but social construction or falling into facile misinterpretations of Jacques Derrida's famous phrase "*Il n'y a pas de hors-texte.*" When this phrase is simplified to "There is nothing outside the text," it implies there is no real world. A similar controversy occurred in mental health around sociologist Thomas Scheff's (1966) early use of "labeling theory" of mental difference to critique mainstream psychiatry. Scheff was often understood through an antipsychiatry lens to mean that mental illness diagnoses are a "myth" because social labels cause mental illness and there is nothing outside language involved.

On the surface, it might seem that mad studies would agree, and indeed we often talk about the social dynamics of mental health labeling at different points of this book. But it is important not to lose sight of a key difference here. From a mad studies perspective, language does not exist in isolation any more than biology does. A social construction model or a biological model can be valuable for certain tactics and strategies of life–either for individuals or for activists. But there is a difference between being valuable for certain uses and being a singular truth–which would imply an antipsychiatry logic that everything else is myth. Mad studies scholarship undermines dogmatic singular "truths" of mental difference, whether they be biological or sociological, but not because they are "myths." It criticizes singular truths because of the way they leave out diverse possibilities of experience and lived practice and the way they close down questions of epistemic justice. Who is included (or excluded) in the making of "truths" and through what power dynamics are they included (or excluded)?

Thus, when mad studies uses interdisciplinary circuits of culture to articulate diverse possibilities and ask questions of epistemic justice, it matters that mad studies' approach to "culture" is complex and expansive. Cultural theorist Johan Fornäs (2017) does a nice job summarizing what this expanded notion of culture looks like through the articulation of five theses for cultural work:

> Thesis 1: Culture is meaning-making practice involving creative imagination.
> Thesis 2: Culture relies on communicative mediation between texts, subjects, and contexts.
> Thesis 3: Besides words and writing, meanings emerge through images, music, and other modes of communication.
> Thesis 4: Besides cognitive thoughts and images, meanings also involve an affective dimension of culture and of culturalization.
> Thesis 5: Culture is a dynamic interface of meaning and materiality.

The first thesis highlights the creative imagination that goes into all cultural work. This includes the arts discussed in Part 1 of this reader and other human meaning-making activities, such as political activism, religion, humanities, and science. The second thesis highlights the centrality of hermeneutics or meaning-making for cultural work. The third thesis makes sure that we don't understand this hermeneutic process as only about words or linguistics so that multiple mediums are equally part of cultural work. The fourth thesis expands the meaning-making process beyond cognition to include the body and affect and the important work that has emerged in affect studies. Finally, the fifth thesis centers the way that meaning-making is always in relation to and grounded in the real, in materiality, and in nature. The power dynamics of meaning-making involve not just humans and culture; nature and the material world too are active participants in the way meaning is made.

Because this expanded understanding of cultural work includes an opening to "the real," it is important to also say a word about the role of science in mad studies. Although much of mainstream mental health and psychiatry legitimizes itself through problematic appeals to science and scientific evidence, that does not mean that mad studies is exclusively "antiscience" any more than it is exclusively "antipsychiatry." We say "exclusively" here because there are people in the mad studies community who continue to champion the value of antipsychiatry worldviews, and this is a form of meaning-making that mad studies respects and values for particular people and particular purposes (Burstow, 2014). But mad studies cultural work, as a whole, is not about a blanket criticism of science or mental health care or psychiatry, it is about the cultural work of reducing sanism and the multiple structural alliances of sanism as these show up in a variety of places—including science, mental health care, and psychiatry. This is not antiscience. There can clearly be scientific work that is attentive to questions of epistemic justice, structural hegemony, and anti-oppression advocacy and that brings these concerns into the creation of research funding, design, method, and empirical practice. Such a methodological stance in scientific inquiry means that science can be, and indeed must be, included in cultural work for the role it can play in countering sanist stereotypes and biases that masquerade as objectivity in questions of mental difference (Ali, 2002; Ali & Sichel, 2018).

One of our contributors to the Critical Scholars section, Lennard Davis, has joined with David Morris to develop a "biocultural" approach to mental and bodily difference—indeed to biology and disability studies more broadly—which is similar to the expanded cultural work of mad studies. Like biocultures, mad studies is open to manifesto-style pronouncements and provocations, sound bites and rallying cries, which can be invaluable in the cultural work to reduce sanism. Adapted here are some of the biocultural rallying cries articulated by Davis and Morris (2007):

- Science and humanities are incomplete without each other.
- You can't fully understand the results of a given data set without knowing the historical, social, cultural, and discursive fields surrounding the data.
- Any contemporary research needs more than a cursory background in history and in the history of the concepts it employs.
- If you divide truths in half, you get half-truths.
- If you divide knowledge, your knowledge is divided.
- Nothing human is universal or atemporal.
- Embodiment is necessarily biological, and knowledge is always embodied.
- A fact is a socially produced conclusion.
- Bodies are always cultural and biological.
- Selves today are embodied, biologized, and shaped by medical knowledge.
- The boundary between organic and inorganic is no longer clear.
- Patients and experimental subjects are part of the decision-making process.
- Science can be postmodern; postmodernisms can be scientific.
- Biology, as a science, cannot exist outside culture; culture, as a practice, cannot exist outside biology.

The authors in our Critical Scholars section may or may not agree with all of these rallying cries, but, as a group, these chapters provide an excellent way into the role of mad studies scholarship and its cultural work around mental health. As a group, they are all involved in critiquing mental health discourses that are caught up in larger social structures of sanism while also affirming alternative possibilities for being with and making sense of our differences.

References

Alcott, L. (2005). Foucault's philosophy of science: Structures of truth / structures of power. In G. Gutting (Ed.), *Continental philosophy of science* (pp. 541–556). Blackwell.

Ali, A. (2002). The Convergence of Foucault and feminist psychiatry: Exploring emancipatory knowledge-building. *Journal of Gender Studies, 11*(3), 233–242.

Ali, A., & Sichel, C. E. (2018). Humanizing the scientific method. In N. Way, C. Gilligan, & P. Noguera (Eds.), *The crisis of connection : Roots, consequences, and solutions* (pp. 211–227). New York University Press.

Allen, A. (2017). Power/knowledge/resistance: Foucault and epistemic justice. In J. Kidd, J. Medina, & G. Pohlhaus (Eds.), *The Routledge handbook of epistemic injustice* (pp. 187–194). Routledge.

Burstow, B. (2014). The withering away of psychiatry: An attrition model for antipsychiatry. In B. Burstow, B. LeFrancois, & S. Diamond (Eds), *Psychiatry disrupted: Theorizing resistance and crafting the (r)evolution* (pp. 34–51). McGill-Queen's University Press.

Collins, P. (2017). Intersectionality and epistemic justice. In J. Kidd, J. Medina, & G. Pohlhaus (Eds.), *The Routledge handbook of epistemic injustice* (pp. 115–124). Routledge.

Cosgrove, L., Karter, J. M, Morrill, Z., & McGinley, M. (2020). Psychology and surveillance capitalism: The risk of pushing mental health apps during the COVID-19 pandemic. *Journal of Humanistic Psychology, 60*(5), 611–625.

Davis, L., & Morris, D. (2007). Biocultures manifesto. *New Literary History, 38,* 411–418.

Fanon, F. (1986). *Black skins, white masks*. Pluto Press.

Fornas, J. (2017). *Defending culture: Conceptual foundations and contemporary debate*. Palgrave Macmillan.

Foucault, M. (1972). *The archaeology of knowledge* (A. M. Sheridan Smith, Trans.). Pantheon Books.

Foucault, M. (1980). Truth and power. In G. Gordin (Ed.), *Power/knowledge: Selected interviews and other writings* (pp. 109–134). Pantheon Books.

Foucault, M. (1983). The subject and power. In H. Dreyfus & P. Rabinow (Eds.), *Michel Foucault: Beyond structuralism and hermeneutics* (pp. 208–229). University of Chicago Press.

Klein, N. (2007). *The shock doctrine: The rise of disaster capitalism*. Metropolitan Books / Henry Holt.

Lewis, B. (2006). *Moving beyond Prozac, DSM, and the new psychiatry: The birth of postpsychiatry*. University of Michigan Press.

McKinlay, J. B. (2019). A case for refocusing upstream: The political economy of illness. *IAPHS Occasional Classics, 1,* 1–10.

Morgan, K. P. (1998). Contested bodies, contested knowledges: Women, health, and the politics of medicalization. In S. Sherwin (Ed.), *The politics of women's health: Exploring agency and autonomy* (pp. 83–122). Temple Univ. Press.

Puar, J. K. (2017). *The right to maim: Debility, capacity, disability.* Duke University Press.

Scheff, T. (1966). *Being mentally ill.* Aldine.

Wilkinson, R., & Pickett, A. (2018, October 3). *The inner level: How more equal societies reduce stress, restore sanity and improve wellbeing.* London School of Economics and Political Science. https://www.lse.ac.uk/lse-player?id=4512

Wilkinson, R., & Pickett, A. (2020). *The inner level: How more equal societies reduce stress, restore sanity and improve everyone's well-being.* Penguin Books.

Chapter 13

Theoretical Considerations in Mad Studies

Erica Hua Fletcher

Summary

There has been a blossoming of mad studies scholarship in recent years, like a barren field bursting into color as the spring emerges. The many scholars involved are far from a single voice, nor do they represent a singular theoretical perspective or disciplinary location. This can make the field dizzyingly difficult to articulate and understand. Mad studies scholar Erica Fletcher provides a window into this emergence that organizes some of the diversity while respecting that multiplicity is a key strength of mad studies.

Within this diversity, a key theme is to center the "perspectives and goals of those who have experienced madness, mental difference, altered mental states, and[/or] mental suffering, and those who have felt harmed by psychiatric or psychological treatments." Fletcher articulates a way to do this that embraces "a big-tent perspective that celebrates a growing polyphony of scholars who are increasingly skeptical of academic discourses and applied fields in mental health care that assert reductionist explanations for the cause and treatment of 'mental illness.'" Additional key themes involve questions of structural inequality around mental difference, questions of mad praxis and methodology, and questions around being with madness. As Fletcher concludes:

> The common ground in mad studies is not sameness or perfect agreement, it is the shared interest in these questions, and it is the shared project of creating a less sanist world that is more accessible, supportive, and resource-rich for narrating and navigating mental difference and mental suffering.

*

"Madness" is a slippery concept, term, and reality. "Mad studies" too is similarly slippery. There is not one type of mad studies scholar, nor is there a single theoretical lens or methodological tool through which mad knowledge is produced. In mad studies, we come from various backgrounds and work across disciplines and in

DOI: 10.4324/9781003148456-16

diverse community settings (Diamond, 2013). Formally named "mad studies" can be enacted from multiple standpoints, including by artists, activists, and scholars, but also by psychiatric user/survivors, friends, family members, coworkers, clinicians, concerned citizens, and other allies. And if we are to consider the informal practice of mad studies—that is, being Mad—we must include everyone who experiences or is exposed to short-lived or extended, non-ordinary mental states. The umbrella of mad studies is wide and large, and its ways of thinking about madness are as multifaceted and complex as the subject itself.

Those engaged in mad studies share an interest in mental difference and distress and how such experiences are deeply entangled in personal, physical, familial, social, political, spiritual, artistic, and economic processes. Mad studies seeks to theorize why madness comes to some, how people enter madness and come out of it, and why others experience madness throughout their lives (Jones & Kelly, 2015). Mad studies asks why some people find a sense of peace within their madness, while others lack the tools and resources to do so. Mad studies also recognizes that the practices and infrastructure to support the wellbeing of mad people remain diverse, dynamic, and divergent throughout the world. Indeed, madness escapes easy articulation, explanation, or solution. And for the most part, "cure" is not the aim of our investigations into madness. As a field, we wish to hold on to the complexities of madness and, at the same time, to question a world that is maddening itself.

In what follows, I will describe the diversity of mad studies and then provide an overview of the key theoretical considerations that have structured the field's development, including issues related to mad identities, structural inequities, and their application. I will also describe major points of debate in this dynamic field and list core questions that can serve as sites for further theorization and inquiry. I conclude by considering how holding the complexities and contradictions of madness remains an integral part of the field's resistance to dominant mental health (or psy) knowledge(s). Mad studies, by working against common reductionist approaches to "mental illness," seeks to promote complexity in how we come to understand unusual mental states. Mad studies, in other words, is a process skill—the process of holding together difference and conflict—as much as it is a content skill of being aware of the multiple approaches for grappling with mental difference.

The Diverse Field of Mad Studies

In mad studies, we use a breadth of theoretical lenses and methodological tools to unpack the historical, sociocultural, psychological, and political etiologies of madness and critique current practices related to its treatment. The diversity of starting points for inquiry about madness is impressive. Some mad studies scholars analyze madness throughout history to the present (Hedva, 2016; Torn, 2018; Wang, 2019), while others point to the emergence of Western psychiatry and psychology, which their scholarship critiques (Russo & Sweeney, 2016). Some psychiatric user/survivor researchers of public mental health services contribute to an evidence base as a strategy to spur system reform (Faulkner, 2017; Johnston, 2019; Sweeney, 2016; Sweeney et al., 2009), while others question the utility of incremental reforms, standardized metrics for mental health recovery, and the efficacy of "evidence-based practices," particularly when they do not involve user-led researchers in implementation and evaluation processes (See Corstens et al., 2014; Voronka, 2019). Others aim to abolish all forms of "psychiatric incarceration" and take a pointed stance of resistance against the psy fields (Burstow, 2019). Still others argue that studying madness via theoretical frameworks may obfuscate seeing madness as it presents itself within each person, within their immediate relationships and environments, and in their society; they advocate for a grounded perspective of caring for and understanding madness along with the person experiencing it and for the primacy of lived experience, from which research follows (Crossley, 2004, p. 167).

Members of mad studies communities also hold political ideologies that span from a libertarian or anarchist bent to liberal, socialist, and communist leanings (Diamond, 2013). We also question which challenging experiences with psychiatry "count" for scholars to claim "lived experience" or mental disability and who instead should claim allyship with mad activism and research (Joseph, 2019; Rose, 2017; Spandler et al., 2015; Voronka, 2016). Moreover, given the nature of madness and disability, the elitism and sanism of academia, and the historic privileging of scholarship from the Global North, many of us hold deep interest in mad studies yet lack the pathways to secure training in the field or employment in supportive workplaces (Jones et al., 2021; Leblanc & Kinsella, 2016; Price, 2011; Spandler & Pousanidou, 2019). This prevents many of us from contributing directly within scholarly discourses.

Despite these wildly divergent relationships to theory, praxis, and visions for the future of madness and mental health care, mad studies scholars generally agree that our contributions aim to center the perspectives and goals of those who have experienced madness, mental difference, altered mental states, and mental suffering and of those who have felt harmed by psychiatric or psychological treatments (Spandler & Poursanidou, 2019). We embrace a big-tent perspective that celebrates a growing polyphony of scholars who are increasingly skeptical of academic discourses and applied fields in mental health care that assert reductionist explanations for the cause and treatment of "mental illness" (Diamond, 2013). Moreover, we question the telos of the psy disciplines to achieve service users' mental health "recovery" or "mental health," given that such notions have often been inseparable from societal views on morality, normality, and productivity under late capitalism (Beresford, 2019, 2020; McWade, 2016; Morrow, 2013). By situating individual mental distress as a valid response to spiritual, physical, social, aesthetic, economic, and political issues, we aim to externalize the locus of madness from an atomized, personal level to a societal, environmental, and even planetary level (Lewis, 2021).

Mad Identities: Challenging "Sanity," Challenging the Universal Subject

This chapter describes theoretical frameworks that center on madness as a historical and cultural artifact through which it is lived and by which systems of power and oppression can be analyzed. Centering mad experiences means asking questions such as how does madness feel? How do people make meaning of their experiences? How do families, healers, and communities address mental distress? How do religious cosmologies, governance structures, and economic systems inform understandings of psychic distress? How are sexual and gender norms reified within specific psychiatric diagnoses and treatments? How are notions of mental wellbeing and mental illness (re)produced within society and throughout the world? What are the ideological origins of the psy disciplines and applied professions? Alongside these questions, we can also point to affect theory, critical disability studies theory, queer and feminist theories, indigenous theories, and many other social theories to analyze how madness is felt, discussed, and addressed (see Donaldson, 2018).

Against a growing tide of psy monoculture for categorizing certain behaviors as mental illness, diverse understandings of madness remain throughout the world and counter totalizing frameworks for "treating" mental distress. Mad studies scholars who seek to describe indigenous and other non-Western understanding of altered mental states may examine local sociocultural, spiritual, and religious meanings of madness (Davoine, 2020). For example, as many psychological anthropologists and indigenous auto-ethnographers have noted, local idioms of distress and culturally-bound syndromes may be understood as an ontological disconnect from the land, from ancestors and gods, and from other members of the community, as well as a lack of economic security and political sovereignty (Luhrmann & Marrow, 2016; Million, 2013). Likewise, experiences of mental crisis may be addressed through local customs and rituals, including communal healing and integration practices, as well as familial and communal adaptations to an individual's needs and abilities. Given the current dominance of the Western biopsychiatric paradigm, such scholars also chart how indigenous and non-Western knowledge systems have resisted, adopted, and hybridized Western biopsychiatric and psychological frameworks for understanding and treating altered mental states (Clark et al., 2013; Gone, 2010; Nakamura, 2013; Raju & Penak, 2019).

Mad studies scholars may draw from historians of philosophy to examine how "madness" and its ontological counter, "sanity," have shifted in Western religious, academic, and social domains over millennia and have come to be imposed on indigenous and other non-Western populations (Hacking, 1998; Lawlor, 2012). This historical perspective may begin as far back as an examination of the first recorded oral traditions and written texts grappling with madness, from the ancient Greeks' definitions and distinctions of madness, along with related questions of selfhood, morality, the good life, civic duty, medical ethics, and governance. It extends to mystic and spiritual frameworks of madness during the Medieval period, and onwards to the 12th century's "discovery" of the individual and the subsequent Renaissance humanists' writings on madness (Morris, 1987; Proctor, 1998). Mad studies scholars also draw from the work of social theorists and historians who note societal upheavals in the transition from feudalism to early capitalism, growing schisms between church and state, and later the revolutions toppling monarchies, which reflected changing perspectives about what it meant to be a subject to the church or the state, to one's community and family, and increasingly to oneself (Federici, 2004; Rothman, 2017). This subjectification and excavation of the self coincided with corresponding endeavors to name, rank, and categorize humans and the rest of the natural world, along with other political, economic, religious, and scientific projects to justify colonial conquests of the 15th and 16th centuries (Hedva, 2016; Torn, 2018).

As a part of the changing understanding of selfhood in relation to European society, mad studies scholars cite the work of historians who note spreading beliefs that governments—rather than families or townships—had a role to play in caring for the mad, which led to the creation of the first insane asylums, or madhouses (Scull, 2015). They also point out problematic assumptions made by Enlightenment thinkers—the intellectual progenitors of the psy disciplines, who relied on both an idealized, platonic figure of the "sane" subject and a characterization by those who seemingly mirrored themselves—elite, liberal, rational, productive, heterosexual, and male (Toulmin, 1990). Highly influential intellectuals Emil Kraepelin and Sigmund Freud continued this tradition as they sought to distinguish psychiatric and psychoanalytic disciplines from the other nascent social sciences of the late 1800s. In turn, mad studies scholars pay special attention to the cultural shifts that enabled their own field's theoretical origins in the 1950s as the world grappled with the scientific atrocities of the Holocaust; and classicist, racist, and sexist beliefs about madness; and shifting attitudes towards state asylums, medical expertise, and medical paternalism in the Global North (Crossley, 2006; Morrow, 2017; Roberts, 2011; Showalter, 1985). Even while the failures of eugenics campaigns to eradicate madness and other "undesirable" characteristics and minoritized ethnic groups were laid bare, the psychologization and psychiatrization of cosmopolitan populations gained traction, as people sought solace from social turmoil and turned to psy expertise to cope with the spiritual, existential, and political ills of their time (De Vos, 2013; Herman, 1995; Lasch, 1991; Liebert, 2018). This growing preoccupation with self-improvement, a belief in technocratic expertise to provide solutions, and the development of the first psychotropic medications led biological psychiatry or *biopsychiatry* to gain prominence over psychoanalysis and other psychological modalities of treatment in the second half of the 20th century (Kutchins & Kirk, 1997).

The affirmation of mad identities via mad studies remains a generative site of great contention and debate among scholars and activists (Beresford, 2020; Voronka, 2016). In upholding madness as a culturally-bound experience and as one that can be found across cultures, mad studies scholars struggle with analyzing mad narratives and representing madness in its particularities, and as one that can be summed up and discussed generally enough to abstract and theorize. A focus on madness and mad narratives as sites of scholarship and personal/political engagement can be empowering, but it can also recreate the idea that its inverse—sanity—is also a universal experience that can be codified and determined in an objective, rather than a subjective, manner. When the latter happens, it creates a tautological or paradoxical bind, in which resisting aspects of the psy disciplines' pathologization of "madness" as mental illness may rely on some assumption of "sanity" outside that framework. These enabling/constraining dimensions of mad narratives are further complicated by the narratives we tell about our own personal and professional lives that often serve as a standpoint from which our scholarship emerges and gains traction in mad studies circles. In our own terms, mad studies scholars embrace various forms of strategic essentialism, narrative identification, and critical realism of madness as tactics to engage in necessary political projects, such as mental health services reform, psychiatric abolition, or decolonial resistance (Joseph, 2015; Lewis, 2011; Voronka, 2016).

Efforts to separate the mad from the sane—particularly among elite scholars, powerful governments, and public health practitioners—throughout history leave us with generative questions about mad identity as a theoretical orientation. To this end, mad studies scholars whose research focuses on cultural analysis and critique ask some of these guiding questions about identity, culture, and the construction of madness: Who is considered mentally ill? Who is considered sane? How did certain behaviors become censured and interpreted as mental illness? How is madness socially and culturally constructed, just as it is grounded in biological, psychological, and political processes? How have categories of madness shifted throughout history? What are the ideological origins of the psy disciplines? How may universalizing global mental health discourses clash with local understandings of altered mental states and mental wellbeing? How have culturally-bound understandings of mental distress changed with respect to the growing dominance of Western biopsychiatric frameworks? In what ways do indigenous and other non-Western peoples resist, incorporate, and adopt aspects of Global Mental Health campaigns? How is the strategic essentialism of mad identities deployed in mad studies? What are the cultural and material limits of identity-based politics?

THEORETICAL FRAMEWORKS THAT EXPLORE MAD IDENTITY AS CULTURAL PRODUCTION

Affect: Describes the immediate, pre-verbal sensations (touch, taste, sight, smell, sound) that are entangled with a specific place and time and the many feelings of madness, recovery, and mental wellbeing that arise in relation to complex interpersonal relationships and political processes (Aho et al., 2017; Million, 2013, pp. 56–77).

Critical disability studies: Draw insights on mental disability from broader disability scholarship and activism. It upholds a social model of disability, which affirms communities' roles in creating spaces that are accessible and for adapting systems of care to meet the needs of all people (Castrodale, 2017; Lewis. 2006; Thorneycroft, 2020).

Critical race: Refers to scholarship that recognizes how white supremacy, anti-Black racism, and other forms of race-based violence shaped scientific—including psychiatric and psychological—notions of racial inferiority or race-based diagnoses. Such theorists assert the social construction of racial categories while recognizing the real effects of racial discrimination in mental health services and racial basis in medicine (Meerai et al., 2016; Roberts, 2011; Redikopp, 2021).

Foucauldian: Describes the forms of self-surveillance and self-policing that have become dominant as whole populations have come to view themselves in psychological—and potentially pathological—terms. Such scholars also contextualize the power of psychiatric and psychological expertise that has replaced the traditional authority of the church and the state in late modernity. They note the political and social factors that contributed to the rise and fall of certain psychiatric diagnoses and paradigms for interpreting human behavior (Ben-Moshe, 2020, pp. 5–7; Bracken, 1995; Liebert, 2018).

Indigenous: Interprets mental crisis and spiritual transformation within local beliefs, customs, and rituals, including communal healing practices. Illness—as a spiritual, social, and physical phenomenon—may result from a disconnect from the land, ancestors, and the community. Affirming one's place in a community and culture, acknowledging intergenerational trauma, recognizing the legacy of colonization, and working towards indigenous sovereignty can serve as forms of healing (Burstow, 2019; Clark et al., 2013; Davoine, 2020; Million, 2013; Nielson, 2012).

Narrative theory: Focuses on an individual's experience of madness via their first-person oral or written accounts, visual portrayals, or auto-fictionalized portrayals. Considers the role of metaphors, plot, point of view, and other narrative devices and structures used in storytelling (Lewis, 2011; Netchitailova, 2019; Rashed, 2019, pp. 188–193).

Phenomenological: Studies structures of consciousness and being from the first-hand experience of madness. This is articulated through a close description of the physical sensations and emotions that arise during times of mental crisis and the interactions psychiatric user/survivors have with caregivers, mental health professionals, and institutions (Kafai, 2020; Woods et al., 2014).

Queer theory: Contextualizes psychiatric diagnoses and therapeutic modalities by challenging how notions of sexual deviance and personality disorders are reproduced with the psy disciplines and how social "problems" become narrowly defined and treated in medical terms (Cvetkovich, 2003; Eales & Peers, 2020; Kunzel, 2017; LeFrançois & Diamond, 2014; Spandler, 2017).

Structural Inequities

As the psy disciplines and mental health services have gained traction globally, mad studies scholars are quick to note the vast power and wealth differentials that exist within a global mental health industrial complex (Davar, 2017; Mills, 2014). For example, power differentials between pharmaceutical corporations and individual prescribers, psychiatrists and incarcerated populations, corporate executives and their working-class employees, special interest groups and welfare recipients, politicians and soldiers, manufacturing corporations and the incarcerated populations whose labor they employ—all foster the conditions that recreate present understandings about mental illness and poverty as personal failings rather than societal ones. Such structural inequities come to frame how "madness" is acted upon within systems of care and control (Hunter, 2018), and they serve as an important site of inquiry among mad studies scholars who turn their attention to issues of material scarcity and security, economic mobility, racialized treatment, and working conditions as key factors in the experience of madness and its treatment. Mad studies scholars who examine structural inequities in mental health care ask (a) How did the psy disciplines become a lens through which social ills are now addressed? and (b) How do systems of care and control—such as social welfare programs, educational systems, criminal justice systems, housing opportunities, and mental health care systems—prevent, induce, sustain, or reduce madness?

A historical, materialist perspective on structural inequities enables us to examine systems of colonization and imperialism—including scientific imperialism—that contributed to the uneven psychiatrization and psychologization of certain populations. For example, mad studies scholars explore how settler colonialists deemed native peoples expendable or extractive resources via genocidal and assimilationist policies since the 15th century (Joseph, 2015, 2019). They note that 16th- and 17th-century European colonizers often described indigenous peoples as childlike, naive, and "noble savages" who experienced less madness than Western societies (Mills, 2014). This belief shifted in the Industrial Revolution, as fears of immigrants and belief in the moral and physical degeneration of the human species gained traction (Pick, 1993), when mad, poor, and racialized populations became the targets of public health interventions. Such fears were bolstered by a growing acceptance of social Darwinism and scientific racism at the turn of the 19th century, exemplified by the writings of Sir Francis Galton and Charles Davenport, whose work on eugenics came to justify "mental hygiene" procedures such as lobotomies and forced sterilization campaigns among those deemed mad throughout much of the Western world in the 20th century (Eales & Peers, 2020, pp. 4–8; Lombardo, 2008). Similarly, in the 1950s and 1960s, US CIA-funded mind research programs, such as Project MKULTRA, funded unethical research of psychiatrists who subjected prisoners, soldiers, and psychiatric inmates to scientific experiments (Washington, 2006, p. 356). Throughout this history, the justification of sanist policies, which discriminated against those deemed mad, serve as stark reminders that Western science and medicine have been weaponized to uphold systems of exploitation and oppression for political and economic aims (Joseph, 2015; Liegghio, 2013).

Structural inequities in institutional care and support for those deemed mad remain of great interest to mad studies scholars as they grapple with the economic, scientific, and political motives in play within governments' decisions to allocate funds to mental health services and research. They note how access to mental health care shifted significantly, based on wealth differentials and changing attitudes towards government responsibilities to provide mental health care to structurally vulnerable citizens. For example, psychiatric and psychological professionals in the Global North, whose services were once considered elite services in the late 1800s and early 1900s, began to treat a majority of poor patients in the 1950s (Burstow, 2015). Since this tipping point in the demographics of mental patients, structurally vulnerable and racialized populations have been subject to increased scrutiny and disproportionate diagnoses of mental illness (see Ben-Moshe, 2020; Meerai et al., 2016; Metzl, 2009). Such disparities point to larger inequities concerning access to mental health care, as well as the quality and suitability of such services.

In recent years, mad studies scholars in the Global North have focused their attention on structural inequities within public mental health systems following deinstitutionalization and the roles that psychiatric user/survivor activists and scholars play in system transformation. In many Western countries, the closure of state asylums was not met by sufficient funding of social welfare programs, public housing, food stamp programs, and community mental health systems of care that were originally intended to replace them (Grob, 1994), and many people became homeless or incarcerated due to this lack. Alongside the popularization of psychotropic medications in the 1950s and subsequent decades, psychiatric patients were increasingly expected to "recover" from mental distress via outpatient care and medication adherence yet often lacked the material resources, social support, and skills to do so (Morrow, 2013; see also Braslow, 2013; Jacobson & Curtis, 2000; Myers, 2015). At the same time, psychiatric diagnoses have become increasingly important, as they are often crucial for patients to secure social welfare and other forms of government support (Mills, 2015; Hansen et al., 2014).

Psychiatric user/survivor-led innovations that emerged from the recovery movement and other forms of mad activism following deinstitutionalization have found entry into mental health systems and research. These include mutual-aid networks, peer support, peer respites, and patient-involved research (See Bouchery et al., 2018; Crossley, 2004; Davidson and Guy, 2012; DuBrul, 2014). Despite such gains in democratizing mental health care, such novel approaches to facilitate more equitable relationships between patients and providers, and among service users and researchers, are often subsumed and mainstreamed under medical, neoliberal models for accessing mental health research funds and services (Beresford & Russo, 2016; Faulkner, 2017; Morrow, 2013). Voluntary, community-based mental health support by and for people with lived experience of mental distress remains subject to challenging current market-based demands to prove their efficiency and efficacy. Noting such trends in mental health services research, mad studies scholars articulate disjunctions between the values held by system administrators and funders and mad values and ethics, even as they argue for the inclusion of peer support, peer leadership, and related user/survivor reforms within public mental health systems (Voronka, 2017).

THEORETICAL FRAMEWORKS TO EXAMINE STRUCTURAL INEQUITIES

Anarchist: Challenges the authority of psychiatrists and psychologists in pathologizing certain mental states and upholding an idealized form of mental health. Seeks to empower mad communities to take a do-it-yourself approach to coping with madness, via the formation of mutual–aid peer support communities (DuBrul, 2014; Johnston & Steckle, 2018).

Anticapitalist: Explores the roots of modern madness and the growth of the psy disciplines in social alienation, poor labor conditions, ecological degradation, and other forms of injustice perpetrated by corporations and plutocracies (Aho et al., 2017; Beresford, 2019; Burstow, 2015).

Antipsychiatry: Asserts that psychiatric treatments have often done more harm than good throughout history and that the psy disciplines—as a part of the "therapeutic state"—have great power over populations. Many antipsychiatrists call for involuntary psychiatric commitment and all forms of incarceration to be abolished (Burstow, 2014, 2019).

Feminist: Examines issues of gender, sexuality, class, and power differentials in the creation of psychiatric categories for mental illness, such as psychiatry's historic pathologization of queer and trans people. Feminist theory grounds knowledge production from the standpoint of historically-oppressed populations, and often adopts collaborative methodologies that include the voices and perspectives of those who have suffered social injustice (Blanchette, 2019; Diamond, 2014; Douglas et al., 2021; Friedman, 2017; Morrow, 2007, 2017).

Marxist/socialist: Locates madness as a product of exploitative labor practices throughout the world and vast wealth inequities between the rich and the poor. Examines how governments and quasigovernmental institutions allocate funds and resources to address mental illness and homelessness and how such policies affect societal perceptions of madness and civic duty. This framework rejects the atomizing, biologically reductionist perspective of mental illness as individual pathology and embraces a vision for society in which everyone has access to necessities, shared ownership of their work, and a government that represents and provides for all its inhabitants (Cohen, 2016; Fisher, 2009; Frantzen, 2019; Gong, 2019).

Postcolonial: Historically contextualizes the growth and spread of psychiatry and psychology from the Global North to the Global South and describes cultural, political, and economic shifts associated with the imposition, hybridization, and adoption of Western mental health frameworks on indigenous and other non-Western populations (Bruce, 2017; Eromosele, 2020; Joseph, 2015; Miller, 2018; Raju & Penak, 2019).

Understandably, divergent theories on structural inequities continue to fuel intellectual debate about visions for attending to and understanding madness. For example, anarchist and antipsychiatry perspectives tend to emphasize abolition from mental health systems and all systems of incarceration, as well as the need for free, community-led mutual-aid support networks to take their place. In contrast, mad studies scholars who adhere to socialist theory and politics tend to support reforms to bolster existing public mental health infrastructure and welfare programs. This support of universal, public programs is sometimes at odds with postcolonial scholars, who emphasize the need for unique community support and mental health practices that are culturally representative of specific populations.

While the content of such debates is outside the scope of this chapter, below I have included the following questions, which point to further sites of inquiry: How do governments, healthcare, and social service systems allocate mental health care? Who can access mental health services? Who experiences forced treatment? How have the psy disciplines and the applied fields of mental health services evolved in relation to market demands under late capitalism? In what ways have colonialism, imperialism, nationalism, and globalization affected mental wellbeing and mental health care? What is the impact of psychiatric user/survivor-led reform efforts in mental health services research and public mental health care? How might user/survivor activism be co-opted or mainstreamed? What lessons for cross-movement solidarity and allyship can be learned as mad studies continues to develop? What impact do research funding structures (foundations and institutes) and employment standards play in shaping academic discourses on madness (Jones et al., 2021)? What counts as "evidence" in the health humanities and in mental health services research? To which larger reformist or abolitionist projects or social movements do mad studies scholars consider themselves to be aligned? How are such politics reflected in their theory and methodology?

TRENDS AND CHALLENGES IN GLOBAL MAD STUDIES

Throughout the world, mad artists, activists, and scholars advocate on behalf of those deemed "mad" by questioning the role and function of psychiatric services and the role governments play in providing mental health services, social welfare, and other public services. They critique the exportation of Western psychiatric and psychological frameworks throughout the Global South and indicate the parallels in movement for global mental health with neo-colonialism, neo-imperialism, and the psychiatrization and securitization of the world (Davar, 2017; Leibert, 2018; Mills, 2014). They also highlight the advocacy of organizations such as Bapu Trust and Mad in Asia, as well as the publication of several declarations from the Global South that affirm the need to democratize mental health care in low- and middle-income countries and end involuntary psychiatric treatment (Latin American Network of Psychosocial Diversity, 2018; Pan African Network of People with Psychosocial Disabilities, 2011; Transforming Communities for Inclusion–Asia Pacific, 2018).

As the field grows, many mad studies scholars have expressed caution that the field may replicate systemic inequities in knowledge production and become an elite, Eurocentric, and academic project (Gorman & LeFrancois, 2017; Kalathil & Jones, 2016). Concerning harbingers of this trend include the lack of strategic partnerships with indigenous groups and other historically oppressed groups in the Global North, and of strong academic or activist alliances with the Global South (Beresford, 2020; Bruce, 2017; Joseph, 2015). Given the great diversity of mental health systems, forms of postcolonial governance, and academic interests and commitments of scholars living in the Global South, the future of mad studies theory in low- and middle-income countries remains all but determined.

Mad Praxis

Mad studies' diverse theoretical groundings inform a wide range of community-based methodologies, and, in turn, such methodologies qualify and clarify social theory. From popular education to patient-involved research methods, mad studies scholars infuse community perspectives on madness within their scholarship, methodological approaches, and activism (Faulkner, 2017; Johnston, 2019; Leblanc & Kinsella, 2016; Rose, 2017; Sweeney, 2016). In practice, mad studies scholars have participated in the formation of peer support networks, activist organizations, and other mad-positive programs within and outside of community mental health systems. We have also organized several mad studies reading groups over the last decade, including those formed virtually and internationally. Furthermore, community-based participatory research, public and patient-involved research, and user engagement groups have enabled mad-identified informants to set research priorities and participate in research projects as employed researchers. The development of several undergraduate and graduate courses on mad studies also signal growing acknowledgment and institutional support of this field. Such community-based methodologies highlight the field's theoretical insights to center mad perspectives as a valid, essential way to understand mental differences and distress and to democratize mental health services and research.

Being with Madness

> Doctors try to give us succinct, definite answers, but is there really an answer to the human psyche?
> Should we not retain some mystery?
> Should we not leave some space for the unknown, for something that we cannot really explain?
>
> (Netchitalilova, 2019, p. 1515)

Theoretical inquiry into madness enables us to see madness within complex relationships to communities, institutions, governments, spiritual and aesthetic practices, economies, and the more-than-human world. We can continue to ponder challenging questions that have not been readily resolved within academic discourse and trace the evolution of such debates throughout the centuries. Moreover, we can begin to tease out the contradictions and conflicts associated with the application of theoretical perspectives to current events, as we work to make theory more nuanced and representative of the data, media, or art analyzed and practiced.

As discussed in this chapter, one register for problematizing "madness" lies in cultural critiques of the psy disciplines, their ideological origins, and their current epistemologies. Another lies in unearthing the political and economic drivers that have led to a lack of material resources and social support among those with psychiatric diagnoses, as well as their disproportionate rates of homelessness and incarceration. That being said, culture is entangled in the material conditions that produce it and both must be examined in relation to each other. Together, scholarship on the sociocultural and material conditions that give rise to current understandings of "madness" ultimately highlights systemic inequalities inherent in global capitalism and the exclusion and oppression of people who are unable to conform to societal expectations for productivity and normality. By unearthing the ideological and material origins of psy dominance as well as mad resistance, mad studies scholars can help us imagine alternative futures to create space for madness and resist dominant knowledge(s).

In light of the complexity, slipperiness, and at times contradictions and conflicts within and around the field, it is important to highlight that mad studies activities are about affinity connections and linkages that embrace, rather than erase, difference. In one of its early vision statements, mutual-aid group The Icarus Project (now known as Fireweed Collective) put it this way:

> Together, we seek new space and freedom for extreme states of consciousness. We support alternatives to the medical model and acknowledge the traumatic legacy of psychiatric abuse. We recognize that we all live in a crazy world, and believe that sensitivities, visions, and inspirations are not necessarily symptoms of illness. Sometimes breakdown can be the entrance to breakthrough. We call for more options in understanding and treating emotional distress, and we advocate for everyone, regardless of income, to have access to these choices. We respect diversity and embrace harm-reduction and self-determination in treatment decisions. Everyone is welcome, whether they support the use of psychiatric drugs or not, and whether they identify with diagnostic categories or not.
>
> (DuBrul, 2014, p. 267)

Similarly, the common ground in mad studies is not sameness or perfect agreement, it is the shared interest in these questions, and it is the shared project of creating a less sanist world that is more accessible, supportive, and resource-rich for narrating and navigating mental difference and mental suffering.

References

Aho, T., Ben-Moshe, L., & Hilton, L. J. (2017). Mad futures: Affect/theory/violence. *American Quarterly*, 69(2), 291–302.

Ben-Moshe, L. (2020). *Decarcerating disability: Deinstitutionalization and prison abolition*. University of Minnesota Press.

Beresford, P. (2019). Including our self in struggle: Challenging the neo-liberal psycho-system's subversion of us, our ideas and action. *Canadian Journal of Disability Studies*, 8(4), 31–59. https://doi.org/10.15353/cjds.v8i4.523

Beresford, P. (2020). 'Mad', Mad studies and advancing inclusive resistance. *Disability & Society*, 35(8), 1337–1342. https://doi.org/10.1080/09687599.2019.1692168

Beresford, P., & Russo, J. (2016). Supporting the sustainability of mad studies and preventing its co-option. *Disability & Society*, 31(2), 270–274. https://doi.org/10.1080/09687599.2016.1145380

Blanchette, S. (2019). A feminist bioethical and mad studies approach to resisting an increase in psychiatric paternalism to competent mental health users/refusers. *Journal of Ethics in Mental Health*, (10), 1–18.

Bouchery, E., Barna, M., Babalola, E., Friend, D., Brown, J. D., Blyeler, C., & Ireys, H.T. (2018). The effectiveness of a peer-staffed crisis respite program as an alternative to hospitalization. *Psychiatric Services*, 69(10), 1069–1074.

Bracken, P. (1995). Beyond liberation: Michel Foucault and the notion of a critical psychiatry. *Philosophy, Psychiatry, & Psychology*, 2(1), 1–13. https://doi.org/10.1353/ppp.0.0113

Braslow, J. T. (2013). The manufacture of recovery. *Annual Review of Clinical Psychology*, 9, 781–809. https://doi.org/10.1146/annurev-clinpsy-050212-185642

Bruce, L. M. (2017). Mad is a place: Or, the slave ship tows the ship of fools. *American Quarterly*, 69, 303–308.

Burstow, B. (2014). The withering away of psychiatry: An attrition model for antipsychiatry. In B. Burstow, B. A. LeFrancois, & S. Diamond (Eds.), *Psychiatry disrupted: Theorizing resistance and crafting the (r)evolution* (pp. 34–51). McGill-Queen's University Press.

Burstow, B. (2015). *Psychiatry and the business of madness: An ethical and epistemological accounting*. Palgrave Macmillan.

Burstow, B. (2019). *The revolt against psychiatry: A counterhegemonic dialogue*. Springer International Publishing.

Castrodale, M. A. (2017). Critical disability studies and mad studies: Enabling new pedagogies in practice. *Canadian Journal for the Study of Adult Education*, 29(1), 49–66.

Clark, N., Walton, P., Drolet, J., Tribute, T., Jules, G., Main, T., & Arnouse, M. (2013). Melq'ilwiye: Coming together: Intersections of identity, culture, and health for urban Aboriginal youth. *The Canadian Journal of Nursing Research / Revue Canadienne de Recherche en Sciences Infirmières*, 45(2), 36–57. https://doi.org/10.1177/084456211304500208

Cohen, B. M. Z. (2016). *Psychiatric hegemony: A Marxist theory of mental illness*. Palgrave Macmillan.

Corstens, D., Longden, E., McCarthy-Jones, S., Waddingham, R., & Thomas, N. (2014). Emerging perspectives from the hearing voices movement: Implications for research and practice. *Schizophrenia Bulletin*, 40(Suppl. 4), S285–S294.

Crossley, N. (2004). Not being mentally ill: Social movement, system survivors, and the oppositional habitus. *Anthropology & Medicine*, 11(2):161–80.

Crossley, N. (2006). *Contesting psychiatry: Social movements in mental health*. Routledge.

Cvetkovich, A. (2003). *An archive of feelings: Trauma, sexuality, and lesbian public cultures*. Duke University Press.

Davar, B. V. (2017). Globalizing psychiatry and the case of "vanishing" alternatives in a neocolonial state. *Disability and the Global South*, 1(2): 266–284.

Davidson, L., & Guy, K. (2012). Peer support among persons with severe mental illnesses: A review of evidence and experience. *World psychiatry*, 11(2), 123–128.

Davoine, F. (2020). Encounters with Sioux medicine men. In M. Brown & R. S. Brown (Eds.), *Emancipatory perspectives on madness: Psychological, social, and spiritual dimensions* (pp. 25–34). Routledge.

De Vos, J. (2013). *Psychologization and the subject of late modernity*. Palgrave Macmillan.

Diamond, S. (2013). What makes us a community? Reflections on building solidarity in anti-sanist praxis. In B. A. LeFrancois, R. Menzies, & G. Reaume (Eds.), *Mad matters: A critical reader in Canadian mad studies* (pp. 64–78). Canadian Scholars Press.

Diamond, S. (2014). Feminist resistance against the medicalization of humanity: Integrating knowledge about psychiatric oppression and marginalized people. In B. Burstow, B. A. LeFrancois, & S. Diamond (Eds.), *Psychiatry disrupted: Theorizing resistance and crafting the (r)evolution* (pp. 194–207). McGill-Queen's University Press.

Donaldson, E. (2018). *Literatures of madness: Disability studies and mental health.* Springer International Publishing.

Douglas, P., Runswick-Cole, K., Ryan, S., & Fogg, P. (2021). Mad mothering. *Journal of Literary & Cultural Disability Studies, 15*(1), 39–57.

DuBrul, S. A. (2014). The Icarus Project: A counter narrative for psychic diversity. *Journal of Medical Humanities, 35*(3), 257–271. https://doi.org/10.1007/s10912-014-9293-5

Eales, L., & Peers, D. (2020). Care haunts, hurts, heals: The promiscuous poetics of queer crip. *Journal of Lesbian Studies.* https://doi.org/10.1080/10894160.2020.1778849

Eromosele, F. (2020). Frantz Fanon in the time of mad studies. *World Futures, 76*(3), 167–187. https://doi.org/10.1080/02604027.2020.1730737

Faulkner, A. (2017). Survivor research and mad studies: The role and value of experiential knowledge in mental health research. *Disability & Society, 32*(4), 500–520. https://doi.org/10.1080/09687599.2017.1302320

Federici, S. (2004). *Caliban and the witch.* Autonomedia.

Fisher, M. (2009). *Capitalist realism: Is there no alternative?* John Hunt Publishing.

Frantzen, M. K. (2019). *Going nowhere, slow: The aesthetics and politics of depression.* John Hunt Publishing.

Friedman, M. (2017). Mad/fat/diary: Exploring contemporary feminist thought through *My mad fat diary. Feminist Media Studies, 17*(6), 1073–1087. https://doi.org/10.1080/14680777.2017.1298145

Gone, J. P. (2010). Psychotherapy and traditional healing for American Indians: Exploring the prospects for therapeutic integration. *The Counseling Psychologist, 38*(2), 166–235. https://doi.org/10.1177/0011000008330831

Gong, N. (2019). Between tolerant containment and concerted constraint: Managing madness for the city and the privileged family. *American Sociological Review, 84*(4), 664–689.

Gorman, R., & LeFrancois, B. A. (2017). Mad studies. In B. Cohen (Ed.), *Routledge international handbook of critical mental health* (pp. 108–114). Routledge.

Grob, G. (1994). *The mad among us: A history of the care of America's mentally ill.* Free Press.

Hacking, I. (1998). *Rewriting the soul: Multiple personality and the sciences of memory.* Princeton University Press.

Hansen, H., Bourgois, P., & Drucker, E. (2014). Pathologizing poverty: New forms of diagnosis, disability, and structural stigma under welfare reform. *Social Science & Medicine (1982), 103,* 76–83. https://doi.org/10.1016/j.socscimed.2013.06.033

Hedva, J. (2016, January 19). Sick woman theory. *Mask Magazine.* Retrieved February 11, 2021, from http://www.maskmagazine.com/not-again/struggle/sick-woman-theory

Herman, E. (1995). *The romance of American psychology: Political culture in the age of experts, 1940–1970.* University of California Press.

Hunter, N. (2018). *Trauma and madness in mental health services*. Palgrave Macmillan.

Jacobson, N., & Curtis, L. (2000). Recovery as policy in mental health services: Strategies emerging from the states. *Psychiatric Rehabilitation Journal, 23*(4), 333–341.

Johnston, M. S. (2019). When madness meets madness: Insider reflections on doing mental health research. *International Journal of Qualitative Methods, 18*, 1–13. https://doi.org/10.1177/1609406919835356

Johnston, M. S., & Steckle, R. (2018). Psychiatric post-anarchism: A new direction for insurrection in the mental health system. *Annual Review of Interdisciplinary Justice Research, 7*, 232–257.

Jones, N., Atterbury, K., Byrne, L., Hansen, M. C., Phalen, P., & Carras, M. C. (2021, March 11). Lived experience, research leadership, and the transformation of mental health services: Building a pipeline. *Psychiatric Services*. https://doi.org/10.1176/appi.ps.202000468

Jones, N., & Kelly, T. (2015). Inconvenient complications: On the heterogeneities of madness and their relationship to disability. In H. Spandler, J. Anderson, & B. Sapey (Eds.), *Madness, distress and the politics of disablement* (pp. 43–56). Bristol Policy Press.

Joseph, A. J. (2015). The necessity of an attention to Eurocentrism and colonial technologies: An addition to critical mental health literature. *Disability & Society, 30*(7), 1021–1041. https://doi.org/10.1080/09687599.2015.1067187

Joseph, A. J. (2019). Constituting lived experience discourses in mental health: The ethics of racialized identification/representation and the erasure of intergenerational colonial violence. *Journal of Ethics in Mental Health, 10*, 1–18.

Kafai, S. (2020). Memory seeking: Mad phenomenology as orientation. *Journal of Critical Phenomenology, 3*(2), 27–29.

Kalathil, J., & Jones, N. (2016). Unsettling disciplines: Madness, identity, research, knowledge. *Philosophy, Psychiatry, & Psychology, 23*(3), 183–188.

Kunzel, R. (2017). Queer history, mad history, and the politics of health. *American Quarterly, 69*(2), 315–319.

Kutchins, H., & Kirk, S. A. (1997). *Making us crazy: DSM: The psychiatric bible and the creation of mental disorders*. The Free Press.

Lasch, C. (1991). *The culture of narcissism: American life in an age of diminishing expectations*. W. W. Norton.

Latin American Network of Psychosocial Diversity. (2018). *Locura Latina: Declaration of Lima*. Rompiendo La Etiqueta. http://www.rompiendolaetiqueta.com/declaration?fbclid=IwAR15vRz_z4sjKaBQc4bxL-rAy4zY8k5UAlUpxSEx2Zw0vdFgFw5kC6iPiu4

Lawlor, C. (2012). *From melancholia to Prozac: A history of depression*. Oxford University Press.

Leblanc, S., & Kinsella, E. (2016). Toward epistemic justice: A critically reflexive examination of "sanism" and implications for knowledge generation. *Studies in Social Justice, 10*(1), 59–78.

LeFrançois, B. A., & Diamond, S. (2014). Queering the sociology of diagnosis: Children and the constituting of "mentally ill" subjects. *Journal of Critical Anti-Oppressive Social Inquiry, 1*(1), 39–61.

Lewis, B. (2006). A mad fight: Psychiatry and disability activism. In L. J. Davis (Ed.), *The disability studies reader* (pp. 3–16). Psychology Press.

Lewis, B. (2011). *Narrative psychiatry: How stories can shape clinical practice.* Johns Hopkins University Press.

Lewis, B. (2021). Planetary health humanities—Responding to COVID times. *Journal of Medical Humanities, 42*(1), 3–16. https://doi.org/10.1007/s10912-020-09670-2

Liebert, R. J. (2018). *Psycurity: Colonialism, paranoia, and the war on imagination.* Taylor & Francis.

Liegghio, M. (2013). A denial of being: Psychiatrization as epistemic violence. In B. A. LeFrancois, R. Menzies, & G. Reaume (Eds.), *Mad matters: A critical reader in Canadian mad studies* (pp. 122–129). Canadian Scholars Press.

Lombardo, P. A. (2008). *Three generations, no imbeciles: Eugenics, the Supreme Court, and Buck v. Bell.* Johns Hopkins University Press.

Luhrmann, T. M., & Marrow, J. (Eds.). (2016). *Our most troubling madness: Case studies in schizophrenia across cultures.* University of California Press.

McWade, B. (2016). Recovery-as-policy as a form of neoliberal state making. *Intersectionalities: A Global Journal Of Social Work Analysis, Research, Polity, And Practice, 5*(3), 62–81. https://journals.library.mun.ca/ojs/index.php/IJ/article/view/1602

Meerai, S., Abdillahi, I., & Poole, J. (2016). An introduction to anti-Black sanism. *Intersectionalities: A Global Journal Of Social Work Analysis, Research, Polity, And Practice, 5*(3), 18–35. https://journals.library.mun.ca/ojs/index.php/IJ/article/view/1682

Metzl, J. M. (2009). *The protest psychosis: How schizophrenia became a Black disease.* Beacon Press.

Miller, G. (2018). Madness decolonized?: Madness as transnational identity in Gail Hornstein's *Agnes's Jacket. Journal of Medical Humanities, 39,* 303–323. https://doi.org/10.1007/s10912-017-9434-8

Million, D. (2013). *Therapeutic nations: Healing in an age of Indigenous human rights.* University of Arizona Press.

Mills, C. (2014). *Decolonizing global mental health: The psychiatrization of the majority world.* Taylor & Francis.

Mills, C. (2015). The psychiatrization of poverty: Rethinking the mental health–poverty nexus. *Social and Personality Psychology Compass, 9,* 213–222. https://doi.org/10.1111/spc3.12168

Morris, C. (1987). *The discovery of the individual, 1050–1200.* University of Toronto Press.

Morrison, L. J. (2005). *Talking back to psychiatry: The psychiatric consumer/survivor/ex-patient movement.* Routledge.

Morrow, M. (2007). Critiquing the "psychiatric paradigm" revisited: Reflections on feminist interventions in mental health. *Resources for Feminist Research / Documentation Sur La Recherche Feministe, 32*(1–2), 69–85.

Morrow, M. (2013). Recovery: Progressive paradigm or neoliberal smokescreen? In B. A. LeFrancois, R. Menzies, & G. Reaume (Eds.), *Mad matters: A critical reader in Canadian mad studies* (pp. 323–333). Canadian Scholars Press.

Morrow, M. (2017). "Women and madness" revisited: The promise of intersectional and mad studies frameworks. In M. Morrow & L. H. Malcoe (Eds.), *Critical inquiries for social justice in mental health* (pp. 33–59). University of Toronto Press.

Myers, N. L. (2015). *Recovery's edge: An ethnography of mental health care and moral agency.* Vanderbilt University Press.

Nakamura, K. (2013). *A disability of the soul: An ethnography of schizophrenia and mental illness in contemporary Japan*. Cornell University Press.

Netchitailova, E. (2019). The mystery of madness through art and mad studies. *Disability & Society, 34*(9–10), 1509–1515. https://doi.org/10.1080/09687599.2019.1619236

Nielsen, K. E. (2012). *A disability history of the United States*. Beacon Press.

Pan African Network of People with Psychosocial Disabilities. (2011). The Cape Town declaration. Reprinted in *Disability and the Global South (2014), 1*(2), 385–386. https://disabilityglobalsouth.files.wordpress.com/2012/06/dgs-01-02-10.pdf?fbclid=IwAR2DuwRBhH8inVbgVfbS0V4A2CQW_wqYpFiOu5dd6jmD6qqi09_Pc2GkrKg

Pick, D. (1993). *Faces of degeneration: A European disorder, C.1848–1918*. Cambridge University Press.

Price, M. (2011). *Mad at school: Rhetorics of mental disability and academic life*. University of Michigan Press.

Proctor, R. E. (1998). *Defining the humanities: How rediscovering a tradition can improve our schools with a curriculum for today's students*. Indiana University Press.

Raju, P., & Penak, N. (2019). Indigenizing the narrative: A conversation on disability assessments. In A. Daley, L. Costa, & P. Beresford (Eds.), *Madness, violence, and power: A critical collection* (pp. 136–149). University of Toronto Press.

Rashed, M. A. (2019). *Madness and the demand for recognitions: A philosophical inquiry into identity and mental health activism*. Oxford University Press.

Redikopp, S. (2021). Out of place, out of mind: Min(d)ing race in mad studies through a metaphor of spatiality. *Canadian Journal of Disability Studies, 10*(3), 96–118. https://doi.org/10.15353/cjds.v10i3.817

Roberts, D. (2011). *Fatal invention: How science, politics, and big business re-create race in the twenty-first century*. New Press.

Rose, D. (2017). Service user/survivor-led research in mental health: Epistemological possibilities. *Disability & Society, 32*(6), 773–789.

Rothman, D. J. (2017). *The discovery of the asylum: Social order and disorder in the new republic*. Taylor & Francis.

Russo, J., & Sweeney, A. (2016). *Searching for a rose garden: Challenging psychiatry, fostering mad studies*. PCCS Books.

Scull, A. (2015). *Madhouses, mad-doctors, and madmen*. University of Pennsylvania Press. https://doi.org/10.9783/9781512806823

Showalter, E. (1985). *The female malady: Women, madness, and English culture, 1830–1980*. Pantheon Books.

Spandler, H. (2017). Mad and queer studies: Shared visions. *Asylum: The Magazine for Democratic Psychiatry, 24*(1), 5–6.

Spandler, H., Anderson, J., & Sapey, B. (2015). *Madness, distress, and the politics of disablement*. Bristol University Press.

Spandler, H., & Poursanidou, D. (2019). Who is included in the mad studies project? *The Journal of Ethics in Mental Health, 10*, 1–20. ISSN 1916-2405.

Sweeney, A. (2016). Why mad studies needs survivor research and survivor research needs mad studies. *Intersectionalities: A Global Journal of Social Work Analysis, Research, Polity, and Practice, 5*(3), 36–61.

Sweeney, A., Beresford, P., Faulkner, A., Nettle, M., & Rose, D. (2009). *This is survivor research*. PCCS Books.

Thorneycroft, R. (2020). Crip theory and mad studies: Intersections and points of departure. *Canadian Journal of Disability Studies, 9*(1), 91–121. https://cjds.uwaterloo.ca/index .php/cjds/article/view/597

Torn, A. (2018). Medieval mysticism to schizoaffective disorder: The repositioning of subjectivity in the discourse of psychiatry. In B. Cohen (Ed.), *Routledge international handbook of critical mental health* (pp. 126–132). Routledge.

Toulmin, S. (1990). *Cosmopolis: The hidden agenda of modernity.* University of Chicago Press.

Transforming Communities for Inclusion—Asia Pacific. (2018). *Bali declaration. TCI Asia.* https://www.tci-asia.org/bali-declaration/

Voronka, J. (2016). The politics of "people with lived experience": Experiential authority and the risks of strategic essentialism. *Philosophy, Psychiatry, & Psychology 23*(3), 189–201. https://doi.org/10.1353/ppp.2016.0017

Voronka, J. (2017). Turning mad knowledge into affective labor: The case of the peer support worker. *American Quarterly, 69*(2), 333–338. https://doi.org/10.1353/aq .2017.0029

Voronka, J. (2019). Slow death through evidence-based research. In A. Daley, L. Costa, & P. Beresford (Eds.), *Madness, violence, and power: A critical collection* (pp. 80–96). University of Toronto Press.

Wang, E. W. (2019). *The collected schizophrenia.* Graywolf Press.

Washington, H. A. (2006). *Medical apartheid: The dark history of medical experimentation on Black Americans from colonial times to the present.* Doubleday.

Woods, A., Jones, N., Bernini, M., Callard, F., Alderson-Day, B., Badcock, J. C., Bell, V., Cook, C. C. H., Csordas, T., Humpston, C., Krueger, J., Laroi, F., McCarty-Jones, S., Moseley, P., Powell, H., Raballo, A., Smailes, D., & Fernyhough, C. (2014). Interdisciplinary approaches to the phenomenology of auditory verbal hallucinations. *Schizophrenia Bulletin, 40*(Suppl. 4), S246–S254. https://doi.org/10.1093/schbul/ sbu003

Chapter 14

Obsession in Our Time

Lennard Davis

Summary

This chapter provides a nimble discussion of the very idea of doing a history of mental "disease." Davis argues against a naive realist perspective which takes the *DSM-III*–style clinical category "obsessive compulsive disorder" (OCD) as the Truth of obsession independent of the cultural, historical, and social context. He highlights that the science of obsession and clinical category making in general necessitates a linguistic practice and that "the language we use to understand madness is … a layered pentimento of concepts and terms that have arisen, been useful, become outmoded, and yet still persists" (p. 24).[1] At the same time, however, and this point is equally important, Davis's discursive approach argues forcefully against an ideological perspective reminiscent of the earlier antipsychiatry genre. "I want to say now very clearly that I am not denying the existence of OCD as a disease … I have no doubt that OCD is real to people suffering from it and real to doctors trying to help those people" (pp. 6–7).

Davis's disability studies background allows him to keep this tension between the real and the constructed without collapsing his argument to one side of the binary or the other. Like disability studies more broadly, he recognizes that the social history of human categories does not contradict the realness of those categories for lived experience and cultural engagement with the material world. What we think of as categories of "mental illness" notoriously defy our attempts to pin them down to a single description or a single causal story. This means, as Davis shows here, that we need to open our study of mental and physical difference to interdisciplinary perspectives beyond biology. One can see, through this perspective, how much synergy there is between disability studies and mad studies.

*

Obsessive Me

When I was around six or seven, I began to have thoughts about death and dying that I couldn't push out of my mind. I realized that I was mortal and would die. I'd lie in bed and panic, sweat, and thrash around wrestling with the inevitability of my

DOI: 10.4324/9781003148456-17

personal demise. To get those thoughts out of my mind, I developed certain rituals. I would try to envision in my mind's eye a black kitten that I had actually earlier brought home and was allowed to keep only until nightfall. That mental image comforted me, as did the vision of a white and cleanly wrapped loaf of Silvercup bread, whose advertising campaign had no doubt made me feel the comfort of food and the safety of home. But mostly, I would lie in bed at night and look out my window at the apartment building next to mine. I decided that I had to count every single window that was illuminated, and once the thought occurred to me, I began to do it compulsively. Since the building was substantial, the count took a fair amount of time. After I had arrived at a total number of illuminated windows, I would begin to doubt whether I had counted correctly. I would then recount. Then it would occur to me that someone might have turned their lights on or off. So another recount was necessary. I did this for hours until I was exhausted.

In the morning my mother worried about the dark circles under my eyes. I assured her everything was fine, since it would be pointless to explain what I had been doing and thinking. On the way to school, I might hit my shoe against a curb by mistake, so of course I had to scuff the other shoe to keep things symmetrical. When I arrived at the traffic light, I had a formula I had to say to myself—"I defy justice. Light change!"—over and over again until the light changed. I also had a compulsion to swallow coins, mostly pennies and dimes, but there were the nickels as well, which I did on a regular basis, with the subsequent visual delight of seeing these gleaming circles emerge from me shiny and cleaned by the acid of my digestive system. When I ate elbow macaroni, I would slide each elbow on the tine of a fork, so that the utensil contained four straightened tubes of pasta, and then I would swallow each one whole. Continuing on the culinary front, I divided my food into absolute and irrevocable sections that must never mix or touch one another. Also, in eating mashed potatoes or any moldable foods, I would create a circle, divide it into four quadrants, eat one quadrant, and then completely remake the food into a slightly smaller circle. And then I would repeat the whole process, as the circle got asymptotically smaller and smaller. In illustrating Zeno's paradox three dimensionally with my food, I was always satisfied, and endlessly caught in my web of complex rituals.

While I was doing that, my father and brother were compulsively washing their hands and surviving through their own developed rituals. Every night my father checked and rechecked the locks on the doors, the faucets, and gas jets while closing and rechecking all the kitchen cabinets, accompanied all the while by repetitive throat clearings and nasal sniffles. My brother lathered himself up so much that he eventually developed a skin rash. My mother was strangely untouched by all these machinations. In the 1950s and in an immigrant, working-class, and under-educated family, we didn't have a name for these kinds of activities. We didn't know we were engaged in obsessional and compulsive activities. We were just doing what came naturally to us in our time and place.

Obsessive You

I am sure as I write these words that countless people all over the country are doing similar things. They are engaged in obsessive-compulsive activities like cleaning and checking, fighting off intrusive thoughts, addictively thinking about sex, food, alcohol, drugs as well as acting on these addictions. People are also working at their jobs addictively and obsessively and then playing hard in an extension of their workday. Many folks are addicted to their nightly television shows, to collecting things, or to obsessing about that someone who is unattainable or lost forever. And not only people, but also our pets are engaged in such activities, as a recent issue of *Cat Fancy* magazine suggests in its cover story "Is This Normal? Recognize Your Cat's Obsessive Behavior."

Indeed, we live in an age of obsession; or more to the point, an age that is obsessed with obsession. No hot romance movie is complete without the idea that the lovers are obsessed. No scientist or musician's reputation is safe without the word "obsessed" tacked to his or her occupation. A perfume seductively carries the name. Talk-show listeners describe themselves as addicted to twenty-four-hour news and discussion. A *New York Times Magazine* special supplement on people obsessed with home design began with a surprising confession from the editor—"You're probably not going to believe this, but I don't have an obsession I may not be obsessed, but I'm grateful for those who are."[2] As the editor pointed out, "Obsession is a commitment; you have to believe in it, because it soon takes you over." To be without an obsession is, according to this view, something extraordinary. The article focuses on "three of the obsessives who are featured in this issue. If the others are working on a smaller scale, no matter. Their passions are just as grand, and their stories just as compelling."

At the beginning of the twenty-first century, obsession is seen both as a dreaded disease and as a noble and necessary endeavor. And that is the point of this book [chapter]. How can a disease also be, when you use a different lens, a cultural goal? Another way of asking this question is, can a disease have a biography? Can there be a genealogy of collective and personal behaviors? How did we get to the point where our diseases are our obsessions and our obsessions are our diseases?

The Dark Side

Obsession can be a cultural trait devoutly to be wished, but it also has a darker side. When I mention obsession to most people, I get a nudge and a wink. They assume that I am really talking about the kinky world of the erotic. Indeed, obsession has a kind of poetic darkness written into its phonemes, and a quick tour of the library catalog will produce a welter of fiction with suggestive titles like *Dark Obsession, Murder and Obsession, Deadly Obsession, A Haunting Obsession, Secret Obsession, Passionate Obsession, Intimate Obsession,* and so on. In the world of the erotic, obsessions have their special place. Some might claim that love isn't love unless it is obsessive. One author of a book on the subject writes.

I should make it clear that I am talking about one particular kind of love: romantic, obsessive love, the hot thing we fall into, the love we're all expected to experience and that we call true love. Think of novels like *Wuthering Heights* and *Dr. Zhivago,* or films like *Casablanca* and *The English Patient.* ... What they have in common is this: two people obsessed with each other while all the ordinariness of life, its consolations and diversions, vanishes.[3]

An entire range of literature and film is devoted to the proposition that in the world of relationships no obsession should go untried. With hand-cuffs, leather, whips, hot wax, toys, oils, latex and leather jumpsuits, nudity, and blindfolds, sex—anal, oral, acrobatic, submerged, drugged, drunk, gay, multipartnered, dangerous, anonymous—seems to need obsessions. This true, hot love is contrasted with the domestic mundane love of ordinary people—sexual convolutions versus Mom and Pop missionary alignments. In order to have a Heathcliff and Cathy or a Humbert and Lolita, you need to have an Ozzie and Harriet or the Waltons providing a baseline of nonobsessive, companionate couplehood. And mere affection pales by comparison with stalking-induced rapture.

Obsessive love is dangerous, and in fiction often leads to murder and mayhem. Yet it provides a kind of fantasy standard that advertising and commercial interests need to promote. The idea behind the product so advertised is that it will provoke in others an obsessive desire for one's own too well known and unexceptional body. The aura of the obsessive hovers over one's ordinary flesh like a mirage of desire over a parched desert. A Gallup Poll analysis of the ad campaign for Calvin Klein's perfume Obsession turned up the reaction of one consumer who said, "Use Obsession for a great sex life? I used it and nothing happened. I'm not having a great sex life."[4] This reader needed obsession either in herself or those within sniffing distance of her. Products like these ask us whether we can bear to live lives of quiet respiration devoid of infatuated chaleur.

We live in a culture that wants its love affairs obsessive, its artists obsessed, its genius fixated, its music driven, its athletes devoted. We're told that without the intensity provided by an obsession things are only done by halves. Our standards need to be extreme, our outcomes intense. Winners never quit and quitters never win. Emily Martin has recently shown how even corporations are trying to exploit the energy and focus of aberrant mental states, like obsession, for their own purposes.[5] Obsessives play obsessively on the streets, in the bars, and in the clubs, stay late in the offices, crank out the articles, novels, books, music, and films of our driven culture. To be obsessive is to be American, to be modern.

Thinking Obsession Through

It is then perhaps coincident that obsessive-compulsive disorder rose to greater public attention in the 1990s, becoming one of the dominant forms of mental distress. A cavalcade of books on OCD have appeared in the past ten years, along with more books on antidepressants like Prozac and their use with OCD. More and more characters in television shows and film are people with OCD. In addition, anorexia, bulimia, and other obsessive and compulsive behaviors, like addiction, stalking, compulsive shopping, compulsive eating (or noneating) are plaguing and at the same time defining us. These are the other darker sides of obsession—the rooted-in-the-blood, bone, and mind forms of the fascination our culture has for the obsessive.

But was it always this way? The aim of this book [chapter] is to show us how we got to this state of affairs—how it is that obsession now defines our culture. It is easy to say that people have always been obsessed or that the desire to find something and focus on it is a universal feature of human life. You couldn't build the pyramids or come up with *The Iliad* unless someone were obsessed enough to do so. True enough, but there is a moment in the Western world when obsession becomes itself something so problematic that people begin to write about it, study it, turn it into a medical problem, and then try to cure it. That defining moment, beginning in the middle of the eighteenth century in England and France, is worth looking at. Before that divide, some people were seen either as eccentrics, or in a more religious mode as "possessed." After that time, the age of obsession begins as a secular, medical phenomenon.

It may be objected that what I've just highlighted isn't obsession in a psychiatric sense, but more properly concerns an interest, a preoccupation, a fixation, or perhaps just a hobby. Indeed, in recent lectures I have given to psychotherapists, psychiatrists, and psychoanalysts, several objected that I was using the term "obsession" in a rather loose way. One insisted that the notion of an obsession, from a psychoanalytic perspective, was specifically about a recurring thought whose content had become disconnected from its original significance while the repetitive, recurring mental intrusion had come to predominate. Another found himself very irritated with me, saying that I was confusing a cultural activity with a brain-induced, life- and- death issue, and that he himself had a patient with OCD who might die within a few weeks. How could I equate a perfume with this kind of real suffering?

So I want to say now very clearly that I am not denying the existence of OCD as a disease. I follow the lead of the discussions of whether a disease is "real" or not from the work of Ian Hacking and Charles E. Rosenberg, among others.[6] Hacking recounts the many psychiatric disorders that come and go over time, and he says that the question of whether an illness is actually real doesn't fully do justice to the complexity of the situation. The assumption of the realness of a disease is taken out of any worldly or societal context. The assumption is that if a doctor and a patient elaborate a disease entity, then it isn't real. But scholars like Rosenberg emphasize that "a time- and place-specific repertoire of such agreed-upon disease categories has, in fact, always linked laypersons and medical practitioners and thus has served to legitimate and explain the physician's status and healing practice."[7] I have no doubt that OCD is real to people suffering from it and real to doctors trying to help those people. I also have no doubt that the search for a biological basis for OCD is a real search that aims to find specific brain functions, chemical interactions, and genetic locations that can help us understand how OCD manifests itself. But none of that prevents us from asking how certain behaviors came to be linked to a disease, how a society at large can influence which behaviors are seen as symptoms, and how researchers arrived at their own ways of organizing knowledge and developing protocols. Our problem comes when we try to deny that diagnosis is a complex process that aims to freeze in a moment the moving target of individual bodies and their processes interacting with psyches, environments, and social, institutional, and cultural milieus. In other words, OCD is real, and so are the circumstances that surround it and bring it into our clinical and social focus.

To make this point a little clearer, let's think about money. Money isn't a naturally occurring thing. It is a totally human-made invention, and yet it is real. Its rules are socially constructed, and its effects can be radical. People without money suffer in a real way. Economists can study how money circulates and gains or loses value. It is a genuine object of study, but it is completely socially constructed. It exists physically in the world, but it also has a symbolic existence. If you hold expired currency, it is still real, but it has lost its value by an abstract process. In asking whether money is real or not, we miss the point. Likewise disease. Disease exists to the extent that humans identify it and learn how it works. That learning can be of a medical kind, and that learning can extend to many other areas, from theoretical to common sense. I will talk more about how we come to know a disease, particularly a psychiatric disease, but I want to make clear at this point that the old saws of "nature or nurture" and "real or constructed" are not the ones I want to be hewing with right now.

Categorizing Obsession

Psychiatrists take their definition of obsession from the *DSM-IV TR,* the diagnostic manual used by practitioners to define and categorize affective and cognitive conditions. Obsessive-compulsive disorder is listed as one of several anxiety disorders. Its diagnostic number is 300.3, and it is described in this way:

> OCD is characterized by uncontrollable intrusive thoughts and action that can only be alleviated by patterns of rigid and ceremonial behavior. Symptoms frequently cause considerable distress and interference with daily social or work activities. There may be a major preoccupation with the smallest of details in daily life. Obsessive ideas frequently involve contamination, dirt, diseases, germs, real/imagined trauma, or some type of frightening/unpleasant theme. People recognize their obsessive ideas do not make sense but are unable to stop them. These obsessive thoughts frequently lead to compulsive behaviors as the person tries to prevent or change some dreaded event. They frequently repeat activities over and over again. (E.g., washing hands, cleaning things up, checking locks.)[8]

In making this type of definition, the common practice is to separate obsessions (thoughts) from compulsions (actions). To complicate the definition a bit further, there is also something called "obsessive-compulsive personality disorder," which is distinguished from the anxiety disorders. Its diagnostic number is 301.4, and it is described this way:

> Obsessive-Compulsive Personality Disorder is characterized by perfectionism and inflexibility. A person with an Obsessive-Compulsive Personality becomes preoccupied with uncontrollable patterns of thought and action. Symptoms may cause extreme distress and interfere with a person's occupational and social functioning.[9]

The former (OCD) is characterized by anxiety, while the latter is not a disorder but a personality type who may function quite well without anxiety or distress. If you have OCD, you do or think things you don't like doing, which makes you unhappy or distressed. If you have an obsessive-compulsive personality disorder, you may do the same things, but you may not mind. In fact, you may like doing or thinking such things.[10]

These are the types of categories concerning obsession that clinicians and practitioners use. Their definitions are useful to them as people whose job it is to diagnose and help cure people who present themselves as suffering from the obsessions and compulsions that are now called OCD. Indeed, one of the stated purposes of the *DSM* is to foster agreement among practitioners by providing common diagnostic categories. I don't wish to deny the utility of such descriptions or the benefits of the cures that have been developed. But I do wish to challenge what we might call the professional jurisdiction over the term "obsession." In some sense, the function of this book [chapter] is to provide the broadest historical and cultural account of obsession to help explain how clinicians got to their profession-specific definition—how the split arose between the undesirable disease and the desirable cultural goal, between the formation of a pathological entity and the coming to be of a desired and necessary trait.

One could say more about obsessions as they are described clinically. There are obsessional thoughts, impulses, and images. Examples of obsessional thoughts are "Did I kill the old lady?" "Christ was a bastard." "Do I have cancer?" Obsessional impulses include: "I might expose my genitals in public." "I am about to shout obscenities in public." "I feel I might strangle a child." Unwanted obsessive images could include mutilated corpses, decomposing fetuses, a family member involved in a serious accident, unconventional sex with an unlikely person. One study ranked the content of obsessional material into five broad categories in order of frequency: dirt and contamination, aggression, orderliness of inanimate objects, sex, and religion.[11] Obsessive thoughts, according to one expert, fall into three main themes—aggressive, sexual, and blasphemous.[12] Another analysis lists "contamination, pathologic doubt, aggressive and sexual thoughts, somatic concerns, and the need for symmetry and precision."[13] Compulsions fall into three major categories—cleaning, checking, and counting.

Obsession as Culture?

What I have just presented is the clinical definition of obsession, but it hardly accounts for what I hope to show is a continuing and serious cultural, historical, and social continuum. That is not to say that the clinical definition is not of interest to us all and does not provide us with a somewhat clear set of guidelines for choosing a particular kind of diagnosis and treatment. Indeed, some practitioners are willing to see connections between the clinical and the popular, as do Stanley Rachman and Ray Hodgson, who write that the popular usage of obsession "retains its utility."[14] What interests me in this project, therefore, moves beyond the desire to diagnose a patient and develop a set of treatments for that patient, which are necessary and valuable activities. Rather, I am more interested in how it came to be that someone on one side of the desk gets to perform a series of judgments and activities and the person on the other side of the desk gets to accede to those judgments and activities when both can be said to be obsessive. Or rather, how does the collaboration go on between the self-reporting patient and the category-giving doctor? In this particular case, one could argue that the physician who uses the *DSM-IV TR* is himself or herself using an obsessive text (obsessive in the sense of taxonomic and categorical—but more on that later)[15] to study with a single-minded fixation the patient who displays obsessive behavior.

As to the objection from clinicians that what I am talking about is not really OCD but more in the line of what one might call a focused activity, an idée fixe or simply a preoccupation, let me agree in the largest sense. But that distinction is also what I want to consider. I am interested in what makes a particular human activity worthy of study by other humans. I will argue, later in the work, that the kind of behavior that the eighteenth century regarded as eccentricity, curiosity, or fascination became, in a rather short period, something that split off into two parallel activities. One was the behavior, and the other was the study of the behavior. In other words, obsession became an illness, and the obsessive study of obsession became a profession. As this split happened, medicine—notably psychiatry and neurology—came into its own, and part of its professional agenda was the establishment of taxonomies and categories whose effect it was to separate out varieties of behavior into a signifying group of the pathological on the one hand and the heuristic on the other.

Fine Distinctions

It will be reasonable, at this point, to object to several things. Am I really saying that there is no difference between a man who cannot stop thinking about sheep and a man who intently studies the physiology of sheep? Is the man who must touch every lamppost really the same as the worker in an automobile assembly line who must paint every door that goes by him? Is a mother who worries obsessively about the safety of her child the same as a mother who just worries about her child? Surely there is a matter of degree, and in the case of the pathological, also a matter of logic. It makes sense to worry about your child, but it doesn't make sense to worry all the time about your child, especially when the child is asleep in the next room.

Of course it is foolish to think that all of these kinds of activities and thought patterns are the same. One wants to make distinctions, to separate the pathological from the normal. But if we simply accede to the reasonableness of the previous sentence, are we unthinkingly signing on to a kind of *doxa*? In my earlier book on the development of the concept of normality I raised questions about the obviousness of the normal.[16] Here, too, I want us to think about the way that human life gets sorted out into categories. Take, for example, the previously stated commonplace distinction between compulsions and obsessions. The *DSM-IV TR* makes a clear distinction. Obsessions are defined as "thoughts or impulses that are distressful, persistent and recurrent. These thoughts or impulses must not just be worries of real-life problems. The person must be aware that these thoughts or impulses are only a product of his/her own mind and they must be actively trying to suppress, ignore, or neutralize them with other actions." Compulsions "must show repetitive behavior, physical or mental, that cannot be controlled. (E.g., washing hands, checking locks, praying over and over again, counting or saying words repeatedly.) These actions must be aimed at trying to prevent or reduce some distressful situation."

The neat distinction between actions and thoughts are [sic] of course not as neat as they seem. Even the definition of compulsions includes the notion of "repetitive behavior, physical or mental." Mental behavior, in this case, includes praying, counting, or saying words mentally, that is, a kind of action within consciousness. But then, is thinking a nonmental activity? Is thinking a kind of mental doing? The fact that very few people have compulsions (only 9 percent in one study of obsessives) indicates that the neat line between obsession and compulsion has more to do with diagnostic categories than it might seem.[17] And obsessions can loop back into compulsions and vice versa, notably, for example, the obsession of doubting following the compulsive act of checking. I make this quibble because I want to highlight the fixation or infatuation behind the seemingly clear and neutral diagnostic criteria. But further, the demarcation between normal behavior and clinical categories is sometimes hard to determine. As Rachman and Hodgson note, "no one has offered a systematic statement of the necessary and sufficient conditions for deciding when and whether a reported experience is an obsession and when and whether a behavioral pattern should be described as compulsive."[18]

The Problem of Obsession

This work has a complex and difficult set of aims. On a simple level, it is an attempt to describe the history of a disorder that was often considered a disease. But I think it is important to understand that no disease exists outside its cultural context. Even cholera, the gold standard for a "real" disease, means one thing in one culture and another in a different culture. Susan Sontag has shown us that disease is about metaphors.[19] So thinking of obsession as simply a disease is a mistake. Obsession is something that becomes a problem for Western culture at a certain moment in history—a problem because it is both the object of study and the way that we study that object. As with the problem of the mind—you can't study the mind with the mind—obsessive investigation of obsessive activity is bound to run into a problem. Our dilemma with obsession—our need for it and our fear of it—is a result of a series of unresolved issues that has haunted our culture since the middle of the eighteenth century.

The simple point of this work is that our obsession with obsession didn't just appear during our own time. This is a fascination and/or a disease that has a history. So this work fits into the larger project of the social history of medicine. But obsession isn't simply a medical category; it is a category of existence. There are obsessives, and there is obsession. Obsessives, if their obsessions are too obsessive, will be treated by medical doctors, particularly if they happen to be born after 1850; if not too obsessive, they will be humored or even admired. In saying that the problem isn't solely medical, I am saying that it is *biocultural*. That term, coined by David Morris, and expanded upon by others, including myself, is used to call into question the range of occurrences, experiments, statements, and discourses that have worked in the past by bracketing science on the one side and the humanities on the other. The goal of a biocultural project is to redeploy culture into the sciences and medicine so that a new synergy and wholeness can illuminate these complex projects.[20]

Biocultural View of Obsession

One must not take a phenomenon like OCD in isolation. The danger of a clinical perspective is that it tends to define the disease entity in universal terms, such that a patient with a particular disease will have these particular symptoms and outcomes in all situations at all times. But in the case of obsessive activity, one wants to begin to see how the activity fits into cultural paradigms and even into the same paradigms that the practitioner uses for observation, diagnosis, and treatment. To construct an artificial discontinuity between practitioner and patient is to fall into a kind of fallacy generated by the observational mechanism itself. Take for example the characteristics of a compulsive activity as described by Rachman and Hodgson: "precise … repetitive, unchanging, mechanical behavior."[21] The first question one might want to pose is, how much of such behavior is a result of a transformed culture?

One begins to see obsessional behavior as a cultural problematic that starts with modernity. This isn't to say that such behavior did not exist before, but it was not seen as problematic before except in the major area of religion. Religious scrupulosity and obsessive thoughts were more clearly problems for earlier times, although the medicalization of scrupulosity is of very recent occurrence.[22] Obsessive thoughts were more clearly tied to possession by the devil until the end of the seventeenth century when, at least in England, demonic possession was legally banned, since it was seen as tied up with Catholicism and popery. So, by the time the eighteenth-century man of letters Samuel Johnson walked down the street touching every light post, his peers noted the behavior and thought it was eccentric but without further consequence. No one called an exorcist. Yet almost a hundred years later when Macaulay noted Johnson's behavior, he saw it as part of a pattern of insanity. And now in the twenty-first century, when clinicians talk about Dr. Johnson, they retrospectively diagnose him as having Tourette syndrome. Each of these eras, including our own, felt they had the explanation down pat.

When an industrial culture evolves to emphasize and rely on a greater sense of precision, repetition, standardization, and mechanization, that same culture will perhaps regard those attributes differently, and members of that society will mime, imitate, embody, internalize, and exaggerate those qualities. Likewise, those members who called themselves scientists might well engage in those behaviors and focus their gaze on what they perceive as aberrations of such behavior. Take for example the following description of attempts to classify obsessional behavior:

> Kringlen … reported that over 50 per cent of the 91 obsessional patients included in his series complained of phobic symptoms. Kringlen subdivided the obsessional patients into four categories and concluded that one-third of the group had a mixture of obsessional thoughts, acts, and phobias while 19 per cent had "predominantly or solely phobias." The stability of the phobic symptoms is attested to by the fact that when

the follow-up investigation was carried out, an average of 16 years after admission to the hospital, no less than 69 per cent of the remaining 84 patients complained of phobic symptoms.[23]

Of course this is the quantified language of science and research, but one notes what we might call the obsessive use of numbers in repetition, which provide a patina of incontrovertibility and learning to a discourse that is characterized by its single-minded focus on a specific group of people—obsessives.[24]

Obsession as Modern Consciousness

Rachman and Hodgson note that the criteria for thinking of behavior as compulsive is "an experienced sense of pressure" and an accompanying sense of "unwillingness to comply," since without the latter, the person would not have a sense that he or she indeed had a problem. For an idea, impulse, or image there is needed intrusiveness, internal attribution, unwantedness, and difficulty of control.[25] This would mean that the person could not keep the idea out of his or her consciousness, realized that the idea was coming from his or her own mind, didn't want the idea to keep arising, yet could not control the idea.

One thing that is striking about this set of conditions is how closely it compares with Michel Foucault's notion of societal control of individuals. Foucault elaborates on a transition in the eighteenth century from a society that controls externally through the use of direct force to one that controls by internalized self-regulation. Could we perhaps see obsession as the visible end of a regulatory mechanism gone wrong? Indeed, the internalization of societal rules, especially when it had been accompanied by the decline of a religious structure that might include mechanisms, like confession or expiation, could indeed cause a kind of massive, cultural building up of a collective superego, as it were. Rachman notes that what makes thoughts, often occurring to most people, obsessive comes with the labeling of those thoughts as repugnant and unacceptable:

> Patients afflicted by recurrent obsessions commonly attach exaggerated significance to these thoughts and regard them as horrific, repugnant, threatening, dangerous. ... Various patients have described their obsessional thoughts, impulses, or images as: immoral, sinful disgusting, revealing, dangerous, threatening, alarming, predictive, insane, bewildering, and criminal. At a higher level, they interpreted these thoughts, impulses, or images as revealing important but usually hidden elements in their character, such as: these obsessions mean that deep down I am an evil person; I am dangerous; I am unreliable; I may become totally uncontrollable ...; I am weird, I am going insane (and will lose control?); I am a sinful person; I am fundamentally immoral.[26]

While it is possible to describe this list in various ways, it is perhaps tempting to think of it as a taxonomy of modern consciousness. People in the past may well have had these feelings and sensations, but there does seem to be something uniquely contemporary about the litany of self-accusations. Although Foucault never discussed the internal psychological mechanism by which the process of self-regulation occurred, it is possible for us to raise the point that the mechanism might look a lot like the obsessive-compulsive motor we have been describing. We might think of the nineteenth century in Europe as rapidly reformulating its rules for behavior and thought. Science and medicine provided a venue for this reformulation, and theories of eugenics, degeneration, evolution, and so on created new and hierarchical categories of the human based on biometrics and psychometrics. Racialized, nationalized, eugenicized, and gendered theories singled out the "good" and the "bad" in human behavior and mentality. As the bar was raised on what the self was and how it should behave, as the scientific gaze framed and measured the desired norms, deviation, whether physical or mental, took on the guilty pallor of transgression. Given this raising of the bar, we can speculate that a culture of obsession began to develop, perhaps as a secular concept of "unwanted" or "repugnant" thoughts and feelings were inscribed into the societal narrative. Nineteenth-century literature, art, and culture were filled with accounts of obsessive behavior—seen as both unacceptable and yet typical of the human condition. Raskolnikov, Bartleby, Kurtz, Dupin, Sherlock Holmes, and Ahab, to name only a few, became cultural icons of the dangers and attractions of obsessive acts and ways of being. Freud, then, could be seen as simply someone who laid bare the problem that was more or less obvious to everyone—the reality that obsessive behavior was the underlying substrate of neurosis. Freud simply obsessed about obsessives, as we will later see.

Dirt, Sex, Blasphemy, Violence

When we consider the content of obsessions and compulsive activities we have some more clues to the societal element in the constellation.[27] Obsessional thoughts are, according to one study, primarily focused on dirt and contamination (59 percent of cases in one study), followed by aggressive thoughts around homicide or suicide (25 percent), impersonal/ orderliness (23 percent), religion (9 percent). Sexuality, which one would assume was a big issue for obsessive activity, was rated as uncommon in one study and at 9 percent in another.[28] A more recent study indicates that one fourth of people with OCD had sexual obsessions within their lifetime, but in any current moment 13.3 percent had such obsessions.[29] Another study sees contamination in the obsessions of 45 percent of patients, repetitive doubts in 42 percent, somatic obsessions in 36 percent, need for symmetry in 31 percent, aggressive impulses in 28 percent, and repeated sexual imagery in 26 percent.[30] For compulsive activities, the most common are activities related to cleaning and checking. Contrary to the psychoanalytic perspective, which sees the particular obsession as a distraction from the central psychodynamic conflict, we might hope to glean some reasons why these particular activities are so common. Is there a reason why cleaning is the most frequent activity?

Cleaning is very often related to fears of contamination—whether through spreading germs or making contact with chemicals. Checking is by and large an act of securing oneself or family members against some danger. Cleanliness and security then are the aims of the majority of compulsive activities. One could argue that it is only with the development of the germ theory and an awareness of toxic chemicals in the environment that one could have developed the kind of contagious fear that motivates a compulsive cleaner. Likewise, only with some idea of domestic security, the creation of a special firewall between inside and outside, and with the advent of modern conveniences and dangers (like gas, electricity, pollutants, chemicals, computers, identity theft, and so on) could checking become a useful and then irrational activity. In other words, a certain set of societal and cultural preconditions are necessary, and an accompanying sense of protecting oneself or family, in order for those activities to be highlighted and themselves worried about. In fact, as I will mention later, worrying itself, as indicated by the use of the word "worry" in the modern sense, came into the English language during the nineteenth century.

Another area of note in obsessive behavior is what is called "primary slowness." This type of behavior is one in which a person will take an enormously long time to perform an activity like dressing, performing a household chore, or getting ready to go out. Of course, such slowness must be placed in comparison with other kinds of cultural activities. In a culture defined by speed, efficiency, and multitasking, primary slowness is in fact contrary to the very pulse and tone of modernity. When George Beard invented the concept of neurasthenia in the nineteenth century, he saw it as a disease in which weakness and enervation resulted from the fast-paced existence of modern life—the new sense of speed created by the railway, the telegraph, industrialization, and urban life. The aim of people like Frederick Taylor, who applied time and motion studies to the factory floor, was to speed up the lapidary and casual slowness of traditional workers, bringing them up to the rapid pace of the machine age. Primary slowness incorporates an awareness of this uptick in pacing, acting as a shocking counterpoint to the speed of modern life. However, in its deliberateness and aim at perfection, an aim also incorporated into the compulsive activity of cleaning and checking which seeks to eliminate any doubt or anomaly in the environment, primary slowness also serves the notion of perfectibility in modernity. If you get it slowed down enough, you can finally get it right. Indeed, nineteenth-century ideas of progress, eugenics, and civilization are unimaginable without an ethos of perfectibility.

Normality and Obsession

The line between normality and obsession is one of the most interesting aspects of this study. In a way, the diagnostician must create a firewall between normality and pathology in order to develop a set of tools and treatments. Where this firewall shows up is in the *DSM-IV TR* distinction between OCD and obsessive personality disorder. In the former, a set of behaviors interferes with the quality of a life. In the latter, people have an obsessive personality with rigid components, but they are generally happy with themselves and their lives. The difference between these two diagnoses disappears in the area of insight and compliance. The rigid personality is not necessarily aware of any problem, and does not mind complying with compulsions and thoughts. While some make this distinction for diagnostic purposes, what interests me is the continuity.[31] The pathological form of obsession is

OCD, particularly when it dominates the life of the person involved. But that same domination, when it is used to constructive ends, can be the root and bole of genius and creativity. As Rachman notes, "when people with creative energy succeed in putting their obsessional personality traits to constructive use, everyone benefits."[32]

In the requirement that the behaviors produce "marked distress" in the person, how one arrives at distress is crucial. The same behaviors in different cultures might produce different results. In other words, it takes a community, a culture, a family to make an obsessive. If your behavior, say the meticulous lining up of objects, is seen as an oddity, you will be distressed that you do it. If it is seen as the useful quality of a master bricklayer then you will not be distressed. In other words, "marked distress" is not a quality itself but rather a socially defined reaction. The other problem is that the neat distinction between the personality disorder (the person doesn't mind being obsessive) and the disorder (the person minds) is, even in the *DSM-IV* definition, confused by an acknowledgment that in some cases people "with OCD" won't be distressed by what they are doing or may even think that what they are doing is actually helpful or valuable. But in that case, they may be seen as having "poor insight."[33] Poor insight itself is a very socially dependent notion—if you agree you have the disorder, you have good insight; if you dispute this point or don't recognize yourself as having the disorder, then you might have poor insight.

One of the areas of concern to clinicians is that the cure rate for people with obsessive-compulsive disorders is not particularly good. In fact, one study notes that the group that fares the best is the one that is untreated, and generally outcome is unrelated to treatment.[34] More optimistic accounts, including ones with behavioral-cognitive therapy, can be found in the literature, but often they are based on assessments by the practitioner, which will always be more positive than a double-blind survey, which is largely impossible with this type of illness. With the advent of the use of drugs that affect serotonin levels in the brain like Prozac or Paxil, treatment outcomes have improved, although it is hard to say if this is really the case or just the result of the general optimism after the initial use of these drugs along with modified notions of cure and improvement. We will have to recall that drug choices in various epochs are tied to the viewpoints of those times. The widespread use of antianxiety drugs in the sixties proved useful to people with OCD, at least for a while, as did the use of antidepressants in the subsequent years. Psychosurgery, including lobotomy, was advocated for people with severe obsessional disorders, and that advice was discounted when psychosurgery went into decline as psychopharmacology picked up. Now that serotonin-increasing drugs, referred to as SSRIs (selective serotonin re-uptake inhibitors) have taken over the role of regnant chemical for affective disorders, we need to be aware of the epochal nature of such interventions. Also, new research using functional MRIs (fMRIs) and PET scans has produced data that may lead to new kinds of treatment.

The general point is that obsessive disorders are in some sense endemic, part of what it means to be human in the modern world. In Rachman and Hodgson's view, "Overall, it would appear that the outlook for obsessional patients is slightly worse than that for people suffering from other types of neurotic disorder."[35] Perhaps the attempt to cure OCD will be regarded by our successors as the equivalent to treating homosexuality or masturbation in the past—those pandemic diseases that proved so intractable to cure. Perhaps the current explanations—that the illness is dissociated from its times and that its victim is the object of a capricious set of brain activities or crossed wires or neurotransmitter imbalances—are not right.

Method for Madness

The methodological problem in this book [chapter] is a considerable one. A researcher approaching the history of mental disorders, particularly those in the eighteenth and nineteenth centuries, is faced with a bewildering collection of pamphlets and books by a variety of practitioners. Unlike the study of literature, in which one author is very likely to have read the preceding body of novels or poems, and genuine tradition can be counted upon, in medicine, strangely enough, the approach is far less systematic. While certain doctors' works have great currency, say the work of Pinel, Charcot, or Freud, the majority of practitioners, even if they publish, are essentially unknown to each other. Only with the growth and development of professional medical organizations and their resulting journals and congresses do we begin to see the attempt of the medical profession to create and normalize diagnoses and treatments. Those organizations provide kinds of linearity, although such organizations also tend to reflect the whims, fancies, trends, and, yes, obsessions of their own times. Further, since the causes of and cures for mental illness are extremely uncertain and obscure, even in our own time, it is very difficult for any single practitioner to prove his or her approach correct. The history of the treatment of mental illnesses is a veritable sideshow, mountebank performance, and medicine show in which a raft of treatments floats through a sea of mental illnesses. The most respected practitioners have relied on and used the most astounding set of treatments imaginable from (literally) bromides of doubtful to pernicious value, from the use of hot or cold water baths, the use of restraints, electricity, heavy metals, hypnosis, purges, pain, poultices, bloodletting, irritants, fresh air, and on and on. Even with the current use of SSRIs, we have no assurance that the treatment is working, will continue to work, and is the final way of dealing with a condition. So there is no true unanimity, no solid ground, for a social and cultural research methodology into an area like obsession.

Then there is the problem of reliability and accuracy of sources. As with any history, the documents one deals with are themselves biased and of their time. Is there, then, a solid footing on which the medical historian can stand concerning a mental state and a set of diagnostic conditions? Is there a location of sanity and objectivity from whose heights one can survey the mad terrain? The answer is, not very likely. In addition, different camps will take differing positions on the nature of obsession, its definition, and the way in which the term can be applied. Psychologists will see the term one way, psychoanalysts another, cultural historians a different way. My hope is that this work will open a discussion about something that is all around us and for that reason appears somewhat mysterious, somewhat obvious, and completely blurred by its very proximity. As Marshall McLuhan once famously noted, "Whoever discovered water, it wasn't the fish." And so in this rediscovery of the obsession that is all around us, may we hope that we aren't exclusively of the finny breed.

I am well aware of the pitfalls of the genre of study I am about to engage in—the historical and cultural study of what is seen as a "new" phenomenon. Such a study has familiar contours. First is the model that relies on a strong sense of then and now—showing how things were different in the past and how by a certain date a new mode of thinking, acting, feeling, or doing had arisen. Second, in this genre the author argues for the invention of something new in culture and society and then goes on to show how that new thing then proliferated in the Western (or whatever) world. Finally, the author shows how important and all encompassing this phenomenon is and has been.

The pitfalls of this approach are obvious. Can one say that heterosexuality or sexuality or masturbation or fatigue or attention or scientific management of labor began on a particular date? To do so, one has to ignore to some extent or explain previous instantiations of what seem like sexuality or masturbation or whatever. Then one has to scour the literature for all occurrences of the new phenomenon. That task alone is herculean and necessarily arbitrary. How do we know that we have all the texts? Can one additional text change everything that one has assumed before? One has to make all kinds of categorical claims and disregard the sneaking evidence that might confound one's large claim. In writing my own history of obsession, I will of course enter into this genre, engage in some of these tactics, but I hope that by being aware of its pitfalls and limitations, I may be able to avoid the most egregious hazards of this kind of endeavor.

Nevertheless, the reader will be asked tentatively to go along with a set of assumptions that I have made. First and foremost is to accept the idea that while I am using the term "obsession" I could as easily have used "hysteria," "mania," "neurosis," or any of the other large categories of mental distress that have had various heydays in psychiatric discourse. I am drawn to the idea of obsession because it seems to characterize best the complexity of any medicalized way of thinking about the mind-body connection and a set of rules or norms supposed to apply to the way that the affects, thoughts, sentiments, and judgments are said to be interconnected. As I hope to show, the term "obsession" was applied to a loose set of behaviors that had been called various things at various times. The continuing interest, however, in obsessive behaviors has a complex set of instantiations and rebirths through the period from the eighteenth century to the present moment.

Disease Entities

Therefore, a logical second assumption that I will ask readers to adopt is that both disease entities and treatments are very much products of the explanatory systems used and the times in which they arise. It might be controversial to assume that there aren't diseases as such but, rather, there are instead what have been called "disease entities." "Disease entities" might be the more complex way of describing the formerly discrete and unchallenged category of disease.[36] The concept of disease entities allows us to move away from the positivist kind of descriptive categories of disease and to think of diseases not as discrete objects but as ranges of bodily difference and reaction. To think about diseases in this way is not simply an intellectual fad.[37]

The justification for this way of thinking is most particularly applicable to psychiatric disorders. In general medicine, or what might be called "classical" medicine, on which psychiatric medicine has tried to model itself, disease definitions often took their contours from somewhat consistent trends and manifestations of infectious diseases, which appeared to have relatively stable durations and symptoms, and a predictable set of outcomes.[38] Cholera, tetanus, influenza, plague, and so on can generally be put in fairly distinct taxonomic categories, and therefore they set the model for the modern scientific idea of disease, although there was a considerable body of medical literature around the idea of disease as a state, literally, of dis-ease, most readily translated as being out of sorts. That school of medicine considered the holistic, as we now say, state of health and therefore looked at disease as general rather than specific. Yet the dominant trend of European and American medicine came to focus on the life cycle, as it were, of specifically delimited infectious diseases caused by (later) identifiable bacteria or viruses.

But psychological disorders that include affective elements are quite another thing. Indeed, contemporary critics of psychiatry, many of whom were or are users of psychiatric services, have tried to call attention to the problematics of the medical model by refusing to call themselves "mental patients," preferring instead to use the term "mental health services users" or "consumers," and eschewing "mental illness" for the less medicalized "mental distress."[39] I will refer later to the way that medical doctors came to see obsession as within their purview. Another more provocative way of saying this is that doctors took over behaviors like obsession and came to see them as analogous to other "classical" diseases. As Michel Foucault even more provocatively noted of nineteenth-century practices, "psychiatry only has an imaginary relationship with scientific knowledge."[40] One might elaborate on what seems to be Foucault's mere denigration (although I believe he is using the notion of the imaginary in the Lacanian sense) in implying that the level of proof for nineteenth-century psychiatry cannot be equated with the level of proof in an ideal scientific experiment. The nineteenth century's notion of science would barely pass muster now, especially with notions of double-blind, randomized studies. In addition, psychiatrists were of course simply following along in a bourgeoning consumer culture that came to define being ill and going to the doctor as one more in a series of acts consumers might perform.

In saying this, let me caution again that I am not claiming that there are no diseases, that people with schizophrenia do not have a mental disorder, that people who are depressed are simply adopting a trendy mode of being in the early twenty-first century. I am, however, following along in the thinking of people like Ian Hacking, who explains very well the concept of what he calls "transient mental illness." Hacking notes that "mental illnesses," for example, fugue states, hysteria, anorexia, or attention deficit disorder, arise in society at given historical moments and then may as well disappear within twenty or thirty years. He notes that such illnesses are "real" but also notes their provisional status. And he highlights the feedback loops between diagnoses and diseases. The point is that we must consider that diseases, particularly ones as complexly envisioned as those we call mental illnesses, are distinctly tied to the historical moment, the set of expected behaviors and norms in society, and the paradigms of the observers and the observed. Juliet Mitchell, for example, notes the similarities between *saka,* a disease of the Taita people in Kenya, and hysteria, and claims that while hysteria is universal, it also changes through different historical periods and therefore "resists any such constraints or classification."[41]

I therefore assume the necessity for being aware of the way disease entities and corresponding explanatory systems arise in synchrony. Obsession is not a thing in itself. Indeed, one could argue that mental conditions can never be seen as discrete things apart from the nosological categories that form them. The cure system that helps define and change the mental or emotional condition is deeply linked to society in its broad and complex being, out of which the triggering behavior was selected.

A final assumption, and a fairly major one, that I will make in this book [chapter] is that science, scientific medicine, and academic specialization—all of which achieve a kind of dominant formation in the nineteenth century in the Western world—are themselves not objective positions of knowledge but in fact aspects of the new problematics of obsession. This new method of knowledge requires all the hallmarks of obsessive behavior—fixation on one thing, repetitive interest in that thing, fixed attention to the details, copious notes, observations, repetitive and focused habits of study, and a strong compulsion to do all this. We can see in nineteenth-century literature a popular awareness that there is something strange and mad about science and scientists. Works like Mary Shelley's *Frankenstein,* Wilkie Collins's *Heart and Science,* Jules Verne's *20,000 Leagues under the Sea,* and Robert Louis Stevenson's *Dr. Jekyll and Mr. Hyde,* feature the visions of "mad scientists," driven to distraction by the obsessive nature of their work. Aware of this vision, the claim in this book [chapter] is that science and by extension knowledge become, to some degree, the socially acceptable face of a culture of obsession, while the obsessive, the monomaniac, the neurasthenic, the sexual pervert, among others, become the extrojected object, selected for observation, by those engaged in the scientific study of obsessive behaviors.

In speaking this way, we need to consider a long and complicated approach to understanding a phenomenon like obsession, because in talking about categories of madness we are speaking of phenomena that have always been understood in different ways at different times. Even under the most favorable conditions we are talking about multiple states and shifting symptoms. Therefore, we have to posit a specific time and place where "obsession," as a shifting term, is understood one way, and then another specific time and place when it is understood another way. And so on through places and times. The result will not be, as is found in most psychiatric texts, that we arrive at the present, where we clearly understand what madness is and the past is all a confusing prolegomenon to a clear present and even clearer future. The truth probably is that madness remains as murky today as it has been in the past. Our contemporary paradigms and treatments are based on different kinds of measures and groupings than were used in the past, but we are by no means certain that the way we view things now is the way they actually will be twenty-five—let alone a hundred—years from now.

Obsessing about Language

The problem is further convoluted by the fact that the language we use to understand madness is itself a layered pentimento of concepts and terms that have arisen, been useful, become outmoded, and yet still persist. Since the words we use will predetermine the object of study, we have to be careful that when we speak of obsession, or madness, or other like terms, we understand that the objects so described through language may not correspond exactly to states of cognitive or emotional distress. Although we are always looking at people, we describe what we see through words.

On a popular level, we talk comfortably about insanity, madness, and mental illness as though each of those terms describes the same thing. We feel capable of judging, at least informally, the level of sanity, neurosis, nervousness, or depression among our friends, family, and selves. Indeed, it is family and friends who will often be the first to diagnose, suggest treatment, and also initiate legal action on behalf of a possible patient. Concepts of madness begin at home. Commonly, we can produce the phrases: "I'm nervous." "He's crazy." "She's neurotic." "They're depressed." "He's a lunatic." No one challenges us in ordinary life to define our terms, and there is a community of opinion within a culture about human behavior that sees all of these behaviors as part of something we have come to call, again without much difficulty or thought, "mental illness." But, as we will see, the exact discourse that should have jurisdiction over madness has never been certain. The set of circumstances that allow a family member to be concerned, seek professional help, and ultimately agree to have a distressed relation brought in for assistance will always be based, circuitously, on the norms and expectations that have been developed mutually over time by practitioners, patients, moralists, politicians, novelists, filmmakers, religious advisers, and so on.

Even our notion of being nervous is part of a long history of overlapping terms and explanations. When the various functions of the nervous system were discovered from the eighteenth through the nineteenth century, people changed the way they spoke of their emotional states. Nerves began to predominate and people began to think of themselves as "nervous" rather than "humorous." "Nervous energy," another term we still use, was seen as a measurable way to discuss slack or tightened nerves. When we say "my nerves were strained to the utmost" we mean that we are "nervous wrecks." But the two meanings join only at the word itself. Strained nerves relate to nerves as sinews, as John Milton, for example meant when he wrote of Samson in 1646 that he was "straining all his nerves" in pushing down the walls. The use of "nervous wrecks," in the sense of an emotional disaster, like a shipwreck, began to be used at the end of the nineteenth century. This comparison shows that when we now use what we are thinking of as a relatively coherent linguistic system to explain our nervousness, we really aren't. What we see is an example of at least two overlapping meaning systems in regard to the body and the mind that we have come to use interchangeably through the persistence of language but the absence of sense.

When George Beard popularized the idea of neurasthenia in his 1881 book *American Nervousness,* he was taking advantage of the nerve as a location of energy and emotions. If your nerves were overly excited you were nervous; if your nerves were weak or exhausted (as in nervous exhaustion) you were neurasthenic. This model of medicine, in turn, was a product of a new way of seeing the body based on a model of balance in which too much or too little of something caused a disease, while the mean or norm was considered good health.[42] Every time we use the word "nervous" we signal the complex and confusing history of the body in relation to culture—the biocultural. So any discussion of obsession as a nervous disorder will reawaken many sleeping myths about the body and the mind.

Obsession Viewed through Technology

At various historical moments, people had to ask of madness, Is this subject a medical one? A psychological one? A physiological one? A philosophical one? One of the points of this study is to trace the problematic of obsession as it moves through these different spheres of knowledge. It will be important to note the changes in the perception of obsession, as well as the perceivers of obsession, as both extend into different ways of knowing. Our current line of thinking is that all psychiatric states are a result of neurochemistry and brain activity. The general assumption is that "mind is what brain does."[43] So some clinicians and researchers who have miraculously persisted in reading my introduction up to this point will all the while have been shaking their heads at the ignorant insouciance of my project. They will tell you with certainty that it may be well and good to describe the social and cultural world surrounding disease, but that at core, at rock-hard base, is the reliable and now visualizable world of fMRI, PET, and various other imaging devices. They will tell you that they are on the verge of finding the place in the brain (the caudate nucleus of the basal ganglia or the cingulum or the prefrontal and orbitofrontal lobes) where OCD resides. These images are intriguing, but their outcome isn't as certain as the scientists might claim. We are in the very early days of understanding the neurochemical and electrical activity of the brain. And, as a recent study has shown, simply providing images from fMRIs will increase acceptance among observers of even deliberately false and illogical explanations about brain function.[44] Technologies themselves will spawn new diagnoses[45] but in the long run we have seen that diagnoses may in fact change with further technologies. In other words, the seeming fixity and specificity of diseases can be buttressed by information provided by new technologies. But therefore, by definition, they can't be fixed or unchanging if they are dependent on a specific kind of technology, which itself can change or become obsolete.

A rather simple question that often gets lost in the very valid work being done in brain imaging and research into brain chemistry is, are the changes we are seeing a result of the disease or the cause of the disease? In other words, are people sad because they have low serotonin, or do people have low serotonin because they are sad? No one doubts that the brain changes and those changes can be measured, but is the OCD brain like that because the person is worrying and compulsive, or is the person obsessing and compulsive because of specific activities and chemistries independent of any individual will? This isn't merely a philosophical question but one with the utmost significance for this discussion of OCD.

In the end, many of psychiatry's assumptions are just assumptions. Mental distress is not easy to treat, nor can success rates be measured so easily. In looking at psychiatric disorders, we are not looking at an area of grand success. One study of OCD shows that without any treatment about a third of the patients get better, a third worse, and a third remained the same.[46] Chemical treatment of mental illness is currently the preferred mode, but we should not make the mistake of thinking that we have finally arrived at a solution through the psychopharmacological modality. Recent retrospective studies are casting serious doubts on the efficacy, safety, and utility of the recent fascination with SSRIs. Indeed, psychotherapists, behavioral therapists, psychoanalysts, and other researchers have made compelling arguments that talking cures and behavior modification can also create measurable changes in brain chemistry and electrical activity.[47] The history of mental distress in medicine shows us that there is a constant alternation among those who see madness as a larger intrapsychic experience, those who see it as a fundamentally physiological one, and those who see it as a combination of both. Of course, there is the additional perspective that comes and goes about the specific nature of distress—linking it to social and historical conditions. There is too the oscillating debate over whether drugs are the cure or whether talking and persuasion are the best methods to bring about a cessation of symptoms. Even talking cures are in debate at the moment, and there is much disagreement about whether psychotherapy should be a standardized practice based on scientific studies or whether it should be an intuitive and theoretical one.[48] While chemicals can and do affect the brain and behavior, the question remains whether mental illness is a chemical phenomenon, how well the chemicals work over a long haul, and how long-term use of and compliance in taking drugs will pan out. And of course, genetic arguments now abound as well.

But should obsession be considered a part of mental illness? That question is predicated on a notion that the thing we call mental illness is what it is—a medical phenomenon. Yet obsession seems both to partake of mental illness and to be separate from it. Indeed, there was a time when obsession was not considered an illness at all. In order to understand obsession, we will have to trace the development of obsession from where it begins as demonic possession and moves to a secularized fascination or curiosity and thence into obsession, the diseased state, and to do that, we have to look at the discourses surrounding obsession that would place it in a disease category.

Notes

1 Davis, L. (2008). *Obsession: A history*. Chicago University Press.
2 Pilar Viladas, "Obsession," *New York Times Magazine* (October 13, 2002), 65.
3 Rosemary Sullivan, *Labyrinth of Desire: Women, Passion, and Romantic Obsession* (Toronto: Harper*Flamingo*, 2001), 2.
4 http://www.gallup-robinson.com/essay65.html.
5 "The Culture of Mania," in *Subjectivity and Experience Transformed*, ed. Joao Biehl, Byron Good, and Arthur Kleinman (Cambridge: Harvard, 2005).
6 Ian Hacking, *Rewriting the Soul: Multiple Personality and the Science of Memory* (Princeton: Princeton University Press, 1995), pp. 8–20; and *Mad Travelers: Reflections on the Reality of Transient Mental Illnesses* (Charlottesville: University of Virginia, 1998), pp. 1–2; 51–102. Charles E. Rosenberg, "The Tyranny of Diagnosis: Specific Entities and Individual Experience," *Milbank Quarterly* 80:2 (2002), 237–60. 10.1111/1468-0009.t01-1-00003
7 Rosenberg, 241.
8 http://www.psyweb.com/Mdisord/AnxietyDis/ocdl.html.
9 http://www.psyweb.com/Mdisord/ocpd.html.
10 The further revision incorporated into the *DSM-V* may in fact eliminate obsessive-compulsive personality as a diagnostic category.

11 Stanley J. Rachman and Ray J. Hodgson, *Obsessions and Compulsions* (Englewood, NJ: Prentice-Hall, 1980), 10.

12 Stanley J. Rachman, *The Treatment of Obsessions* (Oxford: Oxford University Press, 2003), 5.

13 Steven A. Rasmussen and Jane L. Eisen, "The Epidemiology and Clinical Features of Obsessive-Compulsive Disorder," in Michael Jenike, Lee Baer, William Minicheillo, *Obsessive-Compulsive Disorders: Practical Management* (New York: Mosby, 1998), 25.

14 Rachman and Hodgson, 3.

15 For more on the *DSM* in this regard see Geoffrey C. Bowker, *Sorting Things Out* (Cambridge, MA: MIT Press).

16 Lennard J. Davis, *Enforcing Normalcy: Disability, Deafness, and the Body* (London: Verso, 1995).

17 Rachman and Hodgson, 12.

18 Rachman and Hodgson, 13.

19 Susan Sontag, *Aids and Its Metaphors* (New York: Random House, 1979).

20 Lennard Davis and David Morris, "Biocultures Manifesto," *NLH* 38 (Fall 2007), 411–18. 10.1353/nlh.2007.0046

21 Rachmand and Hodgson, 18.

22 See William Van Ornum, *A Thousand Frightening Fantasies: Understanding and Healing Scrupulosity and Obsessive Compulsive Disorder* (New York: Crossroads, 1997).

23 Rachman and Hodgson, 94.

24 There is a further critique to make of the prejudice toward the use of numbers in a statistical mode. And we will want to keep alert to the rise of statistics as a phenomenon of the very same modernity we are ourselves regarding. In this context, we should recall that the founding of the Statistical Society in London began with the assemblage of a group of men, all of whom were eugenicists, who inaugurated a mode of thinking that has become very common now, but which carried with it an entire set of presuppositions about human life and its relation to numbers.

25 Rachman and Hodgson, 21.

26 Rachman, 15.

27 I should note that from a psychoanalytic perspective, the content of the obsession is relatively irrelevant. The principal is that obsessional neurosis is characterized by a divorce of the symptom from the cause, a defense in which the activity provided by obsession is a diversion or a distraction from the motivating cause. In this line of thinking the obsessional activity does not particularly matter and is chosen for its arbitrary distance from the originating cause of unwanted sexual or aggressive impulses. However, most practitioners now disregard a psychoanalytic explanation of OCD.

28 Rachman and Hodgson, 254.

29 John E. Grant, Anthony Pinto, Matthew Gunnip, et al., "Sexual obsessions and clinical correlates in adults with obsessive-compulsive disorder," *Comprehensive Psychiatry* 47:5 (September–October 2006), 325–29. 10.1016/j.comppsych.2006.01.007

30 Naomi Finberg, Donatella Marazziti, Dan J. Stein, eds., *Obsessive Compulsive Disorder: A Practical Guide* (London: Dunitz, 2001), 7.

31 There is an institutional history to the distinction between personality type and disorder. Freud noted the distinction between the anal type of personality and the obsessive neurotic. Ernest Jones and Karl Abraham reiterated the distinction. In the 1960s Joseph Sandler developed tests to distinguish between the personality type (which he called

Type A) and the disorder (which he called Type B). The *DSM-IV-TR* followed that distinction, although there is an indication that the *DSM-V* will abandon the personality type as a pathological entity. Eric Hollander and others have reversed the trend of firewalling distinctions between these types by introducing the notion of an OCD continuum.

32 Rachman and Hodgson, 58.

33 Dana J. H. Niehaus and Dan J. Stein, "Obsessive-Compulsive Disorder: Diagnosis and Assessment" in Eric Hollander, ed., *Obsessive-Compulsive Disorder: Diagnosis, Etiology, Treatment* (London: Informa, 1997), 4.

34 Rachman and Hodgson, 98.

35 Rachman and Hodgson, 99.

36 See David Morris, *Illness and Culture in the Postmodern Age* (Berkeley: University of California Press, 2000).

37 Indeed, the more we learn about genomics, the more we realize that while humans are very similar, significant individual differences in our DNA can make us react quite differently to the same environment.

38 Obviously, even with these physical diseases, there is a large range of variation which observers have smoothed out in order to create agreed-upon diagnostic categories.

39 See Bradley Lewis, *Moving Beyond Prozac, DSM, and the New Psychiatry: The Birth of Postpsychiatry* (Ann Arbor: University of Michigan Press, 2006).

40 Sylvere Lotringer, ed., *Foucault Live: Collected Interviews, 1961–1984* (New York: Semiotexte, 1996), 197.

41 Juliet Mitchell, *Mad Men and Medusas: Reclaiming Hysteria* (New York: Basic Books, 2000), 13.

42 See Georges Canguilhem, *On the Normal and the Pathological*, trans. R. Fawcett (New York: Zone Books, 1991).

43 See for example Nikolas Rose, "Neurochemical Selves," *Society* (November/December 2003), 46–59. 10.1007/BF02688204

44 D. S. Weisberg, F. C. Keil, J. Goodstein, and J. Grey, "The Seductive Allure of Neuroscience Explanations," *Journal of Cognitive Neuroscience* (forthcoming); paper available at http://pantheon.yale.edu.proxy.library.nyu.edu/~dis73/Assets/Weisberg-neuro%20explanations.pdf.

45 Rosenberg, 248.

46 Edith Rüdin, "Ein Beitrag zur Frage der Zwangskrankheit insbesondere ihrer hereditären Beziehungen," *Archiv für Psychiatrie und Zeitschrift Neurologie* 191 (1953), 14–54; 10.1007/BF00345572 cited in Paul Adams, *Obsessive Children* (New York: Penguin, 1973), 209. Actually, although this is impossible to prove, many studies end up with this tri-part conclusion, which is perhaps a function of bell-curve results in poorly planned protocols.

47 See for instance L. R. Baxter, J. M. Schwartz, K. S. Bergman, M. P. Szubba, B. H. Guze, J. C. Mazziotta, et al., "Caudate Glucose Metabolic Rate Changes with Both Drug and Behavior Therapy for Obsessive-Compulsive Disorder," *Archives of General Psychiatry* 49 (1992), 681–89; 10.1001/archpsyc.1992.01820090009002 or J. Schwartz, P. Stoesse, L. Baxter, K. Martin, and M. Phelps, "Systematic Changes in Cerebral Glucose Metabolic Rate after Successful Behavior Modification Treatment of OCD," *Archives of General Psychiatry* 53 (1996), 109–13. 10.1001/archpsyc.1996.01830020023004

48 Benedict Carey, "For Psychotherapy's Claims, Skeptics Demand Proof," *New York Times*, August 10, 2004, F1.

Chapter 15

A (Head) Case for a Mad Humanities

SULA'S SHADRACK AND BLACK MADNESS[1]

Hayley C. Stefan

Summary

Stefan's chapter continues and builds on recent scholarship at the intersection of disability studies and mad studies. Toward this goal, Stefan traces a genealogy of mad studies and argues for the development of mad humanities and mad literary studies. Stefan provides an example of mad literary studies by analyzing the character of Shadrack in Toni Morrison's *Sula* (1973). Stefan understands Shadrack as a complex figure whose characterization resists flattened readings of Black madness. The novel's scholarly history, while rich in disability studies readings, makes evident persistent societal neglect of mentally distressed characters—especially distressed characters of color—as peripheral or symbolic. The chapter uses critical race theory, disability studies, and trauma studies to form an intersectional inquiry into the material and lived conditions of mad individuals of color. In so doing, the chapter demonstrates the significant possibilities of intersectional and interdisciplinary methodology for understanding mental difference.

*

In December 2017, as political tensions surrounding the Trump administration intensified, *New York Times* writers Gail Collins and Bret Stephens asked readers, "Is Trump Crazy Like a Fox or Plain Old Crazy?" Their ostensibly tongue-in-cheek title spoke to ongoing public and legislative discussion about the president's mental and emotional abilities, a question, too, that many answered. The title of Michelle Goldberg's December op-ed column declared, "Trump Is Cracking Up" (2017). *The New Republic*'s Steven Beutler offered his readers "A Medical Theory of Donald Trump's Bizarre Behavior" (2017). Meanwhile, *Washington Post* opinion writer Dana

DOI: 10.4324/9781003148456-18

Milbank told readers, "President Trump actually is making us crazy" (2017). The pathologization of the president came less than two years after media uproariously criticized the same man for verbally and gesturally mocking reporter Serge F. Kovaleski, who is a disabled individual. Public reaction to the recorded video clip of Trump's depiction of Kovaleski on the campaign trail considered Trump's choice a "gaffe" (Graham 2018), his "worst offense" (Carmon 2016), and a sign that the then-candidate "looked like he was done for" (Taylor 2018). The sharp hypocrisy between anger at mocking disabled individuals and ongoing sarcastic jokes about mental or emotional disabilities speaks to an issue that extends beyond political writers to academics: we still do not know how to talk about mental and emotional disability.

As fields, literary and cultural studies have done much work to further Disability Studies' critiques, yet our critical engagement with mental and emotional disability in literature and academia more broadly has been less thorough. Recent scholarship, such as the work of Therí A. Pickens (2017a, 2017b) and Margaret Price et al. (2017), affirms the need to critically reconsider how the humanities discuss, theorize, and validate distress and madness. Scholarship invested in race and disability, especially, including recent formative work on Black Disability Studies by Pickens and others, are foundational to conversations about madness in and within the humanities. As Pickens writes, "The discourse of ability lurks as an undercurrent within the academy, sometimes creating a riptide between the turbulent waters of superior thinking and the threat of madness" (2017b, 243). Pickens speaks to the ways in which scholars who are able to, as she says, "safely embrace their 'crazy'" (243), do so only within networks of support that regularly exclude people of color, LGBTQ individuals, women, and physically disabled individuals. Concurring with Pickens, I argue that the humanities must "embrace the crazy" within academic and public forums. In so doing, I call for a Mad humanities that centralizes literature and cultural studies within "real" experience. In this article, I review influential scholarship guiding this inquiry and sketch a framework for initial analyses. I then apply this framing of a Mad literary studies approach to Morrison's *Sula*, calling attention as I do so to how such a reading offers new insight and builds upon existing formative scholarship on the ostensibly peripheral character of Shadrack and the text overall.

■■■

A still developing subfield, Mad Studies calls attention to the social, medical, and legal systems through which mental "illness" is constructed and stigmatized. Writing for the *Mad Studies Network* site, Lucy Costa defines Mad Studies as "an area of education, scholarship, and analysis about the experiences, history, culture, political organising [sic], narratives, writings and most importantly, the PEOPLE who identify as: Mad; psychiatric survivors; consumers; service users; mentally ill; patients, neuro-diverse; inmates; disabled—to name a few of the 'identity labels' our community may choose to use." In their introduction to the significant 2013 text *Mad Matters: A Critical Reader in Canadian Mad Studies*, Brenda A. LeFrançois, Robert Menzies, and Geoffrey Reaume elaborate upon this, articulating Mad Studies as

> incorporat[ing] all that is critical of psychiatry from a radical socially progressive foundation in which the medical model is dispensed with as biologically reductionist whilst alternative forms of helping people

experiencing mental anguish are based on humanitarian, holistic perspectives where people are not reduced to symptoms but understood within the social and economic context of the society in which they live.

(2013, 2)

As these conceptualizations make clear, Mad Studies is inchoate and amorphous, and there are as yet no stable or universally agreed upon boundaries of its interests or the tenets of its methodology, nor of its location based in activism, academe, anti-psychiatry, or other forums. It is inherently interdisciplinary as both a field and a framework.

At its broadest, Mad Studies refers to a methodological focus on cultural constructions of distress or mental disability, as well as the archival resurrection or support of work by scholars who identify as any of the varying terms under the "mad" umbrella: distressed; disabled; mad-identified (Reville 2013, 170); consumer, survivors, and/or ex-patients of the psychiatric system (c/s/x) (Price 2011, 10; Burstow 2013, 87); or, the less often reclaimed, "mentally ill" (LeFrançois, Menzies, and Reaume 2013, 5).[2]

Notably, while some of these monikers gesture toward the pathologization of distress and mental disability, several reject medicalized terms that characterize the speaker or subject as "afflicted with" or "victim to" diagnoses like post-traumatic stress disorder.[3] Instead, these labels privilege subjective experience and acknowledge resistantly how the subject has been positioned within a psychologized system. Thus, while "distressed" and "disabled" may speak to the social constructionist model of Disability Studies, c/s/x and mad-identified already presage the dialogue between the subject and the biomedicalized model of disability, in which the speaker's identity or status is defined by another. In this way, the mad individual dismisses a hierarchy of knowledges in which biomedical research speaks for or over lived experiential knowledge. This tense distrust of clinical language and models may be one reason for the potential to cultivate Mad Studies scholarship outside of the medical humanities.

Such self-naming seeks to recast the long history of symbolic, often negative, interpretation of distressed or disabled people, including that of the critic, the sage, and the criminal (Foucault 2006, xvi; 109). Madness continues to accumulate different meanings across time, but it oscillates between what Michel Foucault calls "[t]his double movement of liberation and enslavement [which] forms the secret foundations of all that makes up the modern experience of madness" (460). This restriction of agency and the supposition that madness is defined and siloed rather than experienced drives many mad-identified and -allied scholar-activists to appropriate madness for self-identification as well as challenge the various relationships (e.g., doctor/patient, state/ward, public/"mentally ill") that resign the mad-identified to a position of subordination (Price 2011, 11; Beresford 2000, 169). These challenges triangulate a common issue of seeing madness as biologically "Other," inherently negative and deviant, often further compounded by additional systems of oppression. Summarizing mad activist Anne Plumb's formulation of madness, Peter Beresford writes, "the definition/diagnosis of survivors is associated with dissent and the perception of their behaviours [sic] and perceptions as deviant" (170). That is, madness and distress historically have been considered by some as malevolently purposeful rather than biological or even socially constructed, such that to experience distress always already opposes social order.

Resisting this paradigm of sanist superiority, mad scholars and activists foment alternative intersectional conversations of madness. These discussions cull from methodologies of Disability and trauma studies, while attending to the unique ways that madness has been and continues to be viewed and legislated. Yet, because of its specific histories, studies of madness do not neatly fit within the frameworks of either of these methodologies. Arguably, trauma studies utilizes a biomedical or psychologized framing of distress, understandably given its emergence out of psychoanalysis (Berger 2004, 564). Although such an approach identifies and, in some ways, seeks to rationalize or "explain" traumatic symptoms, it often does not explore the way lived experience and social systems influence one another aside from *causing* such distress. While some scholar-activists see Mad Studies as embedded within Disability Studies, some recent work argues that the movements are adjacent and interrelated rather than equivalent. This untethering of Mad Studies from Disability Studies—and their equivalent activist movements—arises out of the differing embodied experiences of mentally distressed and physically disabled persons,[4] as well as disagreement and discomfort surrounding the use of the term "impairment" and the disability/impairment binary (McWade, Milton, and Beresford 2015, 306; Beresford 2000, 168). While the social model of disability regards society as defining impairment (embodied experience) in terms of disability (relation to access), this binary is complicated by the differing experiences of mental and emotional disability or distress, prevailing stigmas about the same, as well as medical and social interpretation of these experiences.

Definitions of impairment within Mad Studies scholarship are fluid and varied but unite in their investment in discussions of subjective experiences, such as pain, confusion, and suffering. In their works on depression, Anna Mollow and Ann Cvetkovich argue that acknowledging and analyzing "suffering" is a necessary part of scholarship (Mollow 2006, 87; Cvetkovich and Wilkerson 2016, 502). Alison Kafer locates such an opportunity to rethink impairment in terms of access in the ongoing conversation in higher education regarding trigger warnings, which she theorizes as "opening[s] that acknowledge trauma and its effects" (2016, 18). Kafer writes that trigger warnings at their worst can function as censors for important practical and theoretical discussions of systemic oppression; at their best, frank conversations about "triggers" encourage us to consider how we interact with ideas and people (12, 15). The debate centers on how we "deal with" trauma as an active impairment that potentially can be mitigated. Kafer's analysis of the avoidance of trauma within higher education analogizes concurrent discussions of pain and debility in Disability Studies by Alyson Patsavas (2014) and Jasbir Puar (2017), among others. As the permeable borders of these fields shift and expand, what it means to be mad-identified or to interpret distressed experiences must always return to the individual, since agreement with medical, psychological, and social models fluctuates among these scholars. To employ a Mad Studies framework at this early stage of the subfield thus demands that scholars treat all models with circumspection.

Recent scholarship interpreting the intersectional relationship between madness and other positionalities demonstrates the potential of Mad Studies as a methodological frame. These include work on madness in higher education, such as Price's *Mad at School: Rhetorics of Mental Disability and Academic Life* (2011), as well as madness in gender and sexuality studies, including what Mollow (2013) calls "Mad Feminism" and Cvetkovich's work on queer affect and depression (2012). Significant research querying mental and emotional disabilities has come from scholars in critical race theory and cultural studies, especially within the field of Black Disability Studies. Important texts such as Nirmala Erevelles' *Disability and Difference in Global Contexts: Enabling a Transformative Body Politic* (2011) and Sami Schalk's *Bodyminds Reimagined: (Dis)ability, Race, and Gender in Black Women's Speculative Fiction* (2018) consider how, in the words of Erevelles and Michael Gill, "race and disability are not oppositional categories but are instead categories of difference that are mutually constitutive of each other" (Gill and Erevelles, 2017, 125). Mining this intersection of race and disability, scholars such as Pickens and Erevelles look at the political, social, and cultural implications of disability and race upon each other. Erevelles' work explores how the material conditions of disability and race inform each other, making possible treatments, education, labor choices, and, to some extent, recognition of the self in the neoliberal capitalist society (2011, 16–17). Pickens attends to a rhizomatic history and development of Black Disability Studies in her crucial introduction to the 2017 special issue of *African American Review*. Pickens collates a non-exhaustive list of disciplines and fields from which critical work on race and disability emerge, including Black feminist literature, trauma studies, critical prison or carceral studies, and cultural studies (2017a, 95). In retracing the importance of foundational work, including Christopher M. Bell's "Introducing White Disability Studies: A Modest Proposal" (2011), Pickens is emphatic that such genealogies obscure what "are and should be very messy" (2017a, 95) histories. She echoes others' calls to resist narratives of resolution and to engage, instead, the complex overlay of systems which "allow this tension to rest uneasily at the surface" (97). Importantly, then, these writers conceive of distress and disability as social constructions, within larger ecologies of embodied existence including dynamics of race, ethnicity, gender, and sexuality. As Black Disability Studies scholars like Pickens have insisted, the multiplicity of these models investigating the networks through which mad individuals identify themselves or are interpellated highlights tensions and possibilities worth further exploration.

Significantly, such Mad Studies approaches extend analysis to how material conditions affect madness and influence lived experience and care. These discussions of material conditions attest to the complex heterogeneous relationships that scholars and activists in Mad Studies have with the medical field and industry. While there is relative unanimity against biomedicalized definitions and restrictions of experience, the Mad community is not centered around rejecting medical care all together. This is evident in the differing terminology and approaches of scholars analyzing madness, whose adherence to a pathologization of madness or mental disability depends on the aims of the project.[5] Mollow (2006) writes that intersectional analyses of mental or emotional disability and distress are both social and political. She argues that literary studies of depression must be informed by lived experience, social constructions, and the interstices that define relationships to medical care (including access, affordability, and racialized medicalization). In many cases, Erevelles notes, "it is the lack of access to economic resources and, consequently, to health care that also contributes to the creation and proliferation of disability" (2011, 17). Picking up Erevelles' argument in the first year of the Trump administration, Puar posits that, as the Republican-majority U.S. government lobbies for more restrictive health care options, "access to health care may well become the defining factor in one's relationship to the non-disabled/disabled dichotomy" (2017, xvi). Indeed, as Tanja Aho, Liat Ben-Moshe, and Leon J. Hilton write in their discussion of *American Quarterly*'s 2017 "Mad Futures" forum, "the impetus to police, surveil, imprison, control, and normalize bodyminds is always bound up with ableist and sanist forms of erasure and death" (299). Investigating these intersecting and overlapping means of legislating and (in) validating experience is imperative for the continuation of literary studies, academe, and the real lives of mad-identified individuals everywhere.

These diverse readings offer a preliminary sketch of a Mad Studies methodology. Like Disability Studies, Mad Studies queries the epistemology and impact of language used to describe people and experiences. Also in the vein of Disability Studies, Mad Studies pushes back against social constructions of mental and emotional "health" and "illness" which effectively restrict who participates in various activities, events, and careers.[6] Mad Studies, however, more directly problematizes the way that social constructions of disability and distress animate discussions about the impairment/ disability paradigm in Disability Studies. This focus on the theoretical and practical experiences of debility, pain, and suffering directly invoke the material conditions that can generate and/or legislate distress—and therefore which individuals are more likely to be consigned to various roles along a "mad" spectrum, from violent to quirky. Consequently, Mad humanities scholarship attends to the following:

- Embodiment—including "visible" and "invisible" mental, affective, and physiological experiences;
- Intersectional social interpretations of madness as applied to characteristics and behavior indexed by race, gender, citizenship, sexuality, and other catalogs of oppression; as well as
- The various institutional systems which (de)legitimize mad living, e.g., citizenship, education, law, medicine, and psychology.

Inherently, then, Mad Studies is a radical approach which affirms the humanity of diverse mad-identified individuals while calling out (and working against) the sanist and ableist rhetorics that intersect with and implicate other systems of oppression.

In the subsequent sections, I model a Mad literary studies approach by examining the character Shadrack from Toni Morrison's *Sula*. The novel tracks Sula and her close friend Nel in the Bottom, the close-knit part of Medallion in which the Black community lives, entering into their lives briefly, with chapters labeled for their corresponding year in time. Nel and Sula encounter racist violence, early romance, and deadly accidents together, their friendship acting as a sort of refuge from each other's families. Sula leaves town after Nel marries her husband, Jude, and upon her return, she refuses to fit into any category, embracing her free will and sexuality in the face of town gossip. Her friendship with Nel ends when Sula and Jude have sex, but years later when Sula is ill and dying, Nel tries to care for her. After Sula dies, the townspeople rejoice in the death of their pariah, joining another town outsider, Shadrack, on his annual National Suicide Day parade, during which many end up drowning.

Described as "[b]lasted and permanently astonished," "ravaged" (1973, 7), and "crazy" (15), Shadrack traditionally has been regarded as a peripheral character, significant primarily as metaphor or symbol. However, the character's function in opening and closing the plot as well as the novel's unique dual portrayal of Shadrack's mental distress through his own experiences and the opinions of others encourage further interrogation of how the text and its readers characterize mental distress. In what follows, I walk the reader through a Mad literary studies approach, attending to Morrison's introduction to Shadrack and signaling what types of scholarship and material conditions could support a more thorough exploration of his role. After this, I use this prefatory sketch to further examine the material conditions of his madness that influence the character, Morrison's conception of him, and the text's reception history. Mad Studies' goals of generating alternate readings of what it means to live with distress or "madness" beg reinterpretation of novels like *Sula* whose extant scholarship has focused primarily on physical disability rather than mental or emotional experience. Because of the significance of Morrison's *Sula* within literary Disability Studies—especially through the character of Eva Peace— rereading the novel through the lens of Mad Studies with specific focus on Shadrack presents a unique opportunity to consider the relationship between these closely related fields.

Approaching *Sula* through Mad Studies

Morrison's 1973 novel follows Sula, her grandmother Eva, and other inhabitants of the Bottom in chronological segments from 1919 to 1965. Eva has been widely interpreted through a Disability Studies lens, most notably in Rosemarie Garland-Thomson's *Extraordinary Bodies* (1997), but also across various works which expand upon and counter Garland-Thomson's arguments. Garland-Thomson writes that Eva's amputation of her own leg for money to provide for her children "is an act of self-production that at once resists domination and witnesses oppression's virulence" (1997, 116). That is, Eva's disability evidences her own resourcefulness and strength at the same time as it testifies to the physical effects of white oppression. Garland-Thomson reads Eva's self-amputation as both generative and metaphorical, and this interpretation of Eva is by many measures accurate. Her amputated missing lower leg seems to make the remaining foot, consistently adorned and cared for, that much more beautiful (Morrison 1973, 41). Indeed, while Eva's disability perhaps inhibits her chances of saving her daughter Hannah from burning to death, her body asserts its own power throughout the novel. Morrison writes that even though "adults, standing or sitting, had to look down at her [...] they didn't know it. They all had the impression that they were looking up at her" (31). This reaction may be due in part to the narrative of her disability, which enigmatically entertains, as a tale of magic realism (in which "the leg got up by itself one day and walked on off") or of cunning adventure, in which Eva exchanges her leg for money (30–31). In this performance, her body testifies to her wit and strength; performing her disability affords Eva acceptance and respect in the community. Her disability is legible through the narrative of white oppression of the Black community: her body, like so many before hers, must be subjugated and mutilated to survive.

Shadrack's experiences as a World War I veteran attest to his own position as a victim of white systemic violence. After the introduction, a history of National Suicide Day opens the novel, offering the reader alongside it a history of its creator Shadrack, a seemingly omnipresent but ignored townsperson. Morrison takes the reader to the moment at which the uncanniness of Shadrack's war experience leads to him black out, later waking in a mental hospital:

> He ran, bayonet fixed, deep in the great sweep of men flying across this field. Wincing at the pain in his foot, he turned his head a little to the right and saw the face of a soldier near him fly off. Before he could register shock, the rest of the soldier's head disappeared under the inverted soup bowl of his helmet. But stubbornly, taking no direction from the brain, the body of the headless soldier ran on, with energy and grace, ignoring altogether the drip and slide of brain tissue down its back.
>
> (1973, 7)

The terrifying image of the "headless soldier" refracts Shadrack's character throughout the text; he is described as a "young man of hardly twenty, his head full of nothing" (7). The adult Shadrack is "uncoordinated" (12), yet his actions are memorable, eventually gathering many behind him in the final Suicide Day march.

In a hospital in "1919," the reader reunites with Shadrack, who has presumably blacked out after witnessing the gruesome scene above. The reader learns of no extensive physical injury experienced by Shadrack, leaving the reader to assume that his hospitalization is mental or emotional in nature. While not legible upon his body, Morrison illuminates Shadrack's distress for the reader. Shadrack envisions his hands involuntarily growing wildly (1973, 8; 9) and becoming endlessly tangled with his shoelaces, effectively immobilizing him (15). In addition to feeling unable to move, Shadrack "suffer[s] from a blinding headache" (13) and physically reacts by trying to "fling off and away his terrible fingers" (9). These experiences then are not merely visual or mental, but physical for him. Moreover, these moments of distress generate unapologetically physical reactions from others, including being strapped into a straightjacket and the police later "pull[ing] his hands away" from his shoes and "lock[ing] him in a cell" (13), before ultimately "escort[ing] him to the back of a wagon" (14). Each of the interactions Shadrack has during these moments of distress result in an individual of authority physically restraining or moving him. Thus, his distress as disability is spatially present in so far as it is contained and made punishable by others, and his bodily autonomy, while ostensibly not impaired, is lost.

The treatment Shadrack receives at the hands of doctors and police officers— as well as the treatment he does *not* receive—are characteristic of the way Black veterans returning home from war were treated. In her research on treatment of Black veterans, Carlos Clarke Drazen notes that health care and support for Black

World War I veterans were ostensibly available because of legislation that should have provided for veteran health care and education (2011, 151). In reality, assumptions about race impeded health care access. This particularly affected veterans like Shadrack, whose experiences in *Sula* evidence both maltreatment and an enforced subjugation in which he is given no information about his diagnosis or methods of care. According to K. Walter Hickel, whom Drazen quotes, the lacuna between legislation and racist practice led to a state in which a racialized interpretation of mental and physical health determined who or what was ill and what it meant to be healthy. Hickel writes, "physicians routinely applied not medical criteria but cultural and racial values.... Such cultural and racial views of disease, through medical fictions, had real consequences...physicians invalidated the disability claims of many black veterans" (qtd. in Drazen 2011, 152). In the instances Hickel references, the rejected legal claim of disability effectively invalidates physical, emotional, and especially social experiences of distress. Resultantly, people of color experiencing distress could be deemed healthy enough to return to service or other labor without treatment or support, such that subsequent changes in labor were seen as racialized character flaws rather than evidence of systemic abuse and neglect.

For Shadrack and many others, this lack of veteran health care was compounded by racist assumptions about Black madness, including the long-held racist pseudo-scientific assumption that people of color were less mentally capable and could not experience mental distress (Jarman 2011, 9–10). This racial stereotype in the guise of medical knowledge undergirded additional stereotypes of Black Americans as lazy, ignorant, or mentally inferior. Moreover, as Mollow notes, many of the stereotypes imposed upon Black Americans correspond with symptoms of depression or disability (2006, 73). Structural racism is therefore buffeted by medical scholarship, which simultaneously declare Black embodied experience a screen for moral inferiority and restrict access to health care and other resources.[7] The doctors treating Shadrack attest to this screen through their condescending treatment of him, referring to him as "Private" rather than by his name, repeating themselves angrily, saying, "We're not going to have any trouble today, are we?" and "Nobody is going to feed you forever" (1973, 9). Such speech—a veiled threat and an unironic reminder about the lack of structural support for (mad) Black (veteran) Americans—recasts the relationship as one not of care, but of punishment uniquely applied to Shadrack as both Black and distressed.

This discrimination lodged against the "mutually constituted" position of Black madness subsequently affects the way Black Americans recognize and seek treatment for their own mental or emotional disability and distress. Mollow's analysis of the racialized biopolitics of distress in Meri Nana-Ama Danquah's memoir *Willow Weep for Me* is a small, but formative part of the larger body of scholarship critiquing a medico-racialized model. Josh Lukin (2013) and other scholars of Disability Studies and madness like Bell (2011) and Michelle Jarman (2011) argue that disability in general and madness in particular have historically been under- and misdiagnosed in people of color because of a fear that such "deviance" would be read as a racial moral failure (Lukin 2013, 312; Bell 2011, 3–4; Jarman 2011, 20–21). Citing research by Jennifer James, Lukin writes that attempts to assert Black humanity, especially during and following the twentieth-century Civil Rights movement, historically eschewed ideas of the Black individual as vulnerable or impaired, seeking to refute and distance these comparisons (2013, 312). Lukin reads this deflection of social stereotypes alongside the Black community's hesitation to acknowledge the disabled within it. This rejection, born out of fear and oppression, may account for the ostracization of Shadrack by the townspeople of the Bottom, from whom no acts of communal care are shown. The townspeople generally ignore Shadrack: on his National Suicide Days "the grown people looked out from behind curtains as he rang his bell; a few stragglers increased their speed, and little children screamed and ran" (1973, 15). They fear, ignore, mock, and hide from his madness until it corresponds with their own desire to perform a sense of "mad" joy following Sula's death.

Beyond resisting ideas (and people) which seemingly align with racist assumptions about Black ability, perceivable Black madness was—and remains—incredibly dangerous for Black individuals, especially Black men (Erevelles 2011, 4). Madness historically has been a method of Othering and of delimiting agency (Foucault 2006, 156), as it represented non-normative performativity and reason, which were both malevolent and violent. The "threat" of madness catalyzes broader racist assumptions about Black violence. In her essay, "Coming Up from Underground: Uneasy Dialogues at the Intersections of Race, Mental Illness, and Disability Studies," Jarman notes that exhibits of "madness" are distinctly threatening "for black people, who are also in particular danger of being arrested, treated violently, and even shot if they are seen in public acting 'crazy'" (2011, 21). Hilton additionally argues that the mentally disabled and/or neurodivergent individual of color is cast in terms that legitimize their restrictions and surveillance, making the mad Black body "hypervisible" (2017, 226). However, as Gill and Erevelles point out, this intersection of Black madness is also a space of erasure (2017, 126–27). The dual position of hypervisibility and erasure flattens Shadrack and other mad Black individuals. Shadrack is hospitalized presumably because his distress is abnormal and medical care is ostensibly available; he is ejected from the hospital because his Blackness characterizes his distress in racialized terms (the repeated "Private" standing in for the long-used racist "Boy"), which reads his madness as a racial defect outside the purview of care. In the Bottom, Shadrack is both singular and normal. "The only black who could curse white people and get away with it" (Morrison 1973, 62), Shadrack was different and strange to the people of the Bottom and the larger community, but he was also unobtrusive, having been "absorbed," like his holiday, "into their thoughts, into their language, into their lives" (15).

This liminality of Shadrack as a character has informed much of the scholarship about *Sula*, which often reads him as contextualizing the novel through allusion to World War I and shell shock, or post-traumatic stress disorder (PTSD).[8] Scholars conventionally have wed Shadrack as symbol to his role in the text as a prophetic figure who potentially foresees the mass drowning and continued white violence against the Black community and recognizes Sula's anxieties. Therein, his madness is absurd, prophetic, and metaphoric of socioeconomic, racial, or militarized traumas. Thus, across a selection of 20 pieces of scholarship on *Sula*, with publication dates ranging from 1978 to 2017,[9] 13[10] either directly describe or allude to Shadrack as a metaphor or symbol, and ten[11] described him as prophetic, divine, or psychic, replicating stereotypes about madness. These readings of Shadrack repurpose his embodied experience of distress in order to critique some of the systems they see oppressing him and perhaps, extenuating his experiences. This framing of madness as primarily symbolic for other issues is admittedly fraught as it characterizes the deflection of mad-identified individuals across history. However, while recognizing madness as individual experience is not the focus of such articles, scholars who interpret Shadrack as victim to systemic racism and militarized violence highlight that experiences like Shadrack's were and continue to be common.

The above outline helps to illuminate Shadrack as a figure whose presence in the text and fictional experiences offer a reading of *Sula* in which Morrison makes visible, and to some extent foregrounds, the liminality of mad Black individuals. Below, I delve into these various networks of oppression, depicted above, which influence Shadrack and the text overall, specifically, Shadrack's veteran experiences and competing conceptions of Black madness as gestures of state violence. Following approaches by Erevelles, Jarman, and Mollow, I extend my analysis beyond how the text depicts madness to the systems that define and legislate mad lives. Reading against a typical rejection of mental disability or distress as metaphor, Jarman notes that the tethering of slavery to madness "reminds readers of the long history of racist misappropriations of 'madness,' not only to justify social oppression, but to perpetuate the so-called rationality of slavery itself" (2011, 16). Building upon their productive work as well as adjacent readings of Shadrack through trauma studies, I offer alternate readings of his character as resisting solely metaphoric interpretations and as a significant portrayal of mad Black lives.

Shadrack's Agentic Madness

The dual manner in which Shadrack's distress is physicalized—through his own experience and the intervention of others—contrasts the otherwise distant portrayal of the character in the narrative. As a peripheral character, the reader is not privy to larger characterization of Shadrack as they are with Sula or Eva. Additionally, after "1919" the narrative perspective in the scenes in which he is present approximates his thoughts only briefly before extending outward to how the townspeople see him. For instance, while the reader experiences Shadrack's initial distress in the hospital alongside him, the narrative then moves outward to how others in the Bottom interpreted his distress. Thus, "once the people understood the boundaries and nature of his madness, they could fit him, so to speak, into the scheme of things" (Morrison 1973, 15). This is not the voice of Shadrack hoping to be "fit into the scheme of things," but those in the Bottom or a distant narrator considering the process. This move away from Shadrack's perspective is demonstrated by a visual break in the page; however, during the 1941 Suicide Day parade it is less clear to the reader from whose perspective they watch as it seems to shift between sentences (159). The result is disorienting and perhaps an attempt on Morrison's behalf to represent the experience from Shadrack's equally "befuddled" and "frightened" position (159). The reader, therefore, experiences Shadrack's distress through him, but interprets his reactions to it alongside the townspeople.

The narrator's and townspeople's descriptions of Shadrack return again and again to negative associations of madness, loss, and neglect, replicating the language used to describe mental distress and madness across the nineteenth and twentieth centuries. In *Sula* alone, Shadrack is "crazy" (Morrison 1973, 15), "ravaged" (7), at once reflective (14) and "hysteri[c]" (12); he is "uncoordinated" (12), disorderly, as well as meticulously structured and "unthreatening" (62). "The nature of his madness" (15), as Morrison's narrator describes it, includes Shadrack's physical appearance (whose "eyes were so wild, his hair so long and matted") (15). Shadrack seems not to care whether he adheres to (or recognizes) the boundaries of bodily conduct, as Sula describes him as the "terrible Shad who walked about with his penis out, who peed in front of ladies and girl-children" (62), but simultaneously Shadrack seems unsexualized in that the townspeople say he "never touched anybody, never fought, never caressed" (15). The variation in the way the text frames Shadrack highlights his position as tabula rasa for the Bottom's—and perhaps, the reader's— assumptions about mental distress. Eva's partially agentic role in her disability and her performance of it mark her as resistant, strong, and cunning, while Shadrack in his supposed submission makes evident the violence of war, racialized medical mistreatment, and white oppression.[12]

In much scholarship analyzing *Sula*, Shadrack's performative madness is metonymic of these systems. His body recalls and represents, and such representations are integral to research in African American Studies and American Studies for the archival work they encourage and pursue. This scholarship points toward the demand to recognize Shadrack as a complex figure. Inherently, this compels us to read his body not merely as symbolic, but as living, inhabiting, and negotiating social norms through mental distress or madness. His creation of National Suicide Day acts as a means of self-therapy, yes, but it also implicates the medical and socioeconomic neglect of madness of and by the Black community. This emphasis on Shadrack as symbol has two main effects for the way the character and the novel are read. First, it seems to elide lived experience of mental distress with its visibility or the possibility of witnessing it, thereby Othering madness as witnessed rather than lived, as well as neglecting the importance of madness as disability. Second, it situates Shadrack's distress in line with a traumatic reaction that can be explained through the war alone and not followed through and compounded by daily embodied experience both within and outside of his community. Instead of reviewing how Shadrack's disability is made visible, then, I turn to the spaces in which the narrator approximates Shadrack's perception of his own experiences to see how they point out and refute various systems of oppression.

Sula's publication in 1973 in the midst of the American wars in Vietnam, Laos, and Cambodia implicates the history of the construction of madness alongside state violence.[13] As wounded veterans returned home without conventional, visible bodily harm, mental distress and disability became mediated through both academic and public spheres. Shadrack's mistreatment by the medical community and others in the Bottom speaks to contemporaneous discussions about the health of Black men in the U.S., instigated in part through the 1965 Moynihan Report as well as ongoing discussions of racial liberalism and the Civil Rights Movement. The novel's publication and narrative dates, then, invite dialogue between Shadrack's World

War I experiences and those of contemporary veterans as their timelines correspond with each other, highlighting the sustained practice of pathologizing and segregating mad-identified individuals of color.

Sula thus enters into pre-existing conversations about traumatic war experience as well as debates in racial liberalism about the socioeconomic problems affecting the Black American family. The first of these issues would culminate in part soon after the novel's publication in 1980 with the addition of PTSD to the *Diagnostic and Statistical Manual of Mental Disorders-III* (*DSM-III*) (Wessely 2006, 208, 269). Prompted in part by mid-1960s discussion about racial inequality publicized further after the 1965 *The Negro Family: The Case for National Action* (commonly called the Moynihan Report), the latter concern very much continues in present-day works which address the social and structural acts of oppression against people of color in the U.S. Through Shadrack, Morrison is in dialogue within these intersecting vectors of pathologizing mental distress and race. Morrison's portrayal of Shadrack, as Manuela López Ramírez, Trevor Dodman, and Chuck Jackson point out, does correspond with symptoms of World War I victims of shell shock and later twentieth-century PTSD. Pamela Thurschwell extends this connection in her analysis of *Sula*, writing

> Along with World War I, Vietnam also hovers behind the political landscape of *Sula*. Shadrack's complete lack of understanding of the war in which he finds himself, Plum's heroin addiction, and the background noise of the history of Black soldiers in America required to fight for a nation which granted them only grudging, nominal rights and citizenship, all remind readers that *Sula* is a novel of 1973.
>
> (114)

Thurschwell here articulates the lineage of U.S. militarized violence which both employed and abused Black soldiers. As she gestures at the end of this quotation, these acts of militarized violence abroad belie state and social violence against Black Americans at home.

Morrison signals these connections to the reader through the continuous presence of Shadrack in the Bottom across time. His entry into the text in 1919, the final Suicide Day parade in 1941, and his last appearance in 1965, each mark moments of high conflict in U.S. history: the end of World War I, the U.S.'s entry into World War II following the attacks on Pearl Harbor, and the escalation of U.S. combat in Vietnam (Appy 2015, 132). This contextualization of international and domestic conflicts reminds the reader of the sustained effects of war and violence in collective experience, despite the ostensible dates that confine them. By extension, these dates also mark progressions in the biomedicalization of mental distress as it coalesces into contemporary nosology—one instantiation of it develops from World War I shell shock to the Vietnam War's PTSD. Subject to these moments of state-imposed violence as a soldier, Shadrack's distress makes him further susceptible to acts of state control and negligence. Writing on race and mental health, Frank Keating, echoing Mollow, connects these overtly: "The medicalisation [sic] of mental illness means that containment, control and compliance become essential features of mental health practices [… which] resemble some BME [black and minority ethnic] communities' experiences in everyday life" (2015, 128). Keating's pattern of regulation recalls

Foucault's identified model of "liberation and enslavement," in which the mad individual—and in this case, the mad individual of color—can access state services only in moments of extreme distress, not to be cared for, but rather "protectively" contained. Shadrack's primary experience of distress in 1919 speaks to this, as his psycho-emotional responses result in his being restrained in a straitjacket and later arrested (Morrison 1973, 9, 13).

Shadrack's experiences are compounded by U.S. practices of militarized intervention and racialized medical care. Contemporaneous discussions of the inequality of Black Americans worsened this racialization of the biomedical model of distress, as the Moynihan Report, popular culture, and public policy propagated myths pathologizing Black Americans.[14] Writer of the report Daniel Patrick Moynihan promoted economic development to support the Black American family, with specific attention on the Black man and father (Geary 2011, 53, 58). According to the report, the crux of the socioeconomic disparity facing Black families was due to the un- or underemployment of Black men, the breakdown of the family, and the matriarchal society which led to the disempowerment of the Black father (U. S. Dept. of Labor 1965, 25, 34). Moynihan writes, "the object should be to strengthen the Negro family so as to enable it to raise and support its members as do other families. After that, how this group of Americans chooses to run its affairs, take advantage of its opportunities, or fail to do so, is none of the nation's business" (U. S. Dept. of Labor 1965, 47–48). Moynihan's articulation of the state's responsibility for Black families marks out the supposed limits of state support and gestures toward blaming Black Americans for the structural oppression to which they have been and continue to be subject. The report garnered much pushback from those who argued that it recycled stereotypes about Black Americans (Geary 2011, 60). While essentially placing the onus of socioeconomic success on Black Americans, the report also disregarded the consistent lack of care given to Black Americans as well as the fact that they were largely excluded from discussions about public policy, social science, and medical care (60). We might read Shadrack's origination of National Suicide Day as a challenge to that exclusion, as it functions as a sort of municipal day of care. The narrator describes Shadrack's motivation to create the day in terms of care, too, stating that Shadrack "hit on the notion that if one day a year were devoted to [the unexpectedness of death and dying], everybody could get it out of the way and the rest of the year would be safe and free" (Morrison 1973, 14). Shadrack's encouragement of suicide, while polemical, speaks to a need to recognize pain, whether through actual suicide or symbolic acknowledgement by marching with him. Embracing the ambiguity of Morrison's framing of the day, we might also read National Suicide Day as a recognition of what Harold Braswell calls "end-of-life autonomy" (Braswell 2011). The "holiday" then is not only an act of self-care or "self-soothing," but also evidences the creation of local institutions to satisfy needs neglected by the state.

Indeed, Shadrack's actions throughout the text speak to his attempts to care for others. In his encounter with Sula after she and Nel accidentally cause Chicken Little's death, his response of "always" (Morrison 1973, 62)—so threateningly obtuse to Sula—is an act of comfort. In Sula Shadrack sees a comrade also fearing death, what is left over when the face flies off. Responding empathetically, he tried to think of something to say to comfort her, something to stop the hurt from spilling out of her eyes. So he had said "always," so she would not have to be afraid of the change—the falling away of skin, the drip and slide of blood, and the exposure of bone underneath. He had said "always" to convince her, to assure her, of permanency.

(157)

Reflecting upon this after Sula's death, Shadrack acknowledges that helping her has benefitted himself as well. In fear after losing Chicken Little, Sula goes to his home following a period of intense distress for Shadrack, during which he stops his meticulous cleaning, does not note the passage of time, and feels increasingly lonely (156). Her arrival seems, to him, to renew his existential purpose, in a sense. Sula "wanted something—from him. Not fish, not work, but something only he could give" (156). This reference to Shadrack's other roles selling fish or doing odd jobs around town indicates his legibility via his labor and indicates that Shadrack has not felt valued aside from the labor he produces. His acts of communal care rebut racist pseudo-scientific arguments, as in the Moynihan Report, of the unproductiveness or incapacity for family life of Black American men. He asserts an alternative family model, declaring Sula "his visitor, his company, his guest, his social life, his woman, his daughter, his friend" (157). In these myriad ways, he rejects a model of liberalism that locates its work in the "freeing" of bodies of color through violence and reaffirms communal and self-love in the Black community of the Bottom.

In focusing on the way the narrative constructs Shadrack as mad—through experiencing his distress and visualizing it as Other—the above reading points to how distress is regarded by assumedly white authorities as that which needs to be contained and penalized, and by the Black community as something to be avoided or feared. In these sections Morrison zooms into moments of Shadrack's distress, valuing and rendering his own experiences as significant. Although Shadrack is an arguably minor character, the persistence of misreading or metaphorizing his experiences of mental distress replicates and perpetuates harmful rhetorics that regard madness as a personal or racial deficiency. Minor characters often become placeholders for madness in literature, as Taylor Donnelly points out, "embody[ing] issues of marginalization and dependency" (2012, 33) and "gestur[ing] toward the realm beyond their flattening and metaphorization, in a direction of other stories, subjectivities, and lived experiences" (60). Rereading the small selections of the novel in which Shadrack is present not only makes evident how scholars have constructed their analyses of him as demonstrating the effects of structural racism, but moreover reaffirms the need to still combat racist paradigms of Black madness, in medical as well as literary fields.

■■■

At the climactic moment of Toni Morrison's *Sula*, the townspeople of the Bottom parade to their deaths on National Suicide Day, while the day's founder Shadrack stands transfixed and disregarded by society, his own traumatic stress and his still ringing bell resonating metaphorically as a funeral toll (1973, 162). Shadrack spends much of the book and has spent much of the book's literary history being read as a symbol: of PTSD, the treatment of Black World War I veterans, or the mysteriously wise town "lunatic." The Bottom's treatment of Shadrack—its discomfort at standing or looking closer—continues in the treatment of mad-identified people, especially those of color in the U.S. today. Given that *Sula* remains a popular text for scholarly analysis and perhaps a useful teaching tool for modeling Disability Studies readings, the text is ideal for highlighting the lack of scholarly engagement with madness—and changing it. Equally important, *Sula*'s structure as a novel and its literary history demonstrate the continued marginalization of mad-identified people of color.

More broadly, this analysis works against continued sanist and ableist paradigms that inflect discourse within and outside of the academy. Grounded within real, lived experience, Mad Studies scholarship rejects the confines of "traditional" academic materials and forums, and the development of a Mad humanities demands the same. As the continuing media stereotypes linking presidential political inadequacy and mental distress (perceived as "illness") demonstrate, investment in (literary) Mad Studies dialogues must be taken on within a public humanities.

A Mad humanities—in academic and public scholarship—then, supplements the already productive work done in Disability Studies and activism and draws attention to potential places of growth in intersectional work, as in critical race theory and trauma studies. Perhaps the best justification for moving away from a universalized, biomedical interpretation of distress is that it has not yet been successful in addressing the concerns of mad-identified individuals, especially mad-identified persons of color, who are further implicated in concatenated systems of oppression. Rethinking the language and frameworks we apply to literature—and use in our pedagogies— has great effect upon individual life experience within and outside of academe[15] (Burgett 2014; Griffin 2014; Heiland and Huber 2015; Shumway 2016). Such a reconceptualization will be messy and asks us as scholars to move within different frames; as Bradley Lewis notes, "it is very possible to tell a story about oneself using psychiatric diagnostic metaphors and plots for the purposes of gaining disability benefits and resources, while at the same time seeing these same diagnostic metaphors and plots as incomplete, inadequate, or even harmful....we do not have to have a mono-story of our mental difference" (2017, 206). A public, Mad humanities compels us to investigate the influence scholarly and popular representations of madness have.

As such, literary and cultural studies scholars need to be aware not only of what we theorize, but how. Engaging in discussions of mental or emotional disability and distress in the humanities reaffirms our global neurodiversity and recognizes the rights and dignity of mad individuals while also advocating for more accurate descriptions of actions like those of President Trump as ableist discrimination and harassment. Extending beyond the classroom, public Mad humanities thus identifies and criticizes the racist, ableist effects of the Trump administration's attempts to dismantle the Affordable Care Act and defund Title X, which directly affect the material conditions and access to care of all mad people and mad people of color, in particular.[16] Calling out those actions in others compels us to do the same for ourselves. As such, an overtly Mad humanities aligns with other methodologies and fields, such as Disability Studies, critical race theory, or Native American and Indigenous Studies, in asking how our own pedagogies, scholarships, and daily acts buttress systemic violence by privileging some ways of knowing over others.

Notes

1 Originally printed in: *Disability Studies Quarterly*, Vol. 38, No. 4 (2018). Reprinted with Permission.

2 See Burstow's "A Rose by Any Other Name: Naming and the Battle against Psychiatry" and Price's *Mad at School: Rhetorics of Disability and Academic Life* (2011) for expanded discussions of public and self-identification regarding mental disability or madness.

3 Importantly, the use of umbrella terms like "mad" does not mean that people outright reject biomedical or clinical diagnoses or possible care through various medical venues. Many scholar-activists, including Merri Lisa Johnson (2015) and Mollow (2006), note that identifying with clinical terms and diagnoses can also empower the individual and enable self-advocacy. The choice to personally or publicly reject or identify with clinical language is unique and frequently complicated by various material and political factors that enable an individual to access care.

4 While it is outside the scope of this article to enumerate the differences between experiences of mad and/or disabled individuals, an example may help clarify Beresford's and others' call for the field. For instance, the relative non-visibility of madness or distress often requires that an individual disclose their experiences to others to improve their access—an action that comes with no small risk. Those identified, by themselves or others, as mad may subsequently risk forced hospitalization, medical consumption, segregation through education or political access, as well as the social effects of stigmas about madness.

5 For instance, madness is labeled and understood differently within the following selection of recent titles: Celia Malone Kingsbury's 2002 *The Peculiar **Sanity** of War: **Hysteria** in the Literature of World War 1*, Charley Baker et al.'s ***Madness** in Post-1945 British and American Fiction* (2010), and Michel Bérubé's *The Secret Life of Stories: From Don Quixote to Harry Potter, How Understanding **Intellectual Disability** Transforms the Way We Read* (2016) (emphasis my own).

6 See, for instance, Price's discussion of how the privileging of some characteristics on the academic job market implicitly marks distressed or disabled candidates as underperforming or subpar ("The Essential Functions of the Position: Collegiality and Productivity" in *Mad at School* 2011).

7 I retain the present tense here to acknowledge that such medicalized racism persists today. Dr. William Lawson reports having been taught as a professor of psychiatry that Black Americans could not be subject to mental illness. This medico-racialized interpretation of distress and disability, he says, was "actually published in papers in 1970s, 1980s, and the issue is still arising, and occasionally you see it in the 1990s and even in the 21st century" (NPR Talk of the Town). In her introduction to the special issue of *African American Review*, Pickens places recent and past work on Black disability in conversation, offering several lines of inquiry to this research. Her endnotes, which she describes as "an accessible way into this text" (2017a, 95), also offer a minor bibliography of important work discussing racist underpinnings of U.S. medical history (see 100n6, for example).

8 For some writers, Shadrack is "symbolically made effeminate by the war" (Thurschwell 2013, 113); "symbolizes the nihilistic and suicidal tendencies of twentieth-century man with his World Wars" (Ogunyemi 1979, 132); "metaphorically symbolizes the black community's struggle to survive in the face of racial discrimination and oppression" (Ramírez

2016, 144); and, along with Sula "represent[s] black sons and daughters of America who would be more at home in Africa" (V. Lewis 1987, 92).

9 While *Sula* scholarship is much more expansive, the texts chosen for this archive each discuss Shadrack's character at length rather than or in addition to the major characters of Sula and Nel.

10 See Ogunyemi (1979, 132), Willis (1982, 39), V. Lewis (1987, 92), Montgomery (1989, 129), Bryant (1990, 734; 736; 743), Bergenholtz (1996, 95), Novak (1999, 187), Thurschwell (2013, 113), Ramírez (2016, 132; 140; 144), and Idol (2017, 61).

11 See Ogunyemi (1979, 133), Willis (1982 39), V. Lewis (1987, 92), Montgomery (1989, 129; 136), Bryant (1990, 744), Hunt (1993, 450), Mayberry (2003, 531), Ramírez (2016, 139), and Idol (2017, 57).

12 Though outside the scope of this study, their competing portrayals of disability in the novel provide additional space for an extension of Garland-Thomson's gendered reading of disability. The characters' treatment also is influenced by gendered perceptions of survival, motherhood, and bodily autonomy.

13 Puar's 2017 *The Right to Maim: Debility, Capacity, Disability* offers a crucial and thorough analysis of the relationship between disability and state violence via debilitation.

14 Gregg Santori (2012) also reads *Sula* as responding to the Moynihan Report, with an emphasis on what he calls "maternal violence." See his "*Sula* and the Sociologist: Toni Morrison on American Biopower after Civil Rights," *Theory & Event* 15 (1).

15 See, for instance, much of the work by the National Endowment for the Humanities, including the series *Ideas Matter: Checking in with the Public Humanities* by WAMC Northeast Public Radio and the state humanities councils of Connecticut, Massachusetts, New Hampshire, New Jersey, New York, Pennsylvania, and Vermont: http://wamc.org/term/ideas-matter.

16 This is not to suggest that health care prior to the Trump administration was comprehensive or equitable. For points in the larger discussion regarding changes to the Affordable Care Act and access to mental health care, see Jones et al. (2018). Title X administers federal funding for reproductive and sexual health care and education. Mad individuals and scholars have long noted the disparities with which mad and/or disabled individuals are restricted from access to reproductive and sexual health care information. For more information on the medical ethics of Title X and madness or disability, see Waxman (1994) as well as Stein and Dillenburger (2016).

References

Aho, Tanja, Liat Ben-Moshe, and Leon J. Hilton. 2017. "Mad Futures: Affect/Theory/Violence." *American Quarterly* 69 (2): 291–302. https://doi.org/10.1353/aq.2017.0023

American Psychiatric Association. 1987. *Diagnostic and Statistical Manual of Mental Disorders: DSM-III R*. Washington, DC: American Psychiatric Association.

Appy, Christian G. 2015. *American Reckoning: The Vietnam War and Our National Identity*. New York: Viking.

Bell, Christopher M., ed. 2011. *Blackness and Disability: Critical Examinations and Cultural Interventions*. East Lansing: Michigan State University Press and LIT Verlag.

Beresford, Peter. 2000. "What Have Madness and Psychiatric System Survivors Got to Do with Disability and Disability Studies?" *Disability & Society* 15 (1): 167–72. https://doi.org/10.1080/09687590025838

Berger, James. 2004. "Trauma without Disability, Disability without Trauma: A Disciplinary Divide." *JAC* 24 (3): 563–582. https://www.jstor.org/stable/20866643.

Bergenholtz, Rita A. 1996. "Toni Morrison's *Sula*: A Satire on Binary Thinking." *African American Review* 30 (1): 89–98. https://doi.org/10.2307/3042096

Beutler, Steven. 2017. "A Medical Theory for Donald Trump's Bizarre Behavior." *The New Republic*, February 17. https://newrepublic.com/article/140702/medical-theory-donald-trumps-bizarre-behavior.

Braswell, Harold. 2011. "Can There Be a Disability Studies Theory of "End-of-Life Autonomy?" *Disability Studies Quarterly* 31 (4). https://doi.org/10.18061/dsq.v31i4.1704

Bryant, Cedric Gael. 1990. "The Orderliness of Disorder: Madness and Evil in Toni Morrison's *Sula*." *Black American Literature Forum* 24 (4): 731–745. https://doi.org/10.2307/3041799

Burgett, Bruce. 2014. "The Future of the (Public) Humanities." *Public: A Journal of Imagining America* 2 (1). http://public.imaginingamerica.org/blog/article/essay-the-future-of-the-public-humanities/.

Burstow, Bonnie. 2013. "A Rose by Any Other Name: Naming and the Battle Against Psychiatry." In *Mad Matters: A Critical Reading in Canadian Mad Studies*, edited by Brenda A. LeFrançois, Robert Menzies, and Geoffrey Reaume, 79–90. Toronto: Canadian Scholars' Press, Inc.

Carmon, Irin. 2016. "Trump's Worst Offense? Mocking Disabled Reporter, Poll Finds." *NBC News*, August 11. https://www.nbcnews.com/politics/2016-election/trump-s-worst-offense-mocking-disabled-reporter-poll-finds-n627736.

Collins, Gail, and Bret Stephens. 2017. "Opinion | Is Trump Crazy Like a Fox or Plain Old Crazy?" *The New York Times*, December 5, sec. Opinion. https://www.nytimes.com/2017/12/05/opinion/is-trump-crazy-like-a-fox-or-plain-old-crazy.html.

Costa, Lucy. 2014. "Mad Studies—What It Is and Why You Should Care." *Mad Studies Network*. https://madstudies2014.wordpress.com/2014/10/15/mad-studies-what-it-is-and-why-you-should-care-2/.

Cvetkovich, A. 2012. "Depression Is Ordinary: Public Feelings and Saidiya Hartman's *Lose Your Mother*." *Feminist Theory* 13 (2): 131–46. https://doi.org/10.1177/1464700112442641

Cvetkovich, A., and A. Wilkerson. 2016. "Disability and *Depression*." *Bioethical Inquiry* 13: 497–503. https://doi.org/10.1007/s11673-016-9751-z

Dodman, Trevor. 2011. "'Belated Impress': River George and the African American Shell Shock Narrative." *African American Review* 44 (1): 149–166. https://doi.org/10.1353/afa.2011.0023

Donnelly, Taylor. 2012. "Vogue Diagnoses: The Functions of Madness in Twentieth-Century American Literature." University of Oregon, PhD dissertation. https://scholarsbank.uoregon.edu/xmlui/bitstream/handle/1794/12366/Donnelly_oregon_0171A_10353.pdf?sequence=1&isAllowed=y.

Drazen, Carlos Clarke. 2011."Both Sides of the Two-Sided Coin: Rehabilitation of Disabled African American Soldiers." In *Blackness and Disability: Critical Examinations* and *Cultural Interventions*, edited by Christopher M. Bell, 149–162. East Lansing: Michigan State University Press and LIT Verlag.

Erevelles, Nirmala. 2011. *Disability and Difference in Global Contexts: Enabling a Transformative Body Politic.* New York: Palgrave MacMillan. https://doi.org/10.1057/9781137001184

Foucault, Michel. 2006. *History of Madness.* Translated by Jean Khalfa. Abingdon: Routledge.

Garland-Thomson, Rosemarie. 1997. *Extraordinary Bodies: Figuring Physical Disability in American Culture and Literature.* New York: Columbia University Press.

Geary, Daniel. 2011. "Racial Liberalism, the Moynihan Report & the 'Dædalus' Project on 'The Negro American.'" *Dædalus* 140 (1): 53–66. https://doi.org/10.1162/DAED_a_00058

Gill, Michael, and Nirmala Erevelles. 2017. "The Absent Presence of Elsie Lacks: Hauntings at the Intersection of Race, Class, Gender, and Disability." *African American Review* 50 (2): 123–37. https://doi.org/10.1353/afa.2017.0017

Goldberg, Michelle. 2018. "Opinion | Trump Is Cracking Up." Accessed March 13. https://www.nytimes.com/2017/12/01/opinion/trump-is-cracking-up.html.

Graham, David A. 2018. "Gaffe Track: Donald Trump Mocks a Disabled Reporter - The Atlantic." Accessed March 13. https://www.theatlantic.com/notes/2015/11/gaffe-track-donald-trump-mocks-a-disabled-reporter/418008/.

Griffin, Farah Jasmine. 2014. "Public Humanities: Crisis and Possibility." *Profession.* https://profession.mla.org/public-humanities-crisis-and-possibility/.

Heiland, Donna, and Mary Taylor Huber. 2015. "Building Capacity for Civic Learning and Engagement: An Emerging Infrastructure in the Academic Arts and Humanities in the United States." *Arts and Humanities in Higher Education* 14 (3): 260–273. https://doi.org/10.1177/1474022215583946

Hilton, Leon J. 2017. "Avonte's Law: Autism, Wandering, and the Racial Surveillance of Neurological Difference." *African American Review* 50 (2): 221–235. https://doi.org/10.1353/afa.2017.0023

Hunt, Patricia. 1993. "War and Peace: Transfigured Categories and the Politics of *Sula.*" *African American Review* 27 (3): 443–459. https://doi.org/10.2307/3041934

Idol, Kimberley. 2017. "Contemplating the Void: How Narrative Overcomes Anonymity in Toni Morrison's *Sula.*" *Interdisciplinary Literary Studies* 19 (1): 48–68. https://doi.org/10.5325/intelitestud.19.1.0048

Jackson, Chuck. 2006. "A Headless Display: Sula, Soldiers, and Lynching." *MFS Modern Fiction Studies* 52 (2): 374–392. https://doi.org/10.1353/mfs.2006.0048

Jarman, Michelle. 2011. "Coming up from Underground: Uneasy Dialogues at the Intersections of Race, Mental Illness, and Disability Studies." In *Blackness and Disability: Critical Examinations and Cultural Interventions*, edited by Christopher M. Bell, 9–30. East Lansing: Michigan State University Press and LIT Verlag.

Johnson, Merri Lisa. 2015. "Bad Romance: A Crip Feminist Critique of Queer Failure." *Hypatia* 30 (1): 251–67. https://doi.org/10.1111/hypa.12134 Bad Romance: A Crip Feminist Critique of Queer

Jones, Audrey L., Susan D. Cochran, Arleen Leibowitz, Kenneth B. Wells, Gerald Kominski, and Vickie M. Mays. 2018. "Racial, Ethnic, and Nativity Differences in Mental Health Visits to Primary Care and Specialty Mental Health Providers: Analysis of the Medical Expenditures Panel Survey, 2010–2015." *Healthcare* 6 (2). https://doi.org/10.3390/healthcare6020029

Kafer, Alison. 2016. "Un/Safe Disclosures: Scenes of Disability and Trauma." *Journal of Literary & Cultural Disability Studies* 10 (1): 1–20. https://doi.org/10.3828/jlcds.2016.1

Keating, Frank. 2015. "Linking 'Race," Mental Health and a Social Model of Disability: What Are the Possibilities?" In *Madness, Distress, and the Politics of Disablement*, edited by Helen Spandler, Jill Anderson, and Bob Sapey. Bristol: Policy Press, 127–138. https://doi.org/10.2307/j.ctt1t898sg.14

LeFrançois, Brenda A., Robert Menzies, and Geoffrey Reaume, eds. 2013. *Mad Matters: A Critical Reading in Canadian Mad Studies*. Toronto: Canadian Scholars' Press, Inc.

Lewis, Bradley. 2017. "Postmodern Madness on Campus: Narrating and Navigating Mental Difference and Disability." In *Negotiating Disability: Disclosure and Higher Education*, edited by Stephanie L. Kerschbaum, Laura T. Eisenman, and James M. Jones, 191–210. Ann Arbor: University of Michigan Press.

Lewis, Vashti Crutcher. 1987. "African Tradition in Toni Morrison's *Sula*." *Phylon* 48 (1): 1–97. https://doi.org/10.2307/275004

Lukin, Josh. 2013. "Disability and Blackness." In *The Disability Studies Reader*, edited by Lennard J. Davis, 308–315.

Mayberry, Susan Neal. 2003. "Something Other than a Family Quarrel: The Beautiful Boys in Morrison's *Sula*." *African American Review* 37 (4): 517–533. https://doi.org/10.2307/1512384

McWade, Brigit, Damian Milton, and Peter Beresford. 2015. "Mad Studies and Neurodiversity: A Dialogue." *Disability & Society* 30 (2): 305–9. https://doi.org/10.1080/09687599.2014.1000512

Milbank, Dana. 2017. "Opinion | President Trump Actually Is Making Us Crazy." *Washington Post*, September 22, sec. Opinions. https://www.washingtonpost.com/opinions/president-trump-actually-is-making-us-crazy/2017/09/22/a6f3d76c-9fb1-11e7-9083-fbfddf6804c2_story.html.

Mollow, Anna. 2006. "'When Black Women Start Going on Prozac': Race, Gender, and Mental Illness in Meri Nana-Ama Danquah's *Willow Weep for Me*." *MELUS* 31 (3): 67–99. https://doi.org/10.1093/melus/31.3.67

Mollow, Anna. 2013. "Mad Feminism." *SocialText Online: Periscope*. https://socialtextjournal.org/periscope_article/mad-feminism/.

Montgomery, Maxine Lavon. 1989. "A Pilgrimage to the Origins: The Apocalypse as Structure and Theme in Toni Morrison's *Sula*." *Black American Literature Forum* 23 (1): 127–137. https://doi.org/10.2307/2903996

Morrison, Toni. 1993. *Playing in the Dark: Whiteness and the Literary Imagination*. 1st Vintage Books ed. New York: Vintage Books.

Morrison, Toni. 1973. *Sula*. New York: Knopf.

Novak, Phillip. 1999. "'Circles and Circles of Sorrow': In the Wake of Morrison's *Sula*." *PMLA* 114 (2): 184–193. https://doi.org/10.2307/463390

NPR Talk of the Town. 2012. "Behind Mental Health Stigmas in Black Communities." https://www.npr.org/2012/08/20/159376802/behind-mental-health-stigmas-in-black-communities.

Ogunyemi, Chikwenye Okonjo. 1979. "Sula: 'A Nigger Joke'." *Black American Literature Forum* 13 (4): 130–133. https://doi.org/10.2307/3041477

Patsavas, Alyson. 2014. "Recovering a Cripistemology of Pain: Leaky Bodies, Connective Tissue, and Feeling Discourse." *Journal of Literary & Cultural Disability Studies* 8 (2): 203–218. https://doi.org/10.3828/jlcds.2014.16

Pickens, Therí A. 2017a. "Blue Blackness, Black Blueness: Making Sense of Blackness and Disability." *African American Review* 50 (2): 93–103. https://doi.org/10.1353/afa.2017.0015

Pickens, Therí A. 2017b. "Satire, Scholarship, and Sanity; or How to Make Mad Professors." In *Negotiating Disability: Disclosure and Higher Education*, edited by Stephanie L. Kerschbaum, Laura T. Eisenman, and James M. Jones, 243–254. Ann Arbor: University of Michigan Press.

Price, Margaret. 2011. *Mad at School: Rhetorics of Mental Disability and Academic Life.* Ann Arbor: University of Michigan Press. https://doi.org/10.3998/mpub.1612837

Price, Margaret, et al. 2017. "Disclosure of Mental Disability by College and University Faculty: The Negotiation of Accommodations, Supports, and Barriers." *Disability Studies Quarterly* 37 (2). https://doi.org/10.18061/dsq.v37i2.5487

Pruitt, Claude. 2011. "Circling Meaning in Toni Morrison's *Sula*." *African American Review* 44 (1–2): 115–129. https://doi.org/10.1353/afa.2011.0009

Puar, Jasbir. 2017. *The Right to Maim: Debility, Capacity, Disability.* Durham: Duke University Press. https://doi.org/10.1215/9780822372530

Ramírez, Manuela López. 2016. "The Shell-Shocked Veteran in Toni Morrison's *Sula* and *Home*." *Atlantis: Journal of the Spanish Association of Anglo-American Studies* 38 (1): 129–147.

Reville, David. 2013. "Is Mad Studies Emerging as a New Field of Inquiry?" In *Mad Matters: A Critical Reading in Canadian Mad Studies*, edited by Brenda A. LeFrançois, Robert Menzies, and Geoffrey Reaume, 170–180. Toronto: Canadian Scholars' Press, Inc.

Schalk, Sami. 2018. *Bodyminds Reimagined: (Dis)ability, Race, and Gender in Black Women's Speculative Fiction.* Durham: Duke University Press.

Shumway, David R. 2016. "Why the Humanities Must Be Public." *University of Toronto Quarterly: A Canadian Journal of the Humanities* 85 (4): 33–45. https://doi.org/10.3138/utq.85.4.33

Stein, Sorah, and Karola Dillenburger. 2016. "Ethics in Sexual Behavior Assessment and Support for People with Intellectual Disability." *International Journal on Disability and Human Development* 16 (1): 11–17. https://doi.org/10.1515/ijdhd-2016-0023

Taylor, Jessica. 2018. "11 Times Donald Trump Looked Like He Was Done For." *NPR.org.* Accessed March 13. https://www.npr.org/2016/12/28/506342901/11-times-donald-trump-looked-like-he-was-done-for.

Thurschwell, Pamela. 2013. "Dead Boys and Adolescent Girls: Unjoining the Bildungsroman in Carson McCullers's The Member of the Wedding and Toni Morrison's Sula." *ESC: English Studies in Canada* 38 (3–4): 105–28. https://doi.org/10.1353/esc.2013.0002

U.S. Department of Labor. 1965. *The Negro Family: The Case for National Action.* Washington, DC: GPO.

Waxman, Barbara Faye. 1994. "Up against Eugenics: Disabled Women's Challenge to Receive Reproductive Health Services." *Sexuality and Disability* 12 (2): 155–71. https://doi.org/10.1007/BF02547889

Wessely, Simon. 2006. "Twentieth-Century Theories on Combat Motivation and Breakdown." *Journal of Contemporary Literature* 41 (2): 269–286. https://doi.org/10.1177/0022009406062067

Willis, Susan. 1982. "Eruptions of Funk: Historicizing Toni Morrison." *Black American Literature Forum* 16 (1): 34–42. https://doi.org/10.2307/2904271

How to Go Mad without Losing Your Mind: Notes toward a Mad Methodology[1]

La Marr Jurelle Bruce

Summary

La Marr Jurelle Bruce begins this chapter with an imaginative and evocative link between Michel Foucault's work on early modernity's ship of fools and Hortense Spiller's work on the slave ships of the Middle Passage. Both ships are historical emblems of othering and exclusion that shore up the identities of those who are left on shore. As Foucault (2009) reminds us, using a quote from Dostoevsky: "It is not [or should not be] by locking up one's neighbor that one convinces oneself of one's own good sense" (xxvii). Bruce brings these ships together in our imagination to help us see the intersectional roots of sanism and racism as they converge in the discursive practices of early Euromodernity: "According to the era's emergent anti-Black and antimad worldviews, both of these ships were floating graveyards of the socially dead. Both ships were imagined to haul inferior, unReasonable beings who were metaphysically adrift amid the rising tide of Reason."

Bruce enters the fray of this fraught legacy, where social constructions of difference and hierarchical relations of difference inextricably comingle with real-life consequences, exclusions, treatments, and otherings. As Bruce puts it, "On the one hand, madness is a floating signifier and dynamic social construction that evades stable definition. On the other hand, or maybe on the same hand, madness is a lived reality that demands sustained attention." Bruce engages this complexity through the creation of a "mad methodology" that is agile enough to keep these tensions alive.

DOI: 10.4324/9781003148456-19

He teases out four overlapping meanings of "madness" that commonly intersect and interact with each other whenever we try to think of mental difference: (1) the lived experience of an "unruly mind"; (2) the psychiatric category of "serious mental illness"; (3) the emotional state also known as "rage"; and (4) any drastic deviation from psychosocial norms. By keeping these multiple meanings alive, Bruce creates an approach to mental difference in which the psychosocial work regarding madness—responding to, critiquing, and moving beyond norms—does not simply collapse into biopsychiatric categories of pathology. At the same time, he does not forget the real consequences of all these comingled meanings.

*

> Confined on the ship, from which there is no escape, the madman is delivered to the river with its thousand arms, the sea with its thousand roads, to the great uncertainty external to everything. He is the Passenger par excellence: that is, the prisoner of the passage. And the land he will come to is unknown—as is, once he disembarks, the land from which he comes. He has his truth and his homeland only in that *fruitless expanse* between two countries that cannot belong to him.
>
> —Michel Foucault, *Madness and Civilization: A
> History of Insanity in the Age of Reason*, 1961

> Those African persons in "Middle Passage" were literally suspended in the "oceanic." ... [R]emoved from the indigenous land and culture, and not-yet "American" either, these captive persons, without names that their captors would recognize, were in movement across the Atlantic, but they were also *nowhere at all*.
>
> —Hortense Spillers, "Mama's Baby, Papa's Maybe:
> An American Grammar Book," 1987

Prelude: Mad Is a Place

HOLD TIGHT. THE WAY TO GO MAD WITHOUT LOSING YOUR MIND IS SOMETIMES UNRULY. It might send you staggering across asylum hallways, heckled by disembodied voices—or shimmying over spotlit stages, greeted by loving applause. It might find you freewheeling through fever dreams, then marching toward freedom dreams, then scrambling from sleep, with blood and stars in your eyes, the whole world a waking dream.[2] But for now, we begin in a liquid void, among ominous ships.

The epigraphs above, culled from the French philosopher Michel Foucault and the black feminist theorist Hortense Spillers, are our floating signposts. They point us to the intersection of a "fruitless expanse" and "nowhere at all": an unmappable coordinate where a ship of fools crosses a slave ship, where imprisoned madness meets captive blackness in a groundless vastness. I shudder and flounder as I wonder: What vertigo does a body undergo, caught between treacherous waters below and treacherous captors above, with "nowhere" outside? How does it feel to be forcibly moved across the sea while forcibly stagnated on the ship—to endure a cruelty in motion that is also a cruelty of stillness? What is it like to be utterly enclosed on the ship and utterly exposed to the whim and will of its captor captain? What noise might ring out if the sound of a laughing "fool" joined the sound of a weeping "slave"—and would the weeper and laugher commiserate? How does one keep time, or discern direction, or remember the way home from "nowhere at all," with no familiar beacon to behold ahead or behind? It seems to me that neither imagination nor historiography is apt to apprehend the seasickness of spirit, the existential dread, and the feverish homesickness that might menace a mad prisoner or black captive trapped at sea.

An unimaginable scene may seem a strange place to launch a study of radical imagination. Likewise, a fruitless expanse makes a bleak backdrop for pondering the fruit of mad black creativity. And furthermore, unanswerable questions may sound odd when opening a work of careful inquiry. But there are lessons to learn from those who make homeland in wasteland, freedom routes to chart that start in a ship's hull, debris of mad and black life to retrieve from the sea, mad black worlds to make that rise from a ship's wake, and questions that refuse answers but rouse movements.[3] And besides, if the anticolonial psychiatrist Frantz Fanon is right, if there is "a zone of nonbeing … an utterly naked declivity where an authentic upheaval can be born,"[4] then "nowhere at all" may be an especially auspicious place to commence. By beginning at this curious crossing, I also hope to orient the reader—which requires that I *disorient* the reader—for the errant, erratic routes to come. Remember that the way is sometimes unruly.

Those opening epigraphs are passages of prose conjuring cataclysmic passages of persons across temporal, spatial, and metaphysical gauntlets. In the first epigraph, Foucault chases a "ship of fools" as it crisscrosses early modern Europe. To have him tell it, ships of fools were fifteenth-century nautical vessels whose lunatic occupants were deemed nuisances to their communities, expelled from home, made wards of sailors, and consigned to those ships as they drifted along European rivers and seas. When Foucault declares that the mad seafarer has "his truth and his homeland only in that fruitless expanse between two countries that cannot belong to him," the words evoke a *mad diaspora*: a scattering of captives across sovereign borders and over bodies of water; an upheaval and dispersal of persons flung far from home; and an emergence of unprecedented diasporic subjectivities, ontologies, and possibilities that transgress national and rational norms.

To a scholar of black modernity, Foucault's account may ring uncannily familiar. It brings to my mind many millions of Africans abducted from their native lands by slave traders in the fifteenth through nineteenth centuries. These stolen people were stacked in the putrid pits of slave ships; made "prisoner of the passage" called the Middle Passage; uprooted from solid "truth" and stable "homeland"; drenched, instead, in oceanic uncertainty; dragged across a "fruitless expanse"; discharged onto a land that, arguably, "cannot belong to" them; and cast into restlessness and rootlessness that persist in many of their descendants.

In the second epigraph, Spillers describes the Passage, and her words bear repeating: "Removed from the indigenous land and culture, and not-yet 'American' either, these captive persons, without names that their captors would recognize, were in movement across the Atlantic, but they were also *nowhere* at all." Some pessimists claim that the progeny of slaves are still not American, still vainly awaiting recognition as citizen and affirmation as human, still existentially captive, still suspended in that void.[5] Wherever blackness dwells—slave ship, spaceship, graveyard, garden, elsewhere, everywhere—those captives accessed what Spillers calls a "richness of *possibility*."[6] They would realize black diasporic mobility, sociality, kinship, creativity, love, and myriad modes of being that flourish in their marvelously tenacious heirs. In a "fruitless expanse," the enslaved bore fruit. The pit held seeds, as pits sometimes do.

Both the ship of fools and the slave ship provoke historiographic dispute. Regarding the ship of fools, many historians insist that Foucault mistook an early modern literary and visual motif for a material vessel.[7] As for the slave ship, it incites crises of calculation about the number of Africans who made it to *the other side*—by which I mean *the Americas* and/or/as *the afterlife*—and about the depth of the wound that the Middle Passage inflicts on modernity.[8] Both ships defy positivist history: the ship of fools because it was likely unreal; the slave ship because it is so devastatingly real that it confounds comprehension, resists documentation, and spawns ongoing effects that belie the purported *pastness* of history. It is no wonder that when Spillers wanted to address the historical and ontological functions of the Middle Passage and its ripples across modernity, particularly black female modernity, she realized that "the language of the historian was not telling me what I needed to know."[9] (Perhaps the language of the mad methodologist, who I will introduce shortly, can better speak to Spillers's concerns.) Spillers further characterizes the Middle Passage as a "dehumanizing, ungendering, and defacing project"—and I would add *deranging* to that grave litany.[10] To *derange* is to throw off, to cast askew, "to disturb the order or arrangement of" an entity. The Middle Passage literally deranged and threw millions of Africans askew across continents, oceans, centuries, and worlds.[11] I use *derange* also to signal how the Atlantic slave trade, and the antiblack modernity it inaugurated, cast black beings as always already wild, subrational, pathological, mentally unsound, mad.

Although it is unlikely that a slave ship ever crossed a ship of fools in geographic space,[12] these vessels converged in the discursive domains and cultural imaginations of early Euromodernity. According to the era's emergent antiblack and antimad worldviews, both of these ships were floating graveyards of the socially dead. Both ships were imagined to haul inferior, unReasonable beings who were metaphysically adrift amid the rising tide of Reason. For the purposes of this study, I distinguish *reason* (lowercase) from *Reason* (uppercase). The former, *reason*, signifies a generic process of cognition within a given system of logic and the "mental powers concerned with forming conclusions, judgments, or inferences."[13] Meanwhile, *Reason* is a proper noun denoting a positivist, secularist, Enlightenment-rooted episteme purported to uphold objective "truth" while mapping and mastering the world. In normative Western philosophy since the Age of Enlightenment, Reason and rationality are believed essential for achieving modern personhood, joining civil society, and participating in liberal politics.[14] However, Reason has been entangled, from those very Enlightenment roots, with misogynist, colonialist, antiblack, and other pernicious ideologies. The fact is that female people, indigenous people, colonized people, and black people have been violently excluded from the edifice of Enlightenment Reason—with Reasonable doctrines justifying those exclusions.[15]

Regarding the hegemony of Reason, political theorist Achille Mbembe remarks that

> it is on the basis of a distinction between reason and unreason (passion, fantasy) that late-modern criticism has been able to articulate a certain idea of the political, the community, the subject—or, more fundamentally, of what the good life is all about, how to achieve it, and, in the process, to become a fully moral agent. The exercise of reason is tantamount to the exercise of freedom.[16]

While Mbembe names "passion" and "fantasy" as examples of "unreason," a third entry belongs on this list: madness itself. If those late-modern critics claim that Reason is requisite for "becoming a fully moral agent," they also imply the inverse—that unReason entails moral deficiency and ineptitude. (This is why throes of *passion*, flights of *fantasy*, and bouts of *madness* are thought inimical to one's moral sense.) Likewise, insofar as "late-modern criticism" insists that "the exercise of reason is tantamount to the exercise of freedom," it also insinuates the inverse—that the condition of unReason is commensurate with the condition of unfreedom. While Mbembe's point of reference is late modernity, Enlightenment-era philosophers like David Hume, Immanuel Kant, Thomas Jefferson, and Georg Wilhelm Friedrich Hegel also asserted that unReasonable beings are suited for unfreedom, that the unReason of Africans ordained them for enslavement.[17] Within white supremacist and antiblack master narratives that calcified in the seventeenth and eighteenth centuries, to be white-*cum*-rational was to inherit modernity's pantheon and merit freedom; to be black-*cum*-subrational was to be barred from modernity's favor and primed for slavery. The modern European affirmed "his" Reason and freedom, in part, by casting the black African as his ontological foil, his unReasonable and enslaved Other.

In staging this encounter between the slave ship and ship of fools, I do not intend to imply a simplistic analogy between the two. Rather, I want to suggest that the slave ship (icon of abject blackness) commandeers the ship of fools (icon of abject madness), tows the ship of fools, helps orient Western notions of madness and Reason, and helps propel this turbulent movement we call modernity.[18]

How to Go Mad: Theory and Methodology

My critical account of madness in modernity proceeds from two premises. On the one hand, madness is a floating signifier and dynamic social construction that evades stable definition. On the other hand, or maybe in the same hand, madness is a lived reality that demands sustained attention. Accounting for these exigencies, I forward a model of madness that is theoretically agile enough to chase floating signifiers and ethically rooted enough to hold deep compassion for madpersons. Thus primed, I propose that madness encompasses at least four overlapping entities in the modern West.

First is *phenomenal madness*: an intense unruliness of mind—producing fundamental crises of perception, emotion, meaning, and selfhood—as experienced in the consciousness of the mad subject. This unruliness may induce distress, despair, exhilaration, euphoria, and innumerable other sensations. In elaborating this mode of madness, I favor a phenomenological attitude attuned to whatever presents itself to consciousness, including hallucinations and delusions that have no material basis. Most important, phenomenal madness centers the lived experience and first-person interiority of the mad subject, rather than, say, the diagnoses imposed by medical authority.

Such diagnoses are the basis of *medicalized madness*, the second category in this schema. Medicalized madness encompasses a range of "serious mental illnesses" and psychopathologies codified by the psy sciences of psychiatry, psychology, and psychoanalysis. These "serious" conditions include schizophrenia, dissociative identity disorder, bipolar disorder, borderline personality disorder, and the antiquated diagnosis of medical "insanity," among others.[19] I label this category medical*ize*d madness—emphasizing the suffix *-ize*, meaning *to become* or *to cause to become*—to signal that mental illness is a politicized *process*, epistemological *operation*, and sociohistorical *construction*, rather than an ontological *given*.

Even forms of medicalized madness that are measurable in brain tissue physiology, neuroelectric currents, and other empirical criteria are infiltrated (and sometimes constituted) by sociocultural forces. The creation, standardization, collection, and interpretation of psychiatric metrics take place in the crucible of culture. Likewise, clinical procedures are designed and carried out by subjective persons embedded in webs of social relations and ideological dispositions. In short, psychiatry is susceptible to ideology. Exploiting that susceptibility, various antiblack, proslavery, patriarchal, colonialist, homophobic, and transphobic regimes have wielded psychiatry as a tool of domination. Thus, acts and attributes such as insurgent blackness, slave rebellion, willful womanhood, anticolonial resistance, same-sex desire, and gender subversion have all been pathologized by Western psychiatric science.[20] Beyond these overt examples of hegemonic psychiatry, I want to emphasize that no diagnosis is innocently objective. No etiology escapes the touch and taint of ideology. No science is pure.[21]

The third mode of madness is *rage*: an affective state of intense and aggressive displeasure (which is surely phenomenal but warrants analytic distinction from the unruliness above). Black people in the United States and elsewhere have been subjected to heinous violence and degradation, but rarely granted recourse. Consequently, black people have plenty of reasons to be mad. Alas, when they articulate rage in American public spheres, black people are often criminalized as threats to public safety, lampooned as angry black caricatures, and pathologized as insane. That latter process—the conflation of black anger and black insanity—parallels the Anglophone confluence of *madness* meaning anger and *madness* meaning insanity. In short, when black people get mad (as in *angry*), antiblack logics tend to presume they've gone mad (as in *crazy*).

The fourth and most capacious category in this framework is *psychosocial madness*: radical deviation from the *normal* within a given psychosocial milieu. Any person or practice that perplexes and vexes the psychonormative status quo is liable to be labeled *crazy*. The arbiters of psychosocial madness are not elite cohorts of psychiatric experts, but rather the vast constituency of public spheres whose members abide by psychonormative common sense. Thus, psychosocial madness reflects how avowedly sane majorities interpellate and often denigrate difference. What I have already stated about medicalized madness also applies to psychosocial madness: acts and attributes such as insurgent blackness, slave rebellion, willful womanhood, anticolonial resistance, same-sex desire, and gender subversion have all been ostracized as *crazy* by sane majorities who adhere to Reasonable common sense. Whereas phenomenal madness is an internal *unruliness of mind*, psychosocial madness might be described as an *unruliness of will* that resists and unsettles reigning regimes of the normal.

In its psychosocial iteration, madness often functions as a disparaging descriptor for any mundane phenomenon perceived to be odd and undesirable. An unconventional hairstyle, unpopular political opinion, physical tic, indecipherable utterance, eccentric outfit, dramatic flouting of etiquette, apathy toward money and wealth, or experience of spiritual ecstasy might be coded as *crazy* in psychonormative discourse. Yet it seems to me that psychosocial madness reveals more about the avowedly sane society branding an object crazy than about the object so branded. When you point at someone or something and shout *Crazy!*, you have revealed more about yourself— about your sensibility, your values, your attentions, your notion of the normal, the limits of your imagination in processing dramatic difference, the terms you use to describe the world, the reach of your pointing finger, the lilt of your accusatory voice—than you have revealed about that supposedly mad entity.[22]

These four categories are not all-encompassing and do not cover every possible permutation of madness. Furthermore, these four categories are not mutually exclusive; in fact, they often intersect and converge. *Rage*, for example, is always also *phenomenal*. Discourses of *medicalized* madness attempt to make sense of *phenomenal* symptoms and inevitably harbor *psychosocial* biases. When black people articulate *rage* at unjust social conditions are often coded as *psychosocial* others (and sometimes diagnosed as *medically* unsound). The spillage of these categories into one another reminds us that madness is too messy to be placed in tidy boxes and too restless to hold still for rigid frameworks.

Beyond approaching madness as an object of analysis, I adapt madness as methodology. As I propose and practice it, *mad methodology* is a mad ensemble of epistemological modes, political praxes, interpretive techniques, affective dispositions, existential orientations, and ways of life.

Mad methodology seeks, follows, and rides the unruly movements of madness. It reads and hears *idioms of madness*: those rants, raves, rambles, outbursts, mumbles, stammers, slurs, gibberish sounds, and unseemly silences that defy the grammars of Reason. It historicizes and contextualizes madness as a social construction and social relation vis-à-vis Reason. It ponders the sporadic violence of madness in tandem and in tension with the structural violence of Reason. It cultivates critical ambivalence[23] to reckon with the simultaneous harm and benefit that may accompany madness. It respects and sometimes harnesses "mad" feelings like obsession and rage as stimulus for radical thought and practice. Whereas rationalism roundly discredits madpersons, mad methodology recognizes madpersons as critical theorists and decisive protagonists in struggles for liberation. To be clear, I am not suggesting that madpersons are always already agents of liberation. I am simply and assuredly acknowledging that they can be, which is a remarkable admission amid antimad worlds. I propose a mad methodology that neither vilifies the madperson as evil incarnate, nor romanticizes the madperson as resistance personified, nor patronizes the madperson as helpless ward awaiting aid. Rather, mad methodology engages the complexity and variability of mad subjects.

Regarding anger, Audre Lorde asserts that it is "loaded with information and energy."[24] Mad methodology is rooted in the recognition that phenomenal madness, medicalized madness, and psychosocial madness, like angry madness, are all "loaded with information and energy." Mad methodology proceeds from a belief that such information can instruct black radical theory and such energy can animate black radical praxis.

Most urgently, mad methodology primes us to extend *radical compassion* to the madpersons, queer personae, ghosts, freaks, weirdos, imaginary friends, disembodied voices, unvoiced bodies, and unReasonable others, who trespass, like stowaways or fugitives, in Reasonable modernity. Radical compassion is a will to care for, a commitment to feel with, a striving to learn from, and an openness to being vulnerable before a precarious other, though they may be drastically dissimilar to yourself. Radical compassion is not a naïve appeal to an idyllic oneness where subjectivities converge and difference is blithely effaced. Nor is it a smug projection of oneself into the position of another, consequently displacing that other.[25] Nor is it an invitation to walk a mile in someone else's shoes and amble, like a tourist, through their lifeworld, leaving them existentially barefoot all the while. Rather, radical compassion is an exhortation to ethically walk and sit and fight and build alongside another whose condition may be utterly unlike your own. Radical compassion works to impart care, exchange feeling, transmit understanding, embolden vulnerability, and fortify solidarity across circumstantial, sociocultural, phenomenological, and ontological chasms. It persists even and especially toward beings who are the objects of contempt and condemnation from dominant value systems. It extends even and especially to those who discomfit one's own sense of propriety. Indeed, this book [chapter] sometimes loiters in scenes and tarries with people who may trouble readers. I hope that this book [chapter] also models the sort of radical compassion that persists through the trouble.

I characterize mad methodology as a parapositivist approach insofar as it resists the hegemony of positivism. (As a philosophical doctrine, positivism stipulates that meaningful assertions about the world must come from empirical observation and interpretation to generate veritable truth. However, when engaging the phenomenal, the spiritual, the aesthetic, the affective, and the mad, we must frequently deviate from the logics of positivism.[26]) As a parapositivist approach, mad methodology does not attempt to wholly, transparently reveal madness.[27] How could it? Madness, after all, resists intelligibility and frustrates interpretation. Conceding that I cannot fully understand the meaning of every madness I encounter, I often precede my observations with the qualifiers *maybe*, *it might be*, and *it seems*. In studying madness, I have come to accept and embrace uncertainty and irresolution. I heed poet-philosopher Glissant's insistence that "the transparency of the Enlightenment is finally misleading. ... It is not necessary to understand someone—in the verb 'to understand' [French: *comprendre*] there is the verb 'to take' [French: *prendre*]—in order to wish to live with them."[28] I want to *live with* the madpersons gathered in this study, but I do not need or want to *take* them. I strive to *pursue* madness, but not to *capture* it. Recall that I began this chapter by warning you to *hold tight*. Mad methodology also, sometimes, entails *letting go*: relinquishing the imperative to know, to take, to capture, to master, to lay bare all the world with its countless terrors and wonders. Sometimes we must hold tight to steady ourselves amid the violent tumult of this world—and sometimes we must let go to free ourselves from the stifling order imposed on this world. I am describing a deft dance between release and hold, hold and release. In short, mad methodology is how to go mad without losing your mind.

Drapetomaniacal Slaves and Rebels

Some of those captives in slave ships leaped from the decks of those vessels and into the Atlantic Ocean, choosing biological death over the wretchedness that sociologist Orlando Patterson deems "social death."[29] Psychiatry tends to label such acts *suicide* and pathologize them as the outcome of utter hopelessness and absolute self-abnegation. While the frame of psychopathology is apt for apprehending why some people take their own lives, it cannot hold all those Flying Africans. Amid the misery of the Middle Passage, suicidal ideation might be a mode of radical dreaming, an urge to escape to a distant elsewhere in an afterlife, otherworld, ancestral gathering place, heaven, or home. For the captive on the ship, suicide might be an act of radical self-care, intended to relieve and leave the hurt of the ship's hold and expedite arrival in that elsewhere.[30] Sometimes the leap was not a plummet to doom, but a launch into flight; not an outcome of self-abnegation, but an act of self-assertion; not a descent to a bog of hopelessness, but an outburst of radical hope hurled into another world. To be clear, I do not glibly romanticize suicide; I know and ardently assert that each life is sacred, singular, precious, miraculous, and should be treated with ineffable care. At the same time, I acknowledge that there are conditions of unbearable duress where taking one's own life might be a critical, ethical, radical act—albeit dreadful and woeful, too. *How to Go Mad* attends to people and practices who, like those Flying Africans, will not be captured by normative Reason.

By the nineteenth century, the slave ship gave way to the plantation as the paradigmatic site of black abjection and confinement in the Western Hemisphere. Meanwhile, the ship of fools, if it ever existed, was succeeded by the prison house and later the asylum as the West's preferred receptacle for the allegedly insane.[31] Amid these shifts, the association of blackness and madness remained. In antebellum America, that association manifested in the similar logics used to justify the plantation and the asylum. Literary and cultural historian Benjamin Reiss writes that

> both institutions revoked the civil liberties of a confined population in the name of public order and the creation of an efficient labor force, and both housed a purportedly subrational population … with the asylum's triumph over madness paralleling the white race's subduing of the black.[32]

The plantation and asylum were forums in which arbiters of antebellum Reason rehearsed methods of domination and developed logics of justification.

I want to linger at the site of the asylum to highlight the salience of space and movement in modern notions of madness. Within Anglophone idiom, subjects *go* crazy, as though mad is a place or constellation of places. The ship of fools, the insane asylum, the psychiatric hospital, the carnival, the wrong side of the supposed line between genius and madness, and even the continent of Africa are frequently mapped as mad places within Western discourse. It is as though madness is a metaphysical zone, a location outside the gentrified precincts and patrolled borders of Reason. Or maybe madness is a mode of motion occasioned in treacherous terrain: a wavering, trembling, swelling, zigzagging, brimming, bursting, shattering, or splattering movement that disrupts Reason's supposedly steady order and tidy borders. It seems to me that madness, like diaspora, is both location and locomotion. Madness, like diaspora, is both place and process.[33] Madness, like diaspora, transgresses normative arrangements—of the sane and sovereign, in turn.

The transgressive motion of fugitive slaves was framed as madness-as-kinesis by proslavery psychiatry. In 1851, the prominent Confederate physician Samuel Cartwright coined *drapetomania*, which he described as "the disease causing Negroes to run away" from their God-ordained place at the foot of the slaveholder in the muck of the plantation.[34] As formulated by Cartwright, drapetomania is a racialized diagnosis that exclusively afflicts "Negroes"-as-slaves, reflecting an antebellum antiblack insistence on conflating *blackness* and *slaveness*.[35] Of course, this discursive conflation was allied with the material, legal, and existential yoking of blackness and slaveness in chattel slavery.

Cartwright further argues that "the cause in the most of cases, that induces the negro to away from service, is as much a disease of the mind as any other species of mental alienation, and much more curable, as a general rule." He suggests that drapetomania can be cured if the slaveholder upholds a dual role as disciplinarian master (with the use of the whip, so that slaves will fearfully obey) and paternalistic protector (so that slaves will be made agreeable by bonds of affection and the incentive of protection).[36] In pathologizing black self-emancipation, Cartwright joins a proslavery, antiblack conspiracy against black freedom: antiblack slave codes criminalized black freedom; antiblack religion demonized black freedom; antiblack philosophy stigmatized black freedom; and antiblack slaveholders and vigilantes terrorized black freedom. It is no wonder, then, that antiblack medicine would pathologize black freedom. Under the obscene regime and episteme of antebellum slavery, black freedom was crime, sin, stigma, liability, and sickness, too.

Whereas drapetomania supposedly compelled black people to flee servitude, Cartwright coined another psychopathology to ail them once they found freedom. He writes that "Dysaesthesia Aethiopica is a disease peculiar to negroes, affecting both mind and body. ... [I]t prevails among free negroes, nearly all of whom are more or less afflicted with it, that have not got some white person to direct and to take care of them." Cartwright claims that black people are constitutionally unfit for freedom, sickened by it, and that they are mentally and physically healthier when enslaved. To have Cartwright tell it, the motley symptoms of dysaesthesia aethiopica include cognitive decline, lethargy, lesions, and skin insensitivity. In a flourish of melodramatic antiblackness, he decrees that to "narrate [dysaesthesia aethiopica's] symptoms and effects among them would be to write a history of the ruins and dilapidation of Hayti, and every spot of earth they have ever had uncontrolled possession over for any length of time."[37] He names the first free black republic as ground zero in a sort of hemispheric epidemic of dysaesthesia aethiopica. If mad is a place, according to Cartwright, it might be "Hayti."[38]

The notion that slavery was salutary for black people also infused antebellum political rhetoric. John C. Calhoun, an eminent nineteenth-century politician whose career included stints as US Secretary of State and US Vice President, offered this justification for antiblack chattel slavery circa 1840: "Here is proof of the necessity of slavery. The African is incapable of self-care and sinks into lunacy under the burden of freedom. It is a mercy to him to give him the guardianship and protection from mental death."[39] Calhoun claims that freedom will career Africans into lunacy, into a helpless and mindless oblivion that he deems "mental death." If slavery was social death and freedom was mental death, those Africans were caught in a deadly double-bind—doomed one way or another. Within the wicked machinations and pernicious logics of antebellum antiblackness, black people, whether enslaved or free, were the living dead.

Beyond *discursive* conflations of blackness and madness, slavery induced *lived* convergences of blackness and madness. It perpetrated systematic trauma, induced mental distress, and ignited crises of subjectivity—which is to say, it produced phenomenal madness—in black people both enslaved and free. Regarding black women in colonial and antebellum America, for example, Nobel laureate and novelist Toni Morrison explains that

> black women had to deal with post-modern problems in the nineteenth century and earlier. ... Certain kinds of dissolution, the loss of and the need to reconstruct certain kinds of stability. Certain kinds of madness, deliberately going mad ... "in order not to lose your mind." These strategies for survival made the truly modern person.[40]

Morrison suggests that "going mad" was sometimes a strategy to doggedly clutch hold of one's mind when Reason would steal or smash it. If Reason is benefactor of white supremacy, proponent of antiblack slavocracy, and underwriter of patriarchal dominion, an enslaved black woman might fare better by going insane instead. Rather than remain captive behind the barbed fences of slavocratic sanity, she might find refuge—however tenuous, vexed, and incomplete—in the fugitivity of madness.

In Anglophone idiom, *to snap* is to break, to come undone, to lose control, to go crazy; *to click* is to come together, to fall into place, to make sense. Much as the sounds of physical snaps and physical clicks are sometimes indistinguishable to the ear, the processes signified in these idioms are sometimes indistinguishable to critical interpretation. Sometimes coming undone is precisely how one falls into place. Sometimes a breakdown doubles as a breakthrough. Sometimes a snap is a click. *Sometimes.* I recognize and reckon with occasions where madness entails pain, danger, terror, degradation, and harm for those who experience it and those in its vicinity. But I hasten to mention that Reason may entail pain, terror, abjection, and harm, too. In fact, far more modern harm has been perpetrated under the aegis of Reason—I have in mind chattel slavery, colonialism, imperialism, genocide, war, and other evils both momentous and mundane—than committed by rogue madpersons.[41] And if antiblack Reason constitutes the "normal" and "proper" function of antiblack modernity, than we might choose to mount a pathological disruption and derangement of that system.

As we work to destigmatize madness, including the medicalized madness of mental illness, it is also crucial that we resist romanticizing it. While simplistic metaphors may be rhetorically expedient, they come at grave ethical cost if they distort and objectify people. With these cautions in mind, I center representations of madness that illuminate, rather than efface, its lived experience.

No matter how carefully I qualify my mobilization of madness, and despite my work to avoid romanticizing it, this study might incite the ire of a cohort I call *rationalist readers*. Analogous to the moral reader hailed in slave narratives and sentimental novels, the rationalist reader—and more broadly, the rationalist audience—is the presumed paradigmatic consumer of psychonormative culture. Such a reader possesses psychonormative sensibilities, adheres to Reason's common sense, and shuns madness as categorically detrimental. Some rationalist readers may fear that my focus on mad blackness reinforces myths of black savagery and undermines the "respectable" project of Reasonable blackness. The latter project puts faith in Reason, a structure that I approach with well-warranted skepticism. Rather than integrate black people into the pantheon of Reason, or seek a place for them at its hallowed table, I want to interrogate the logics that undergird that pantheon and prop up that table. I am especially interested in artists who refuse to have a seat, but would rather flip the table and carry their meals outside.

Notes

1 This essay is adapted from the first chapter of La Marr Jurelle Bruce, *How to Go Mad without Losing Your Mind: Madness and Black Radical Creativity* (Durham, NC: Duke University Press, 2021).

2 Epigraphs: Michel Foucault, *Madness and Civilization: A History of Insanity in the Age of Reason*, trans. Richard Howard (New York: Vintage, 1988), 11; emphasis mine; Hortense Spillers, "Mama's Baby, Papa's Maybe: An American Grammar Book," *Diacritics* 17, no. 2 (Summer 1987): 72.

   The phrase *freedom dreams* comes from Robin D. G. Kelley's theorization of black radical thought in *Freedom Dreams: The Black Radical Imagination* (Boston: Beacon Press, 2002).

3 Christina Sharpe theorizes the "wake" of the slave ship—and its various historical and existential effects—in her book, *In the Wake: On Blackness and Being* (Durham, NC: Duke University Press, 2016).

4 Frantz Fanon, *Black Skin, White Masks*, trans. Charles Lam Markmann (London: Pluto Press, 1986), 2.

5 Regarding the Afropessimistic perspective, see Frank B. Wilderson III, *Red, White, and Black: Cinema and the Structure of U.S. Antagonisms* (Durham, NC: Duke University Press, 2010).

6 Spillers, "Mama's Baby, Papa's Maybe," 72; emphasis in original.

7 See Winifred B. Maher and Brendan Maher, "The Ship of Fools: Stultifera Navis or Ignis Fatuus?," *American Psychologist* 37, no. 7 (1982): 756–61.

8 Concerning these controversies over the number dead and the harm done in the Middle Passage, see Maria Diedrich and Henry Louis Gates Jr., eds. *Black Imagination and the Middle Passage* (New York: Oxford University Press, 1999); Herbert S. Klein, Stanley L. Engerman, Robin Haines, and Ralph Shlomowitz, "Transoceanic Mortality: The Slave Trade in Comparative Perspective," *William and Mary Quarterly* 58, no. 1 (2001): 93–117; Patrick Manning and William S. Griffiths, "Divining the Unprovable: Simulating the Demography of African Slavery," *Journal of Interdisciplinary History* 19, no. 2 (1988): 177–201.

9 Hortense Spillers, Saidiya Hartman, Farah Jasmine Griffin, Shelly Eversley, and Jennifer L. Morgan, "'Whatcha Gonna Do?': Revisiting 'Mama's Baby, Papa's Maybe: An American Grammar Book,'" *Women's Studies Quarterly* 35, nos. 1/2 (2007): 308.

10 Spillers, "Mama's Baby, Papa's Maybe," 72.

11 Marcus Rediker generates an extensive cultural and social history of the slave ship in *The Slave Ship: A Human History* (New York: Penguin, 2007).

12 According to Foucault's account, ships of fools peaked in prevalence during the fourteenth and fifteenth centuries (*Madness and Civilization*, 8). Meanwhile, slave ships began to proliferate after the 1452 issuance of the papal bull *Dum Diversas*, which sanctioned Catholic nations in perpetual enslavement of "pagan" peoples and granted moral license to Portugal to take its place at the vanguard of the Atlantic slave trade. If Foucault's account of the ship of fools is historically accurate, the two sorts of vessels overlapped in time. A packed slave ship and a ship of fools would scarcely encounter each other in space, though, since laden slave ships primarily traversed the Atlantic Ocean, while ships of fools, if they physically existed, commuted primarily along Europe's internal rivers and canals.

13 Wordference.com, *reason* from *Random House Unabridged Dictionary* 2020.

14 See V. B. Shneider, "What Is It to Be Rational?" *Philosophy Now: A Magazine of Ideas* 1, no. 1 (Summer 1991), https://philosophynow.org/issues/1/What_Is_It_To_Be_Rational; Achille Mbembe, *Necropolitics* (Durham, NC: Duke University Press, 2019); and James Bohman and William Rehg, eds., *Deliberative Democracy: Essays on Reason and Politics* (Cambridge, MA: MIT Press, 1997).

15 Regarding the exclusions of nonwhite people from Enlightenment ideals, see Emmanuel Chukwudi Eze, ed., *Race and the Enlightenment: A Reader* (Malden, MA: Blackwell, 1997). Eze compiles key passages on race authored by David Hume, Thomas Jefferson, and Immanuel Kant, and other philosophers. Essays excerpted include David Hume, "Of the Populousness of Ancient Nations" and "Of National Characters"; Immanuel Kant, "Geography" and "On National Characters"; and Thomas Jefferson, "Notes on the State of Virginia."

   Concerning the exclusion of women from Enlightenment ideals, see, for example Susanne Lettow "Feminism and the Enlightenment," in *Companion to Feminist Philosophy*, ed. Ann Gary, Serene Khader, Alison Stone (London: Routledge, 2017), 94–107.

   Regarding the exclusion of poor people from Enlightenment ideals, see Fred Powell, "Civil Society History IV: Enlightenment" in *International Encyclopedia of Civil Society*, ed. Helmut Anheier and Stefan Toepler (New York: Springer, 2010).

16 Mbembe, 67.

17 See Eze.

18 In his own articulation of the centrality of black slavery to the invention of Western modernity, Paul Gilroy designates the slave ship as the "central organizing symbol." He announces that "getting on board [the slave ship] promises a means to reconceptualise the orthodox relationship between modernity and what passes for its prehistory." Paul Gilroy, *The Black Atlantic: Modernity and Double Consciousness* (London: Verso, 1993), 17.

19 Though the term *insanity* has been disavowed by the Anglophone medical establishment since the 1920s, its clinical connotation endures in its current legalistic and colloquial usage. See Janet A. Tighe, "'What's in a Name?': A Brief Foray into the History of Insanity in England and the United States," *Journal of the American Academy of Psychiatry and the Law* 33, no. 2 (2005): 252–58.

20 Concerning the pathologization of blackness, see, for example, Jonathan Metzl, *The Protest Psychosis: How Schizophrenia Became a Black Disease* (Boston: Beacon Press, 2009). Concerning the pathologization of (rebellious) femininity, see Maria Ramas, "Freud's Dora, Dora's Hysteria: The Negation of a Woman's Rebellion," *Feminist Studies* 6, no. 3 (1980). Regarding the pathologization of transness, see Cecilia Dhejne, Roy van Vlerken, Gunter Heylens, and Jon Arcelus, "Mental Health and Gender Dysphoria: A Review of the Literature," *International Review of Psychiatry* 28, no. 1 (2016): 44–57. Concerning the pathologization of homosexuality, see Ronald Bayer, Homosexuality and American Psychiatry: The Politics of Diagnosis (Princeton, NJ: Princeton University Press, 1987). Concerning the pathologization of poverty, see Helena Hansen, Philippe Bourgois, and Ernest Drucker, "Pathologizing Poverty: New Forms of Diagnosis, Disability, and Structural Stigma under Welfare Reform," *Social Science and Medicine* 103 (2014): 76–83.

21 For an especially eloquent discussion of how hegemonic judgments impact the so-called objectivist realm of science and medicine in the United States, see Steven Epstein, *Impure Science: AIDS, Activism, and the Politics of Knowledge* (Berkeley: University of California Press, 1996). My declaration that "no science is pure" is inspired, in part, by Epstein's study.

22 In *Disturbers of the Peace: Representations of Madness in Anglophone Caribbean Literature*, Kelly Baker Josephs arrives at a similar conclusion. She observes, "While mad can define a person, situation, or event, it more often describes the person attempting to define said person, situation, or event. That is, the term says as much, if not more, about the subject employing it as about the object it attempts to label." Kelly Baker Josephs, *Disturbers of the Peace: Representations of Madness in Anglophone Caribbean Literature* (Charlottesville: University of Virginia Press, 2013), 8.

23 Regarding "critical ambivalence," I have written elsewhere that "Sometimes it is useful, even crucial, to tarry in the openness of ambiguity; in the strategic vantage point available in the interstice (the better to look both ways and beyond); in the capacious bothness of ambivalence; in the sheer potential in irresolution … Lingering in ambivalence, we can access multiple, even dissonant, vantages at once, before pivoting, if we finally choose to pivot, toward decisive motion. To be clear, I am not describing an impotent ambivalence that relinquishes or thwarts politics. Rather, I am proposing an instrumental ambivalence that harnesses the energetic motion and friction and tension of ambivalent feeling. Such energy might propel progressive and radical movement." La Marr Jurelle Bruce, "Shore, Unsure: Loitering as a Way of Life," *GLQ* 5, no. 2 (2019): 357.

24 Audre Lorde, "The Uses of Anger: Women Responding to Racism" in *Sister Outsider: Essays and Speeches* (Berkeley: Crossing Press, 1984), 127.

25 In *Scenes of Subjection: Terror, Slavery, and Self-Making in Nineteenth-Century America*, Saidiya Hartman unpacks the epistemic violence wrought by hegemonic "empathy." She writes:

"Properly speaking, empathy is a projection of oneself into another in order to better understand the other" or "the projection of one's own personality into an object, with the attribution to the object of one's own emotions." Hartman further writes that "by exploiting the vulnerability of the captive body as a vessel for the uses, thoughts, and feelings of others, the humanity extended to the slave inadvertently confirms the expectations and desires definitive of the relations of chattel slavery … empathy is double-edged, for in making the other's suffering one's own, this suffering is occluded by the other's obliteration." Saidiya Hartman, *Scenes of Subjection: Terror, Slavery, and Self-Making in Nineteenth-Century America* (New York: Oxford University Press, 1997), 18–19.

26 For further information on positivism as a philosophical tradition and orientation, see Seth B. Abrutyn, "Positivism" in *Oxford Bibliographies in Sociology* (Oxford, UK: Oxford University Press, 2013).

27 I am grateful to the audience at the 2018 Harold Stirling Lecture at Vanderbilt University for encouraging me to center this *unknowability*. Special thanks to Robert Engelman for his important comments on this matter.

28 Édouard Glissant, *The Collected Poems of Édouard Glissant* (Minneapolis: University of Minnesota Press, 2005), xxxii–xxxiii. Bracketed definitions in original.

29 Sociologist Orlando Patterson suggests that the status of the slave is one of "social death," which entails three primary characteristics: violent subjection, natal alienation, and general dishonor. See Orlando Patterson, *Slavery and Social Death: A Comparative Study* (Cambridge, MA: Harvard University Press, 1982), 1–16.

30 For an extended account of suicide as a mode of agency among slaves, see Terri L. Snyder, *The Power to Die: Slavery and Suicide in British North America* (Chicago: University of Chicago Press, 2015).

31 Concerning the campaign of confinement that swept Europe in the seventeenth and eighteenth centuries—and in particular the treatment of purportedly violent madmen—Foucault writes that "those chained to the cell walls were no longer men whose minds had wandered, but beasts preyed upon by a natural frenzy. … This model of animality prevailed in the asylums and gave them their cagelike aspect, their look of the menagerie" (Foucault, *Madness and Civilization*, 72). Alas, Foucault does not connect the "animality" imputed to the insane and the animality concomitantly ascribed to Africans; does not note any resemblance between "cagelike" asylum technology and cagelike slave ship and plantation technology. Foucault fails to critically engage the matter of blackness—especially considering the importance of blackness as foil to whiteness in the drama of Western modernity, and also considering the worldwide colonial and racial upheavals concurrent with his composition of *History of Madness*.

32 Benjamin Reiss, *Theaters of Madness: Insane Asylums and Nineteenth-Century American Culture* (Chicago: University of Chicago Press, 2008), 15.

33 For a rich exegesis of diaspora as process, see Brent Hayes Edwards, *The Practice of Diaspora: Literature, Translation, and the Rise of Black Internationalism* (Cambridge, MA: Harvard University Press, 2003).

34 Samuel Cartwright, "Diseases and Peculiarities of the Negro Race," *DeBow's Review: Southern and Western States* 11 (1851): 331.

35 Frank Wilderson suggests that black people in modernity are subjected to relentless and categorical social death, which categorically positions them as slaves. Insisting that their abjection as slaves is the foundation upon which the modern world is built, Wilderson writes "Blackness and slaveness cannot be dis-imbricated, cannot be pulled apart" in

"Blacks and the Master/Slave Relation" in *Afro-pessimism: An Introduction* (Minneapolis: Racked and Dispatched, 2017), 15–30, https://rackedanddispatched.noblogs.org/files/2017/01/Afro-Pessimism2.pdf.

36 Cartwright, 332.

37 Cartwright, 333.

38 Regarding such pathologization of black freedom, Barbara Browning writes that "the terrifying contagion which the United States really feared in 1793 [amid the Haitian Revolution] was the contagion of black political empowerment." See Barbara Browning, *Infectious Rhythm: Metaphors of Contagion and the Spread of African Culture* (New York: Routledge, 1998), 82.

39 Robert W. Wood, *Memorial of Edward Jarvis, M.D.* (Boston, American Statistical Association, 1885), 11.

40 Toni Morrison quoted in Paul Gilroy, "Living Memory: A Meeting with Toni Morrison," in *Small Acts* (Essex, UK: Serpent's Tail, 1993), 178. Morrison's insight about "deliberately going mad in order, as one of the characters says, 'in order not to lose your mind,'" helped inspire the title of the present book.

41 According to the landmark MacArthur Violence Risk Assessment Study, mental illness alone does not correspond to a statistically significant increased likelihood of committing violent crimes. However, they are significantly more likely to be victims of violent crimes. See John Monahan et al, *Rethinking Risk Assessment: The MacArthur Study of Mental Disorder and Violence* (Oxford: Oxford University Press, 2001). See also MacArthur Research Network on Mental Health and the Law, "The MacArthur Violence Risk Assessment Study: September 2005 Update of the Executive Summary," MacArthur Research Network, http://www.macarthur.virginia.edu/risk.html.

Editor's Reference

Foucault, M. (2009). *History of Madness*. Routledge.

Chapter 17

Commercialized Science and Epistemic Injustice

EXPOSING AND RESISTING NEOLIBERAL GLOBAL MENTAL HEALTH DISCOURSE

Justin M. Karter, Lisa Cosgrove, and Farahdeba Herrawi

Summary

In this chapter, scholars Justin Karter, Lisa Cosgrove, and Farahdeba Herrawi explore the commercialization of psychiatric science and demonstrate its many damages, including the devaluation of the knowledges and agency of individuals with lived experience. By reinforcing a medicalized understanding of emotional distress, science has constructed a system of epistemic injustice that privileges the perspectives of the very institutions, individuals, and organizations that benefit from the field's profit-enhancing strategies. This is not a coincidence: through interwoven practices and policies that empower a deeply commercialized industry of "care," psychiatry has created a knowledge base that ignores those who suffer systematic oppression and—in a global context—the violation of human rights. This chapter warns us of the dangers of colluding in this commercialization and the effects of these practices on those who continually suffer as a result of persistent corruption in the mental health industry.

*

Commercialized Science and Epistemic Injustice: Exposing and Resisting Neoliberal Global Mental Health Discourse

Mental health research and practice has faced sustained critiques on many fronts. Critics of the psy-disciplines have taken the field to task for a myriad of issues, such as the lack of validity of prominent diagnostic constructs (Phillips et al., 2012; Karter

DOI: 10.4324/9781003148456-20

& Kamens, 2019), the medicalization of emotional distress and over-diagnosis and over-treatment (Moncreiff & Crawford, 2001; Frances, 2013), and the undue influence of the pharmaceutical industry and the resulting corruption of research and clinical practice guidelines (Cosgrove et al., 2018). Some of the most powerful critiques have come from the field of Mad Studies, where differently positioned and diverse people with lived experience have documented the pathologization and disempowerment of those engaging with mental health services (Crepaz-Keay & Kalathil, 2013) and the complicity of the psy-disciplines with oppressive social systems and ideologies (Russo & Beresford, 2015). This is why Mad Studies as "a project of inquiry, knowledge production, and political action [is] devoted to the critique and transcendence of psy-centered ways of thinking, behaving, relating, and being" (LeFrancois, Reaume, & Menzies, 2013, p. 13). These critiques embody Hacking's (2002) observation that "lively scholars do not stay still."

In this chapter, we focus on how the commercialization of science reinforces psychiatrized ways of understanding emotional distress, which leads to epistemic injustice and the systemic devaluation of the knowledges and agency of "Mad people(s)." Additionally, we discuss how this manipulation of the scientific discourse in the psy-disciplines is enabled by neoliberalism. Neoliberal policies and practices empower industry actors to pursue profit-enhancing strategies through the corruption of the scientific discourse while simultaneously undermining an appreciation for the upstream causes of ill-health. Taking the Global Mental Health (GMH) movement as a case example, we discuss the current debates within the movement and show how the concepts of structural violence and vulnerability provide pathways to increasing epistemic humility (Cosgrove & Herrawi, 2021). We also explore how the structural and conceptual competency movements may advance an appreciation for the "global burden of obstacles" to mental health (Pūras, 2017).

Global Mental Health and Madness

> The dominant criteria of valid knowledge in Western modernity, by failing to acknowledge as valid kinds of knowledge other than those produced by modern science, brought about a massive epistemicide, that is to say, the destruction of an immense variety of ways of knowing that prevail mainly on the other side of the abyssal line—in the colonial societies and sociabilities.
>
> (De Sousa Santos, 2018, p. 8)

> An emergent discipline entitled "global mental health," backed by the WHO, the US National Institute of Mental Health, and the drug industry, is establishing itself in universities and on the ground. The discipline's literature concedes the social and economic determinants of poor mental health, but the thrust is on the global deployment of Western biomedical models of mental disorder.
>
> (Summerfield, 2013, p. 346)

The GMH movement has been met with criticism from cross-cultural and critical psychiatrists and psychologists, as well as psychiatric survivors, service-users/consumers, and psychosocial disability advocates, for reifying Western conceptions of mental disorders and diverting resources from the social determinants of mental health (Mills, 2014; Beresford, 2018). However, there are efforts to transform the GMH from a top-down, individualized, and treatment-oriented approach, toward a rights-based conception that accounts for the cultural, political, and economic conditions that produce distress and disability (Davar, 2008, 2017; Rose, Carr, & Beresford, 2018). By emphasizing the importance of equity issues (rather than focusing on the need to "scale-up" individualized medical and therapeutic interventions), the writing and activism of people with lived experience of mental distress provide a powerful counter-discourse to the rhetoric evidenced in mainstream summits and reports (Rose, 2018). Thus, the debates within the GMH movement often center around those who argue for increased access to treatment for underserved populations, and those who focus on the socio-political determinants of health and the problems with Western psychiatry's capture of the movement (Whitley, 2015).

For example, terms such as "mental illness," "mental disorder," and "brain disorder" are common in the literature on GMH that is produced by the WHO, the World bank, and the Lancet Commission (Mills, 2018). It is therefore not surprising that the interventions emphasized in these reports and promotional campaigns reveal a conception of rights that allows for a "right to treatment" while the rights of service-users to determine the terms under which this treatment occurs are not considered. This omission is one of the reasons that the term "madness" is sometimes preferred by many mental health advocates with lived experience; it is a term with deep historical roots that refers to a broader conception of experiences of distress than are captured using a medical lens. As Scull (2015, p. 14) notes:

> Madness has much broader salience for the social order and the cultures
> we form part of and has resonance in the world of literature and art and
> of religious belief, as well as in the scientific domain.

The broader focus is important; although the term "madness," may be seen as stigmatizing by some, it is often favored by psychiatric survivors and those who resist a reductive medical approach (Faulkner, 2017). Indeed, this is why Foucault (1967, 1977) invoked the term—to challenge the notion that madness is primarily a property of individual consciousness. He showed that there is a nuanced interplay between individual psyches and social formations, subjectivity, and discourse. In so doing, he revealed the historical and cultural contingency of conceptions of madness, as different discursive formations have taken precedence at different times with marked changes occurring through epistemic shifts.

More recently, the term "psychosocial disability" has emerged from those engaging in global mental health activism (see e.g., PANUSP, 2011; TCI Asia-Pacific, 2018a) in order to show how the psy-disciplines continue to exert power over knowledge production and are dismissive of alternative epistemic cultures (Russo & Wooley, 2020). Unfortunately, within the GMH movement there has been resistance to incorporating the voices and scholarship of people who identify with the Mad Studies movement and those who identify as psychosocial disability activists (Cosgrove, Morrill et al., 2020; Cosgrove, Mills et al., 2020). In fact, when the Lancet Commission released its latest report on GMH in October of 2018, the Commission emphatically called for scaling up mental health care globally (Patel et al., 2018) to "close the treatment gap," while facing criticism for failing to meaningfully include the perspectives and participation of people with psychosocial disabilities. Not surprisingly, coalitions of activists and service-users organized open letters detailing their concerns with the report (Beresford, 2018; National Survivor User Network (NSUN), 2018). In these letters, the lack of representation and participation of important stakeholders in the development of the report was noted. Additionally, another central issue raised was by TCI Asia-Pacific, a coalition of disabled people's organizations (DPOs) working to advance the rights of persons with psychosocial disabilities. They critiqued the report for continuing to advocate for a "North driving the South" approach to mental health care, which is especially problematic given the colonial legacy of mental health services and psychiatry in many parts of the world (TCI Asia-Pacific, 2018).

Commercialization and Epistemic Injustice: What's Neoliberalism Got to Do with It?

> Measurement is a potent moment in the construction of scientific knowledge.
>
> (Barad, 2007, p. 166)

> Neoliberalism perpetuates the colonial notion of "ideal bodies", docile ones predicated on a normalized able-bodiedness driven by productive output and measurable indicators. Disabled people are again (re)constructed as those who are not integrated in the market economy, part of the problem, who need to be corrected or removed, as disability continually falls outside the normative remits of utility, economic growth, and development indicators.
>
> (Grech & Soldatic, 2015, p. 15)

Commercialized science—the use of science primarily to meet industry needs—is a pernicious problem in medicine. It is now widely recognized that industry influences the biomedical field in a multitude of ways—not only by funding clinical drug trials but also through the process of "ghost management" (i.e., when pharmaceutical companies design the trials, draft the manuscript, and disseminate the results; see Sismundo, 2008, 2009). Industry's capture and colonization of psychiatry has led both the public and a growing number of researchers, clinicians, and mental health activists to raise concerns about the trustworthiness of psychiatric research and practice (Porter, 2015). Additionally, the commercialization of psychiatric research undermines an appreciation for epistemic diversity; it is impossible to genuinely respect diverse idioms of distress when human experience is understood predominantly in terms of a biomedical model. The resulting "professionalization of suffering" sustains the authority of psychiatrists and other mental health professionals over people with lived experience (Kleinman & Kleinman, 1997).

In contrast to the psychiatrization of lived experience, Fricker's (2007) concept of epistemic injustice provides a useful framework for analyzing and challenging the subjugation of Mad knowledge(s). Scholar activists within the field of Mad Studies have argued that a refusal to value the perspectives of those living with madness is so entrenched in Western social practices and discourses (Rimke & Brock, 2012) that epistemic injustice is often perpetuated without consideration of potential social harm (Perlin, 2003). Unfortunately, the increase in neoliberal policies and practices creates a perfect storm for strengthening, rather than dismantling, epistemic injustice, and the commercial influence in organized psychiatry and in the GMH movemen.

To more fully understand how neoliberalism and the commercialization of science are implicated in epistemic injustice, it is important to remember that neoliberalism should not be conflated with deregulation or a conservative political agenda (Cosgrove & Karter, 2018). Following Mirowski (2009) and Nik-Khah (2014), we see neoliberalism as a worldview that reflects (an often invisible) market-based logic. As such, neoliberalism may be described as an attitude toward science, knowledge making, and subjectivity. Hence, the implications of medical neoliberalism are profound; a market-based logic makes it easy to re-cast human suffering in a disease framework and focus on the economic fallout incurred by psychiatric disorders (Peters, 2019). It is noteworthy that in the late 1990s, the WHO made a deliberate decision to re-label "International Health" as "Global Health" when it became apparent that the World Bank was moving in this direction under the leadership of neoliberal economist Jeffery Sachs (see, e.g., Brown, Cueto, & Fee, 2006). It was at this point that global mental health began to be conceptualized in biological and economic terms (Bemme & D'Souza, 2014).

The disability-adjusted life years (DALY) metric and, relatedly, the focus on calculating the global burden of disease, are perhaps the most paradigmatic examples of conceptualizing mental health in biological and economic terms. The market-based logic and rhetoric in the DALY are evident in the metric's attempt to quantify at the population level the total years of life lost, not only to early death but also to the years of life lived with any health condition that reduces functioning (Chen et al., 2015). This metric, which was developed by the World Bank and the World Health Organization, is thus used to prioritize health conditions and make recommendations for resource allocation. As Parks (2014) notes, the DALY became instrumental in economically justifying "biomedical sovereignty." Within the last ten years, there has been increasing attention focused on the global burden of mental disorders, and concomitantly, the economic burden that these "brain disorders" are imposing on countries. In fact, the WHO estimates that depression is the leading cause of disability worldwide (WHO, 2017).

Despite these dire predictions, and the growing acceptance and use of the DALY, there have been longstanding critiques of this metric on philosophical grounds for monetizing and commodifying the worth of people. For instance, it has been pointed out that the DALY explicitly devalues the lives of disabled people (Arnesen & Nord, 1999), and is "epistemologically lamentable" (Summerfield, 2017, p. 52). Additionally, the DALY calculations and disease burden estimates have been critiqued on methodological grounds. Brhlikova, Pollock, and Manners (2011) identified the data sources used in the Global Burden of Depression estimates (GBDep) and assessed these sources in terms of completeness and representativeness (e.g., data were not drawn from a nationally representative population). The authors found poor compliance with GBDep inclusion criteria, concluding:

> Poor quality data limit the interpretation and validity of global burden
> of depression estimates. The uncritical application of these estimates
> to international healthcare policy-making could divert scarce resources
> from other public healthcare priorities.
>
> (Brhlikova, Pollock, & Manners, 2011, p. 25)

Despite these critiques, the GMHM continues to be embedded in a medical neoliberal framework. The connection between the treatment of mental health issues and neoliberal economic interests was evident in the GMH campaigns that were developed by the WHO in collaboration with the World Bank on depression (WHO, 2017). The campaigns, which were designed to increase attention to (and funding for) mental disorders, framed the problem in economic terms and emphasized the loss of human capital (see Figure 17.1).

Framing the problem in economic terms not only reinforced the dominance of a biomedical model but also allowed the pharmaceutical industry to exploit this framing. For example, in 2014, the pharmaceutical company Lundbeck, for whom the antidepressant Celexa was the "cornerstone for the company's international expansion" (Lundbeck, 2021), co-sponsored with the Economist a global summit on depression titled, *The Global Crisis of Depression: The Low of the 21st Century?* In a press release announcing the conference, the company described the depression as a global issue in need of innovative solutions:

> Lundbeck is sponsoring a one-day forum to examine the burden of
> depression as well as a variety of national responses to it, bringing in
> cross-sector stakeholders who are trying to tackle a problem that has
> become a leading cause of illness. The event will take a multi-faceted
> approach, gathering together policymakers, healthcare providers, the
> pharmaceutical industry, academia, employers and patient groups.
>
> (Lundbeck, 2014)

The following year, Lundbeck, together with Otsuka, disseminated materials internationally to patient advocacy groups, policymakers, and other stakeholders calling on nations for greater investments in depression, a "chronic, recurring and progressive disorder" that is "predicted to become the leading cause of burden by 2030." The materials also claim that "gains made by improved productivity at work can offset the costs of treatment for depression by 45–98%" and that global investments in these treatments "should match the burden of disease" (Lundbeck & Otsuka, 2015). Lundbeck has also developed a website, Progress in Mind—The Psychiatry and Neurology Resource Center. The primary goal of this website is "to communicate and spread greater awareness of the massive economic and societal burden posed by psychiatric and neurological disorders" (Progress in Mind, 2021).

Lundbeck is not alone in strategically developing a discourse around "the global burden of brain disorders" to make a case for greater investment in their products. The pharmaceutical industry's involvement in promoting the view that that mental disorders are a significant, costly, and growing international problem in need of immediate attention, and can be seen in Table 17.1. In this table, we identify some influential population-based studies, all of which conclude that the economic burden

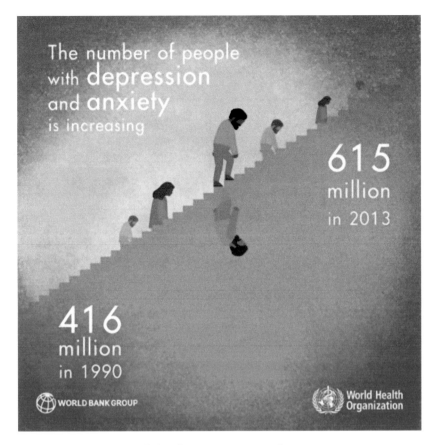

Figure 17.1   Depression let's talk: Campaign essentials.
World Health Organization (2017). Retrieved from: https://www.who.int/news-room/events/detail/2016/04/13/default-calendar/out-of-the-shadows-making-mental-health-a-global-development-priority.

of mental disorders is staggering and that scaling up treatment is urgently needed. We also detail the evidence of significant financial conflicts of interest from their own disclosures. The authors of these studies were either employees of pharmaceutical companies that manufacture psychotropic medications, had financial ties to these companies, or the study was paid for by industry.

As can be seen in the table, by shifting the discourse around global mental health toward a "brain disorders" model, industry is reinforcing the hegemony of a biomedical approach to emotional distress. In turn, this allows for the dissemination of a powerful (and industry-friendly) message: (1) mental disorders are a growing problem, not only at the individual level, but in terms of economic loss to nations and (2) this problem can be solved, in a cost-effective way, by increasing access to mental health diagnosis and treatment, especially with psychopharmaceuticals. As one leading psychiatrist noted almost a decade ago, the discipline of "global health" and the movement for GMH are, "in effect, selling … the products of the Western mental health industry to the non-Western world" (Summerfield, 2013, p. 346).

Table 17.1 Influential Studies Sponsored by Pharmaceutical Industry That Advance "Global Burden" and "Brain Disorders" Discourse

Article	FCOI	Conclusion
The economic burden of depression and the cost-effectiveness of treatment (2003) https://doi.org/10.1002/mpr.139	Unrestricted educational grant from Wyeth Pharmaceuticals. "Preparation of this chapter was supported, in part, by … an unrestricted educational grant from Wyeth Pharmaceuticals as part of the Global Research on Anxiety and Depression Network (GRAD) through an unrestricted educational grant by Wyeth-Ayerst Pharmaceuticals." (p. 30)	This study highlights the economic impact of depression and emphasizes cost-efficient treatment interventions to reduce the economic impact of depression. "Depression is clearly associated with enormous economic burden, the largest component of which derives from lost work productivity. Although efficacious and tolerable treatments exist, the widespread inadequate, and insufficient use of treatment of patients with depression compounds the economic burden of depression. Enhanced care of patients with depression is needed and should include as core features aggressive outreach and improved quality of treatments." (p. 29)
Depression in the workforce: The intermediary effect of medical comorbidity (2011) https://doi.org/10.1016/S0165-0327(11)70006-4	The authors received an honorarium from Bristol-Myers Squibb for writing this manuscript. "Dr. McIntyre and Dr. Taylor each received an honorarium for writing this manuscript. There was no interference from the sponsor (Bristol-Myers Squibb; BMS), which was not involved in the collection, analysis and interpretation of data, or in manuscript preparation. Dr. McIntyre has participated on advisory boards, and/or in, continuing education activities for numerous pharmaceutical companies, including Astra Zeneca, Bristol-Myers Squibb, Eli Lilly, GlaxoSmithKline, Janssen-Ortho, Lundbeck, Organon, Pfizer, Wyeth. Dr. Taylor has participated on advisory boards, and or in, continuing education activities for: Astra Zeneca, Bristol-Myers Squibb, Eli Lilly, GlaxoSmithKline, Janssen-Ortho, Wyeth." (p. 534)	This study suggests that increased screening, treatment, and prevention initiatives are needed to reduce workforce disability. "Major depressive disorder is associated with decreased health-related quality of life, productivity (absenteeism/presenteeism), and increased short- and long-term disability. Interventional studies have documented the salutary effects of chronic disease management on workforce disability." (p. 533) "Sufficient evidence justifies screening for depression and associated medical conditions, ensuring that available resources can provide further evaluation and treatment." (p. 534)

(Continued)

Table 17.1 Influential Studies Sponsored by Pharmaceutical Industry That Advance "Global Burden" and "Brain Disorders" Discourse (*Continued*)

Article	FCOI	Conclusion
Cost of disorders of the brain in Europe (2010) https://doi.org/10.1016/j.euroneuro.2011.08.008	The overall Task Force project received an unrestricted educational grant supported by H. Lundbeck A/S and from the European College of Neuropsychopharmacology "We gratefully acknowledge the unrestricted financial support from the European College of Neuropsychopharmacology, the European Federation of Neurological Societies and from H. Lundbeck A/S." (p. 71)	Every year over a third of the total EU population suffers from mental disorders. The true size of "disorders of the brain" including neurological disorders is considerably larger. Disorders of the brain are the largest contributor to the all-cause morbidity burden as measured by DALY in the EU. "In total we come to the conclusion in our current report that the cost of disorders of the brain amounts overall to a staggering €798 billion in Europe in 2010 or more than the double of our previous estimate." (p. 42)
The societal cost of depression: Evidence from 10,000 Swedish patients in psychiatric care (2013) https://doi.org/10.1016/j.jad.2013.03.003	Written by three employees of AstraZeneca. Other co-authors were on the AZ board and received speaker fees from AZ. "While the work on this study was performed, Mattias Ekman (ME) was an employee of Optum Insight (formerly i3 Innovus) and Ola Granström (OG) was an employee of AstraZeneca. ME is now an employee of AstraZeneca and OG of Gilead Sciences. Johanna Jacob is an employee of AstraZeneca. Mikael Landén is on the advisory board for AstraZeneca and Lundbeck, and has received speaker's fees from AstraZeneca, Eli Lilly, Lundbeck, Wyeth, and Servier. Sead Omérov has declared no conflicts of interest." (p. 796)	This study suggests that the societal costs of depression in Sweden are substantial. "This study suggests that the societal costs for depression in Sweden are substantial. We found total costs to be considerably higher for patients who had been hospitalized compared with those who had not. Furthermore, costs were substantially higher during active depressive episodes, in patients with comorbid symptoms such as psychosis, and in patients with low global functioning as assessed with GAF." (p. 796)
The prevalence and burden of mental and substance use disorders in Australia: Findings from the Global Burden of Disease Study 2015 (2018) https://doi.org/10.1177/0004867417751641	The author(s) declared no potential conflicts of interest with respect to the research, authorship, and/or publication of this article. However, Baune has reported elsewhere (see for example, Baune & Falkai, 2021; Baune et al., 2019) that he received honoraria from AstraZeneca, Bristol-Myers Squibb, Lundbeck, Pfizer, Servier, Wyeth, and Otsuka; research grants from private industries or nonprofit funds from AstraZeneca and Sanofi-Synthélabo.	This study noted that the leading burden of mental and substance use disorders has remained unchanged and suggests interventions for change. "MSDs are significant contributors to the total burden of disease in Australia. Despite decades of policy attention accompanied by increased treatment rates, the burden has remained unchanged over the 25 years to 2015. The sector needs to develop more efficacious interventions and pay increased attention to prevention if the burden of MSDs is to be reduced." (p. 489)

Industry commercialization of the psy-disciplines has advanced reductive biomedical understandings of emotional distress and "madness" to the exclusion of epistemologies that are grounded in experiential knowledge (LeFrançois, et al., 2013)

Sites of Resistance: The Psychosocial Disability Framework and a Rights-Based Approach

> They said ... that he was so devoted to Pure Science ... that he would rather have people die by the right therapy than be cured by the wrong.
>
> (Sinclair Lewis, 1926, p. 137)

Organizations of psychiatric survivors, people with lived experience, and service-users, among others, campaign for full legal equality for people labeled mad and call for protection from coercive practices within the psy-disciplines, such as forced treatment, but also from discriminatory practices in employment and other social institutions (Sayce, 2017). Similarly, scholars working in critical disability studies argue that social and structural changes are necessary for inclusion and that full inclusion necessitates a transformation of normative standards (Dirth & Adams, 2019). While tensions and philosophical differences exist between Mad Studies and disability theory, the emergent psychosocial disability framework leverages international human rights law to challenge and improve current practices (Cresswell & Spandler, 2016; Spandler & Anderson, 2015).

In addition, the psychosocial disability framework was central to the development of the United Nations Convention on the Rights of Persons with Disabilities (CRPD), the "first comprehensive and legally binding international framework for psychosocial disability" (Drew et al., 2011, p. 2). The formal adoption of the CRPD by the United Nations in 2006 marked an important shift in the expectations on governments with regard to their policies on persons living with psychosocial disabilities from recipients of welfare to people entitled to equality and protection under the law (Hoffman, Sritharan, & Tejpar, 2016). Consistent with this approach, the UN Special Rapporteur on the right to health (August 2014-July 2020), Lithuanian psychiatrist Dainius Pūras, has called for a radical and global shift in approach to the treatment of mental health issues. In a report to the UN in 2017, he urged policymakers to address the "social determinants and abandon the predominant medical model that seeks to cure individuals by targeting 'disorders'" (Puras, 2017, p. 19). Pūras offers policy recommendations for confronting global mental health challenges from a rights-based perspective, including measures to establish meaningful participatory frameworks toward the inclusion of people with psychosocial disabilities in mental health research, policy, and treatment delivery.

The psychosocial disability and rights-based discourse challenges commercialized psychiatry on both conceptual and structural grounds. That is, an understanding of psychosocial disability as arising in a complex interaction between individuals and their environmental contexts, cultural attitudes, and societal barriers has the potential to disrupt the acontextual account of emotional distress that is evidenced in the GMH movement. It also shifts the ethical and legal responsibility for disability away from an individual deficit (to be overcome through medical intervention) and toward the forces of structural oppression that differentially afford health and illness (Dirth & Adams, 2019). A perspective on global mental health that takes social and collective distress as its object, rather than individual pathology, can differentiate thriving communities from distressed communities. Therefore, rather than focus predominately on "scaling up" access to individual treatment, the emphasis is on identifying the structural and environmental risk factors for collective distress (Campbell & Burgess, 2012). The rights-based approach to GMH contradicts the "global burden" and "brain disorder" framework advanced by commercialized science as it actively resists a neoliberal and industry-friendly discourse that isolates distress and locates it within individual brains. Additionally, the international legal frameworks can be leveraged to oppose pharmaceutical industry conferences and think tanks that do not actively empower and invite the participation of the people who are ultimately the subjects of their studies.

Altering Practice: Structural and Conceptual Competency Approaches

> Inequality is the enemy of knowledge … and … epistemic injustice is inextricably linked to social injustices.
>
> (Medina, 2012, p. 27)

Structural and conceptual competency movements have been developed in an effort to identify the upstream causes of physical and emotional ill-health. In particular, the structural competency framework can be useful in training clinicians to have a greater appreciation for how structural violence—unfair social arrangements that cause harm—perpetuates inequity. When studying structural violence, the focus is on examining the ways that social structures (economic, political, medical, and legal systems) can have a disproportionately negative impact on particular groups and communities, and how histories of marginalization and oppression are implicated in the presentation of individual distress.

Specifically, the structural competency framework trains mental health professionals to consider how "institutions, neighborhood conditions, market forces, public policies, and health care delivery systems shape symptoms and diseases, and to mobilize for correction of inequalities as they manifest both in physician-patient interactions and beyond the clinic walls" (Metzl & Hansen, 2017, p. 115). Explicit in this approach is an emphasis on the ways in which social structures impact those who are likely to experience distress and come under the purview of psychiatric treatment. For instance, Metzl and Hansen (2018) highlight how drug marketing strategies differentially impact different communities and lead to disproportionate rates of psychiatric diagnoses. A structurally competent provider is thus able to recognize these structural factors and go beyond individualized care to engage in community-based advocacy for systemic change. The structural competency framework has been applied to the GMH movement, where it can be useful in developing global mental health trainings that "recognize the complex forces at work in a place, seek the expertise of those with deep experiential knowledge of the community, and collaborate with them in structural interventions" (Gajara et al., 2019, p. 4).

Relatedly, the conceptual competence framework provides important challenges to the dominant discourses in the mental health professions by questioning prevailing assumptions about both psychiatric diagnosis and treatment. The aim is to bring an "epistemic humility" to the clinical encounter by shedding light on the limitations of the current knowledge systems in the psy-disciplines. In so doing, this framework highlights the epistemic injustice that results from embracing Western biomedical approaches to emotional distress. By using an ecological model for synthesizing the major debates about psychiatric diagnostic taxonomies, there is an opportunity to enhance critical consciousness in mental health professionals (Karter & Kamens, 2019). For example, in their conceptual competence curriculum, Aftab and Watermen (2020) include training on the unsettled philosophical debates, and they help clinicians incorporate these debates into their clinical practice. In this way, the conceptual competence framework opens up space for the knowledge and expertise of those with lived experience. The conceptual competence framework explicitly addresses how the psy-disciplines' diagnoses, treatments, and research methods are indelibly shaped by larger historical and political-economic forces, such as colonialism and neoliberalism, as well as more immediate financial incentives of the pharmaceutical industry and for-profit healthcare companies (Karter, 2019).

Conclusion

He/she/they that control language also control resources and manipulate the sources of hope. Culture at large, not doctors alone, should define normal and hopefully celebrate many variants of it. Give more power to clients, families and communities as well as to nurses and social workers (and other providers) and less to those who think our genes and biologies define our humanity rather than our stories and our relationships.

(Whitehouse in Aftab, 2020)

The commercialization of science and the related capture of psychiatry by industry reinforces epistemic injustice through the production of a neoliberal mental health discourse—one that casts emotional distress as economically burdensome "brain disorders." Neoliberal policies that serve industry interests have been prioritized in the GMH movement, to the near-total exclusion of "mad" epistemologies. This promotion of a medicalized understanding of distress is accomplished through the exercise of cultural and ideological power that shapes dominant conceptual frameworks within the psy-disciplines. Moreover, when people choose to enter mental health systems, there is the risk that epistemic injustice will be perpetuated if service-providers do not remain open to a critique of the tools of the psy-disciplines or if they deny alternative ways of knowing presented by service-users.

Indeed, it is clear that taking emotional suffering out of its moral, ethical, and political context (Kleinman, 2019) creates challenges for appreciating the diversity of emotional experiences and reproduces epistemic injustice. However, emerging frameworks such as structural and conceptual competency movements, together with powerful international institutions, including the United Nations, provide possible sites of resistance for Mad activists and scholars. As we have discussed in this chapter, the psychosocial disability and rights-based mental health approaches prioritize the inclusion and full participation of people with lived experience. In so doing, they open up political opportunities for transforming GMH policies from within.

References

Aftab, A. (2020). Social constructionism meets aging and dementia: A conversation in critical psychiatry with Peter J. Whitehouse, MD, PhD. *Psychiatric Times.* https://www.psychiatrictimes.com/view/social-constructionism-meets-aging-and-dementia

Aftab, A., & Waterman, G. S. (2020). Conceptual competence in psychiatry: Recommendations for education and training. *Academic Psychiatry,* 1–7.

Arnesen, T., & Nord, E. (1999). The value of DALY life: Problems with ethics and validity of disability adjusted life years. *BMJ, 319*(7222), 1423–1425.

Bemme, D., & D'souza, N. A. (2014). Global mental health and its discontents: An inquiry into the making of global and local scale. *Transcultural Psychiatry, 51*(6), 850–874.

Beresford, P. (2018). A failure of national mental health policy and the failure of a Global Summit. *British Journal of Mental Health Nursing, 7*(5), 198–199.

Brhlikova, P., Pollock, A. M., & Manners, R. (2011). Global Burden of Disease estimates of depression--How reliable is the epidemiological evidence?. *Journal of the Royal Society of Medicine, 104*(1), 25–34. https://doi.org/10.1258/jrsm.2010.100080

Brown, T. M., Cueto, M., & Fee, E. (2006). The World Health Organization and the transition from "international" to "global" public health. *American journal of public health, 96*(1), 62–72.

Campbell, C., & Burgess, R. (2012). The role of communities in advancing the goals of the Movement for Global Mental Health. *Transcultural psychiatry, 49*(3–4), 379–395. ISSN 1363-4615. DOI: 10.1177/1363461512454643

Chen, A., Jacobsen, K. H., Deshmukh, A. A., & Cantor, S. B. (2015). The evolution of the disability-adjusted life year (DALY). *Socio-economic planning sciences, 49,* 10–15.

Cosgrove, L., & Herrawi, F. (2021). Beware of equating increased access to mental health services with health equity: The need for clinical and epistemic humility in psychology. *The Humanistic Psychologist, 9*(2), 338–341.

Cosgrove, L., & Karter, J. M. (2018). The poison in the cure: Neoliberalism and contemporary movements in mental health. *Theory & Psychology, 28*(5), 669–683.

Cosgrove, L., Morrill, Z., Karter, J. M., Valdes, E., & Cheng, C. P. (2021). The cultural politics of mental illness: Toward a rights-based approach to global mental health. *Community Mental Health Journal,* 57(1), 3–9. https://doi.org/10.1007/s10597-020-00720-6.

Cosgrove, L., Mills, C., Karter, J. M., Mehta, A., & Kalathil, J. (2020). A critical review of the lancet commission on global mental health and sustainable development: Time for a paradigm change. *Critical Public Health, 30*(5), 624–631.

Cosgrove, L., Peters, S. M., Vaswani, A., & Karter, J. M. (2018). Institutional corruption in psychiatry: Case analyses and solutions for reform. *Social and Personality Psychology Compass, 12*(6), e12394.

Crepaz-Keay, D., & J. Kalathil. (2013). Personal narratives of madness: Introduction (Companion website fulford Et Al: The Oxford handbook of philosophy and psychiatry). http://global.oup.com/booksites/content/9780199579563/narratives/

Cresswell, M., & Spandler, H. (2016). Solidarities and tensions in mental health politics: Mad Studies and Psychopolitics. *Critical and Radical Social Work, 4*(3), 357–373.

Davar, B. V. (2008). From mental illness to psychosocial disability: Choices of identity for women users and survivors of psychiatry. *Indian Journal of Women's Studies.* https://doi.org/10.1177/097152150801500204.

Davar, B. V. (2017). Globalizing psychiatry and the case of 'vanishing' alternatives in a neocolonial state. *Disability and the Global South, 1*(2), 266–284.

de Sousa Santos, B. (2018). *The end of the cognitive empire: The coming of age of epistemologies of the South.* Duke University Press.

Dirth, T. P., & Adams, G. A. (2019). Decolonial theory and disability studies: On the modernity/coloniality of ability. *Journal of Social and Political Psychology, 7*(1), 260–289.

Drew, N., Funk, M., Tang, S., Lamichhane, J., Chávez, E., Katontoka, S., … Saraceno, B. (2011). Human rights violations of people with mental and psychosocial disabilities: An unresolved global crisis. *The Lancet, 378*(9803), 1664–1675.

Faulkner, A. (2017). Survivor research and Mad Studies: The role and value of experiential knowledge in mental health research. *Disability & Society, 32*(4), 500–520.

Foucault, M. (1967). *Madness and civilization: A history of madness in the age of reason.* Translated by R. Howard. Random House.

Foucault, M. (1977). *Power/knowledge: Selected interviews and other writings, 1972–1977.* Vintage.

Frances, A. (2013). *Saving normal: An insider's revolt against out-of-control psychiatric diagnosis, DSM-5, Big Pharma, and the medicalization of ordinary life.* William Morrow & Co.

Fricker, M. (2007). *Epistemic injustice: Power and the ethics of knowing.* Oxford University Press.

Gajaria, A., Izenberg, J. M., Nguyen, V., Rimal, P., Acharya, B., & Hansen, H. (2019). Moving the global mental health debate forward: how a structural competency framework can apply to global mental health training. *Academic Psychiatry*, 1–4. https://doi.org/10.1007/s40596-019-01073-3 (Link)

Hoffman, S. J., Sritharan, L., & Tejpar, A. (2016). Is the UN Convention on the Rights of Persons with Disabilities impacting mental health laws and policies in high-income countries? A case study of implementation in Canada. *BMC International Health and Human Rights, 16*(1), 28.

Karter, J. M. (2019). An ecological model for conceptual competence in psychiatric diagnosis. *Journal of Humanistic Psychology.* DOI: 10.1177/0022167819852488.

Karter, J. M., & Kamens, S. R. (2019). Toward conceptual competence in psychiatric diagnosis: An ecological model for critiques of the DSM. In S. Steingard (Ed.), *Critical psychiatry: Controversies and clinical implications* (pp. 17–69). Springer.

Kleinman, A. (2019). *The soul of care. The moral education of a husband and a doctor.* Penguin.

Kleinman, A., & Kleinman, J. (1997). Moral transformations of health and suffering in Chinese society. In A. Brandt & P. Rozin (Eds.), *Morality and health.* (pp. 101-118) London, UK: Routledge. .

LeFrançois, B. A., Menzies, R., & Reaume, G. (Eds.). (2013). *Mad matters: A critical reader in Canadian mad studies*. Canadian Scholars' Press.

Lewis, S. (1926). Arrowsmith. Starbooks Classics.

Lundbeck, H. (2021). About Us: Facts and background. Retrieved April 18, 2021, from https://www.lundbeck.com/global/about-us/facts-and-background

Lundbeck, H. (2014). Lundbeck puts depression on the global mental health agenda, November 2014. www.lundbeck.com/global/about-us/features/2014/lundbeck-puts-depression-on-the-global-mental-health-agenda.

Lundbeck, H., & Otsuka. (2015). Investments made in depression should match the burden of disease: Infographic developed by Otsuka Pharmaceutical Europe Ltd. and H. Lundbeck A/S from published literature and endorsed by the European Depression Association. PARC/4958/OPEL0715/BREX/1038d. Retrieved from: https://www.lundbeck.com/upload/global/files/pdf/about-us/features/Infographic_MDD_300915.pdf

Medina, J. (2013). *The epistemology of resistance: Gender and racial oppression, epistemic injustice, and the social imagination*. Oxford University Press.

Metzl, J. M., & Hansen, H. (2018). Structural competency and psychiatry. *JAMA psychiatry*, 75(2), 115–116.

Mills, C. (2014). *Decolonizing global mental health: The psychiatrization of the majority world*. Routledge.

Mills, C. (2018). From 'invisible problem' to global priority: The inclusion of mental health in the sustainable development goals. *Development and Change*, 49(3), 843–866.

Mirowski, P. (2009). Defining neoliberalism. In P. Mirowski & D. Plehwe (Eds.), *The road from Mont Pèlerin: The making of the neoliberal thought collective* (pp. 417–450). Harvard University Press.

Moncrieff, J., & Crawford, M. J. (2001). British psychiatry in the 20th century—Observations from a psychiatric journal. *Social Science & Medicine*, 53(3), 349–356.

National Survivor User Network (NSUN). (2018). Open letter to the organisers, partners and delegates of the global ministerial mental health summit, London 9th and 10th October, 2018. Accessed 24 October 2018. https://www.nsun.org.uk/news/global-ministerial-mental-health-summit-open-letter

Nik-Khah, E. (2014). Neoliberal pharmaceutical science and the Chicago School of Economics. *Social Studies of Science*, 44(4), 489–517.

Pan African Network of People with Psychosocial Disabilities (PANUSP). (2011). Cape town declaration of 16 October 2011. Retrieved September 22, 2020, https://disabilityglobalsouth.files.wordpress.com/2012/06/dgs-01-02-10.pdf.

Parks, R. (2014). The rise, critique and persistence of the DALY in global health. *The Columbia Journal of Global Health*, 4(1), 28–32.

Patel, V., Saxena, S., Lund, C., Thornicroft, G., Baingana, F., Bolton, P., ... Herrman, H. (2018). The lancet commission on global mental health and sustainable development. *The Lancet*, 392(10157), 1553–1598.

Perlin, M. L. (2002). You have discussed lepers and crooks: Sanism in clinical teaching. *Clinical Law Review*, 9, 683.

Peters, S. M. (2019). Medical neoliberalism in rape crisis center counseling: An interpretative phenomenological analysis of clinicians' understandings of survivor distress. *Journal of Social Issues*, 75(1), 238–266.

Phillips, J., Frances, A., Cerullo, M. A., Chardavoyne, J., Decker, H. S., First, M. B., … Zachar, P. (2012). The six most essential questions in psychiatric diagnosis: A pluralogue part 1: Conceptual and definitional issues in psychiatric diagnosis. *Philosophy, Ethics, and Humanities in Medicine, 7*(1), 1–29.

Porter, D. (2015). Colonization by/in psychiatry: From over-medicalization to democratization. *Journal of Ethics in Mental Health Open, 1*, 1–7.

Progress in Mind. (2021). *Welcome to progress in mind.* The Psychiatry & Neurology Resource Center. Retrieved from: https://progress.im/en/page/welcome-progress-mind-%E2%80%94-%C2%A0psychiatry-neurology-resource-center

Pūras, D. (2017). *Report of the Special Rapporteur on the right of everyone to the enjoyment of the highest attainable standard of physical and mental health* (Report A/HRC/35/21). United Nations. Retrieved September 22, 2020, from https://documents-dds-ny.un.org/doc/UNDOC/GEN/G17/076/04/PDF/G1707604.pdf?OpenElement.

Pūras, D. (2019). *Right of everyone to the enjoyment of the highest attainable standard of physical and mental health—Report of the special rapporteur on the right of everyone to the enjoyment of the highest attainable standard of physical and mental health* (Report A/HRC/41/34). United Nations. Retrieved September 22, 2020, from https://documents-dds-ny.un.org/doc/UNDOC/GEN/G19/105/97/PDF/G1910597.pdf?OpenElement.

Rimke, H., & Brock, D. (2012). The culture of therapy: Psychocentrism in everyday life. In M. Thomas, R. Raby and D. Brock (Eds.), *Power and Everyday Practices* (pp. 182–202). Toronto: Nelson.

Rose, N. (2018). *Our psychiatric future.* John Wiley & Sons.

Rose, D., Carr, S., & Beresford, P. (2018). 'Widening cross-disciplinary research for mental health': What is missing from the Research Councils UK mental health agenda? *Disability & Society, 33*(3), 476–481.

Russo, J., & Beresford, P. (2015). Between exclusion and colonisation: Seeking a place for mad people's knowledge in academia. *Disability & Society, 30*(1), 153–157.

Russo, J., & Wooley, S. (2020). The implementation of the convention on the rights of persons with disabilities: More than just another reform of psychiatry. *Health and Human Rights, 22*(1), 151.

Sayce, L. (2017). *It's time for full legal equality: Without it, it will never be fully OK to talk about mental health.* National Survivor User Network. Retrieved from: https://www.nsun.org.uk/its-time-for-full-legal-equality

Scull, A. (2015). *Madness in civilization: A cultural history of insanity from the Bible to Freud, from the madhouse to modern medicine.* Thames and Hudson/Princeton: Princeton University Press, London.

Sismondo, S. (2008). How pharmaceutical industry funding affects trial outcomes: Causal structures and responses. *Social science & medicine, 66*(9), 1909–1914.

Sismondo, S. (2009). Ghosts in the machine: Publication planning in the medical sciences. *Social Studies of Science, 39*(2), 171–198.

Soldatic, K., & Grech, S. (Eds.). (2017). *Disability and Colonialism:(dis) encounters and Anxious Intersectionalities.* Routledge.

Spandler, H., & Anderson, J. (Eds.). (2015). *Madness, distress and the politics of disablement.* Policy Press.

Summerfield, D. A. (2013). "Global mental health" is an oxymoron and medical imperialism. *BMJ, 346.*

Summerfield, D. A. (2017). Western depression is not a universal condition. *The British Journal of Psychiatry, 211*(1), 52–52.

Transforming Communities for Inclusion Asia Pacific (TCI Asia-Pacific). (2018a). *Bali declaration*. Retrieved March 22, 2021, from: http://tciasiapacific.blogspot.com/2018/09/bali-declaration-2018.html

TCI Asia-Pacific. (2018b). *Open letter to the organisers, partners and delegates of the global ministerial mental health summit*. Retrieved October 9 and 10, 2018, from: http://tciasiapacific.blogspot.com/2018/10/open-letter-to-organisers-partners-and.html

Whitley, R. (2015). Global mental health: Concepts, conflicts and controversies. *Epidemiology and Psychiatric Sciences, 24*(4), 285–291.

World Health Organization. (2017). Depression: Let's talk says who, as depression tops list of causes of ill health. Retrieved January 7, 2019. https://www.who.int/news/item/30-03-2017--depression-let-s-talk-says-who-as-depression-tops-list-of-causes-of-ill-health

Chapter 18

"Structural Competency" Meets Mad Studies

RECKONING WITH MADNESS AND MENTAL DIVERSITY BEYOND THE SOCIAL AND STRUCTURAL DETERMINANTS OF MENTAL HEALTH

Nev Jones

Summary

This chapter offers a valuable critique of the structural competency framework, urging those in the fields of psychiatry and psychology to interrogate their own role in "power-knowledge hierarchies that subordinate those deemed mad." Structural competency describes an invaluable approach to medicine and psychiatry that focuses, beyond the individual, on systemic causes of morbidity and mortality. Structural competency locates structural racism, violence, and inequity as root causes of many illnesses and health disparities. Building on this work, Jones foregrounds the need for us to move beyond structural competency toward an epistemic justice—challenging reductionist narratives of mental disability/difference, "complicating disorder," and asking "Who has (historically) and continues to (contemporaneously) generate institutionally sanctioned knowledge about psychiatry and disorder?" Jones encourages clinicians and researchers to move past a goal of "structural humility" toward a larger goal of "overall humility." This goal lets survivors speak for themselves and cultivates clinicians' ability to listen and hear even, or especially, when it counters core assumptions about mental health, mental illness, and psychiatry as a whole.

*

Since the publication of Metzl (2012) and Metzl and Hansen's (2014) foundational conceptualizations of "structural competency" (SC) roughly a decade ago, a steadily

DOI: 10.4324/9781003148456-21

growing number of medical schools have implemented some form of SC training and/or curriculum. In their seminal 2014 paper, Metzl and Hansen define SC as:

> the trained ability to discern how a host of issues defined clinically as symptoms, attitudes, or diseases (e.g., depression, medication "non-compliance," trauma, psychosis) also represent the downstream implications of a number of upstream decisions about such matters as health care and food delivery systems, zoning laws, urban and rural infrastructures, medicalization, or even about the very definitions of illness and health.

Departing from the more individualistic orientation behind the older "cultural competency" movement, SC thus explicitly foregrounds underlying structural and institutional forces that shape service users' lives, the systems of care in which clinical interactions unfold, and ultimately individual and population health outcomes. While the ideas behind SC function as a powerful corrective across fields of medicine, when we turn to psychiatry—perhaps the most contested of the medical fields—work under the SC umbrella has so far failed to more meaningfully engage with critical scholarship and activist contestations spanning disability studies, mad studies, user/survivor research, and organizing. Major, perhaps unintended, consequences explored in this chapter include tacit naturalization of "symptoms" and "disorder," failure to more radically displace a "medical" or clinical model of madness and attendant "interventions," and inattention to multifaceted epistemic inequalities already present in operative conceptualizations of "mental illness" and potential alternatives. Above all, key structural competency texts habitually position states and affects such as anger, grief, and long-term madness as negative or unwanted outcomes of the structural determinants in questions, leaving madness' messy, polyvalent potential to challenge and transform what we are and how we think, unspoken, unthought, and unrealized.

Structural Competency and Its Disjunctions

Aligned with public and population health emphases on social and structural rather than individual determinants of health, SC has called for a significant shift in medical education and training involving much greater emphasis on learned "recogn[ition] of the] structures that shape clinical interactions;" the "rearticula[tion of] cultural formulations in structural terms;" and pursuit of "structural interventions" and "structural humility" (Metzl & Hansen, 2018).

While Metzl's work on psychosis and race has generally been welcomed and even applauded by the user/survivor community (cf Madness Radio, 2010), foundational writings on SC have for the most part failed to engage deeper—equally structural—critiques of psychiatry, instead engaging in what we might understand as a kind of partial task-shifting: emphasizing extra-individual (rather than individual) social determinants of access, care, and outcomes, including structural racism, poverty, and regional geopolitics, while leaving many core assumptions about mental illness (qua biopsychosocial disease or disorder) intact. Long-standing epistemic inequities in the production and consolidation of psychiatric knowledge go largely unaddressed;

the SC literature, that is, says little about the extent to what we (think we) know about "mental illness" and intervention is in fact shaped by an evidence base that has been and continues to be overwhelmingly premised on the exclusion of those described and targeted, in all their intersectional complexity.

As one example, we might turn to Metzl and Hansen's (2018) introduction to a series of viewpoints on structural competency in *JAMA Psychiatry*, one of the world's most influential psychiatry journals. In addition to a compilation of viewpoints that include only MDs as authors—none of whom, to the best of my knowledge, has disclosed personal experience of, for example, homelessness, incarceration or treatment for "serious mental illness"—the authors ground the importance of structural competency in a series of observations that center structurally patterned inequalities spanning symptoms, disorders, treatment, and outcomes, while leaving conventional assumptions about the nature and definition of "mental illness" and health fully intact:

> Stressful social and economic conditions <u>exacerbate mood and anxiety disorders</u>. Substance use <u>disorders</u> such as opioid <u>dependence</u> are shaped by upstream forces such as federal regulations, drug marketing strategies, law enforcement, and racialized societal beliefs about whose pain is worthy of treatment. The <u>diagnosis and treatment of conditions ranging from schizophrenia to eating disorders to postpartum depression</u> have been shown to differ by race, ethnicity, and socioeconomic status based on unspoken institutional practices. Meanwhile, structural factors such as the geographical concentration of incarceration and the lack of housing, transportation, and safe, walkable space in low-income communities of color carry profoundly negative implications for mental health.

Meanwhile, exemplars of structural competency training or intervention, such as those described in the viewpoint series, limit the involvement and invocation of "peers" to community navigation and bridging roles, rather than centering them as primary drivers of SC pedagogy and design. And while it is always possible that evidence of greater involvement was simply omitted due to word count limitations (perhaps community members/peer workers in question did in fact *co-design* the SC "interventions" in question), these omissions, like the unproblematized use of the language of disorder and diagnosis deployed above, is itself telling. That is, whose perspectives and what positionalities were present among special series authors (and knowledge generators), if reflected on, were putatively not important enough to (publicly and visibly) reflect on and discuss.

In subsequent sections of this chapter, I will take this critique further; for now, suffice to say that my overarching concern is that even as a "learned ability" to identify structural determinants is put forward, simultaneously—performatively, in and through the stories structural competency leaders publicly tell—the (epistemic) marginalization of particular actors and agents goes unchallenged and is tacitly reinscribed. And this is a problem: if what we aspire to do is in fact performatively (or enactively) challenge the structural status quo.

Users and Survivors Push Back: Complicating "Disorder" and Its Prevention

Stretching back at least to the mid-1900s, psychosocial disability activists (variously identified as (ex-)patients, service users, survivors, and/or persons with lived experience) have frontally challenged reductionist narratives of mental disability/difference, including frameworks that *assume* that "mental illnesses" or disorders represent undesirable mental conditions would ideally be "prevented" or "eradicated," that ignore or minimize positive dimensions of mental and/or neuro-diversity, and/or disregard "social model" approaches that conceptualize disability as a product of socially imposed barriers rather than an intrinsic consequence of particular conditions (cf Dubrul, 2014; Rashed, 2019; Rosvqist et al., 2020; Spandler et al., 2015; Schrader et al., 2010). Rather than disavowing the suffering that disability/difference can involve—as is sometimes charged—activists have often gone to great lengths to acknowledge the challenges and suffering involved, while nevertheless emphasizing a much more complex and multifaceted picture of "madness" (see eg Jones & Kelly, 2015; Rashed, 2019; Spandler & Poursanidou, 2019). In the Icarus Project's grounding metaphor, for example, the "story of Icarus' wings" is invoked to, as they put it:

> remind us that sometimes the most incredible of gifts can also be the most dangerous. With our double-edged blessings we have the ability to fly to places of great vision and creativity, but like the mythical boy Icarus, we also have the potential to fly dangerously close to the sun—into realms of delusion and psychosis—and crash in a blaze of fire and confusion. (Icarus Project, 2013)

Alternately, the British collective Recovery in the Bin *centers* the reality of long-term mental health challenges, while critiquing neoliberal self-management approaches and calling for both a "robust 'social model of madness and distress' and greater access to 'non-medicalized alternatives'" (RITB, 2017).

A second common counter to activist discourse holds that those activists and activist-scholars who speak out in the above ways, do not "represent" the more authentically suffering patient, who, it is claimed, does not celebrate madness but instead wants to be free of it; wants to be cured. And to be sure, some do; many others, however—over half of individuals diagnosed with schizophrenia, if researchers focused on "lack of insight" are to be believed—reject both explicit "mad pride" *and* "get me a cure" positionalities. Many individuals, that is, who have been labeled with "lack of insight" tied to psychosis, mania, or dissociation, reject *either* of these labels as valid descriptions of experiences they instead directly *occupy* (e.g., see the narratives of TJ and Jorge below)—and ultimately not just the labels but the deeper ontological and epistemological frames in which they are embedded.

I also reflect, repeatedly, on actual statistics regarding "disengagement" from mental health services, which in psychosis run upwards of 50%. Half, no small margin, of service recipients, that is, reject the services they receive, hardly an indication that the reductive medicalization we see in fact succeeds en masse. Most often, said disengagement is attributed to lack of insight and/or "treatment resistant" symptoms—symptoms which putatively render the individual incapable of a thoughtful rejection of what has been offered. And while inattention to structural disadvantage is clearly a problem in mainstream services (Jones et al., 2019, 2021), this inability to listen and hear is arguably even more fundamental.

In addition to far-reaching implications with respect to "treatment"—discussed further below—a multivalent reframing of disability/difference also calls for a rethinking of assumptions about "prevention" discourse. Described by many critical disability scholars as a "new eugenics" (Rembis, 2009; Reinder et al., 2019), efforts to prevent various forms of disability through biological or social intervention tend to import (and strengthen) social and political judgments about the conditions in question: that they are undesirable and burdensome, and that not only individuals but also families and communities would be "better off" were they eradicated. These sentiments in turn readily reinforce existing structural and social stigma: by what logic can (or could) we "celebrate" identities or differences best eliminated?

Neoliberal economic arguments also frequently undergird prevention efforts, with policy makers framing the benefits of prevention in terms of reduced healthcare and social welfare "costs" and increased worker productivity (both at the individual and family level, due to the "freeing up" of individuals otherwise engaged in caregiving). Somewhat notoriously, the centering of cure and prevention also tends to undermine support for (or redirect it away from) supportive programs and interventions (Mathis, 2019). This logic has repeatedly played out in the budgetary distributions of the National Institute of Mental Health and other major research funders—namely, a huge imbalance in funding dedicated to cure-driven biological and biogenetic research rather than clinical and services projects (Braslow, 2021; Patel, 2020; Torrey et al., 2020, 2021; Woelbert et al., 2020).

Ironically, perhaps, discourse on the prevention of disorder grounded in "social and structural determinants" also risks over-writing the narratives of (actual) ethnoracialized individuals with "serious mental illness" in the guise of an emancipatory "structural competency." I reflect, for example, on the actual narratives of recent minoritized participants from qualitative research projects on early psychosis. For example, one participant, a young Black man whom I will call TJ, acknowledged a background featuring the worst of structural oppression in the United States: removed from his biological family in early childhood and moved from foster care placement to foster care placement; repeatedly abused, hospitalized, and arrested; finally funneled into a specialized early psychosis service and then an "adult" residential group home. TJ expresses full awareness of just how structurally oppressive these systems have been. But his critique also takes quite a different form from SC discourse: namely, his "psychosis"—or rather the beliefs and problems attributed to his psychosis—reflects reality, not thought disorder. And the determination that he is "psychotic" or "schizophrenic," the medical records that inscribe him as such, and the consequent way in which interlocutors dismiss his experiences as "disorder," and that subject him to forms of state-sanctioned violence (involuntary injections, court-ordered treatment) are, in his mind, the real manifestations of structural racism:

> *You got to understand, you got to understand what it's really about … all it is, is like the genocide [of Black people]. It's about keeping us on watch. In the later days, because I woke up to it, that's why I don't want to be a part of this psychiatric system … You can easily drug somebody up with some pills that's going to at least turn down a specific blood count in they body to make them act this way, act that way: so we see that you a mad motherfucker. So what we going to do is, we're going to give you some medicine that's going to pretty much lower that blood count that goes through your cell that deals with your muscle, your metabolism. We see you like to prove people wrong, so what we going to do is we going to get you some medicine. They absorb my behaviors in these treatment facilities. It's like a cage, man. And then that report [medical records/psychiatric history] … [when they see it] they look at you, and they'll just dope your ass up. … And I don't believe in psychosis. That shit [what I've experienced] is <u>real</u>. You know what I'm saying?*

A "structurally competent" psychiatrist, to make this point another way, who nevertheless understands TJ's experiences as schizophrenia, as disorder, even if resulting from structural vectors, would still miss the deeper point, still end up engaging in epistemic silencing and violence.

Another interviewee, "Jorge," a young Latinx man who came to the US from Mexico to live with his grandparents at the age of 12 or 13, first apologizes that I am interviewing someone for a psychosis study that does not and has never experienced "psychosis" ("just know that I don't actually meet your criteria"), then explains to me what he *has* experienced. After qualifying for a prestigious summer program on nano-technology as teen, applying and get admitted to major research universities in his senior year, "*[one day] I felt like a magnetic field in my hand: my whole body was like a magnetic field. … And there were charged nano-particles in the water and food, and the magnetism in my hand repelled them.*"

Over the ensuing months, he explains, all those whom he interacted with—hospital staff, the police, the local early psychosis team—told him that his experiences were not real, that he was "crazy," or, he notes, did not actually tell him this but were clearly thinking it. Didn't believe him; discounted his experiences.

And so, in the isolation of his own room, he reads and watches documentaries to try and understand what's going on. "*There's all this mind control stuff that I read,*" he expands; "*I went to so many articles and histories of people and … it gave me ideas, not just of looking at it through a bad view, but looking at the positive view. … It has pushed me to becoming more like a cybersecurity [expert]. I am trying to think about possible ways to protect people.*" People who, he emphasizes, will only believe "once it's too late," and whom he therefore needs to protect from their own lack of present awareness. (They don't know what big tech firms are working on, they don't understand the dangers that lie in the future.) Eventually, he takes out his phone and pulls up a series of patents—for nanobots that can move through the human bloodstream, sonic wave blasters, technology related to mind control. The patent holders are Google, Microsoft, and Lockheed Martin. *"There's a lot of things going on that people don't know about, he continues, but there is—[it's real]—you can see it right here,"* and he holds up his phone.

> "Have you showed these patents to your therapist?" I ask—"How did she respond."
> *"She didn't believe it...she said she doesn't believe it."*
> "Do you feel like," I follow up, "ideally, people would respond to your experiences and the arguments you're making differently?"
> *"Uhm...uh,"* he pauses, *"I just know that people will never believe me no matter what they tell me."*

And so, he explains, he has to walk the path on his own, with commitments that exceed what a clinician—even a bilingual and bicultural clinician—can or is willing to accept, refashioning a more conventional immigrant narrative of mobility—his earlier immigrant story of immigrant-Mexican-youth-who-goes-to-prestigious-university—with mobility (and social justice) on his own terms. As for his therapist, he describes her as sweet; he cares about her. *"She's like the kind of girl I'd like to marry."* But therapy? *"Since I don't have psychosis, it's obviously not something I need."*

We might then ask how a conventional structural competency approach would understand and frame TJ and Jorge's experiences and their narratives. Whether there is in fact any deeper consideration of the epistemic injustice inherent in the normalized disbelief in (and reductionistic pathologization) of their experiences; whether SC discourse instructs the providers who work with such youth not just to center structural determinants but also their political agency. That, perhaps above all, explicitly challenges the *automatic* coupling of psychiatry (or psychiatric subjects) and "illness." While progressive SC theorists would likely concede a co-constitutive relationship between anti-Black racism and "stigma" involving dangerousness, unpredictability, and violence, it is less clear that SC would embrace either TJ's claims regarding pathologization and medication-medicalization themselves as forms of racialized social control (cf Meerai et al., 2016; White, 2021) or Jorge's rejection of the "psychosis" label and need for psychopharmacological "help."

If We Wanted to Engage More Deeply, What Questions Would We Actually Ask? Epistemic Reflexivity as a Foundation of Anti-Sanist "Structural Competence"

Although Foucault himself ultimately abandoned methodology described in *Archaeology of Knowledge*, its chapters of *Archaeology* pose numerous questions beyond those we tend to find in structural competency discourse, questions, as Foucault puts it "[of] the already-said at the level of its existence," beneath the consciousness of any individual subject. Questions that re-orient the reader to underlying assumptions, conditions of possibility, of what is said. In the sections that follow, these questions form the inspiration for a deeper interrogation of decisions and relations that are not explicitly claimed within structural competency writings, but structure and undergird those claims that are more explicitly made.

Who Is Authorized to Speak, in What Institutional Sites of Discourse

Reflecting both on historical discourse about "psychiatric disorder"—where we have come from—and contemporary structural competency writings—the ostensibly progressive place at which some psychiatrists have now reached—Foucault's *Archaeology* might be read as asking us to pause and ask who, across SEX texts, is in fact authorized to speak, and on what grounds: about psychiatry, about disorder, about "structural violence" against, or affecting, the "mentally ill"? Unquestionably, within SC, the primary speakers, the *experts*, are psychiatrists and physicians. Certainly, there is no explicit questioning of these positionalities, that is, no stated commitment to either co-production or the more radical de-centering of conventional psychiatric (or medical) expertise. Indeed, the term competency, much critiqued for this reason in the context of "cultural competency," tends to center acquisition of knowledge, skills, and "expertise over" rather than critical reflexivity, humility, and attention to complex power hierarchies in medicine (cf Kumagai & Lypson, 2009; Tervalon & Maria-Garcia, 1998). "Decolonization" also provides a helpfully instructive contrast to SC: Buyum and colleagues (2020), for example, in a large part through displacement and decentering, rather than "competency"; or, to quote them directly "an agenda of repoliticising and rehistoricising health through a paradigm shift, a leadership shift and a knowledge shift." In Buyum et al's formulation, the paradigm shift engendered by "decolonization"—a radical reorientation to underlying structural vectors—comes closest to SC, while the "leadership shift" (leadership "reflecting the diversity of people the [systems or institutions in question] are intended to serve") and "knowledge shift" (reciprocal learning, centering knowledge generated locally) represent a stronger departure.

Thus, in SC, we see little or no *explicit* questioning of the kind that concerns the absence of those on the receiving end of psychiatric services as equal or even more central "experts" (except, perhaps, in a limited or pejorative sense, as we unpack below); nor reflection on the ironies of medicine's (and psychiatry's) starkly hierarchical position over disciplines and professional fields that have in fact long-centered structural conditions and person-in-environment (as in, for example, social work; Germain, 1973; Kemp et al., 1997). This place (or institutional site) of "structural competency"—the medical school, psychiatric residency or fellowship, clinic—that is, like the question of who the institutionally designated "experts" in fact are, goes almost entirely unremarked. As do the complex disciplinary histories and hierarchies that continue to play out (in many states, the singular place of physicians to approve involuntary psychiatric holds, for example; or to undertake forensic assessments or determine capacity).

Assumptions Regarding Epistemology

The epistemology—how we know what we (think) we know—underlying structural competency qua competency also goes largely uninterrogated. Epistemic politics, that is, are not thematized, except perhaps insofar as conventional psychiatric knowledge has allowed "structural factors" to drop out and racism and classism (in a certain sense) to shape clinical interactions. There is, however, no sustained attention to what Foucault—outside *Archaeology* in this case—famously termed "subjugated knowledges":

> [those] knowledges that have been disqualified as inadequate to their task or insufficiently elaborated: naive knowledges, located low down on the hierarchy, beneath the required level of cognition or scientificity … unqualified, even directly disqualified knowledges (such as that of the psychiatric patient, of the ill person…).

Or perhaps we should say, little or no attention to the *politics* of the subjugation in question, more so than its simple presence. And thus, one might fairly infer, silence on the extent to which "structural competency," no less than "cultural competency" or "evidence-based practice," might come to operate as a particular kind of "knowledge regime" or privileged institution in which "policy relevant ideas are generated and percolate" (Campbell & Pederson, 2007). A regime, to riff on Tanenbaum, then, in which inevitably "some knowledge" and "some knowers" are privileged in both "the consulting room and policy arena" Tanenbaum, 2005, p. 163).

What Positions the Psychiatric (or Psychiatrized) Subject Is Allowed or Authorized to Occupy

Perhaps tellingly, in the one example provided across Metzl and Hansen's 2018 special section on structural competency training interventions in which "peers" or service users are present, they play an extremely limited role. Per the article, which does not make any direct service user involvement in authorship explicit, psychiatric residents in the training in question work with peer "liaisons" or "navigators" who introduce them to the ostensible structural realities of the latter's communities and associated systems of social welfare (or control). Seemingly not far from the roles we see peer support workers occupy in the broader mental health system, these individuals appear empowered to convey individual or localized knowledge about place and structure, and yet this empowerment is clearly circumscribed. To quote the philosopher Jose Medina, there are in fact still:

> problems of epistemic justice in treating someone only as an informant, for there is no full and equal epistemic cooperation when that is the case. When one is allowed to be an informant without being allowed to be an inquirer, one is allowed to enter into one set of communicative activities—those relating to passing knowledge and opinions—but not others, precisely those others that are more sophisticated, happen at a higher level of abstraction, and require more epistemic authority: formulating hypotheses, probing and questioning, assessing and interpreting opinions, and so forth. Giving people "epistemic subjectivity" instead of treating them as mere objects does not guarantee that "their general status as a subject of knowledge" may not be constrained or minimized

Meanwhile in their counseling take on structural competency, Ali and Sichel (2014) depart from psychiatric SC in some respects (using distress in lieu of illness or disorder, for example), and explicitly recommend "partnering with clients." It is nevertheless striking that the only reference in Ali and Sichel's dedicated section on "partnering" is to Open Dialogue (an arguably progressive but in other ways conventionally clinician-developed and led approach); Mad Studies or work within Mad Studies is not mentioned; the work of psychiatric survivors is not mentioned. The International Network to Advance Recovery's (INTAR's) work is presented as providing a window into "alternative strategies" for addressing distress, but not alternative conceptualizations that seek to reclaim mad-positive and disability-positive identities, or link to alternative histories which foreground the richness, complexity and depth of voices, visions, and extreme states beyond "suffering," "distress," or "disablement" (LeFrancois et al., 2013; McCarthy-Jones, 2012; Woods, 2013; Schrader et al., 2013). Nor is there discussion of what Joseph Gone (2013, 2019, 2021) among others have described as the neocolonialism of "therapy culture" (cf Furedi, 2013; Foucault, 1990). In other words, even here, it is questionable to what extent critical user/survivor/mad and/or intersectional discourse with its claims to epistemic and collective self-determination and justice beyond psychologized "healing" is recognized, much less explicitly centered.

Risk, Determinants, Distress, Illness, Madness

A broader trend, spanning many SC publications but also broader discourse on the "social determinants of mental health" is the often heavy-handed conflation of experiences and conditions as diverse as grief, hopelessness, anger, 'dysfunctional behavior,' cognitive challenges, depression, mania, and schizophrenia. Framed in epidemiological terms, social and structural determinants are then construed as conferring risk for the development of illness, disease, or undesired outcomes, often without distinguishing between *expectable* emotional states (anger because of racism; grief after a loved one has died), responses to the social and institutional *sequelae* of being labeled as "mentally ill" (shame, anger, hopelessness), reactions to material consequences of institutionalization and disablement (i.e., struggles tied to poverty, lack of access to housing, material needs that may masquerade as "disorder"), and long-term psychosocial disabilities and/or forms of "madness," which for many are experienced as co-extensive with sense of self. And for some, including TJ and Jorge, all of the above categories may be refused, and experiences labeled as mad or psychotic understood and experienced straightforwardly as *real* and precisely not psychological in *any* sense (cf Gone, 2019, 2021).

For SC in particular, the failure to make such distinctions explicit suggests that either the authors are unaware of these distinctions (unlikely?) or that they do not find them sufficiently politically and socially salient. De facto conflation of these differences, alongside a de facto pathologization and/or clinicalization of "illness" and "disorder," risks positioning madness and Mad folk most centrally as the "negative" and undesired outcome of oppressive social and structural determinants (perhaps in combination with biogenetic factors). Other possible social identities—and agency within them—are tacitly written out, as is the potential for distress, righteous anger, and mental diversity to inspire, transform, deepen, and enrich. Even when the madness in question is the most challenging—especially when it is the most challenging.

Conclusion

Structural competency, and more broadly the science of the social and structural determinants of mental health, foreground critical dimensions of social injustice, including racism, income inequality, poverty, and segregation. Addressing these sources of injustice is critical for any democratic society. As this chapter has argued, however, a major form of structural oppression is in fact reified if social determinants and structural competency writings do not explicitly and visibly interrogative their own role in power-knowledge hierarchies that subordinate those deemed Mad, leave the reduction of madness to pathology unchallenged, and fail to deeply engage with user/survivors and the alternative social identities and "knowledges" they have painstakingly forged.

All of this matters—perhaps particularly much—in the context of structural competency because the latter is widely perceived as progressive and even paradigm-shifting. And yet by leaving so much unspoken and unchallenged, the risk of the reification and further sedimentation of the foreclosures noted in this chapter is substantial. The mad movement does need allies, but they must be real allies; it does need pedagogy but it must be a pedagogy that consistently and substantively disrupts, and in disrupting, opens space for a deeper reimagining. This is what I personally wish and hope to see. But I also hold that it is what any deeper notion of social justice demands of us; all of us.

I give the final word to agitators for justice and solidarity, old and new: Martin Luther King Jr and the Latin American Network of Psychosocial Diversity.

> I am cognizant of the interrelatedness of all communities and states. I cannot sit idly by in Atlanta and not be concerned about what happens in Birmingham. Injustice anywhere is a threat to justice everywhere. We are caught in an inescapable network of mutuality, tied in a single garment of destiny. Whatever affects one directly, affects all indirectly. (King, Letter from Birmingham Jail, 1964)
>
> We denounce the pathologization and medicalization of our diversity, and all other forms of discrimination and abuse from psychiatry, psychology and other specialties in the name of "mental health" and "normality." We demand the construction of a new paradigm … which accepts "psychosocial diversity" as a fact and a principle derived from human diversity and recognizes us as experts by experience. (Declaration of Lima, 2016)

References

Ali, A., & Sichel, C. E.(2014). Structural competency as a framework for training in counseling psychology. *The Counseling Psychologist, 42*(7), 901–918.

Braslow, J. T. (2021). Psychosis without meaning: Creating modern clinical psychiatry, 1950 to 1980. *Culture, Medicine, and Psychiatry, 45*(3), 429–455.

Büyüm, A. M., Kenney, C., Koris, C., Mkumba, C., & Raveendran, Y. (2020). Decolonising global health: if not now, when?. *BMJ Global Health, 5*(8), e003394.

Campbell, J. L., Pedersen, O. K. (2007). Knowledge regimes and comparative political economy. *Socio-Economic Review, 13*(4), 679–701.

Cohen, B. M. (2014). *Passive-aggressive: Māori resistance and the continuance of colonial psychiatry in Aotearoa New Zealand. Disability and the Global South, 1*(2), 319–339.

Corstens, D., Longden, E., & May, R. (2012). Talking with voices: Exploring what is expressed by the voices people hear. *Psychosis, 4*(2), 95–104.

DiPolito, S. A. (2007). Olmstead v. LC-deinstitutionalization and community integration: An awakening of the nation's conscience?. *Mercer Law Review, 58*(4), 14–30.

DuBrul, S. A. (2014). The Icarus Project: A counter narrative for psychic diversity. *Journal of Medical Humanities, 35*(3), 257–271.

Fabris, E. (2012). *Experiences labelled psychotic: A settler's autoethnography beyond psychosic narrative*. University of Toronto.

Foucault, M. (1990). *The history of sexuality: An introduction*. Vintage.

Furedi, F. (2013). *Therapy culture: Cultivating Vu*. Routledge.

Germain, C. B. (1973). An ecological perspective in casework practice. *Social Casework, 54*(6), 323–330.

Gone, J. P. (2013). Redressing first nations historical trauma: Theorizing mechanisms for indigenous culture as mental health treatment. *Transcultural Psychiatry, 50*(5), 683–706.

Gone, J. P. (2019). "The thing happened as he wished": Recovering an American Indian cultural psychology. *American Journal of Community Psychology, 64*(1–2), 172–184.

Gone, J. P. (2021). Decolonization as methodological innovation in counseling psychology: Method, power, and process in reclaiming American Indian therapeutic traditions. *Journal of Counseling Psychology, 68*(3), 259.

Hansen, H., Braslow, J., & Rohrbaugh, R. M. (2018). From cultural to structural competency—Training psychiatry residents to act on social determinants of health and institutional racism. *JAMA Psychiatry, 75*(2), 117–118.

Hart, A. (2020). A new alliance? The hearing voices movement and neurodiversity. In Rosqvist, H. B., Chown, N., & Stenning, A. (Eds.), *Neurodiversity Studies* (pp. 221–225), Routledge.

Hoagwood, K. E., Atkins, M., Kelleher, K., Peth-Pierce, R., Olin, S., Burns, B., ... & Horwitz, S. M. (2018). Trends in children's mental health services research funding by the National Institute of Mental Health from 2005 to 2015: A 42% reduction. *Journal of the American Academy of Child & Adolescent Psychiatry, 57*(1), 10–13.

Hoffman, G. A. (2019). Public mental health without the health? Challenges and contributions from the Mad Pride and neurodiversity paradigms. In *Developments in Neuroethics and bioethics* (Vol. 2, pp. 289–326). Academic Press.

Icarus Project. (2013). Friends make the best medicine. http://nycicarus.org/articles/friends-best-medicine/

Jones, N., & Kelly, T. (2015). Inconvenient complications: On the heterogeneities of madness and their relationship to disability. In *Madness, distress and the politics of disablement* (pp. 43–56). Policy Press.

Jones, N., Godzikovskaya, J., Zhao, Z., Vasquez, A., Gilbert, A., & Davidson, L. (2019). Intersecting disadvantage: Unpacking poor outcomes within early intervention in psychosis services. *Early Intervention in Psychiatry, 13*(3), 488–494.

Jones, N., Kamens, S., Oluwoye, O., Mascayano, F., Perry, C., Manseau, M., & Compton, M. T. (2021). Structural disadvantage and culture, race, and ethnicity in early psychosis services: International provider survey. *Psychiatric Services, 72*(3), 254–263.

Kemp, S. P., Whittaker, J. K., & Tracy, E. M. (1997). *Person-environment practice: The social ecology of interpersonal helping.* Transaction Publishers.

King Jr, M. L. (1964 / 2003). Letter from Birmingham jail. In, Roger Gottliebe (Ed.), *Liberating faith: Religious voices for justice, peace, & ecological wisdom* (pp. 177–187). Rowman & Littlefield.

Kumagai, A. K., & Lypson, M. L. (2009). Beyond cultural competence: Critical consciousness, social justice, and multicultural education. *Academic Medicine, 84*(6), 782–787.

Latin American Network of Psychosocial Diversity (2016). Declaration of lima. https://rompiendolaetiqueta.com/declaration

LeFrançois, B. A., Beresford, P., & Russo, J. (2016). Destination mad studies. *Intersectionalities: A Global Journal of Social Work Analysis, Research, Polity, and Practice, 5*(3), 1–10.

LeFrançois, B. A., Menzies, R., & Reaume, G. (Eds.). (2013). *Mad matters: A critical reader in Canadian mad studies.* Canadian Scholars' Press.

Longden, E. (2010). Making sense of voices: A personal story of recovery. *Psychosis, 2*(3), 255–259.

Longden, E., Madill, A., & Waterman, M. G. (2012). Dissociation, trauma, and the role of lived experience: Toward a new conceptualization of voice hearing. *Psychological Bulletin, 138*(1), 28.

Madness Radio. (2010). Schizophrenia and black politics: Interview with Jonathan Metzil. Accessed at https://www.madnessradio.net/madness-radio-schizophrenia-and-black-politics-jonathan-metzl/

Madrid, J. C. C., & Parada, T. C. (2018). Locura y neoliberalismo. El lugar de la antipsiquiatría en la salud mental contemporánea. *Política y sociedad, 55*(2), 559–574.

Mathis, J. (2019). Medicaid's institutions for mental diseases (IMD) exclusion rule: A policy debate—Argument to retain the IMD rule. *Psychiatric Services, 70*(1), 4–6.

McCarthy-Jones, S. (2012). *Hearing voices: The histories, causes and meanings of auditory verbal hallucinations.* Cambridge University Press.

Medina, J. (2012). Hermeneutical injustice and polyphonic contextualism: Social silences and shared hermeneutical responsibilities. *Social Epistemology, 26*(2), 201–220.

Metzl, J. M. (2012). Structural competency. *American Quarterly, 64*(2), 213–218.

Metzl, J. M., & Hansen, H. (2014). Structural competency: Theorizing a new medical engagement with stigma and inequality. *Social Science & Medicine, 103*, 126–133.

Metzl, J. M., & Hansen, H. (2018). Structural competency and psychiatry. *JAMA Psychiatry, 75*(2), 115–116.

Meerai, S., Abdillahi, I., & Poole, J. (2016). An introduction to anti-Black sanism. *Intersectionalities: A Global Journal of Social Work Analysis, Research, Polity, and Practice, 5*(3), 18–35.

Patel, V. (2020). Mental health research funding: Too little, too inequitable, too skewed. *Lancet Psychiatry 8(3),*171–172.

Rashed, M. A. (2019). *Madness and the demand for recognition: A philosophical inquiry into identity and mental health activism.* Oxford University Press.

Recovery in the Bin (RITC). (2017). RITC: Key principles. https://recoveryinthebin.org/ritbkeyprinciples/

Redesfera Latinoamericana de la Diversidad Psicosocial - Locura Latina. (2016). *Declaration of Lima / Declaracion de Lima.* Accessed at https://rompiendolaetiqueta.com/blog/2019/5/8/declaracin-red-locura-latina

Schrader, S., Jones, N., & Shattell, M. (2013). Mad pride: Reflections on sociopolitical identity and mental diversity in the context of culturally competent psychiatric care. *Issues in Mental Health Nursing, 34*(1), 62–64.

Spandler, H., & Anderson, J. (Eds.). (2015). *Madness, distress and the politics of disablement*. Policy Press.

Spandler, H., Anderson, J., & Sapey, B. (Eds.). (2015). *Madness, distress and the politics of disablement* (Vol. 1). Bristol: Policy Press.

Tanenbaum, S. J. (2005). Evidence-based practice as mental health policy: Three controversies and a caveat. *Health Affairs, 24*(1), 163-173.

Tervalon, M., & Murray-Garcia, J. (1998). Cultural humility versus cultural competence: A critical distinction in defining physician training outcomes in multicultural education. *Journal of Health Care for the Poor and Underserved, 9*(2), 117–125.

Torrey, E. F., Center, T. A., Arlington, V., Zdanowicz, M. T. J. D, T. A. C., & Davis, J. M. (2003). *A federal failure in psychiatric research: Continuing NIMH negligence in funding sufficient research on serious mental illnesses*. Treatment Advocacy Center.

White, W. (2021). *Re-writing the master narrative: A prerequisite for mad liberation*. Mad Studies Reader.

Woelbert, E., Lundell-Smith, K., White, R., & Kemmer, D. (2020). Accounting for mental health research funding: Developing a quantitative baseline of global investments. *The Lancet Psychiatry*, 8(3), 250–258.

Woods, A. (2013). The voice-hearer. *Journal of Mental Health, 22*(3), 263–270.

Rashed, M. A. (2019). *Madness and the demand for recognition: A philosophical inquiry into identity and mental health activism*. Oxford University Press.

Rembis, M. A. (2009). (Re) Defining disability in the 'genetic age': Behavioral genetics, 'new' eugenics and the future of impairment. *Disability & Society, 24*(5), 585–597.

Reinders, J., Stainton, T., & Parmenter, T. R. (2019). The quiet progress of the new eugenics. Ending the lives of persons with intellectual and developmental disabilities for reasons of presumed poor quality of life. *Journal of Policy and Practice in Intellectual Disabilities, 16*(2), 99–112.

Rosqvist, H. B., Chown, N., & Stenning, A. (Eds.). (2020). *Neurodiversity studies: A new critical paradigm*. Routledge.

Spandler, H., & Poursanidou, D. (2019). Who is included in the mad studies project?. *The Journal of Ethics in Mental Health, 10*.

Torrey, E. F., Knable, M. B., Rush, A. J., Simmons, W. W., Snook, J., & Jaffe, D. J. (2020). Using the NIH research, condition and disease categorization database for research advocacy: Schizophrenia research at NIMH as an example. *PLoS One, 15*(11), e0241062.

Torrey, E. F., Simmons, W. W., Hancq, E. S., & Snook, J. (2021). The continuing decline of clinical research on serious mental illnesses at NIMH. *Psychiatric Services, 72*(11), 1342–1344.

Chapter 19

The Neoliberal Project

MENTAL HEALTH AND MARGINALITY IN INDIA

Zaphya Jena

Summary

This article was first published in the Mariwala Health Initiative's *ReFrame III*, which is devoted to "mental health beyond clinical contexts." The Mariwala Health Initiative[1] (MHI) is a grant-making and advocacy organization working on improving mental health in India. Their goal is to foster accessible, affirmative, rights-based, and user-centric mental health care. Part of the challenge of this work is the way India is adopting increasingly globalized mental health models that overmedicate and overpathologize individuals. MHI uses the *ReFrame* series to help change the paradigm of mental health in India and to provide a platform for scholars, activists, clinicians, artists, and other key stakeholders in mental health.

Zaphya Jena's contribution to *ReFrame III* combines a background in counseling psychology with graduate work in humanities and social sciences. She uses this interdisciplinary position to connect the dots between "neoliberal frameworks of health: individualized pathologization (where social suffering is covered up by the veil of individual-level mental illness) and the prescription of free psychotropic drugs." Jena also addresses the ways that neoliberal notions of productivity are reconfiguring the self in India toward a market-economy normalcy based on "individualized responsibility, productivity, and—eventually—success." It is only when we work through these critiques that the disenfranchised can receive care and understanding that underscore the way that "an unjust social order contributes to neuropsychological conditions."

*

DOI: 10.4324/9781003148456-22

Neoliberalism as Paternalism

The increasing prevalence of mental illness amongst Scheduled Tribes (ST) has been a source of worry for community health workers in ST populations; case studies among Adivasis highlight the need for mental health equity. For instance, histories of marginalization have been observed (Sadath et al., 2019) to have had critically adverse effects on the mental health of Adivasis in Wayanad district in the state of Kerala. "Poverty, low living standards and related factors" (Saddath et al., 2018) are risk factors for mental health, and community health workers must attempt to address these health inequalities for historically disadvantaged communities. However, the responses of both the health community and the government often involve a paternalistic form of governance that functions within neoliberal frameworks of health: individualized pathologization (where social suffering is covered up by the veil of individual-level mental illness) and the prescription of free psychotropic drugs. These frameworks involve the "marketization" of healthcare and, with their focus on the individual, may serve to cast a veil over shortcomings in the area of human rights (Kottai, 2018).

The Individual in the Mental Health Marketplace

Scholars drawing from Mudge's conceptualization of neoliberalism's three interconnected spheres argue that neoliberalism and globalization have catalyzed widening health inequities between various communities (Baru & Mohan, 2018). These interconnected faces, namely the political, bureaucratic, and intellectual domains, intersect insidiously to reconfigure the delivery of health services. Baru and Mohan (*ibid.*) go on to highlight how various domains of neoliberalism have led to the commodification of health. The role of the state as provider of health as a public utility has, under late capitalism, been replaced with the marketization and privatization of health, regulating service demand and supply. The rise of philanthro-capitalism, along with neoliberalism's ties with conservative politics, has drastic consequences for marginalized groups, with health governance emerging as a means of social control. Ramifications include scant access to quality health resources, languishing public infrastructure such as sanitation and water supply, poor nutrition, and limited health-seeking behaviour.

Drawing on the above framework, this piece further argues that besides its impact in the sociopolitical, economic, and academic realms, neoliberalism has also aided in the dubious reorganization of the subjective, psychological self. This argument becomes crucial to the analysis of neoliberal ideology and its involvement in psychiatric treatment, given that the psychopharmacological revolution gave birth to an obsession with situating mental illness within the individual, decontextualized from social reality, and how that viewpoint continues to be supported by neoliberal ideologies that gloss over structural inequalities (Esposito & Perez, 2014).

Scholars have also traced how the biomedical discourse dominates health circles, supported by a market rationale that evaluates merit (and notions of normalcy) based on notions of individualized responsibility, productivity, and—eventually—success. This aligns with the psy-disciplines' conventional concepts of mental illness, in which immense value is placed on work and productivity. For example, one of the diagnostic criteria for alcohol use disorder in the *DSM-V* is the failure to fulfill obligations at work, school, or home and the inability to be a productive member of society; similar language is used in the descriptions of other disorders (American Psychiatric Association, 2013). This fetishization of productivity, and the way it dictates notions of normalcy and deviance, has vastly benefited the pharmaceutical industry. Sophisticated prescriptive drugs are able to modify behaviour to make it fit neoliberal notions of the functional person, who is seen to be in primary charge of their own happiness, success, and health. This reconfiguration of the self is strengthened by market forces, notably in the intellectual realm, through the drug industry's blatant sponsorship of motivated medical research—conferences, training seminars, branding, and product placement—that has led to a substantial increase in the number of drugs prescribed (Esposito & Perez, 2014) and, worryingly, an increasingly neurochemical approach to mental illness.

Colonization Makes a Comeback in Mental Health

Categories such as post-traumatic stress disorder (PTSD) and substance abuse are arbitrarily appropriated and applied to mask the social suffering brought about by neoliberal notions of development. For instance, based on physical and symbolic violence perpetrated on the bodies of marginalized caste groups in Kerala, Kottai (2018) traces the way paternalistic governance of mental health practices has led to the categorization of poor, displaced Adivasis as "alcoholic" and "mad." Meanwhile, funds poured into de-addiction centers, rehabilitation homes, and the mechanized dispersal of free drugs and treatment enable narratives of "development" to flourish—not only in the systematic expropriation of tribal lands for neoliberal development, but also in the construction of a "normal" self (as opposed to mad and/or alcoholic) that suits regional and cultural sensibilities (Kottai, 2018). What transpires, then, is not just the colonization of psychiatric nosology (the branch of medical science dealing with the classification of diseases) in Kerala, drawing as it does from Euro-American frameworks, but also involves shaping models of mental health to fit into local subjectivities of normalcy and development.

Philanthro-capitalism further aids in the constructing of good health as a commodity, which makes a right into something that depends on the benevolence of the rich, perpetuating the lack of accountability and power asymmetries in health services (Baru & Mohan, 2018). Non-governmental organizations, too, often rely on certain given scripts of mental illness, both while training mental health practitioners and while treating clients. Such scripts tend to emphasize treatment of the "deviant self" and use workplace productivity as a measure of successful recovery. Besides, when the role of such NGOs includes the rehabilitation of "at-risk" populations through counseling and psychiatric modalities, "vulnerability" is understood, and gets treated, as an individual-level phenomenon removed from its sociopolitical origins.

Similarly, ethnographic research from Nandigram, West Bengal (Carr, 2010), shows how neoliberal policies (manifested, in this case, in dispossessing villagers of their land for the establishment of Special Economic Zones, or SEZs) are fundamentally antipeople, violently causing (Bhatia & Priya, 2018) displacement, a range of suffering, and a sense of betrayal. Euro-American nosology might read the ensuing symptoms as being indicative of PTSD—one of the categories that have colonized our notion of the self. This neoliberal notion of the self-contained self allows for the explaining away of poverty, violence, and discrimination in terms of "individual psychiatric disorders" (Kottai, 2018).

The Way Forward

Where maximization of profit takes precedence, the human brain is perceived as capital. In a world where the capitalistic logic of demand and supply determines the ups and downs of a volatile ecopolitical environment, the onus to transform, in spite of all odds, is placed on the "unhealthy" individual. Humans are, however, not only neuronal but political as well (Malabou, 2009). With mental illness increasingly being used as a means of social control (as the ethnographic evidence outlined above suggests), it is imperative that we ensure that the disenfranchised receive cognitive justice, which would involve explicitly underscoring that an unjust social order contributes to neuropsychological conditions. I offer this criticism not to invalidate advancements made in biomedicine but more to highlight the kinds of cognitive injustice perpetrated in the name of "development." A more compassionate analysis of mental illness, therefore—while remaining wary of certain constructions of health and personhood—is perhaps the way forward for how we categorize, diagnose, and treat mental illness.

Note

1 The Mariwala Health Initiative website can be accessed here: https://mhi.org.in/

References

American Psychiatric Association. (2013). *Diagnostic and statistical manual of mental disorders* (5th ed.). Author.

Baru, R. V., & Mohan, M. (2018). Globalisation and neoliberalism as structural drivers of health inequities. *Health Research Policy and Systems, 16*(1) (Supplement 1), 91.

Bhatia, S., & Priya, K. R. (2018). Decolonizing culture: Euro-American psychology and the shaping of neoliberal selves in India. *Theory & Psychology, 28*(5), 645–668.

Carr, E. S. (2010). *Scripting addiction: The politics of therapeutic talk and American sobriety.* Princeton University Press.

Esposito, L., & Perez, F. M. (2014). Neoliberalism and the commodification of mental health. *Humanity & Society, 38*(4), 414–442.

Kottai, S. R. (2018). How Kerala's poor tribals are being branded as mentally ill. *Economic and Political Weekly, 29*(13), 11117–11123.

Malabou, C. (2009). *What should we do with our brain?* Fordham University Press.

Sadath, A., Kumar, S., Jose, K., & Ragesh, G. (2019). Mental health and psychosocial support program for people of tribal origin in Wayanad: Institute of Mental Health and Neurosciences model. *Indian Journal of Social Psychiatry, 35*(4), 224.

Sadath, A., Uthaman, S. P., & Kumar, T. S. (2018). Mental health in tribes: A case report. *Indian Journal of Social Psychiatry, 34*(2), 187.

Chapter 20

Child As Metaphor

COLONIALISM, PSY-GOVERNANCE, AND EPISTEMICIDE[1]

China Mills and Brenda A. LeFrançois

Summary

This paper mobilizes transdisciplinary inquiry to explore and deconstruct the often-used comparison of racialized/colonized people, intellectually disabled people and mad people as being like children. To be childlike is a metaphor that is used to denigrate, to classify as irrational and incompetent, to dismiss as not being knowledge holders, to justify governance and action on others' behalf, to deem as being animistic, as undeveloped, underdeveloped or wrongly developed, and, hence, to subjugate. We explore the political work done by the metaphorical appeal to childhood, and particularly the centrality of the metaphor of childhood to legitimizing colonialism and white supremacy. The article attends to the ways in which this metaphor contributes to the shaping of the material and discursive realities of racialized and colonized others, as well as those who have been psychiatrized and deemed "intellectually disabled". Further, we explore specific metaphors of child-colony, and child-mad-crip. We then detail the developmental logic underlying the historical and continued use of the metaphorics of childhood, and explore how this makes possible an infantilization of colonized peoples and the global South more widely. The material and discursive impact of this metaphor on children's lives, and particularly children who are racialized, colonized, and/or deemed mad or crip, is then considered. We argue that complex adult-child relations, sane-mad relations and Western-majority world relations within global psychiatry, are situated firmly within pejorative notions of what it means to be childlike, and reproduce multisystemic forms of oppression that, ostensibly in their "best interests", govern children and all those deemed childlike.

*

DOI: 10.4324/9781003148456-23

Introduction

To be childlike is a metaphor that has been used for centuries to denigrate and subordinate certain groups including racialized/colonized others, and/or psychiatrized and disabled people. Erica Burman (2016) states that an important analytic task "is to render explicit the work done by the rhetorical appeal to childhood" (p. 2). Inspired by Burman, the analytic task of this article is to trace the work done by the metaphorical appeal to childhood, specifically in relation to colonialism, madness and disability. We ask: how does the "child" function as metaphor, and what is the performative nature of this metaphor – what does it do both for those deemed childlike, and for actual children (Mills, 2014)? While the metaphorics of childhood in relation to child/colony have been well documented, less attention has been paid to the metaphorics of the child in relation to madness and disability. Thus, this article takes seriously the need to explore the centrality of the child and the metaphor of "childlike" in the development of white supremacy (Levander, 2006), colonialism, sanism, disablism, and ableism.[2]

For Ashis Nandy (2007), the Western worldview of childhood as an imperfect transitional state on the way to adulthood is embedded in ideologies of colonialism and modernity, meaning "the use of the metaphor of childhood [is] a major justification of all exploitation" (p. 59). Accordingly, parentification – or even *in loco parentis* – has been used to justify, and to deem benevolent, interventions used by the powerful to "protect" those who are "childlike". Not so hidden from the surface are the vested capitalist interests as well as the social, political, and psychological agendas of power and control taken on by those in the parental role within these socially constructed and contrived "parent-child" relations. The developmental logic that underlies these power relations legitimizes various regimes of ruling that promote the subordination of certain groups in the name of benevolence. In this article, we demonstrate the ways in which these forced paternalistic encounters, and the infantilization that characterize them, serve not only to debase and erase racialized/colonized, psychiatrized, and/ or disabled adults and children as knowers, but also serve to reinscribe children themselves as incompetent and inferior. Colonial logics intersect with medical and psychiatric logics that enable not just the marking of certain individual bodies as subhuman but also the global categorizing of whole groups of people as being undeveloped, underdeveloped, and/or wrongly developed. Correspondingly, we understand the importance placed within mainstream corporate academia upon the subfields of developmental studies within political science, international development, international relations, economics, geography, child psychology, and medicine, all which serve the same function of maintaining the status quo of (white) supremacy whilst (re)producing majority world people, children, psychiatrized and/or disabled people as childlike (Blaut, 1993). We expose and contest such debasement whilst also disputing the essentialized and adultist meanings contained within the very concept of *childlike*, a concept which emanates from dominant Euro-western and adult-centric constructions of childhood.

Metaphor is "pervasive in everyday life", and is classically understood as structuring the way we think and act, and enabling us to understand and experience "one kind of thing in terms of another" (Lakoff & Johnson, 1980, pp. 3–5). Yet many concepts may not be separate as such, and may be historically entangled with one another. Metaphors are contextually bound and have a performative aspect in that they structure what action we can take (Kövecses, 2015). Understanding something through metaphor may hide aspects of a concept that are not consistent with that metaphor (Lakoff & Johnson, 1980), and thus metaphors can be used to do political and ideological work. We are interested in how certain groups of peoples (colonized, racialized, mad and crip)[3] come to be understood, talked about and acted upon through the metaphor of childhood. Specifically, the pervasive, entangled and co-constitutive nature of metaphors of the child, colony/"savage", mad and crip are explored. The intersections of these metaphors call for an approach attuned to overlaps and not constricted by disciplinary boundaries.

We engage in this analysis through a creative transdisciplinary inquiry that is not discipline-specific but instead brings together knowledges that are rarely understood to coexist and that may at times be in tension with each other (Augsburg, 2014; Leavy, 2006; Mitchell & Moore, 2015; Montuori, 2013). Transdisciplinarity – as contingent and non-essentialized – alerts us to and rejects the politics of differentiation and exclusion, key to the bordering and disciplining practices of social scientific knowledge and their beginnings in the codification of Enlightenment rationality used to justify slavery, colonialism and apartheid (Sehume, 2013). Following Nicolescu (2008), we understand transdisciplinary inquiry to be a form of meaning-making that breaks down the academic hierarchy of epistemological relationships, that is open to different forms of logic including that which is unknown (Augsburg, 2014), and that strives to eliminate epistemic injustice (Leblanc & Kinsella, 2016) or epistemicide (Santos, 2014). Further, our inquiry is informed by mad studies, critical disability studies, critical childhood studies, as well as critical race, transnational and postcolonial theories.

Mad studies transgresses the academy and its disciplines, with its beginnings being located outside the academy and within mad social movements (Gorman & LeFrançois, 2017; LeFrançois et al., 2013; Russo & Sweeney, 2016). A transdisciplinarity lens is consistent with Mad studies, in that it is not only inquiry based but also questions the logics and the very form in which that inquiry may take (Augsburg, 2014), whilst Mad studies may further rebelliously challenge enlightenment and Eurocentric notions of rationality (Blaut, 1993) which underpins and structures knowledge emanating from academic disciplines (Sehume, 2013). That is, at times, Mad studies may be at odds with rationalism as the basis of knowledge production and as the basis of the formation of the academy. As Bruce (2017) notes, "(r)ationalist readers may fear that such a mad study…detrimentally reinforces myths of black savagery and subrationality. Such investment in rationalism presumes that Reason is paramount for fully realized modern personhood" (p. 307). Like Bruce (2017), we reject such investments and presumptions, and our work instead interrogates the adultist, disablist, sanist, colonial, and racist logics that often underpin the conventional academic imaginary. However, debasement of mad people's knowledges does not just occur within the academy but also within the general public (Leblanc & Kinsella, 2016). Mad studies produces knowledge where the meaning-making of mad people is centred, but where other meanings emanating from other sources – academic or otherwise – also can be considered and deconstructed, incorporated, or rejected.

So too do we argue that (critical) childhood studies should also be seen as transdisciplinary (Mitchell & Moore, 2015) and as a direct challenge on 'Reason' as key for children's entrance into a fully realized personhood, given the ways adultist notions of children's inherent irrationality, lack of reason, rule by passion, animism (Scott and Chrisjohn, forthcoming), and their supposed lack of contribution as productive members of (capitalist) society[4] is conventionally inscribed on their bodies and minds in the West. According to Rollo (2018, p. 61) this denigration and subordination of children – misopedy – was in ancient Greece a "form of social and political hierarchy". Here the child functions as the ontological other to reason and politics; children as a group for whom there was seen to be a moral obligation to assist but for whom political claims were seen as impossible. It was this that made possible the framing of violence as necessary and legitimated as being in children's 'best interests'. As these dominant notions of children and childhood not only exist but also shut down discussions of the social construction of childhood within most academic disciplines (child psychology, sociology, social work, medicine, psychiatry, etc), understanding (critical) childhood studies as a direct challenge to this denotes the desire to disrupt and break away from "the governing strictures found within academic modes of dominant knowledge production that both center and reproduce privileged and constraining notions of reason and productivity" (LeFrançois & Voronka, 2022). For the most part, the academy neither acknowledges the existence of nor includes knowledge production emanating from children themselves, whether such contributions mirror dominant (adult) discourses or not, as the concept of "children's contributions" is read through an adultist lens.

This is not to imply that the heterogeneous accounts of children and/or mad people are innocent; it is instead about radically calling into question what the academy counts as knowledge. For those contributions deemed childlike, whether they emanate from children, colonized and racialized peoples, psychiatrized or disabled people, transdisciplinarity coupled with Mad studies may provide a platform for ensuring epistemic justice through both the deconstruction of dominant, racist, sanist, and ableist strictures but also by opening up a wider space for meaning-making beyond such adultist and Euro-western positivism. We argue that the use of child as metaphor operates as a form of epistemicide – what Santos (2014) terms, a "failure to recognise the different ways of knowing by which people across the globe provide meaning to their existence" (p. 111), including different ways of knowing children. This operates as a form "cognitive injustice" often followed by attempts to destroy epistemological diversity with a single story that claims to be universal (Santos, 2014), including a single developmental story about children and those deemed childlike. These concepts are mostly used by Santos in reference to the violent eradication of Indigenous knowledge systems enabled through a colonial framing of irrationality. Yet cognitive injustice is also at work in the dismissal of alternative experiences of reality and alternative cognitions that are classified as 'mad' and intellectually disabled respectively, and hence, marked as incompetency and irrationality.

Child As Metaphor

We are interested in how the child functions as a metaphor for colonized, racialized, psychiatrized and disabled peoples. Literature on the iconography of childhood usually makes a distinction between metaphorical or symbolic and actual "flesh and blood" children (Burman, 2016; Morrigan, 2017). We also make this distinction here by exploring the performative nature of "child as metaphor" for those deemed childlike, and for actual children. However, in making this distinction we do not seek to reify a naturalized and essentialized developmental child. Sánchez-Eppler (2005) notes the entanglement of "childhood as a discourse and childhood as persons", particularly in Euro-western affective deployments of childhood (p. xxiii). Furthermore, we recognize that given the "societally as well as intrapsychically invested character of childhood, arguably all appeals to 'the child' are metaphorical" (Burman, 2016, p. 2; Stainton Rogers & Stainton Rogers, 1992). Our point of departure, then, is the analytic task outlined by Burman (2016) to render "explicit the work done by the rhetorical appeal to childhood" (p. 2), and the task in this article is to trace the work done by the metaphorical appeal to childhood, specifically in relation to colonialism, madness and disability. While we are concerned with the effects of metaphor, we are cognizant that the conceptual basis on which "child as metaphor" functions is largely a Euro-western construction of childhood as an early rung on a linear developmental ladder and a stage marked by a lack of intellectual capacity, dependency, irrationality, animism, emotionality, – or "rule by passion", and economic unproductivity (Blaut, 1993). This is an evolutionary and developmentalist narrative globalized by the West as a universal standard (Nieuwenhuys, 2009) and, as we shall see, a narrative that is deeply entangled with colonialism (Blaut, 1993) and epistemic injustice.

Child / Colony

Multiple colonial texts portray colonized people as children, for instance, as "sullen peoples, Half-devil and half-child" (Kipling, 1899). Nandy (2007) finds that there are a number of "metaphor[s] of childhood that justified colonialism", from James Mill's conception of Britain as an adult guiding the development of India, to Cecil Rhodes' assertion (in Southern Africa) that "the native is to be treated as a child and denied franchise" (p. 58). Here we see evidence that "colonial ideology required savages to be children, but it also feared that savages could be like children" [and indeed that children could be "savage"] (Nandy, 2007, p. 58) – a dual framing of children as at once innocent and dangerous.

Postcolonial theory has long recognized the centrality of "the metaphor of childhood [as] legitimizing colonialism and modernity" (Nandy, 2007, p. 69), where the "child-native" performs a discursive function "foundational to the ideology of imperialism" (Barker, 2011, p. 7). Thus, the "classic connection in the colonial library is, of course, that between the colonized other and the white child" (Eriksson Baaz, 2005, p. 52). Burman (2016) states that "longstanding colonial dynamics link children with the colonised", where child/colony comes to stand as other/ed to the male western industrialized liberal self (p. 10). The construction of colonized peoples as developmentally akin to white children was central to colonialism, yet a key difference here is that, unlike ableist imaginings of the ideal white child, colonized peoples are constructed as permanently childlike and unable to develop further (Barker, 2011) and as stuck within a state of savagery and 'mental infancy' (Scott and Chrisjohn forthcoming). This diverges from Rollo's compelling argument that the child provides the internal structure and logic of the colonial conception of the "Indian"' (2018, 63) meaning the 'child' is a homology, not a metaphor, for settler colonialism. Thus, Rollo concludes it is 'not contingent' but 'necessary that justificatory frameworks of European empire and colonialism depict Indigenous peoples as children' (2018, p. 60). Despite our focus in this paper on metaphor, we acknowledge the need for further discussion as to differences between homology and metaphor, and about what each framing may make visible and foreclose. The metaphoric of child/colony is contingent on patriarchal domination, where the familial ruling of the husband/father is naturalized as a model for colonial domination (McClintock, 1995). It is also contingent on what Melber (1989, as cited in Heinz, 1998) describes as the "colonial view" – a process that reconfigures inequities and difference as modes of evolutionary hierarchy and that represents western white adult males as the highest stage of evolution against which colonized peoples are constructed as inferior. This is evident in some psychoanalytical framings that posit, "the Negro is just a child" (Fanon, 1967, p. 27).

Nandy has commented on the seeming "subsidiary homology between childhood and the state of being colonized" (1983, p. 11), and the "implied homology between the adult-child relationship and the West-East encounter under colonialism" (2007, p. 70). Similarly, it is this "colonial conflation of the colonized with the figure of the child" that, for Nieuwenhuys (2009, p. 149), needs to be interrogated to enable a deconstruction of "childhood as a metaphor for institutionalized violence visited upon humanity in the name of progress". In this way, the trope of the "childlike" functions to reframe violence, to construct it as necessary, legitimate, and even benevolent.

Nelson Mandela (1994) describes the racialization of the South African prison system, in which black African prisoners (unlike white prisoners) were forced to wear shorts because "African men are deemed 'boys' by the authorities" (p. 396). This racist infantilization of Black people persists in both colony and metropole, with black men routinely referred to as "boy" (Burman, 1994). In this way, notes Levander (2006), "the child works to establish race as a central shaping element of ostensibly raceless Western ideals…[Thus] excavating the child's importance to the development of white supremacy is urgently needed" (pp. 2–3). Goerg (2012) argues that colonial logics include an entrenched openly racist paternalism where Africans were infantilized as "child-people" and hence treated like "big children" or as being and living in a "state of childhood". This comparison of colonized people to children was evident in French Africa, the Belgian Congo, as well as the British and Portuguese colonies (Goerg, 2012), while Hegel (1975) said that "Africa proper" was the "land of childhood" (p. 91). Yet, the metaphor of childhood not only impacts on those constructed as childlike but also has had, and continues to have, materially violent effects for colonized and racialized children.

Much in the same way that Piaget (1953, 1967) falsely assessed children as being incapable of abstract thinking – an adultist and markedly masculine Euro-western interpretation of children's abilities (Burman, 1997; Macnamara, 1976; Prout & James, 1997) – so too did white supremacy in the form of colonization lead to the assessment of Africans as having limited ability to engage in abstraction. Colonial authorities saw themselves as protectors of the colonized; people who, like children, were impressionable and immature, unable to exercise critical judgement, had "weak intellects", and were, therefore, in need of guidance. As Goerg (2012) explains, this was exemplified in 1949 when Sudanese officials requested censorship of French and other foreign films that were seen as having a bad influence on their children and young people. This call was echoed by Senegalese officials and others within French West Africa,[5] looking to bolster existing local censorship laws through a stronger decree and the application of consistent compliance. This call for supervision from the West Africans themselves fed into colonial logics of the incompetence of colonial subjects, and the mission to protect peoples who were understood to have, by nature, less intellectual capacity than their white colonizers. As West African adults attempted to shield their young people from what many considered immoral and violent influences of foreign cinema, and perhaps in an effort to resist assimilation of their young people, French authorities readily supported this call, in order to shield themselves from the potential of any radicalization provoked by the subversive content of some of these films. In this example, we see an intertwining of, and a direct connection between, West African parent-child relations and colonizer-colonized relations, and the protectionism that mutually constituted both, with notions of morality, public order and obedience providing the motivation to enforce such a protectionist stance.

At the same time, many colonial administrators romanticized and exoticized those they were colonizing, and felt compelled through racist stereotyping to preserve their (white) image of an unspoilt (black) Africa (Goerg, 2012), much in the same way that the (heterosexual) Western imaginary calls for the preservation of "childhood innocence" (Greensmith & Sheppard, 2017; Morrigan, 2017; Scraton, 1997). However, rather than merely and ostensibly protecting African children and preserving "Black Africa", the colonizers were most concerned with self-protection and maintaining their economic interests within Africa. Indeed, as Goerg (2012) notes, the targeting of West African children and young people for this exercise of control and censorship ensued because they were seen as not only the most vulnerable but also as the most dangerous to colonial power, given that it is the young people who were understood to be more likely to revolt against the violence of colonization and foreign domination. By falsely claiming the right to choose for others, established in the name of moral and intellectual superiority, and often inscribed legally through the "rule of law" imposed in many colonies, political, economic and cultural domination through white supremacy persisted (Goerg, 2012; McBride, 2016). In this example, colonized children were perceived by both colonized and colonizing adults (albeit for very different reasons) as in need of saving from foreign cultural influences, in an attempt to perhaps preserve their "childhood innocence" on the one hand, to preserve African cultures or the "culture of Black Africa" on the other hand, and with a third underhanded agenda on the part of the colonizers to preserve colonial power and authority. West African children themselves appear to have been left silenced on the question of the censorship of foreign cinema by both the racist infantilization of Africa as a whole, and by the adultism that was used to further debase them as West African young people.

According to Valentin and Meinert (2009), the "civilization of the children of the 'savages' in the colonial world was an inherent part of the colonization mission in Africa, the Americas and Oceania in the 19th century" (p. 23). For example, in the settler-colonial context of Canada, huge numbers of Indigenous children were forcibly taken from their families and communities and incarcerated in residential schools, which explicitly aimed to "kill the Indian in the child" (Razack, 2015). Here another powerful use of metaphor is evident in the construction of First Nations, Inuit and Métis peoples as an inevitably "dying race", incapable of self-governance, enabling residential schools to be justified as "saving" Indigenous children from "the death of their race" (Chapman et al., 2014, p. 7; Kelm, 2005). This logic has many similarities to the child apprehension policies within racist/colonialist child protection systems that led to the "sixties scoop" (Chrisjohn & Young, 1997; Blackstock, 2009; LeFrançois, 2013) and, in what is now Australia and Torres Strait, constituted the "stolen generation" (Read, 1981). Continuing since the "sixties scoop", Indigenous children remain vastly over-represented within the Canadian child protection system (Chrisjohn & Young, 1997; LeFrançois, 2013). Here, a difference becomes apparent in the colonial violence enacted on colonized adults who are constructed as childlike and on actual colonized children, constructed as in need of saving both from their Indigenous parents and kin, as well as from their indigeneity.

A key effect of constructing colonized peoples through the metaphor of childhood is to justify governance of the "natives" who are constituted as "immature, childlike beings that need to be subjected to European discipline and control" (Giesebrecht, 1898, as cited in Heinz, 1998, p. 427). In this way, non-Europeans were constructed as:

> ripe for government, passive, child-like…needing leadership and guidance, described always in terms of lack-no initiative, no intellectual powers.; or on the other hand, they are outside society, dangerous, treacherous, emotional, inconstant, wild, threatening, fickle, sexually aberrant, irrational, near animal, lascivious, disruptive, evil, unpredictable.
>
> (Carr, 1985, p. 50)

Moreover, assimilated colonized people in Africa – those who behaved less "native" and acquired the mannerisms of their colonizers – were seen as less childlike, and those who were judged to be, or physically appeared to be, "more black" were seen as more childlike (Georg, 2012). In addition, colonized subjects who outwardly demonstrated their intelligence in ways that could not be denied by the white lens were marked as an aberration or *hors-norme*.

Child/Mad – Child/Crip

In the Eurocentric imaginary, the "colonized were discursively linked and compared not only with women and children, but also mental patients, criminals, and the working-class in Europe", where "'primitives' were equated with children and the mentally disturbed" (Eriksson Baaz, 2005, pp. 53–54). Nandy (2007) reads this fear of childishness as a symptom of psychological insecurity in cultures that use "the metaphor of childhood to define mental illness, primitivism, abnormality, [and] underdevelopment" (p. 65). Disability and madness figure in three key ways within the colonial apparatus: the representation of colonized peoples as childlike and thus impaired and irrational; ableist discourse as central to domination; and the idea that the colony can itself disable and drive white people mad. We discuss madness and disability, and specifically intellectual disability, alongside each other because the distinction between them in much contemporary discourse doesn't hold historically and is also in part a construction of "western" medicalized and psy discourse.

It is not unusual for adults who have been psychiatrized to indicate that they are treated as being childlike by those who work within psychiatric services. This infantilization is evident in Malacrida's (2015) account of Canadian institutions for intellectually disabled people where "inmates regardless of their age were treated as though they were children", not permitted freedom of movement or choice, and were seen as incapable (pp. 90–91). In many ways, being deemed childlike, using denigrating Euro-western understandings of what constitutes a child, is a classic example of the form of sanism (Poole et al., 2012; Meerai et al., 2016) that is deeply rooted within psychiatry and within society generally. The comparison of mad people to children is embedded within historical and current day psychiatric practices. For example, the evolutionary psychiatry dominant in England from 1870 to the First World War posited that insanity constituted an evolutionary reversal - a movement backwards on the assumed evolutionary developmental scale (Showalter, 1985). Sicherman (1977) points out the similarities between infancy and the "enforced dependency" of the rest cure, developed as treatment for white upper-class women diagnosed with neurasthenia, with treatment constituting "childlike obedience" to a male physician. The current day Diagnostic and Statistical Manual (DSM-V) continues to list "childishness" and "childlike behaviour" in adults as a symptom of mental illness. What constitutes childlike behaviour in the DSM includes such things as "silliness", being "disorganized", "clinging" to others, "unpredictable agitation", "self-effacing and docile behaviour" and "gregarious flamboyance with active demands for attention", which can be found as symptoms within the categories of dependent personality disorder, histrionic personality disorder, as well as schizophrenia spectrum and other related psychotic disorders.

Not only do we find here stereotypes of the essentialized child and associated behaviours, but we find also the essentializing of narrowly defined adult behaviours, with those daring to behave differently being deemed mad. The implications of these diagnostic criteria for colonized people are exemplified by Chrisjohn and McKay's (2017) demonstration that despite centuries of the racist infantilization of Indigenous peoples (motivated by capitalist greed and enacted through white supremacy [sic]), by the 1990s Indigenous peoples in Canada began to be labelled as dependent and, thus, psychopathologized with dependent personality disorder. Chrisjohn and McKay (2017) explain:

> [I]t was economic conservatives doing the talking, and they weren't using dependency in any recognizable economic form (you know, as in seizing

the assets and means of production of a whole people and determining the shape and direction of their fundamental economic activities) ... (Instead) (t)hey applied it to us.... We were suffering from "dependency disorder"; or even, from the lack of an "entrepreneurial instinct", such as they themselves possessed. This defect accounted for our absence in the mainstream Canadian political economy, our economic backwardness, our relative joblessness, why we got fired a lot, and why we were always late for appointments. The cure...consisted of cancelling all treaties, ending any social programs and subsidies, taxing Indian reserve lands (and seizing the lands when taxes weren't paid on time).. The self-serving circularity of the whole conception bypassed even a hint of science...: we obviously had the "inner, hidden trait" of dependency.

(pp. 167–168)

Here we see the ways in which the infantilization of generation after generation of Indigenous peoples is then later characterized by psychiatry as a mental illness within those who have been infantilized, in the form of dependency. The source of the violence of colonization, dispossession and genocide is obscured with the psychiatric gaze turning directly onto the colonized rather than the colonizers. Psychiatrization is thus deployed in order to divert attention away from the violence exerted upon colonized peoples (Chrisjohn & McKay, 2017).

The political utility of diagnoses of mental illness is further exemplified in Samuel Cartwright's coining of drapetomania – the so-called mental disease that was said to compel enslaved Africans in the Americas to run away. This too was entangled with the metaphorics of childhood, when Cartwright wrote that "like children, they [slaves] are constrained by unalterable physiological laws, to love those in authority over them. Hence, from a law of his nature, the negro can no more help loving a kind master, than the child can help loving her that gives it suck" (Cartwright, 1851, as cited in Gould, 1981, p. 71). As treatment, Cartwright prescribed continued slavery and the handling of slaves like children, in order to "cure" them from running away.

Throughout colonial texts colonized peoples were represented as limited in intellectual capacity, as behaviourally disordered, as physically degenerate (Barker, 2011) and as animistic (Scott & Chrisjohn, 2018), depicting "the colony not only [as] a child but an oafish child" (Prentice, 1997, p. 71). Scott and Chrisjohn (2018) note that racism (and disablism) fuels the assertion, first declared by cultural anthropologist E. B. Taylor in 1871, that "primitives" like children are inherently animistic: they believe (wrongly) that everything is alive. This assertion designates colonized people, intellectually disabled people, and/or children as having a general lack of attachment to reality, as "backward" and cripped as "simpletons"; and as stuck within a state of savagery and "mental infancy" (Scott & Chrisjohn, 2018). Imperial children are understood to eventually grow out of it, whereas Indigenous peoples are locked into permanent animism. Chrisjohn elaborates*:[6]

When Indians say something like they believe in honouring the spirits in the environment around them, they are childish, unsophisticated animist philosophers who are just wrong and stuck in … (undeveloped) "emotional" or "cultural" faculties. (I)t is racism and it is maybe the biggest part of infantilizing Native people.[7]

This understanding of animism – as a lack of attachment to reality – is also used as justification to psychiatrize and drug people who hear voices and/or who see, feel or communicate with spiritual entities in their midst.

The trope of "disabled child-nation" has its "antecedents in a long colonial history in which childhood and disability contributed substantially to the conceptual apparatus of empire" (Barker, 2011, p. 7). The construction of colonized peoples as "permanently childlike" worked to frame European imperialists as "permanent guardians" (McEwan, 2008, p. 136), masking colonial "ambitions to achieve global sovereignty under the rhetorical banner of a duty of care" (Barker, 2011, p. 7). Barker (2011) shows how this permanent state of childhood is suggestive of disability in a way that mediates the racialized differences between colonized child and colonizer adult. Ableist discourse was central to bolstering colonial and racial domination, where the "subtext of disability" suspended "normal" developmental logic, with colonized peoples seen as unable to fully develop, "producing a model of arrested development that stabilized and consolidated the conditions required for ongoing colonial dependency" (Barker, 2011, p. 8). In this way, "the child, figured as a developing body, has been used in the making of global hierarchies and knowledge" (Castañeda, 2002, p. 13). The expansion of imperialism throughout the mid-19th century fed into and occurred alongside the establishment of developmental norms and the 'science' of eugenics, where cultural differences were equated with biological deficiency. Here normalcy became a benchmark by which children, colonized peoples, and disabled people were judged, meaning that conceptions of normal and pathological behaviour and psychology were made possible through the colonial binary of the "normal" West and the pathological "Rest" (Eriksson Baaz, 2005). For Meekosha (2011) this means that:

> The idea of racial and gender supremacy of the Northern Hemisphere is very much tied to the production of disability in the global South and racialised evolutionary hierarchies constructed the colonised as backward, infantile and animal-like. We cannot meaningfully separate the racialised subaltern from the disabled subaltern in the process of colonisation.
>
> (pp. 672–673)

Alongside seeing colonized people as childlike, the colonies themselves were seen as capable of disabling white children and preventing them from "growing up". It was assumed in Britain that if the colonizer's children were not sent back to Europe from the colonies during the important years of childhood, they would become "stunted in growth and debilitated in mind" (Thomson, 1843, p. 116). In tracing the above history, it becomes possible to see how "childhood and disability have provided interlinked markers of the helplessness, dependency and subnormality of the 'Third World' countries", continuing today within the contemporary development regime, humanitarian rhetoric and developmental psychology (Barker, 2011, p. 7).

Child / Development

Above we traced the co-constitutive histories of imperialism, developmentalism and normalcy, and the centrality of child-colony-mad-crip to this history. Throughout this we see examples of how "savages were made developmentally equivalent to children" (Castañeda, 2002, p. 26), and implications of this in terms of paternalistic colonial dominance. Hence Nandy's (2007) claim that "much of the pull of the ideology of colonialism and much of the power of the idea of modernity can be traced to the evolutionary implications of the concept of the child in the Western worldview" (p. 57). Developmental logic is key to white supremacist narratives of progress linked to the nation state, and used to justify colonialism as a civilizational and economic project (Klein & Mills, 2017). Here the history of the development of Western countries is imagined as a linear trajectory of progress that all countries must pass through in order to "develop". Cultural recapitulation assumes that in their lifetime, an individual body will reproduce the same developmental stages as the development of the species body. This is central to the colonial idea that:

> the adults of inferior groups must be like the children of superior groups, for the child represents a primitive adult ancestor. If adult Blacks and women are like white male children, then they are living representations of an ancestral stage in the evolution of white males. An anatomical theory for ranking races – based on entire bodies – had been found.
> (Gould, 1981, as cited in Mclintock, 1995, p. 51)

This is summarized by the social Darwinist, Herbert Spencer (1895), who said that "the intellectual traits of the uncivilized ... are traits recurring in the children of the civilized" (pp. 89–90). Gould (1981) shows the influence of recapitulation in Freudian and Jungian theories, and within the school curriculum in the United States, where a number of school boards "prescribed the Song of Hiawatha in early grades, reasoning that [white] children, passing through the savage stage of their ancestral past, would identify with it" (p. 114). The Song of Hiawatha, authored by a white man and telling the story of the noble savage and the vanishing Indian, was also taught in residential and industrial schools for Indigenous children throughout the USA and Canada as an attempt to socialize Indigenous peoples into inferior roles (White, 2016). Recapitulation was a central argument in justifying colonial expansion into what was known as "tropical Africa", where Kidd (1898) wrote that African peoples "represent the same stage in the history of the development of the race that the child does in the history of the development of the individual. The tropics will not, therefore, be developed by the natives themselves" (p. 51).

Recapitulation is evident also in Freudian constructions of "the aboriginal [as] Europe's childhood and her children" (Emberley, 2007, p. 97). Castañeda (2002) takes this further, showing how "the now of the primitive was not only placed in the time of childhood, but also in the child-body: the child was seen as a bodily theater where human history could be observed to unfold in the compressed timespan of individual development" (p. 13). This posits a shared global developmental telos of multiple forms of development, from the child to the economy, that positions the "West" as more advanced, with global South countries constructed as needing to catch up and "grow up".

This links closely to the growth of developmental psychology and developmental stage theories that portray child development as a series of distinct naturalized stages, akin to evolution, through which a child passes on a linear pathway. These theories have come to be applied and used to understand diverse areas of life, from the growth of a child to the construction of nation states. Children who don't meet prescribed levels of progress are said to be developmentally delayed (Valdivia, 1999), while whole populations of the global South have been and continue to be framed as underdeveloped or developing societies, and in need of "western" expertise. Interestingly, those deemed mad and/or crip are often framed as being wrongly developed.

Discussion: Infantilization of the Global South and the Fourth World

The centrality of parent-child metaphors to 19th-century colonialist imperialism is well documented in postcolonial scholarship (Ashcroft et al., 1989), where the idea of the child functions to make thinkable the colonial apparatus of "improvement" used to justify subjugation (Wallace, 1994). Linked to the construction of children as the "property" of their parents, "parental care and education have often been a cover for the widespread social and psychological exploitation of children" (Nandy, 2007, p. 60). Like colonial interventions into child saving, child-focused development initiatives often justify the child as site of intervention through appeal to a developmental narrative of early intervention, constructing children as "objects for adult and institutional intervention" (Valentin & Meinert, 2009, p. 23). The framing of whole populations as childlike, and thus as unable to take care of their own children, extends into current day neo-colonial practices of child saving within multiple development projects in the global South. Valentin and Meinert (2009) trace how the idea of "civilizing through children" (p. 29) continues in the global South through child-focused development projects that are heavily reliant on foreign aid. Through global inequalities in power, the global North acts *in loco parentis* of the global South, meaning the "'adult North' can bestow rights and duties on the 'young South', and if the South fails to comply with these, can implement sanctions" (Valentin & Meinert, 2009, p. 24). Indeed, the legal doctrine of *in loco parentis* implies not only the parentification of one individual or group and the infantilization of another, but that there is a responsibility on the part of the former to maintain that status over the latter and to make decisions in their best interest, including exerting discipline. This sense of responsibility, and the professed benevolence that ostensibly informs it, obscures the oppressive and coercive relations that it enforces.

Here populations of the global South are not only being talked about as children, they are being acted upon as if they were children, with global North countries working *in loco parentis* for children of the global South, further serving to infantilize populations of the global South, especially those in receipt of aid (Burman, 1994). This extends to the treatment of Indigenous peoples in current settler-colonies in the Fourth World, and of racialized peoples globally. The doctrine of *in loco parentis* is understood to allow for parental substitutions for children or "incapacitated" adults when their "natural" parents are unable to perform their parental duties. However, in the colonial context this doctrine was used by some settler nation states to make decisions for the colonized groups they deemed childlike and in need of parental guidance, often resulting in economic exploitation and the furthering of the capitalist colonial agenda. In the context of the treatment of Indigenous peoples in Canada, Chrisjohn and McKay (2017) poignantly explain that:

> The Indian Act, for example, on the assumption that we were, essentially, children in grown-up bodies, placed the government in position of control over our economic resources. Search the histories of what royalty deals Canada, *in loco parentis,* made in our name with oil companies, and ask if you want your parents to behave like this.
>
> (p. 167, emphasis in original)

Chrisjohn and McKay (2017) further note that still to this day Indigenous peoples in Canada experience "racism, marginalization, condescension, infantilization, disparagement, and (unidirectional) cultural ignorance" (p. 97). As we have seen, the ways in which the infantilization of Indigenous peoples and the enacting of the doctrine of *in loco parentis* – which in its very construction forcibly fabricates dependent parent-child relations – is then characterized as mental illness in the form of dependency within those who have been infantilized.

Both *in loco parentis* and the related legal doctrine of *in parens patriae* may be used to create a parental substitute for either a child or an "incapacitated" adult and, as we have seen, in relation to colonized peoples as a group. Both historically and in current times, these doctrines have been used to allow the state, or a substitute adult or institution, to act, for example, as the "general guardian of all infants, lunatics, idiots" (Blackstone, 1769) or, for example, in the "role of a parent to a child who is under 18 or 18 years of age or older and incapable of self-care because of a mental or physical disability" (United States Department of Labor, 1993) in many Western countries. In order to further ensure that adults, who have been deemed mad or crip and are seen as incompetent, are unable to make decisions for themselves within health institutions, for example, many countries have also adopted specific legislation around medically assessing capacity, such as the Mental Capacity Act in Canada. We see how the infantilization of colonized, mad, and crip subjects has over time become enshrined within Western legal doctrines and legislation, all the while reproducing the notion that children themselves are naturally incompetent. This locates racialized/colonized children, psychiatrized children, and intellectually disabled children in a particularly dehumanizing space within these white supremacist hierarchical arrangements.

Likewise, in child protection cases, where parents are deemed unable to protect their children from neglect and/or abuse, *in parens patriae* may be invoked to give the state the right to parent, and engage in the associated responsibilities in relation to protecting actual children. As we saw above, with the over-representation of Indigenous children living in Fourth World contexts within neo-colonial child protection systems, as well as the over-representation of black and racialized children within these same racist child protection systems (Clarke, 2011; Pon et al., 2011), the invoking of the legal doctrine of *in parens patriae* is rampantly used against both Indigenous families and black settler families in Canada. If colonial administrators served *in loco parentis* for the adults they were colonizing – as a surreptitious means to engage in economic exploitation at the same time as promoting degradation through infantilization and scientific racism – and then the state served *in parens patriae* for many of the children of those infantilized adults, the implications become stark for generations of actual children whose parents have been deemed as in need of parenting themselves.

Further to Burman's (1994) analysis of infantilization within global North-South relations, we also see, then, how the adult-Western world "benevolently" offers help and knowledge to the infantilized Fourth World, repeating the colonial paternalism inherent to Indigenous-colonizer relations in what is now Canada, formalized in the Gradual Civilization Act (1857) and the British North American Act (1876), amongst other early legislation, which was then consolidated within the Indian Act (1876). This Western "benevolence" was then further cemented more than a century later within children's rights discourse through the United Nations Convention on the Rights of the Child (1989). Pupavac (2001) writes that the export of western child developmental models "in the absence of the universalisation of the conditions upon which the model[s] arose" (p. 103), serves to legitimize western governmental and non-governmental actors behaving in children's "best interests" and on their behalf in the global South, as well as, we argue, within Fourth World communities. This also echoes Nieuwenhuys' (2009) assertion that development agencies (and, we add, child protection agencies) push the global South (and, we add, Indigenous communities located elsewhere) for "the emulation of a kind of childhood that the West has set as a global standard" (p. 148). Here we see a dual epistemic injustice, whereby those deemed childlike and actual children are seen as seen as cognitively subpar, while at the same time other/ed ways of knowing children are actively denigrated by western models – destroying epistemological diversity in relation to children. This results in current day advancing of the longstanding and now deep-rooted (white) Western agenda of assimilation and genocide within both former colonies and current white settler-colonial nation states.

And yet, the kind of childhood that the West has set as the gold standard is one where children are denigrated, which is in striking opposition to the ways in which children are valued within many Indigenous cultures within the Fourth World. For example, the lack of a common understanding of what constitutes childhood led to misunderstandings amongst some of the first Christian missionaries in Canada. With the goal of engaging in the assimilation of the Wendot peoples, referred to as the Hurons, through Frenchification (Jaenen, 1968), Gabriel Sagard, a Recollects missionary, documented his attempts. In his writings from 1623 and 1624 when he lived amongst the Hurons, Sagard notes that the Hurons did not hold a high opinion of French settlers but "in comparison with whom they considered their children wiser and more intelligent, so good a conceit have they of themselves and so little esteem for others" (Wrong, 1939, p. 138). Betrayed in this description is Sagard's projection of the European's lack of esteem for children onto the words of the Wedot people.

As Oneida academic and critical psychologist Roland Chrisjohn explains, the concept of "children" within the Iroquois Federation (of which the Hurons form part) is not the insult that it is from the Euro-western perspective. "Rather, our word (for children) merely implies someone who hasn't been around as long as some other people: 'Someone who is inexperienced with regard to certain things' is what was being implied, not 'someone not to be taken seriously because they have underdeveloped mental skills'".[8] As such, the Hurons may have been communicating to Sagard that the French settlers had less experience living in the bush than the Huron children, which no one would have likely taken issue with at the time. However, so ingrained within the Euro-western mindset that children are in many ways subhuman, the mention of a comparison between the French settlers and children directly connects to the degrading discourse of the time that infantilized all Indigenous people as being childlike and in need of guidance from the colonizers. It appears that the Hurons' words were misunderstood and mischaracterized by Sagard's Euro-western lens. This, however, is not to imply that all non-Western cultural understandings are somehow innocent or not degrading of children, or disabled people (Kolářová, 2016).

Throughout this chapter we have demonstrated the ways in which the concept of child as metaphor functions to denigrate colonized, psychiatrized, and/ or intellectually disabled people, as it reproduces these groups and actual children as being irrational, incompetent, unintelligent, animistic, in need of (parental) guidance, (economically) unproductive, and epistemically void. The use of this metaphor, as we have seen, performs important political agendas inherent to the colonial project, racism, epistemicide, the medicalization of madness and disability, and the subjugating notions of development that underpins each. All this is accomplished by focusing on and imposing a pejorative Western understanding of childhood that may be neither consistent with Indigenous/ non-Western understandings of what constitutes childhood nor consistent with actual children's abilities. Regardless, the material and discursive impact on children has been demonstrated to include multisystemic oppression including the interplay of adultism, colonialism, racism, sanism and dis/ableism, which mutually constitute and complicate each other. This interplay takes place at the level of adult-child relations and the psy-governance of childhood itself, within global North-South-Fourth World relations and the racist infantilization-paretification constructed within them, as well as within sane-mad relations and ableist-crip relations, including the psy and medical domination that governs both.

A transdisciplinary approach has enabled the deconstruction of the co-constitutive metaphors of mad, crip, child, and colony/savage. This has made visible how the psy-disciplines have been constituted through colonialism and so are always already a colonial practice, and how the psy-disciplines and colonialism (even when seemingly operating apart from one another) use similar tools, which are built upon the interlacing metaphors of madness, disability, savagery, and childhood. We suggest that a transdisciplinary (critical) childhood studies must continue to unsettle and reconcile its current and historical attachment both to development (in its various disciplinary and applied forms) and to whiteness by embracing and maturing into a symbiotic interdependence with critical race, feminist, transnational and postcolonial theories (Sehume, 2013). So too do we suggest the need for a greater influence and integration of deconstructed notions of adultism, and the unsettling of adultist forms of knowledge production, within and beyond the academy, including within critical race-informed interventions, cultural studies, and transdisciplinary praxis.

Notes

1 Originally printed in: Child As Metaphor: Colonialism, Psy-Governance, and Epistemicide, World Futures, 74:7–8, 503–524, DOI: 10.1080/02604027.2018.1485438. Reprinted with permision from Taylor and Francis. *This manuscript has had minor updates applied since its original publication.
2 For a discussion of the importance of deconstructing dis/ableism and the distinction between disablism and ableism, see Liddiard (2018).
3 We use the terms "mad" and "crip" as reclaimed signifiers and as concepts that unsettle, contest, and challenge normalcy and biological reductionism (LeFrançois et al., 2013; Liddiard, 2018; McRuer, 2006). The terms "psychiatrized", "mad" and "madness" are used interchangeably in this article, as are the terms "crip", "disabled", "intellectually disabled" and "disability".
4 These are Euro-western understandings of childhood, which not only negate the realities of children's abilities and experiences in the West, but further make invisible the lives of children in the global South, including those who are materially affected by the capitalist exploitation that characterizes child labour practices.
5 French West Africa consisted of Mauritania, Senegal, French Sudan (Mali), French Guinea, the Ivory Coast, Burkino Faso, Benin, Niger, Togo, and parts of Nigeria.
6 Season 5, episode 4, 2017, *The Endling*. See: https://www.springfieldspringfield.co.uk/view_episode_scripts.php?tv-show=the-blacklist&episode=s05e04
7 Personal communication, November 15, 2017.
8 Personal communication, August 14, 2017.

References

Ashcroft, B., Griffiths, G., & Tiffin, H. (1989). *The empire writes back: Theory and practice in post-colonial literatures.* London: Routledge.

Augsburg, T. (2014). Becoming transdisciplinary: The emergence of the transdisciplinary individual. *World Futures, 70*(3/4), 233–247.

Barker, C. (2011). *Postcolonial fiction and disability: Exceptional children, metaphor and materiality.* London: Palgrave MacMillan.

Blackstock, C. (2009). The occasional evil of angels: Learning from the experiences of Aboriginal peoples and social work. *First Peoples Child & Family Review, 4*(1), 28–37.

Blackstone, W. (1769). *Commentaries on the laws of England, Book the Third.* Oxford: Clarendon Press.

Blaut, J. (1993). *The colonizer's model of the world: Geographical diffusionism and Eurocentric history.* New York: Guilford Press.

Bruce, L. M. J. (2017). Mad is a place: Or, the slave ship tows the ship of fools. *American Quarterly, 69*(2), 303–308.

Burman, E. (1994). *Deconstructing developmental psychology.* London: Routledge.

Burman, E. (1997). Developmental psychology and its discontents. In D. Fox & I. Prilleltensky (Eds.), *Critical psychology* (pp. 159–175). Buckingham, UK: Open University Press.

Burman, E. (2016). Fanon's other children: Psychopolitical and pedagogical implications. *Race, Ethnicity and Education, 20*(1), 1–15.

Carr, H. (1985). Woman/Indian, the "American" and his others. In F. Barker, P. Hulme, M. Iversen, & D. Loxley (Eds.), *Europe and its other*, (Vol. 2., pp. 12–27). Colchester, UK: University of Essex Press.

Castaneda, C. (2002). *Figurations: Child, bodies, worlds.* Durham, NC: Duke University Press.

Chapman, C., Carey, A. C., & Ben-Moshe, L. (2014). Reconsidering confinement: Interlocking locations and logics of incarceration. In L. Ben-Moshe, C. Chapman, & A. Carey (Eds.), *Disability incarcerated: Imprisonment and disability in the United States and Canada* (pp. 3–24). New York: Palgrave Macmillan.

Chrisjohn, R., & McKay, S. (2017). *Dying to please you: Indigenous suicide in contemporary Canada.* Penticton, BC: Theytus.

Chrisjohn, R., & Young S. (1997). *The circle game: Shadows and substance in the Indian residential school experience in Canada.* Penticton, BC: Theytus.

Clarke, J. (2011). The challenges of child welfare involvement for Afro-Caribbean families in Toronto. *Children and Youth Services Review, 33*(2), 274–283.

Emberley, J. V. (2007). *Defamiliarizing the Aboriginal: Cultural practices and decolonization in Canada.* Toronto: University of Toronto Press.

Eriksson Baaz, M. (2005). *The paternalism of partnership: A postcolonial reading of identity in development aid.* London: Zed Books.

Fanon, F. (1967). *Black skin, white masks* (C. L. Markmann, Trans.). London: Pluto Press.

Goerg, O. (2012). Entre infantilisation et repression coloniale: Censure cinéematographique en AOF, 'grands enfant' et protection de la jeunesse. *Cahier d Études Afncaines, LII*(I, 205), 165–198.

Gorman, R., & LeFrançois, B. A. (2017). Mad studies. In B. M. Z. Cohen (Ed.), *Routledge international handbook of critical mental health* (pp. 107–114). London: Routledge.

Gould, S. J. (1981). *The mismeasure of man.* New York: WW Norton and Company.

Greensmith, C., & Sheppard, L. (2017). At the age of twelve: Migrant children and the disruption of multicultural belonging. *Children & Society.* doi:10.1111/ chso.12251

Hegel, G. W. F. (1975). *Lectures on the philosophy of world history.* Translated from the German edition of Johannes Hoffmeister from Hegel papers assembled by H. B. Nisbet). Cambridge: Cambridge University Press.

Heinz, A. (1998). Colonial perspectives in the construction of the psychotic patient as primitive man. *Critique of Anthropology, 18*(4), 421–444.

Jaenen, C. J. (1968). The frenchification and evangelization of the Amerindians in the seventeenth century New France. *CCHA Study Sessions, 35,* 57–71.

Kelm, M. E. (2005). Diagnosing the discursive Indian: Medicine, gender, and the dying race. *Ethnohistory, 52*(2), 371–406.

Kidd, B. (1898). *The control of the tropics.* New York: Macmillan.

Kipling, R. (1899, February 10). The white man's burden: The United States and the Philippine Islands (poem). *New York Sun.* Retrieved December 19, 2017, from http://www.bartleby.com/364/169.html

Klein, E., & Mills, C. (2017). Psy-expertise, therapeutic culture and the politics of the personal in development. *Third World Quarterly, 38*(9), 1990–2008.

Kolářová, K. (2016). 'What kind of development are we talking about?' A virtual roundtable with Tsitsi Chataika, Nilika Mehrotra, Karen Soldatic and Kateřina Kolářová. *Somatechnics, 6*(2), 142–158.

Kövecses, Z. (2015). *Where metaphors come from. Reconsidering context in metaphor.* Oxford: Oxford University Press.

Lakoff, G., & Johnson, M. (1980). *Metaphors we live by.* Chicago: University of Chicago Press.

Leavy, P. (2006). *Essentials of transdisciplinary research: Using problem-centered methodologies.* London: Routledge.

Leblanc, S. & Kinsella, E. (2016). Toward epistemic justice: A critically reflexive examination of 'sanism' and implications for knowledge generation. *Studies in Social Justice, 10*(1), 59–78.

LeFrançois, B. A. (2013). The psychiatrization of our children, or, an autoethnographic narrative of perpetuating First Nations genocide through 'benevolent' institutions. *Decolonization: Indigeneity, Education & Society, 2*(1), 108–123.

LeFrançois, B. A., Menzies, R., & Reaume, G. (2013). *Mad matters: A critical reader in Canadian mad studies.* Toronto: Canadian Scholars' Press.

LeFrançois, B. A., & Voronka, J. A. (2022). Mad epistemologies and the ethics of knowledge production. In T. Macias (Ed.), *Un/ethical un/knowing: Ethical reflections on methodology and politics in social science research.* Toronto: Canadian Scholars' Press.

Levander, C. F. (2006). *Cradle of liberty: Race, the child, and national belonging from Thomas Jefferson to W. E. B. DuBois.* Durham, NC: Duke University Press.

Liddiard, K. (2018). *The intimate lives of disabled people.* London: Routledge.

Macnamara, J. (1976). Stomachs assimilate and accommodate, don't they? *Canadian Psychological Review, 17*(3), 167–173.

Malacrida, C. (2015). *A special hell: Institutional life in Alberta's eugenic ears.* Toronto: University of Toronto Press.

Mandela, N. (1994). *Long walk to freedom.* Philadelphia: Little Brown and Co.

McBride, K. (2016). *Mr. Mothercountry: The man who made the rule of law.* Oxford: Oxford University Press.

McClintock, A. (1995). *Imperial leather: Race, gender, and sexuality in the colonial contest.* New York: Routledge.

McEwan, C. (2008). *Postcolonialism and development.* London: Taylor and Francis.

McRuer, R. (2006). *Crip theory: Cultural signs of queerness and disability.* New York: New York University Press.

Meekosha, H. (2011). Decolonizing disability: Thinking and acting globally. *Disability and Society, 26*(6), 667–682.

Meerai, S., Abdillahi, I., & Poole, J. M. (2016). An introduction to anti-black sanism. *Intersectionalities, 5*(3), 18–35.

Mills, C. (2014). *Decolonizing global mental health: The psychiatrization of the majority world.* London: Routledge.

Mitchell, R. C., & Moore, S. A. (2015). Muse, ruse, subterfuge: Transdisciplinary praxis in Ontario's post-secondary bricolage? *Review of Education, Pedagogy, and Cultural Studies, 37*(5), 393–413.

Montuori, A. (2013). The complexity of transdisciplinary literature reviews. *Complicity: An Interdisciplinary Journal of Complexity and Education, 10*(1/2), 45–55.

Morrigan, C. (2017). Trauma time: The queer temporalities of the traumatized mind. *Somatechnics*, 7(1), 50–58.

Nandy, A. (1983). *The intimate enemy: Loss and recovery of self under colonialism*. Oxford: Oxford University Press.

Nandy, A. (2007). Reconstructing childhood: A critique of the ideology of adulthood. In A. Nandy (Ed.), *A very popular exile* (pp. 56–76). Oxford: Oxford University Press.

Nicolescu, B. (2008). In vitro and in vivo knowledge: Methodology of transdisciplinarity. In B. Nicolescu (Ed.), *Transdisciplinarity: Theory and practice* (pp. 1–21). Cresskill, NJ: Hampton Press.

Nieuwenhuys, O. (2009). Is there an Indian childhood? *Childhood*, 16(2), 147–153.

Piaget, J. (1953). *The origin of intelligence in the child*. London: Routledge & Kegan Paul.

Piaget, J. (1967). *Biologie et connaissance*. Paris: Gaillimard.

Pon, G., Gosine, K., & Phillips, D. (2011). Immediate response: Addressing anti-Native and anti-Black racism in child welfare. *International Journal of Child, Youth and Family Studies*, 2(3/4), 385–409.

Poole, J. M., Jivraj, T., Arslanian, A., Bellows, K., Chiasson, S., Hakimy, H., Pasini, J., & Reid, J. (2012). Sanism, mental health, and social work/education: A review and call to action. *Intersectionalities*, 1, 20–36.

Prentice, C. (1997). "Born in a marvellous year"? The child in colonial and postcolonial New Zealand literature. *New Literatures Review*, 33, 65–80.

Prout, A., & James, A. (1997). A new paradigm for the sociology of childhood? Provenance, promise and problems. In A. James & A. Prout (Eds.), *Constructing and reconstructing childhood* (pp. 7–33). London: Falmer Press.

Pupavac, V. (2001). Misanthropy without borders: The international children's rights regime. *Disasters*, 25(2), 95–112.

Razack, S. H. (2015). *Dying from improvement: Inquests and inquiries into Indigenous deaths in custody*. Toronto: University of Toronto.

Read, J. (1981). *The stolen generations: The removal of Aboriginal children in New South Wales 1883 to 1969*. Surrey Hills, NSW: New South Wales Department of Aboriginal Affairs.

Rollo, T. (2018). Feral Children: Settler colonialism, progress and the figure of the child. *Settler Colonial Studies*, 8(1), 60–79.

Russo, J., & Sweeney, A. (2016). *Searching for a rose garden: Challenging psychiatry, fostering mad studies*. Wyastone Leys, UK: PCCS Books.

Sánchez-Eppler, K. (2005). *Dependent states: The child's part in nineteenth-century American culture*. Chicago: University of Chicago Press.

Santos, B. S. (2014). *Epistemologies of the south: Justice against epistemicide*. Boulder, CO: Paradigm.

Scott, S., & Chrisjohn, R. (2018). Inferior minds: The 'psychological science' of dehumanizing Native peoples. In R. Chrisjohn & S. McKay (Eds.), *"… and Indians, too!": Indigenous Peoples and the Canadian form of racism*. (Manuscript in preparation).

Scraton, P. (1997). Whose 'childhood'? What 'crisis'? In P. Scraton (Ed.), *'Childhood' in 'crisis'* (pp. 163–186). London: UCL Press.

Sehume, J. (2013). Transformation of cultural studies into transdisciplinarity. *Critical Arts*, 27(2), 163–181.

Showalter, E. (1985). *The female malady: Women, madness, and English culture, 1830–1980*. New York: Pantheon Books.

Sicherman, B. (1977). The uses of a diagnosis: Doctors, patients, and neurasthenia. *Journal of the History of Medicine, 32*(1), 33–54.

Spencer, H. (1895). *The principles of sociology.* New York: D. Appleton and Company.

Stainton Rogers, R., & Stainton Rogers, W. (1992). *Stories of childhood: Shifting agendas of child concern.* Lewes, UK: Harvester Wheatsheaf.

Thomson, A. S. (1843). Could the natives of a temperate climate colonize and increase in a tropical country and vice versa? *Transactions of the Medical and Physical Society of Bombay, 6,* 112–137.

United States Department of Labor. (1993). *Family and medical leave act.* Washington, DC: Author.

Valdivia, R. (1999). *The implications of culture on developmental delay.* Educational Resources Information Center, ERIC Digest, #E589.

Valentin, K., & Meinert, L. (2009). The adult north and the young south: Reflections on the civilizing mission of children's rights. *Anthropology Today, 25*(3), 23–28.

Wallace, J. A. (1994). De-scribing the water-babies: The child in postcolonial theory. In C. Tiffin & A. Lawson (Eds.), *De-scribing empire: Postcolonialism and textuality* (pp. 171–184). London: Routledge.

White, L. (2016). White power and the performance of assimilation: Lincoln Institute and the Carlisle Indian School. In J. Fear-Segal & S. D. Rose (Eds.), *Carlisle Indian industrial school: Indigenous histories, memories and reclamations* (pp. 106–123). Lincoln: University of Nebraska Press.

Wrong, G. M. (1939). *The long journey to the country of the Hurons* (H.H. Langton, Trans.). Toronto: The Champlain Society.

Chapter 21

Beyond Disordered Brains and Mother Blame

CRITICAL ISSUES IN AUTISM AND MOTHERING[1]

Patty Douglas and Estée Klar

Summary

Clinical models of mental difference extend beyond the clinics to impact individuals, societies, and families. This is true across the spectrum of different labels and diagnoses. In this chapter, Douglas and Klar bring an interdisciplinary perspective that includes feminist disability studies, neurodiversity, and critical autism studies to better understand the impacts of dominant mental health models of "autism" on mothers and families. One key finding is that mothers are often simultaneously blamed and burdened with responsibility while being given limited support. Mother blame can come in the form of overt models of mother causation, such as causal models of "refrigerator mothers," or in the form of blame for not becoming effective "mother therapists." Douglas and Klar give a genealogy of these different forms of mother blame. They work through many of the central issues and debates, and provide new directions for research, support, and understanding.

*

The Centers for Disease Control and Prevention in the United States have called the sharply rising rates of autism diagnosis worldwide an "urgent public health concern" (27). Media images of so-called warrior mothers who cure their autistic child, or, alternately, mothers who abandon or murder their autistic child have become commonplace. Cultural fascination with the strange otherworldliness of autism has peaked in popular television shows such as *Parenthood* and Hollywood movies such as *Roman J Israel, Esq.* This chapter provides an overview of critical issues in autism and mothering in order to shed some light on this complicated terrain. We lay bare

DOI: 10.4324/9781003148456-24

the long histories of mother blame and biomedical regulation of mothers as "fixers" of autism, understood as a negative difference. We suggest instead that autism is an embodied difference that should be accepted, not cured, and consider how mothers have also been key supporters and advocates of this alternative view. More supports that accept autism and that support access to life for both mothers and autistic individuals are urgently needed.

Context and Background

By Way of a Brief History: Introducing Key Themes and Theories

The predominant understanding of autism or autism spectrum disorder in our contemporary moment is a biomedical one. Autism is understood as a neurodevelopmental disorder – a genetic condition that affects brain development and functioning. This is thought to result in three key areas of impairment: communication (e.g., impaired language), social interaction (e.g., difficulty making friends, averted eye gaze), and repetitive movements and behaviours (e.g., hand flapping) ("Autism Spectrum Disorder"). Level of impairment is measured along an axis of severity from level 1 "requiring support" to level 3 "requiring very substantial support" ("DSM-5 Criteria"). Within this view, autism is understood to be the result of both heritability and environmental triggers (Rutter). This prevailing biomedical view of autism is partnered with the biomedical imperative to view disorder and mental difference as unnatural and to remedy it (Michalko). Mothers – who carry the bulk of carework globally – are recruited as the primary agents in remedial autism treatments (Douglas, "As If You Have a Choice"). Guided by biomedical practitioners and self-fashioned expertise as "mother warriors," many mothers access treatments for their child that are intensive and expensive and often have normalization or recovery as their goal (e.g., behavioural therapies). Given today's biogenetic landscape, mothers are also recruited into particular practices of self-governance to "watch" their own actions. Undergoing expensive testing for the "autism gene," for example, or engaging in self-care routines that mitigate epigenetic (inherited) risks of having a child with autism (such as maternal nutrition) have become common routines. Learning to watch for the signs of autism in your developing child, too, has become everyday practice (Douglas, *Autism and Mothering*; McGuire). And yet, things have not always been this way.

Autism emerged as a distinct medical category in the 1940s. Leo Kanner, director of child psychiatry at Johns Hopkins Hospital and a leader in this new field, called this new disorder "early infantile autism." He distinguished it from childhood schizophrenia (Nadesan 11) in that the children he observed were impaired from the start in their ability to communicate, unable to engage in reciprocal social interaction, and engaged in stereotyped behaviours such as rocking or "twiddling" (Kanner). Given the influence of biological psychiatry and mental hygiene in the 1940s, Kanner thought there must be some biological basis for the disorder. However, he also infamously noted the potential influence of parents, describing those in his study as lacking in warmth and affection. Most parents in the study were college graduates and worked outside of the home, and most families were middle-class and white. These children, said Kanner in an interview for *Time*, were "kept neatly in a refrigerator which didn't defrost" ("Medicine: Frosted Children" 78).

Such notions of refrigerator parents alongside the age-old adage of mother blame were quickly swept up within gendered post-war efforts to bolster social stability, reinstate middle-class white mothers in the home, and replace biological psychiatry with relational approaches such as psychoanalysis in an era reeling from the atrocities of the Nazi holocaust and scientific racism (Nadesan). In the work of University of Chicago psychologist Bruno Bettelheim and others, the "refrigerator mother" was born. This so-called cold mother of the 1950s and 1960s (in some cases, up to the 1980s and 1990s) was overtly blamed for her child's autistic withdrawal. It was a mother's innately disordered love and desires – wanting to work outside the home, for example – where the trigger for autism could be found (Douglas, "Refrigerator Mothers"). The image of the autistic child trapped in a fortress emerged during this time when Bettelheim made the disturbing analogy between refrigerator mothers and guards in concentration camps, a fate so intolerable for the child the only recourse was to withdraw completely. Separation from her child through institutionalization and psychoanalytic treatment for mothers was often prescribed by experts as the solution. Ironically, the refrigerator mother emerged as a privileged identity – other "bad" mothers of this era (i.e., black, working-class, unwed) and their children were excluded from this elite category and regulated instead through racist and classist hierarchies (Douglas, "Refrigerator Mothers"; Ladd-Taylor and Umansky 12).

Mothers and parents searching for alternatives in the 1960s and 1970s began to champion emerging biological understandings of autism (Rimland). A prominent theory in cognitive neuropsychology, for example, posits that autistic people lack Theory of Mind (ToM), a cognitive structure thought to be locatable within brains as the precondition for empathy, understood as that which makes us human (Baron-Cohen et al.). The alarming implication of this still-popular theory is that without remediation, autistic people do not fully share in humanity and, indeed, are thought to be "victim-captives" of their neurology (Yergeau 3). Parents, particularly mothers, formed local and national autism advocacy organizations to educate the public about biological views of autism, raise money for scientific research, advocate for public funding and access to public schools and community living supports (Douglas, *Autism and Mothering*; McGuire). Through their efforts, overt forms of mother blame were debunked, new supports for families and their offspring secured, and a nascent form of disability activism forged (O'Toole; Panitch 7; Ryan and Runswick-Cole).

New and intensive behavioural therapies – Applied Behaviour Analysis – emanating from the behaviourist experiments of Ole Ivar Lovaas at University of California Los Angeles on autistic and gender non-conforming children sought to normalize autistic children and their disordered biology/brains through the use of aversives to extinguish autistic behaviours (i.e., shocks from electrified floors) and rewards to shape normative ones (i.e., hugs, food) (Gibson and Douglas; Gruson-Wood). Against the backdrop of neoliberal capitalism and shifting family-state-market relations that pushed care back into the home and community as the primary responsibility of mothers (even as middle-class white mothers entered the workforce in record numbers), the ideology of intensive mothering emerged (Brodie; Hays).

It would be "mother therapists" (Douglas, *Autism and Mothering*) under the guidance of new behaviourists who would be tasked with the "critical exigence" (Yergeau 4) to work intensively to remediate and normalize autism. Mothers were taught to "watch" themselves anew – to love and care for their child through practicing [sic] intensive, scientifically guided behavioural techniques. For those mothers who "failed" to take up these new modes of self-governance – working-class, black, and other disadvantaged mothers – or who did not want to care intensively in this way, this was a new form of covert mother blame that concealed unequal gender, class, and race relations and individualized a mother's failure to remedy her child (Douglas, *Autism and Mothering*; Hays 165; Sousa).

Today, ours is a risk society that understands autism as non-viable and hopeless, a threat to a family's, community's, and nation's economic and emotional well-being. Today's "mother warrior" must work ever more intensively to safeguard her family from the proliferating risk of autism, including from her own genes and potentially poor coping and mothering choices (Douglas, "As If You Have a Choice"; McGuire). Within social scientific studies of autism and mothering, for example, research on coping with the stress and stigma of autism as well as resiliency is predominant (Gray). While vital, possibilities for more autism-accepting and sociopolitical understandings of autism and mothering are elided in this view. Covert mother blame again cloaks mothers' unequal access to resources and is intensified in our time; mothers become powerful curative forces as "warriors" staving off risk through their own choice and resilience (Douglas, "As If You Have a Choice").

Central Issues and Debates

In response to the predominance of biomedical approaches to autism, autistic people, mothers and critical and feminist scholars (not mutually exclusive) have raised a number of important issues and debates: (1) What is autism? Is it a deficit in need of remedy or a human difference? (2) How might mothers care differently, outside a biomedical framework? (3) How do power and privilege shape autism and mothering? (4) What is the role of mothers within disability and autistic self-advocacy movements? (A human rights based movement started in the 1980s by and for autistic people advocating for access and acceptance. See *Autistic Self Advocacy Network*; *Autistics United Canada; Autistics for Autistics*); (5) What should the goal of autism research be? In this section, we introduce alternative frameworks, including feminist disability studies, neurodiversity, and critical autism studies, that illuminate these key issues and debates.

Briefly, the interdisciplinary field of disability studies rethinks disability as a sociopolitical phenomenon and raises questions about how power shapes the meaning we make of human difference. In other words, the field of disability studies is concerned with "not simply the variations that exist in human behavior, appearance, functioning, sensory acuity, and cognitive processing, but, more crucially, the meaning we make of those variations" (Linton 2; also see Michalko and Titchkosky). The marginalized standpoints of disabled persons are centered [sic], and the biomedical view that disability is a *thing* locatable within individual bodies and brains, troubled.

As Lennard Davis articulates, "Disability is not an object – a woman with a cane – but a social process that intimately involves everyone" (2). Rather than a personal tragedy, disability studies understands disability as a legitimate, albeit different, way of being in the world with something of value to teach us about our relationships and our life together (Davis). Lived experiences and the fleshy stubbornness of different bodies become sites of cultural production, resistance, and new knowledge (Douglas et al., "Re-storying Autism"; Rice). Scholars have also signaled [sic] the need for disability studies to take up complex histories and intersections between disability, race, class, gender, sexuality, and other oppressions and struggles for human freedom (O'Toole 297).

Scholars of mothering, care, and disability working at the intersection of feminist and disability studies raise complex questions that attend to such intersections. They point to questions raised by autistic self-advocates, for example, about mothers' (who may also be disabled) troubling implication in histories of ableist violence, oppression, and exclusion toward autistic people such as ABA (Dawson), where care is imagined as a burden on families and mothers in particular. In this view, a mother's care must recover the autistic body to its presumed normative state, that is, to an independent, productive, and contributing body that relies on itself. At the same time, disability studies scholars point out that mothers have, in many instances, been at the forefront of struggles against autistic persons' oppression (Ryan and Runswick-Cole). Mothers are key support persons and advocates for their autistic offspring, a sometimes-unsettling reality for autistic self-advocacy and disability rights movements that have worked hard to distance themselves from patronizing, dehumanizing, and devalued feminized aspects of care (such as dependence) to achieve support and autonomy as their fundamental right (Hughes et al.; Kelly). Beginning from the supposition that care and support are "fundamental to life," feminist disability studies recognizes the mother-child relationship not only as political but also ethical: "caring relationships characteristically carry a jolting, perhaps irresolvable paradox – that of transgressive possibility and coercive constraint, intimate inter-dependence and constraining power, love and violence" (Douglas et al., "Cripping Care" 4–5). Within the relational tension of loving our "different" child, and against the recruitment of mothers to fix that same child through neoliberal capitalist and biomedical logics (that we suggest do violence to difference), new possibilities for supporting and being-with (versus fixing) our child in relation emerges (Douglas, Autism and Mothering; Klar).

Alongside such relational and ethical questions, feminist disability studies scholars trouble the notion of disability as an added care burden for mothers – a common theoretical position in feminist political economy of care. They raise complex questions about interconnections between feminist and disability emancipation within intensive mothering and neoliberal capitalist regimes, for example, pointing out that disability and autistic self-advocates, alongside mothers in positions of privilege, are implicated in transnational capitalist flows of labour given that racialized, disadvantaged and Third World women fill the gap of underpaid carework in Global North neoliberal capitalist economies (Erevelles; Meekosha; Williams). Bridging such ethical, political, and economic tensions to achieve deeper understandings of intersecting oppressions and to work toward disability and feminist liberation is vital (Kelly).

A first move toward bridging these tensions is to attend to emerging research that opens different possibilities and questions around autism and mothering. One important approach emanating from autistic communities is neurodiversity, which is the understanding that human neurology is neither static nor fixed (Walker). In other words, embodied difference is part of life and should be accepted, not cured. This offers an alternative to biomedical views such as Theory of Mind or behaviour therapies that assume autistic behaviour is the result of a disordered neurology, and therefore that it is meaningless and involuntary (Yergeau). Neurodiversity has been a formative concept within autism self-advocacy organizations organized by and for autistic persons, including Autistics United Canada and the Autistic Self Advocacy Network in the United States (*Autistic Self Advocacy Network*, *Autistics United Canada*), as well as for many autistic bloggers,[2] who argue that autism is a viable way of being, and that parent advocacy should not advance a world without autism as its goal (McGuire 105–07). Neurodiversity perspectives shift the understanding of the human so that neuro-normativity (behaviour that conforms to normative expectations) is no longer the measuring stick of what makes a life worth living, and so that neurodivergent identities (any identity counter to neuro-normativity; see Neurodivergent K) are a viable option for people. A second important alternative to biomedical frameworks and curative therapies comes out of the emerging field of critical autism studies. Runswick-Cole et al., for example, call for a troubling of "any of the current accepted understandings that view autism as a biologically based biomedical disorder or brain difference" (7–9). They include neurodiversity in this challenge. These researchers aim to debunk the science of autism, understand how the diagnosis of autism impacts the lives of those who attract it, critique the autism industry, and promote alternative ways to provide service and supports to individuals and families beyond that of diagnosis, labelling, and remediation (8; also see Davidson and Orsini). Neurodiversity and critical autism studies, in different ways, shift the meaning of autism and the purpose of research, opening up new possibilities for being together beyond biomedical frameworks and normalizing regimes.

Controversies and Challenges

We delve more deeply now into two key areas of controversy related to autism and mothering that have particular salience in our contemporary moment. The first controversy is the question of autism treatment, which touches on deeper issues raised earlier around the meaning of autism, power, and privilege (in terms of access to supports as well as whose knowledge about autism counts), and the goal of autism research. We focus our discussion on one recent controversy within parent and autism communities around Applied Behavioral [sic] Analysis (also called Intensive Early Behavioural Intervention); however, our comments also apply to a number of other controversial treatments, which we point to along the way. Applied Behavioural Analysis (ABA) is currently the sole funded treatment in most countries (if any), understood as the only evidence-based intervention proven scientifically to be effective in extinguishing autistic behaviours (i.e., flapping or rocking) and increasing normative ones (i.e., making eye contact, using spoken language) (Gibson and Douglas; Ontario Scientific Expert Taskforce). Its goal is independence and normalization. It is prescribed in intensive dosages (up to thirty or more hours per week), and thought to be most effective if started early, by age two. As its founder Ivar Lovaas puts it, the goal is for treated children to become "indistinguishable from their normal friends" (8). ABA is often offered to mothers at the point of diagnosis as a child's best or only hope for a good life – understood as a life free from autism. Mothers and families have been at the forefront of advocacy efforts for public funding for ABA (Klar, Douglas and McGuire). It is, of course, vital for families and autistic individuals to have access to a variety of supports and therapies to support their well-being and access to life, just as it is for us all. However, when ABA – alongside its goal of independence and normalization – is offered as the only possible hope, this powerfully communicates hopelessness for families who cannot (or do not want to) access ABA due to long waitlists, limited financial resources, or alternative goals for their child (Klar, Douglas and McGuire; also see Gibson and Douglas). It also elides ethical and relational questions about difference (discussed earlier), and supports the view that autism is a problem that must be fixed. When ABA fails to recover or produce a "normal" child, which is most often the case, the dire need for support, and alternative approaches to autism is clear.

Within our contemporary moment, the biomedical imperative to remedy difference (Michalko) arising from the prestige of Western science as the utmost authority on health and disability drives normalizing treatments such as ABA. Many families go into substantial debt to access ABA treatment. Other mothers and parents pursue alternative, sometimes risky and usually expensive and intensive treatments to recover or normalize their child including chelation therapy, gluten-free/casein-free diets, hypobaric oxygen treatment, vitamin treatment, anti-vaccination stances, the list goes on (Nadesan). In this way, parents become part of a booming autism industry that commodifies autism (Mallet and Runswick-Cole) and profits from the "critical exigence" (Yergeau 4) to eliminate difference. For over thirty years, autistic self-advocates, activists, and academics (not mutually exclusive) have articulated harm as a result of undergoing intensive, normalizing treatments such as ABA that use neuro-normativity as the measuring stick of what is considered human and a worthwhile life (Dawson; Sequenzia; Yer-geau). They articulate the need to move beyond dominant biomedical "theories that privilege restrictive notions of what it means to interact and interrelate" (Yergeau 12). The lengthy list of parents who have murdered their autistic child citing hopelessness for their child's future is an urgent signal that access to supports, different therapeutic goals, and positive representations of autistic individuals are urgently needed (McGuire).

This raises a second area of controversy surrounding autism and mothering, namely, mother advocacy and activism, which again touches on deeper issues raised earlier about the meaning of autism, power and privilege, and the goal of autism research. The most powerful and financially affluent parent advocacy organizations today, such as *Autism Speaks* (McGuire 57), advocate and educate, now globally, from within a dominant Western biomedical framework. This framework, to recap, understands autism as a neurodevelopmental problem in need of a biomedical solution. In this view, behavioral [sic] and genetic therapies are interventions that aim to reshape impairments caused by disordered brain development, and a mother's role becomes that of therapist, fixer, and even "warrior." While seemingly a benevolent aim, these efforts export Western culture's understanding of the normative human as non-autistic, white, and Western (Douglas, "As If You Have a Choice"; Mallet and Runswick-Cole; McGuire; Titchkosky and Aubrecht). Other ways of understanding autism and care beyond that of deficit and remedy are marginalized; scientific research agendas target the cause and cure of autism to the exclusion of research to support a good life for autistic individuals. MSSNG, for example, is a collaboration that brings together corporate America (google) with *Autism Speaks* and over fifty academic and research institutions in thirteen countries to "create one of the world's largest databases on autism," the goal of which is to pinpoint different types of autism and biogenetic treatments ("MSSNG"). One important effect of such efforts has been the generation of vast autism research industries invested in biomedical approaches (McGuire) primarily of financial benefit to non-autistic researchers rather than mothers and autistic individuals (Mallet and Runswick-Cole).

The approach of *Autism Speaks* has been criticized by autistic self-advocates, activists, and academics who support a different understanding of autism, autism support, and research. These criticisms raise important questions about whose experience and knowledge of autism matters. The Autistic Self Advocacy Network (ASAN), for example, an influential self-advocacy organization in the United States, points out that most money raised by *Autism Speaks* does not support mothers, families, and autistic individuals but rather scientists' careers and executive salaries. Further, autistic people's voices are marginalized within the leadership of *Autism Speaks*, and awareness and fundraising campaigns turn on promoting negative, stigmatizing, and fearful images of autism ("Before You Donate to Autism Speaks"). ASAN's slogan, "Nothing about us without us!" forwards a vital message that speaks back to dominant approaches and research agendas, suggesting that a different direction for future research is needed.

New Directions for Future Research

Research that brings autistic voices to the centre and considers the ethical and political dimensions of autism and mothering is crucial. We make the following recommendations. First, future research must aim to more deeply understand the lived experiences of mothers and autistic individuals within current neoliberal and biomedical contexts. This understanding must include both the ethical and political dimensions of care so that the supports and services required for a good life for autistic individuals and those who support them – still predominately mothers – can be identified and implemented. Secondly, research agendas must move away from unquestioned views of autism as disordered neurology in need of a mother's curative labour and toward understanding difference as fundamental to life. This shift in perspective opens new possibilities to support access to life for *all* people, including autistic individuals and mothers. Finally, a complex interrogation of interdependence as a key goal and value of relationships and relational support should be at the centre of future research agendas. This aligns with recent calls in feminist disability studies research on disability and care to recentre interdependence

> in ways that bring the perspective of disabled people and the force of political economy to the fore, taking into account gendered, racialized, and classed aspects of care work while sustaining earlier disability critiques of the realities of violence against disabled persons within care relationships.
>
> (Douglas et al., "Cripping Care" 5)

Key questions to guide future research include: (1) How do mothers support their adult autistic children in a social system that demands independence (Klar; Rooy)? (2) How might we reimagine autistic individuals as agential and relational within the mother/child dyad (Klar; Yergeau)? (3) How might we rethink mothering, care, and support vis-à-vis interdependence (Douglas et al., "Cripping Care")?

Conclusion

The history of autism and mothering is one of regulation, whether the regulation of a mother's love and care within biomedical and neoliberal patriarchal capitalist regimes, or the meaning of being human as exclusive of autistic and other difference within powerful research agendas. This chapter has suggested that embodied difference such as autism, as well as care and support – still predominately performed by women and mothers – are "fundamental to life" (Douglas et al., "Cripping Care"). Given this, the need for alternatives to biomedical understandings of difference and care is dire if we are to move beyond a landscape of hopelessness and harm for mothers and autistic individuals alike. Within the current research context, social support for autistic people and mothers remains contingent on subscribing to biomedical understandings of autism. Mothers who understand autism differently, or who seek educational and other opportunities for their autistic child beyond ABA, are left on their own without financial support or access to other resources. Indeed, mothers remain vexed figures, either covertly blamed within biomedical frameworks for failing to normalize their autistic child or criticized within autism communities for enforcing curative therapies. It is by pursuing a deeper understanding of the ethical and political complexities of mothering and autism that new possibilities for being together beyond biomedical frameworks and normalizing regimes might emerge. It is critical that future research attend to such possibilities.

Further Reading

Notes

1 Originally printed in: The Routledge Companion to Motherhood, edited by Lynn O'Brien Hallstein, Andrea O'Reilly and Melinda Giles (2020). Reprinted with Permission from Taylor and Francis.

2 See, for example, Amanda Baggs, https://ballastexistenz.wordpress.com/ and Michelle
   Dawson www. sentex.net/~nexus23/naa_02.html.

Books, Articles, and Videos

"Autism and the Concept of Neurodiversity." *Disability Studies Quarterly* (Special issue on the concept of neurodiversity), vol. 30, no. 1, 2010. http://dx.doi.org/10.18061/dsq .v30i1.

Baggs, Amanda. *In My Language*, 14 Jan. 2007, www.youtube.com/watch?v=JnylM1hI2jc. Accessed 29 Mar. 2018.

Douglas, Patty. "Refrigerator Mothers." *Journal of the Motherhood Initiative for Research and Community Involvement*, vol. 5, 2014, pp. 94–114.

Hanley, J. J. (Producer) and David E. Simpson (Director). *Refrigerator Mothers* [Motion Picture]. Kartemquin Films, 2002.

Jack, Jordan. *Autism and Gender: From Refrigerator Mothers to Computer Geeks*. U of Illinois P, 2014.

Lewiecki-Wilson, Cynthia, and Jan Cellio, editors. *Disability and Mothering: Liminal Spaces of Embodied Knowledge*. Syracuse UP, 2011.

McGuire, Anne. *War on Autism: On the Cultural Logic of Normative Violence*. U of Michigan P, 2016.

Murray, Stuart. *Representing Autism: Culture, Narrative, Fascination*. Liverpool UP, 2008.

Nadesan, Majia Holmer. *Constructing Autism: Unraveling the 'Truth' and Understanding the Social*. Routledge, 2005.

Runswick-Cole, Katherine, et al., editors. *Re-thinking Autism: Diagnosis, Identity and Equality*. Jessica Kingsley, 2016.

Ryan, Sara, and Katherine Runswick-Cole. "From Advocate to Activist? Mapping the Experiences of Mothers of Children on the Autism Spectrum." *Journal of Applied Research in Intellectual Disabilities*, vol. 22, 2009, pp. 43–53.

Silverman, Chloe. *Understanding Autism: Parents, Doctors and the History of a Disorder*. Princeton UP, 2012.

Sinclair, Jim. "Don't Mourn for Us." *Our Voice: The Newsletter of Autism*, vol. 1, no. 3, 1993. www.autreat. com/dont_mourn.html. Accessed 11 Dec. 2017.

Sousa, Amy C. "From Refrigerator Mothers to Warrior-Heroes: The Cultural Identity Transformation of Mothers Raising Children with Intellectual Disabilities." *Symbolic Interaction*, vol. 34, 2011, pp. 220–43.

Yergeau, Melanie. *Authoring Autism: On Rhetoric and Neurological Queerness*. Duke UP, 2018.

Websites

Amy Sequenzia: https://ollibean.com/author/amy-sequenzia/
Aspies for Freedom: www.aspiesforfreedom.com/
Autistics for Autistics https://a4aontario.com/
Autistics United Canada https://www.autisticsunitedca.org/
The Autism Acceptance Project. www.taaproject.com/
The Autism Crisis: http://autismcrisis.blogspot.ca/
The Autistic Self Advocacy Network: http://autisticadvocacy.org/
Enacting Autism Inclusion: http://enactingautisminclusion.ca/

Neurodiversity.com: www.Neurodiversity.com
Positively Autistic: https://positivelyautistic.weebly.com/
Tiny Grace Notes: https://tinygracenotes.blogspot.ca/

Works Cited

"Autism Spectrum Disorder." American Psychiatric Association. www.psychiatry.org/patients-families/autism/what-is-autism-spectrum-disorder. Accessed 11 Dec. 2017.

"Autistic Self Advocacy Network." http://autisticadvocacy.org/. Accessed 2 Feb. 2019.

"Autistics United Canada." https://www.autisticsunitedca.org/. Accessed 27 Sept. 2019.

Baron-Cohen, Simon, et al. "Does the Autistic Child Have a Theory of Mind?" *Cognition*, vol. 21, 1985, pp. 37–46.

"Before You Donate to Autism Speaks: Consider the Facts." Autistic Self Advocacy Network. https://autistic advocacy.org/?s=Before+you+donate. Accessed 31 Jan. 2018.

Bettelheim, Bruno. *The Empty Fortress: Infantile Autism and the Birth of the Self.* The Free Press, 1967.

Brodie, Janine. *Politics on the Margins: Restructuring and the Canadian Women's Movement.* Fernwood, 1995.

Centers for Disease Control and Prevention (CDC). "Prevalence of the Autism Spectrum Disorders (ASDs) in Multiple Areas of the United States, 2004 and 2006." www.cdc.gov/ncbddd/autism/states/ADDMCommunityReport2009.pdf. Accessed 12 Dec. 2017.

Davidson, Joyce, and Michael Orsini, editors. *Worlds of Autism: Across the Spectrum of Neurological Difference.* U of Minnesota P, 2013.

Davis, Lennard J. *Enforcing Normalcy: Disability, Deafness and the Body.* Verso, 1995.

Dawson, Michelle. "The Misbehavior of Behaviorists: Ethical Challenges to the Autism-ABA Industry." *No Autistics Allowed*, 18 Jan. 2004, www.sentex.net/~nexus23/naa_aba.html. Accessed 30 Mar. 2018.

Douglas, Patty. "As If You Have a Choice: Autism Mothers and the Remaking of the Human." *Health, Culture & Society*, vol. 5, 2013, pp. 167–81. https://doi.org/10.5195/hcs.2013.137

———. "Refrigerator Mothers." *Journal of the Motherhood Initiative for Research and Community Involvement*, vol. 5, 2014, pp. 94–114.

———. "Autism and Mothering: Pursuing the Meaning of Care." University of Toronto, PhD dissertation, 2016. /hdl.handle.net/1807/72960.

Douglas, Patty, et al. "Cripping Care: Care Pedagogies and Practices." *Review of Disability Studies*, vol. 13, no. 4, 2017, pp. 3–12.

———. "Re-storying Autism: A Body Becoming Disability Studies in Education Approach." *International Journal of Inclusive Education*, Advance online publication, 4 Jan. 2019. https://doi.org/10.1080/13603 116.2018.1563835

"DSM-5 Criteria." *Autism Speaks.* www.autismspeaks.org/dsm-5-criteria. Accessed 31 Jan. 2018.

Erevelles, Nirmala. "Signs of Reason: Rivière, Facilitated Communication and the Question of SelfDetermination." *Foucault and the Government of Disability*, edited by Shelley Tremain, U of Michigan P, 2005, pp. 45–64.

Gibson, Margaret, and Patty Douglas. "Disturbing Behaviours: O Ivar Lovaas and the Queer History of Autism Science." *Catalyst: Feminism, Theory, Technoscience*, vol. 4, no. 2, 2018, pp. 1–28. https://doi.org/10.28968/cftt.v4i2.29579

Gray, Donald E. "Gender and Coping: The Parents of Children with High Functioning Autism." *Social Science & Medicine*, vol. 56, 2003, pp. 631–42.

Gruson-Wood, Julia F. "Autism, Expert Discourses, and Subjectification: A Critical Examination of Applied Behavioural Therapies." *Studies in Social Justice*, vol. 10, 2016, pp. 38–58.

Hays, Sharon. *The Cultural Contradictions of Motherhood.* Yale UP, 1996.

Hughes, Bill, et al. "Love's Labors Lost? Feminism, the Disabled People's Movement and an Ethic of Care." *Sociology*, vol. 39, 2005, pp. 259–75.

Kanner, Leo. "Autistic Disturbances of Affective Contact." *Nervous Child*, vol. 2, 1943, pp. 217–50.

Kelly, Christine. *Disability Politics and Care: The Challenge of Direct Funding.* UBC Press, 2016.

Klar, Estée. "The Mismeasure of Autism." *Concepts of Normalcy: The Autistic and Typical Spectrum*, edited by Wendy Lawson. Jessica Kingsley Publishers, 2008, pp. 104–29.

Klar, Estée, Patty Douglas, and Anne McGuire. "Autism Strategy Masks Societal Exclusion of Autistic Ontarians." *Ottawa Citizen*, 19 Apr. 2016. http://ottawacitizen.com/opinion/columnists/klar-douglas-and-mcguire-autism-strategy-masks-societal-exclusion-of-autistic-ontarians. Accessed 18 Aug. 2019.

Ladd-Taylor, Molly, and Lauri Umansky, editors. *"Bad" Mothers: The Politics of Blame in Twentieth-Century America.* New York UP, 1998.

Linton, Simi. *Claiming Disability: Knowledge and Identity.* New York UP, 1998.

Lovaas, Ole Ivar. "Behavioral Treatment and Normal Educational and Intellectual Functioning in Autistic Children." *Journal of Consulting and Clinical Psychology*, vol. 55, 1987, pp. 3–9.

Mallet, Rebecca, and Katherine Runswick-Cole. "Commodifying Autism: The Cultural Contexts of "Disability" in the Academy." *Disability and Social Theory: New Developments and Directions*, edited by Dan Goodley et al., Palgrave Macmillan, 2012, pp. 33–51.

McGuire, Anne. *War on Autism: On the Cultural Logic of Normative Violence.* U Michigan P, 2016.

"Medicine: Frosted Children." *Time*, 26 Apr. 1948, pp. 77–78.

Meekosha, Helen. "Decolonising Disability: Thinking and Acting Globally." *Disability & Society*, vol. 26, 2011, pp. 667–82.

Michalko, Rod. *The Difference that Disability Makes.* Temple UP, 2002.

Michalko, Rod, and Tanya Titchkosy. *Rethinking Normalcy: A Disability Studies Reader.* Canadian Scholar's Press, 2009.

"MSSNG: Changing the Future of Autism with Open Science." *MSSNG.* www.mss.ng/#. Accessed 31 Jan. 2019.

Nadesan, Majia Holmer. *Constructing Autism: Unraveling the 'Truth' and Understanding the Social.* Routledge, 2005.

Neurodivergent, K., and Kassiane Sibley. *Radical Neurodivergence Speaking.* timetolisten.blogspot.ca/. Accessed 10 Dec. 2017.

Ontario Scientific Expert Taskforce for the Treatment of Autism Spectrum Disorder. *Evidence Based Practices for Individuals with Autism Spectrum Disorder: Recommendations for*

Caregivers, Practitioners and Policy Makers, Apr. 2017, www.ontaba.org/#&panel1-2. Accessed 31 Jan. 2019.

O'Toole, Corbett Joan. "The Sexist Inheritance of the Disability Movement." *Gendering Disability*, edited by Bonnie G. Smith and Beth Hutchison, Rutgers UP, 2004, pp. 294–300.

Panitch, Melanie. *Disability, Mothers and Organization: Accidental Activists*. Routledge, 2008.

Rice, Carla. *Becoming Women: The Embodied Self in Image Culture*. U of Toronto P, 2014.

Rimland, Bernie. *Infantile Autism: The Syndrome and Its Implications for a Neural Theory of Behaviour*. AppletonCentury-Crofts, 1964.

Rooy, Robert, director. *DEEJ*. Rooy Media LLC and The Independent Television Service, 2017.

Runswick-Cole, Katherine, et al., editors. *Re-thinking Autism: Diagnosis, Identity and Equality*. Jessica Kingsley, 2016.

Rutter, Michael. "Genetic Studies of Autism: From the 1970s into the Millennium." *Journal of Abnormal Child Psychology*, vol. 28, 2000, pp. 3–14.

Ryan, Sara, and Katherine Runswick-Cole. "From Advocate to Activist? Mapping the Experiences of Mothers of Children on the Autism Spectrum." *Journal of Applied Research in Intellectual Disabilities*, vol. 22, 2009, pp. 43–53.

Sequenzia, Amy. "Autistic Conversion Therapy." *Autistic Women and Nonbinary Network*, 27 Apr. 2016, autismwomensnetwork.org/autistic-conversion-therapy/. Accessed 31 Jan. 2019.

Sinclair, Jim. "Don't mourn for us." *Our Voice: The Newsletter of Autism*, vol. 1, no. 3, 1993, www.autreat. com/dont_mourn.html. Accessed 11 Dec. 2017.

Sousa, Amy C. "From Refrigerator Mothers to Warrior-Heroes: The Cultural Identity Transformation of Mothers Raising Children with Intellectual Disabilities." *Symbolic Interaction*, vol. 34, 2011, pp. 220–43.

Titchkosky, Tanya. *Disability, Self and Society*. U of Toronto P, 2003.

Titchkosky, Tanya, and Catherine Aubrecht. "Who's MIND, Whose Future? Mental Health Projects as Colonial Logics." *Social Identities: Journal for the Study of Race, Nation and Culture*, vol. 21, 2015, pp. 69–84.

Walker, Nick. "Throw Away the Master's Tools: Liberating Ourselves from the Pathology Paradigm." *Loud Hands: Autistic People, Speaking*, edited by Julia Bascom, The Autistic Press, 2012, pp. 154–62.

Williams, Fiona. "Towards a Transnational Analysis of the Political Economy of Care." *Feminist Ethics and Social Policy: Towards a New Global Political Economy of Care*, edited by Rianne Mahon and Fiona Robinson, UBC Press, 2011, pp. 21–38.

Yergeau, Melanie. *Authoring Autism: On Rhetoric and Neurological Queerness*. Duke UP, 2018.

Chapter 22

Enacting Activism

DEPATHOLOGIZING TRAUMA IN MILITARY VETERANS THROUGH THEATRE

Alisha Ali and Luke Bokenfohr

Summary

In this chapter, Alisha Ali and Luke Bokenfohr describe their respective work in veteran-led theatre and performances that showcase the real-life stories of veterans who are dealing with trauma and the challenges of reintegrating into civilian life. They describe two projects: *Contact! Unload* (a play that weaves together stories from returning veterans) and DE-CRUIT (a Shakespeare-based program in which veterans construct and perform their own trauma monologues). Across these two projects, the following themes emerge: healing through community, art as a "model of action," and collective experience of emotion. These themes reveal how the emotional act of witnessing these veterans' stories can mobilize audience members toward mental health activism by humanizing the veteran experience and allowing audience members to directly interact with the performing veterans post-performance, thereby building a bridge of trust and healing between the veteran community and civilians.

*

Introduction

The process of healing from trauma is never linear. It involves numerous setbacks and unforeseen challenges that can occur at any time and at any stage in the "recovery" process. For that reason, treatments for the effects of trauma must be adaptable and responsive to the realities confronting those who have suffered trauma and continue to live with its effects. Military veterans are one such population. Veterans not only experience the ongoing impact of military trauma but also the obstacles of reintegrating into civilian society. Statistics indicate that veterans show elevated rates of mental

DOI: 10.4324/9781003148456-25

health problems, suicide, unemployment, incarceration, and homelessness, as well as a suicide rate of over 20 US veterans per day (US Department of Veterans Affairs, 2019). Given these stigmatizing data, it is imperative to understand that veterans' struggles with reintegration and traumatic stress stem not from inner pathologies, but rather from contexts that do not readily support the transition into post-military life.

Evidence also shows that many veterans are dealing with early life traumas that impact their ability to move forward with their lives when they no longer have the routinized structure and camaraderie of military life. It is therefore also important to conceptualize "treatment" for veterans not as a form of fixing defects in the individual, but rather as the construction of systems of processes and people that can together foster healing within a collective environment. This form of *communalization of trauma* has been identified by psychiatrist and author of *Achilles in Vietnam*, Jonathan Shay (1995), as one of the most important elements in trauma treatment for veterans. In this chapter, we describe one approach to utilizing communalization as a treatment modality in working with veterans that encourages sharing and mutual support. Specifically, the focus of this chapter is on the use of theatre as a form of communalized narration that involves not only veterans working alongside other veterans but also the broader community of veterans and non-veterans. We will argue that theatre represents a unique opportunity for healing wherein stories of trauma are articulated, shared, and ultimately taken on by fellow storytellers, performers, and audience members through overlapping mechanisms of humanizing, understanding, and collective growth.

Theatre, Communalization, and Collective Healing

We write this chapter as two authors who have each been closely involved with theatre projects that were designed to help veterans with the process of adjusting to civilian life. Alisha has worked with the US-based DE-CRUIT Veterans Program in the capacity of a researcher, and Luke has worked with the Canada-based *Contact! Unload* project as a military veteran, an actor, and a mental health counselor. Each of these theatre-based programs is connected to the process that veterans go through as they work through the effects of trauma and build lives for themselves as veterans and as community members.

The DE-CRUIT program uses Shakespeare's plays to heal military veterans' trauma. The plays have numerous soldiers, military veterans, and family members of veterans as characters. Additionally, the world of Shakespeare and the Elizabethan Great Chain of Being parallel the rigid hierarchy of military life. In DE-CRUIT, veterans work together to learn the Shakespearian monologue form, and they come to understand that veterans from Shakespeare's time and ever since have suffered psychologically and emotionally in much the same way that they have. The veterans in the program eventually write their own personal trauma monologues that they will "hand off" to a veteran in the group who will perform the monologue and thereby allow the group members and the writer of the monologue to bear witness to the trauma and its effects. This process of communalization continues to the end of the program, which culminates in a performance to friends, family, and community members in which each veteran performs their own trauma monologue as well as a Shakespearian monologue that has been selected to match some aspect of the trauma that is represented in their own personal trauma monologue.

The *Contact! Unload* project originated with firsthand stories from veterans and transformed those stories into a play that has been performed widely to audiences of veterans, civilians, and even politicians, royalty, and world leaders – all with the aim of building a collective movement that supports veterans' re-entry into civilian life. Through the power of storytelling and acting, *Contact! Unload* brings audience members into the veterans' world in a manner that is emotionally difficult but still welcoming. As we will explore, our respective experiences with these theatre-based projects transformed the ways that we think not only about mental health but also about mental health activism.

Alisha's Experience

As a Muslim Canadian woman of color, I never expected that my career trajectory would lead me to specialize in working with US military veterans in post-9/11 New York. Moreover, as a psychologist who trained primarily in medical settings, my understanding of mental health problems was shaped by psychiatry's reliance on the notion of pathology as a means of framing and defining those who suffer psychologically and emotionally. My experience with the DE-CRUIT Veterans Program fundamentally altered that understanding for me. I first learned about the DE-CRUIT program from attending Stephan Wolfert's play "Cry Havoc" (which is excerpted in this volume). "Cry Havoc" is Stephan's personal story of experiencing military trauma and using theatre – specifically Shakespeare – to heal from that trauma. The play is also the basis for the DE-CRUIT program. I eventually came to understand DE-CRUIT, in its use of theatre and the culminating performance of veterans sharing their personal stories, as a form of mental health activism that demonstrated to the civilian community the need to advocate for veterans as they transition back to civilian life. Working with the DE-CRUIT program also introduced me to the work that Luke was doing as part of the *Contact! Unload* team based in Vancouver, Canada. Luke's experience with that program – and the lessons he learned about the power of theatre to foster recovery – exemplify the function of narration through theatre as a path to collective healing and collective action in the realm of mental health.

Luke's Experience

Theatre has long been used as a transformative and meaningful form of expression, communication, and healing. In *The Body Keeps the Score*, Bessel van der Kolk (2014) refers to the military veterans of Ancient Greece performing for crowds of their peers as far back as 2500 years ago, stating that this may have served as a "ritual reintegration for combat veterans" back into society. More recently, theatre has been used as a therapeutic vehicle for modern veterans in their journey toward healing from posttraumatic stress injuries, as well as a platform for mental health advocacy, raising awareness in the public to the cause-and-effect of trauma on service members. In Ancient Greece, as van der Kolk notes, for instance, during the prominence of Greek playwright Sophocles, all adult males were either serving members of the military, as service was mandatory for every adult male citizen, or they were combat veterans of the then-recent Persian wars (van der Kolk, 2014). Since 9/11, many of the citizens of Western countries who had not previously been to war for many decades have seen a marked increase in their own citizens serving in the military and having experienced combat. The veteran populations within these societies will have risen dramatically, as will the rates of traumatic stress injuries. And yet barriers exist to getting help for those affected. Admitting to suffering from the effects of being exposed to trauma can be career suicide within the military. The stigma attached to admitting to mental health problems undoubtedly leads to individuals not coming forward to ask for help and consequently suffering in silence. While public awareness of mental health has increased in the last few years concurrent with the rise of returning veterans from conflict zones, there may be a disconnect between the experiences of veterans and the understanding of the public and the people close to them. Theatre continues to be used as a tool to connect and communicate with the public those raw, visceral experiences and highlight the toll they have taken on servicemen and women. Little did I know when I began my military career 20 years ago that I would be one of the voices trying to share that message.

My own journey from the battlefield to the stage began with my military service, which was non-traditional, in that as a Canadian, I traveled to the United Kingdom and joined the military there, as Commonwealth citizens can do. I served ten years in the British Armed Forces as a front-line infantryman with the Royal Marine Commandos. The five operational tours I took part in included the invasion of Iraq in 2003 and working from a forward operating base in Afghanistan in 2008/2009. That last tour was tougher than the rest. I had placed myself in a situation where, among other incidents, I had to witness several sad events, including the loss of several brothers-in-arms within a combat setting. I was fortunate that I had strong support from my family and friends and within the military organization, which I believe added to my psychological resiliency. Indeed, the absence of strong social networks and preexisting coping skills have been shown to put soldiers at increased risk for developing stress-related injuries (Friedman et al., 1994). Many of my comrades-in-arms were not as lucky to have available to them the same resources I had. I have good friends who to this day still carry the deep emotional wounds from their service. Many of them feel they cannot communicate this pain with those closest to them. I could well relate to this feeling. While I have been able to share most of my own experiences with those closest to me, there were relationships within which this was impossible. When I left the Corps, I was concerned that I would struggle with reintegration back into civilian life, as the military was an all-encompassing life experience in which I had immersed myself completely. My identity, my passion, and my purpose were wrapped up in my role as a serviceman. When I decided to leave that world, I sought out the Veteran's Transition Network (VTN), a Canadian non-profit organization dedicated to helping servicemen and women address adverse effects from their service, including helping them successfully transition from the military to civilian life. I wanted to ensure maximum success in civilian life after so long in the military and drop any "baggage" I might be carrying around because of my service. The program the VTN was offering appeared to be just what I was looking for.

One of the cornerstone therapeutic interventions of the VTN's group therapy programs is therapeutic enactment (TE), a form of trauma-focused group therapy (TFGT). The TFGT model features the affected individual, in this case the veteran, re-experiencing a traumatic event within their own narrative construction, and having the group witness their overt sharing of this event. The TE as an intervention allows veterans to re-create a traumatic event within a safe setting to carefully "re-story" the incident, allowing not only the individual re-experiencing the traumatic event to benefit but also involving the group members who no longer just witness the event but actively participate in the healing process. It was within this group setting that I saw firsthand the power of group therapy and TE to create positive change. While in the VTN's flagship program, the Veteran's Transition Program (VTP), I met a fellow soldier, a younger man who was very obviously bearing the burden of his service. His eyes were glossed over, he stared into the distance, and he was barely a shadow of a man as I spoke with him. He could not focus on an emotion, appearing numb to the world. Within the VTP, I saw this young man brought back to life before my eyes. I watched one of the facilitators of the group, Marv Westwood PhD, seemingly pull this man back into his body from where it had been long hidden. I likened it to a scene in the movie, "Lord of the Rings: The Two Towers," where the wizard Gandalf expels another wizard from the King of Rohan's body, bringing life back into his eyes. Marv is one of the founders of TE as a therapeutic intervention within a clinical setting, and he has facilitated its use within group settings for veterans for over 20 years. It was this sort of "wizardry" that piqued my interest and led me to ask Marv how I could do similar work. Marv made me put my money where my mouth was and, a short time later, I was enrolled in a graduate program at the University of British Columbia (UBC), studying to be a counselor myself.

Fast forward a couple of years and Marv approached me to ask if I'd be willing to be involved in a play about veterans, for veterans, and performed by veterans. I certainly had trepidation at first, as the sum of my acting skills had been limited to taking a high school drama class over 20 years earlier. The play Marv was referring to was to be called *Contact! Unload*. It was a collaboration between academics and veterans and would turn out to have a significant impact on the lives of many. The play would have several contributors but was the initial brainchild of George Belliveau PhD, also from UBC. In his pursuit of research-based theatre, George was seeking to communicate the struggles of veterans through the story of their time in service and the challenges they face when reintegrating back into society. The therapeutic modality of TE would feature prominently in the play.

I wasn't involved in the initial creation of the script, so when I eventually did get involved, I was unprepared when I was emotionally and physically triggered upon reading my lines. One of the lines that caused a tightness in my chest and an increase in my heart rate that sticks with me to this day is: "and the last thing I saw were the soles of his boots." During my tour of Afghanistan in 2009 I had organized the extraction (casualty-evacuation or "casevac") of one of the men under my direct command, a man I considered a friend, from the battle line during a firefight with the Taliban. He had suffered a gunshot wound to the head and I knew he was in a bad way. When he was safely away from the gunfire and before I turned back to rejoin the firefight, I saw him carried away by four soldiers. The last thing I would ever see of Daz were the soles of his boots. In reading this line and remembering that moment I was activated. I asked the group to stop and stay in that moment, and they did. We had all been through the VTP and all possessed a new vocabulary and a new skill set for our own emotional witnessing. There was no stigma attached to sharing my vulnerability and "activation" in that moment, and the group of fellow actors all sat and listened patiently.

I remember speaking with George about his frustration with the pace of rehearsals, that there were many more breaks in the reading of dialogue to explore moments than there would be in a "normal" play. My experience with theatre is limited, but I think all of us understood that this was no normal play and that the process of creation and preparation would be atypical as well. The bond created within the theatre group, especially among the veterans, was immediate and palpable. We had all seen trauma within our service and had all been able to share our stories with each other. What I hadn't expected when embarking on this project with my brothers-in-arms was the effect our performances would have on the audience.

I had no idea when I volunteered to be part of the project how powerful the medium of theatre would be in conveying the lived experience of veterans to the civilian population. I know I'm not alone as a veteran in feeling that there's often a disconnect between what the veteran experiences and what the civilian understands with regard to that. The play was performed for various audiences: veterans, academics, and the general public. I don't remember a single performance where there wasn't a person deeply affected, as evidenced by gestures, commentary, or tears. During post-show panels and informal discussions, the effect of the play on civilians in the audience was raw and intense. There is a sense of immediacy to the medium of theatre: you can't hit a "pause" button – you have to experience the moment along with the performers. All of us were also method actors by design, which gave an authenticity to the experience. This was not our choice but simply the de facto reality of combat veterans performing the roles of veterans. We all intrinsically understood the characters, as a piece of us was evident in each of them. It seemed almost effortless to deliver sincere and expressive performances for our audience. The feedback from the audience supported that belief (Belliveau & Lee, 2020). One spectator stated: "It felt like I was very intimately watching someone experience something that was real. I almost felt like I was intruding on someone's very private moment of healing." Another audience member recounted the emotional impact the play had on them: "I've never been to a play where I've felt like this … it's real life, a unique hybrid of theatre and real life." Over the years, I have come to see more and more clearly the ways that the play has fostered deep empathy with the veteran experience, as well as raising awareness about the depth and complexity of the mental health struggles faced by veterans.

Theatre as Mental Health Activism: Guiding Principles

Through our respective work with these two projects (the DE-CRUIT program and *Contact! Unload*), we have learned that the reach of theatre goes beyond the telling of stories and into the realm of transformation. Much as we have been changed by this work, we have seen audience members and communities changed; becoming more eager to support veterans in the goal of growing through and past their trauma. Both of these forms of theatre are examples of mental health activism. From our reflections on what we have learned, three main themes have emerged, each of which represents an area of future work that we hope to expand upon as these projects reach more and more audiences in Canada, the US, and internationally.

Healing through Community

Hodermarska et al. (2015) have explored the function of *therapeutic theatre* and the broad, society-based role that it can play. They examine the ways that performance can contribute to healing. This healing can occur for performers and audience members alike. Indeed, an aim of the DE-CRUIT program is for the Culminating Performance to create individual healing among the presenting veterans and also a feeling of collective healing among the community members in attendance. Given that the audience members will likely be upset and disturbed by the stories they hear, it is imperative that there is a corresponding element of healing that takes place before the audience members leave the performance space. This aim reveals that there is an ethical imperative at play in this theatre work as well.

Similarly, *Contact! Unload* has been performed to varied audiences, some that are already part of the military or veteran community, and some that are fully civilian. The natural impetus to respond to human suffering affects both of these audiences, and both communities have a part to play in the process of healing. However, by working to bring these communities together, the DE-CRUIT and *Contact! Unload* performances endeavor to create an integrative community of change centered on collective action. It's important to point out that audience members who have come to repeat performances or followed up with project team members sometimes speak of the ways that advocating for veterans serves as a form of emotional healing for them and honors their veteran family members with whom they never spoke about the trauma of war and its aftermath.

Art as a "Model of Action"

In attempting to understand the function of art as a form of mental health activism, we can draw upon the discipline of *relational aesthetics*. In his description of relational aesthetics, Bourriaud (2001) states that art can present "models of action within the existing real" (p. 13). With respect to theatre, the impetus toward social change within a realm of the existing real takes on a compelling tenor when the performed stories come from the lived experiences of those who have suffered. All audience members can understand the fundamental meaning of suffering on some level, and that common ground serves to bridge the veteran-civilian divide in performances in DE-CRUIT and performances of *Contact! Unload*.

Beyond the sharing of stories, these performances by veterans can mobilize audience members toward action by showing them realities in their own world that they had been unaware of until now. The post-performance discussions often reveal that most audience members have a close connection to at least one veteran through blood relations or otherwise. They are encouraged to reach out to veterans in their lives and learn their stories and about their struggles with reintegration into the civilian world. As psychologist Paula Caplan (2016) has explained in her writing about trauma and veterans, the act of simply listening to a veteran's story without interruption can be a moment of activism when entered into with an open heart and an open mind. In addition to this listening, audience members become invested in the lives of the presenting veterans and often come away from performances asking "What can I do to support veterans in my community?" This is the type of action-oriented advocacy that these performances are intended to elicit.

Collective Experience of Emotion

Because the audiences in DE-CRUIT and *Contact! Unload* know that they are witnessing real-life stories, there is a certain air of reverence during the performances and a collective experience of awe, grief, and caring for the veterans. As psychologist Keith Oatley (1992) has elucidated in his psychological research on emotions, our emotions serve a practical function in our lives by directing us to notice and attend to certain stories and details that then begin to matter to us on a deeper level. In keeping with the conventions of theatre-going, the audiences in these performances by veterans hold space and bear witness to their stories of strength and suffering. They do not challenge, question, or confront them about their actions or their decisions; they allow the stories to unfold at a pace that reflects the veterans' lived experiences. In this way, the emotions of the audience come to mimic those of the veterans. That phenomenon reflects Aristotle's concept of mimesis through theatre which Oatley has identified as a simulation of emotions presented on stage that elicits a sympathetic and deeply felt emotional response in audience members. This mimetic encounter can lead to a collective cathartic experience when the subject matter of the shared stories involves personal trauma. Interestingly, Oatley points to Shakespeare's verse as being emblematic of this mimetic experience, and the DE-CRUIT performances certainly benefit from the familiarity of certain lines and phrases from Shakespeare that resonate with the performing veterans and audience members alike.

Another benefit of this emotional engagement with the performances is that audiences are able to suspend preconceived myths about mental health and focus instead on the lived experiences of veterans presented in veterans' words. This is key to mobilizing audiences because it humanizes veterans by making their stories accessible and relatable. This process is heightened by the Q&A and dialogue sessions that follow the performances, which bring the audience even closer to the work and allows them to ask the performing veterans what they can do to be of service to those who have served. This brings into focus not only the emotional element of these programs, but the activist element as well.

Final Thoughts

Given the culture of masculinity and emotional stoicism that pervades the military, it is not surprising that military veterans are often not inclined to share their experiences of mental suffering. Theatre creates a space that is distanced enough from the veterans' day-to-day lives to allow them to perform themselves as a sort of character that they experience as *me* and *not-me* at the same time. This builds a comfort level with the sharing of emotions and thereby provides a glimpse into the inner lives of veterans as they struggle with psychological distress.

These struggles reveal not only individual, personal reflections, but also larger themes of the workings of oppression in veterans' lives. Veterans are a marginalized community and are over-represented in populations of those who are homeless, incarcerated, unemployed, and dealing with various forms of addiction. While these problems are often construed as individual problems, seeing themes across veterans' stories shows the pervasive trends in these experiences and demonstrates an undercurrent of oppression. In the lives of veterans, that oppression is very often rooted in early childhood experiences of trauma, racism, poverty, and abuse. These oppressive factors have been shown in research to set the stage for individuals' decisions to enlist in the military and also to function as predictors of slower recovery from traumatic stress after leaving the military (Ali et al., 2020). By allowing us to see the workings of oppression in veterans' lives, these theatre-based programs can further reveal the need for systemic change beyond simply "treating" traumatic stress as a mental illness.

There are important future directions for the work we have described here. Key among those are continuing relationships between the theatre work and university-based research. *Contact! Unload* is housed within the University of British Columbia's multidisciplinary initiative on theatre-based research, which takes an activist-oriented stance on tackling social issues including mental health and oppression. Similarly, the DE-CRUIT program is partnered with the Advocacy and Community-Based Trauma Studies (ACTS) Lab at New York University, which conducts research on the mental health benefits of theatre. These partnerships are important not only in expanding the scope of the work but also in building an awareness in the academic and scientific communities about the need to understand and publicize the role that the arts can play in individual and collective efforts to build communities of healing.

References

Ali, A., Wolfert, S., McGovern, J., Aharoni, A., & Nguyen, J. (2020). A trauma-informed analysis of monologues constructed by military veterans in a theatre-based treatment program. *Qualitative Research in Psychology, 17*(2), 258–273.

Belliveau, G., & Lee, G. (2020). *Contact! Unload: Military veterans, trauma, and research-based theatre.* Vancouver: UBC Press.

Bourriaud, N. (2001). *Postproduction: Culture as screenplay: How art reprogrammes the world.* New York: Lukas & Sternberg.

Caplan, P. (2016). Vets aren't crazy. War is. In W. Hall (Ed.), *Outside mental health: voices and visions of madness* (pp. 285–286). Madness Radio.

Friedman, M. J., Schnurr, P. P., & McDonagh-Coyle, A. (1994). Post-traumatic stress disorder in the military veteran. *Psychiatric Clinics, 17*(2), 265–277.

Hodermarska, M., Landy, R., Dintino, C., Mowers, D., & Sajnani, N. (2015). As performance: Ethical and aesthetic considerations for therapeutic theatre. *Drama Therapy Review, 1*(2), 173–186.

Oatley, K. (1992). *Best laid schemes: The psychology of the emotions.* Cambridge University Press.

Shay, J. (1995). *Achilles in Vietnam.* New York: Simon & Schuster.

U.S. Department of Veterans Affairs (2019). *National veteran suicide prevention annual report.* Washington, DC: Author.

van der Kolk, B. A. (2014). *The body keeps the score: Brain, mind and body in the healing from trauma.* New York: Viking Press.

Part III. Concerned Clinicians

DOI: 10.4324/9781003148456-26

THIS SECTION TURNS TO THE ROLE that concerned clinicians play in the struggle over meaning-making practices around mental difference. As with artists, scholars, and activists, much of this struggle is around the dominant biomedical model of mental difference, which we call biopsychiatry. The clinical world is far from a totality and the biomedical model is a source of antagonism and struggle within the clinical world. Mad studies-oriented clinicians, whether or not they use the term "mad studies," have been active in critiquing the limits, harms, and sanist risks of biopsychiatry. We say "sanist risks" here because biomedical models, while not inherently sanist, often rely on a pathologizing frame which risks sliding into sanist relationships— where the pathological designation is less a "disease like other diseases" and more of a pathogizing of the person themselves. When we are pathologized by the biomedical model or otherwise, we risk losing our voice, and we risk prejudice, denigration, subordination, and exclusion. We risk losing our human agency and being coerced, manipulated, treated, and/or confined against or without our will. We risk human rights abuses.

Because of these limits and risks, clinicians have been active in developing alternatives to the biomedical model that can provide lines of flight from biopsychiatry for those who need or prefer them. These alternatives open up ways of understanding and being with mental difference beyond pathologizing models and beyond broken brains, chemical imbalances, and neurocircuitry malfunction. To understand this work, it helps to unpack what we mean by "biopsychiatry," to compare mad studies approaches with antipsychiatry approaches, and to articulate alternatives clinicians are taking beyond biopsychiatry.

A good place to begin understanding the biomedical model is with psychiatrists Peter Tyrer and Derek Steinberg's book *Models for Mental Disorder* (2013). Tyrer and Steinberg explain that biopsychiatry, or what they call "the disease model," focuses its attention primarily on impaired brain functioning as a consequence of physical and chemical changes. This focus on biological variables gives the model a deep affinity with science and medicine. From this perspective, the only real difference between medicine and psychiatry comes from the specificity of the "disease." Medicine deals with general malfunctions of the body; psychiatry specializes in malfunctions of the nervous system. As Nobel Prize-winning psychiatrist and neuroscientist Eric Kandell (1998) put it: "All mental processes, even the most complex psychological processes, derive from operations of the brain. The central tenet of this view is that what we commonly call mind is a range of functions carried out by the brain" (p. 460). Following this logic, the biomedical model argues that, since the brain is the organ of the mind, dysfunctions of mind can be reduced to diseases of the brain.

Tyrer and Steinberg (2013) articulate four principles that follow from the psychiatric biomedical model:

1. Mental pathology is always accompanied by physical pathology.
2. The classification of this pathology allows mental illness to be classified into different disorders which have characteristic features.
3. Mental illness is handicapping and biologically disadvantageous.
4. Cause of mental illness is explicable by its physical consequences.

(p. 12)

Following these principles, it makes perfect sense that Nancy Andreasen, former editor of the *American Journal of Psychiatry*, chose to name her bestselling introduction to this model *The Broken Brain* (Andreasen, 1984). The term "broken brain" signifies the diseased, or malfunctioning, brain at the core of mental illness.

Although the term "broken brain" continues to have some purchase, it has gradually been replaced with the more ubiquitous phrase "chemical imbalance." Since broken brains cannot usually be demonstrated in individual cases, the phrase "chemical imbalance" has taken over from "the broken brain" as the popular explanatory metaphor of biopsychiatry. The term "chemical imbalance" is more amorphous than "broken brain," but its implication is more or less the same. In a chemical imbalance, the brain is still broken, but at the subtle level of chemical functioning rather than at the macro level of brain structures. You may not be able to see it in diagnostic studies, but it is broken nonetheless. Thus, the signifiers "broken brain" and "chemical imbalance" are perfect soundbite translations of the biomedical model into everyday language.

William Styron's memoir, *Darkness Visible* (2002), is a paradigmatic example of the biomedical model being brought into lived experience. Styron describes himself as "laid low by the disease," a "major illness" of "horrible intensity," which came on him like a "brainstorm ... a veritable howling tempest in the brain, which is indeed what clinical depression resembles like nothing else" (pp. 114–115). If we leave to side the Anthropocene human caused climate change, this connection between depression and bad weather perfectly captures the disease model of depression as lying outside the frame of human goals, desires, losses, and disappointments. Like the weather, depression comes from the material world of inhuman forces, from physical and chemical interactions. For a strong biomedical model advocate like Styron, it makes no more sense to give human meaning to depression than to tell an atheist that thunder is caused by God's anger toward us. Styron explains how he sees it: "I shall never learn what 'caused' my depression, as no one will ever learn about their own … so complex are the intermingling factors of abnormal chemistry, behavior and genetics" (p. 115).

Styron's embrace of the biomedical model is important to consider for mad studies clinicians because it helps articulate a difference between antipsychiatry and mad studies. Antipsychiatry would likely devalue Styron's perspective on his experience, where mad studies would have a both/and response. Mad studies both respects and values Styron's biomedical perspective on his situation and, at the same time, works to expand the cultural field beyond the biomedical option. An antipsychiatry approach would likely denigrate Styron's form of meaning-making because it blames the brain and removes all other contexts. For antipsychiatry, this ontological reduction is false, a myth, and therefore bad. But, from a mad studies-epistemic justice perspective, the question shifts from assessment of truth to questions of who gets to decide and what structures of exclusion keep people away from the meaning-making table. Styron's narrative identification with the biomedical model may be the best choice for him, and he is able to decide. But, at the same time, individual choices are made under dominant meaning-making conditions. The biomedical model dominates the cultural field because of a coordinated invasion of the media environment with pharmaceutical marketing and ghost research devoted to promoting psychiatric medications.

To see how this works, it helps to unpack some of the details. The most well-known tools of this pharmaceutical marketing invasion are *direct-to-consumer* (DTC) and *direct-to-provider* (DTP) advertising, which now saturate the lay and professional media. The less well-known tools of the marketing blitz are *indirect-to-consumer* (ITC) and *indirect-to-provider* (ITP) promotions. These indirect methods follow the public relations tactic known as the "third man" technique—in which promotion comes indirectly through a seemingly neutral "third man" and therefore sidesteps the usual scrutiny and skepticism people give to direct advertising (Rampton & Stauber, 2002). For consumers, indirect promotion includes press and video news releases, product placement techniques, and setting-up various patient and disease-specific advocacy groups (which allow products to be promoted without seeming as though the promotion comes from the corporations directly). For providers, indirect promotion includes a tidal wave of continuing medical education materials, medical opinion leaders, and medical practice and treatment guidelines. Indeed, even scientific research and subsequent medical education itself have in many ways become a marketing arm of the pharmaceutical companies (Applbaum, 2009; Dumit, 2012; Lewis, 2012; Matheson, 2008; Sismondo, 2007; Sismondo & Green, 2015; Smith, 2005).

Psychiatry, in other words, provides pharmaceutical public relations experts with a corporate "marketer's dream" (Angell, 2005, p. 88). This marketing invasion is so successful that psychiatrists have put their patients on multiple drugs for multiple conditions and drug company profits have soared. To take a single-year example, the global market for pharmaceuticals was 900 billion dollars in 2010, and, after treatment for cancer, psychiatric medications were the second bestselling class of drugs that year—coming to a total of 50 billion dollars (Healy, 2012, p. 10).

For the industry to become this kind of colossus, it has had to create a cultural climate of opinion and desire surrounding the product. Jan Leschly, the former CEO of Squibb pharmaceuticals, explains:

> Suddenly information technology was so essential that we realized we are an information company more than we are a pill company. Because it's the software—all the research, networking, marketing—that's important in a pill. … It's not the pill that costs so much; it's the software. (quoted in Crister, 2005, p. 61)

In Leschly's analogy, the modern colossal drug company does not sell its products, the pills, as much as it sells the information that surrounds their pills. Today's neoliberal pharmaceutical industry has become an information industry, an industry of cultural change, not a pill industry. The lengths to which it will go have become so out of control that Peter Gotzsche (2013), the cofounder of the Cochrane Center dedicated to evidence-based uses of pharmaceuticals, compares pharma's business practices to organized crime. Whether or not one agrees with Gotzsche, it is clear that this avalanche of pharmaceutical promotion results that the field of meaning-making options in mental health that is severely limited and biased in the direction of medication.

It is here that mad studies most strongly criticizes the biomedical model—it has become a monopoly that drowns out other possibilities. Monopoly products are beyond true/false or good/bad and it makes sense that people, like Styron, will use them. The challenge for mad studies clinicians, therefore, is to respect people who find the model useful while at the same time criticizing the biomedical model for its monopoly status and helping create alternatives so that people will have additional options.

When we move beyond the simulacrum of pharmaceutical hype, it's clear that the options for understanding mental difference do not stop with the disease model. The most common alternative models are cognitive behavioral models and psychoanalytic models. Going a little further from the mainstream, we find family therapy models, humanistic models, feminist models, antiracist models, and structural competence models. And, going even further, we find mutual-aid, spiritual, expressive-arts, and political models. These last models can be used inside the mental health system; they can also be used to shrink the need for the mental health system. We can clearly shrink the mental health system by providing additional community and public health supports such as mutual aid, adult education, spiritual practices, community arts, and so on. We can also shrink the mental health system by reducing the social determinants of stress and by building a world with less inequality and less social injustice—which are key drivers of social suffering and social stress. There are also attempts to integrate different approaches. Integrative approaches can happen through models designed specifically for integration, such as mindfulness-based cognitive therapy, neuro-psychoanalysis, or the biopsychosocial model. And even seemingly reductive models can have an integrative dimension; one key example of this is neuroscience itself, particularly neuroscience that adopts more holistic logics of mirror neurons and neuroplasticity. Integration can also happen through eclectic models, narrative models, and person-centered models.

All of this means that the clinical world is far from static. It is deeply engaged in ongoing critique and in the creation of models of understanding and practice. Mad studies clinicians, as we understand the term and as we have collected for this reader, are clinicians who join with mad studies artists, scholars, and activists to open mental health care to greater epistemic justice. This means, on one hand, less sanism and less big-pharma and biotech monopolization. And, on the other hand, it means more mad-positive perspectives, more mutual aid, and more alternatives—including alternatives outside the mental health system.

References

Andreasen, N. (1984). *The broken brain: The biological revolution in psychiatry.* Harper and Row.

Angell, M. (2005). *The truth about drug companines: How they deceive us and what to do about it.* Random House.

Applbaum, K. (2009). Getting to yes: Corporate power and the creation of a psychopharmaceutical blockbuster. *Culture, Medicine, and Psychiatry, 33*(2), 185–215.

Crister, G. (2005). *Generation rx: How prescription drugs are altering American's lives, minds and bodies.* Houghfton Mifflin.

Dumit, J. (2012). *Drugs for life: How the pharmaceutical industry defines our health.* Duke University Press.

Gøtzsche, P. C. (2013). *Deadly medicines and organized crime: How big pharma has corrupted healthcare.* Radcliffe.

Healy, D. (2012). *Pharmageddon.* University of California Press.

Kandel, E. (1998). A new intellectual framework for psychiatry. *American Journal of Psychiatry, 155*(5), 457–469.

Lewis, B. (2012). Recovery, narrative theory, and generative madness. In A. Rudnick (Ed.), *Recovery of people with mental illness: Philosophical and related perspectives.* Oxford University Press.

Matheson, A. (2008). Corporate science and the husbandry of scientific and medical knowledge by the pharmaceutical industry. *BioSocieties, 3,* 355–382.

Rampton, S., & Stauber, J. (2002). *Trust us we're experts: How industry manipulates science and gambles with your future.* Tarcher.

Sismondo, S. (2007). Ghost management: How much of the medical literature is shaped behind the scenes by the pharmaceutical industry? *PLOS Medicine, 4*(9), 1429–1433.

Sismondo, S., & Green, J. (Eds). (2015). *The pharmaceutical studies reader.* John Wiley and Sons.

Smith, R. (2005). Medical journals are an extension of the marketing arm of pharmaceutical companies. *PLoS Medicine, 2*(5), 364–366.

Styron, W. (2002). *From darkness visible.* In N. Casey (Ed.), *Unholy ghost: Writers on depression* (pp. 114–126). Harper Perennial.

Tyrer, P., & Steinberg, D. (2013). *Models for mental disorder: Conceptual models in psychiatry* (5th ed.). John Wiley and Sons.

Chapter 23

Mental Illness Is Still a Myth[1]

Thomas Szasz

Summary

This chapter provides an excellent introduction to Szasz's "two-pronged" critique of psychiatry: (1) conceptual and (2) moral-political. Szasz's *conceptual critique* rests on a strong distinction between literal and metaphorical use of language. He equates "literal" with hard fact and physical evidence, and he equates "metaphorical" with soft imagination and superstitious myth. This equation of metaphor and myth is at the heart of his understanding of mental illness as a myth. For Szasz, "If mental illnesses are disease of the central nervous system (for example, paresis), then they are disease of the brain, not the mind; and if they are names of (mis)behaviors (for example, using illegal drugs), then they are not diseases." For example, "A screwdriver may be a drink or an implement. No amount of research on orange juice and vodka can establish that it is a hitherto unrecognized form of a carpenter's tool."

Szasz's *moral-political critique* rests on a separation of the health system from the legal system. As he puts it, "No physician *qua* medical healer has the right to deprive another of life, liberty or property." The task of taking away people's moral rights and making those people wards of the state should belong to "lay persons (jurors) and judges, not physicians or mental health specialists." In other words, no one should have their liberty deprived without due process of law. This does not mean that the legal system is free of biases and prejudices. But at least the legal system is a sector specifically empowered in this area and does not leave the task to teachers, clergy, coaches, therapists, and the like. This issue has not changed since Szasz wrote. The mental health system of today does have some due process, but it is much less substantial than other areas of the legal system.

Even though many in mad studies have moved beyond Szasz's "myth/truth" critiques, his work continues to be invaluable for many involved in mad studies. Some continue to feel that the "myth" approach is a valuable way to address the limits of mainstream psychiatry. And many continue to feel that psychiatrists, as clinical professionals, should not be able to involuntarily confine or treat people. Taking away civil liberties, from this perspective, should be a legal prerogative, not a medical one.

*

DOI: 10.4324/9781003148456-27

In a memorable statement C. S. Lewis once remarked, "Of all the tyrannies a tyranny sincerely exercised for the good of its victims may be the most oppressive. ... To be 'cured' against one's will and cured of states which we may not regard as disease is to be put on a level with those who have not yet reached the age of reason or those who never will; to be classed with infants, imbeciles, and domestic animals." These words still apply to psychiatry today.

Anyone with an ear for language will recognize that the boundary that separates the serious vocabulary of psychiatry from the ludicrous lexicon of psychobabble, and both from playful slang, is thin and permeable to fashion. This is precisely wherein lies the richness and power of language that is inexorably metaphoric. Should a person want to say something sensitive tactfully, he can, as the adage suggests, say it in jest, but mean it in earnest. Bureaucrats, lawyers, politicians, quacks, and the assorted mountebanks of the "hindering professions" are in the habit of saying everything in earnest. If we want to protect ourselves from them, we had better hear what they tell us in jest, lest the joke be on us.

As far back as I can remember thinking about such things, I have been struck by the analogic-metaphoric character of the vocabulary of psychiatry, which is nevertheless accepted as a legitimate medical idiom. When I decided to discontinue my residency training in internal medicine and switch to psychiatry, I did so with the aim of exploring the nature and function of psychiatry's metaphors and to expose them to public scrutiny as figures of speech.

During the 1950s, I published a score of articles in professional journals, challenging the epistemological foundations of the concept of the mental illness and the moral basis of involuntary mental hospitalization. In 1958, as my book *The Myth of Mental Illness* was nearing completion, I wrote a short paper of the same title and submitted it to every major American psychiatric journal. Not one of them would accept it for publication. As fate would have it——and because the competition between psychologists and psychiatrists for a slice of the mental health pie was then even more intense than now——*The American Psychologist* published the essay in 1960. The following year, the book appeared. I think it is fair to say that psychiatry has not been the same since.

Responses to my work have varied from lavish praise to bitter denunciation. American psychiatrists quickly closed ranks against me. Official psychiatry simply dismissed my contention that (mis)behaviors are not diseases and asserted that I "deny the reality that mental diseases are like other diseases," and distorted my critique of psychiatric slavery as my "denying life-saving treatment to mental patients." Actually, I have sought to deprive psychiatrists of their power to involuntarily hospitalize or treat competent adults called "mental patients." My critics have chosen to interpret this proposal as my trying to deprive competent adults of their right or opportunity to seek or receive psychiatric help. By 1970, I had become a non-person in American psychiatry. The pages of American psychiatric journals were shut to my work. Soon, the very mention of my name became taboo and was omitted from new editions of texts that had previously featured my views. In short, I became the object of that most effective of all criticisms, the silent treatment——or, as the Germans so aptly call it, *Totschweigetaktik*.

In Great Britain, my views elicited a more favorable reception. Some English psychiatrists conceded that not all psychiatric diagnoses designate *bona fide* diseases. Others were sympathetic to the plight of persons in psychiatric custody. Regrettably, that posture rested heavily on the misguided patriotic belief that the practice of psychiatric slavery was less common in England than in the United States.

Not surprisingly, my work was received more favorably by philosophers, psychologists, sociologists, and civil libertarians, who recognized the merit of my cognitive challenge to the concept of mental illness, and the legitimacy of my questioning the morality of involuntary psychiatric interventions. I thus managed to set in motion a controversy about mental illness that is still raging.

When people now hear the term "mental illness," virtually everyone acts as if he were unaware of the distinction between literal and metaphoric uses of the word "illness." That is why people believe that finding brain lesions in some mental patients (for example, schizophrenics) would prove, or has already proven, that mental illnesses exist and are "like other illnesses." This is an error. If mental illnesses are diseases of the central nervous system (for example, paresis), then they are diseases of the brain, not the mind; and if they are the names of (mis)behaviors (for example, using illegal drugs), then they are not diseases. A screwdriver may be a drink or an implement. No amount of research on orange juice and vodka can establish that it is a hitherto unrecognized form of a carpenter's tool.

Such linguistic clarification is useful for persons who want to think clearly, regardless of consequences. However, it is not useful for persons who want to respect social institutions that rest on the literal uses of a master metaphor. In short, psychiatric metaphors play the same role in therapeutic societies as religious metaphors play in theological societies. Consider the similarities. Mohammedans believe that God wants them to worship on Friday, Jews that He wants them to worship on Saturday, and Christians that He wants them to worship on Sunday. The various versions of the American Psychiatric Association's (APA) *Diagnostic and Statistical Manual* rest on the same sort of consensus. How does behavior become illness? By the membership of the American Psychiatric Association reaching a consensus that, say, gambling is an illness and then issuing a declaration to that effect. Thereafter "pathological gambling" is a disease.

Obviously, belief in the reality of a psychiatric fiction, such as mental illness, cannot be dispelled by logical argument any more than belief in the reality of a religious fiction, such as life after death, can be. That is because, *inter alia,* religion is the denial of the human foundations of meaning and of the finitude of life; this authenticated denial lets those who yearn for a theo-mythological foundation of meaning and who reject the reality of death to theologize life and entrust its management to clerical professionals. Similarly, psychiatry is the denial of the reality of free will and of the tragic nature of life; this authenticated denial lets those who seek a neuro-mythological explanation of human wickedness and who reject the inevitability of personal responsibility to medicalize life and entrust its management to health professionals. Marx was close to the mark when he asserted that religion was "the opiate of the people." But religion is not the opiate of the people. The human mind is. For both religion and psychiatry are the products of our own minds. Hence, the mind is its own opiate; and its ultimate drug is the word.

Freud himself flirted with such a formulation. But he shied away from its implications, choosing instead to believe that "neuroses" are literal diseases, and that "psychoanalysis" is a literal treatment. As he wrote in his essay "Psychical (or Mental) Treatment":

> Foremost among such measures [which operate upon the human mind] is the use of words; and words are the essential tool of mental treatment. A layman will no doubt find it hard to understand how pathological disorders of the body and mind can be eliminated by 'mere' words. He will feel that he is being asked to believe in magic. And he will not be so very wrong. ... But we shall have to follow a roundabout path in order to explain how science sets about restoring to words a part at least of their former magical power.

I took up the profession of psychiatry in part to combat the contention that abnormal behaviors are the products of abnormal brains. Ironically, it was easier to do this fifty years ago than today. In the 1940s, the idea that every phenomenon named a "mental illness" will prove to be a bona fide brain disease was considered to be only a hypothesis, the validity of which one could doubt and still be regarded as reasonable. Since the 1960s, however, the view that mental diseases are diseases of the brain has become scientific fact. This contention is the bedrock claim of the National Alliance for the Mentally Ill (NAMI), an organization of and for the relatives of mental patients, with a membership in excess of one hundred thousand. Its "public service" slogan, intoned like a mantra, is: "Learn to recognize the symptoms of Mental Illness. Schizophrenia, Manic Depression, and Severe Depression are Brain Diseases."

Diagnoses Are Social Constructs Which Vary from Time to Time and from Culture to Culture

Psychiatrists and their powerful allies have thus succeeded in persuading the scientific community, the courts, the media, and the general public that the conditions they call "mental disorders" are diseases—that is, phenomena independent of human motivation or will. This development is at once curious and sinister. Until recently, only psychiatrists—who know little about medicine and less about science—embraced such blind physical reductionism.

Most scientists knew better. For example, Michael Polanyi, who made important contributions to both physical chemistry and social philosophy, observed: "The recognition of certain basic impossibilities has laid the foundations of some major principles of physics and chemistry; similarly, recognition of the impossibility of understanding living things in terms of physics and chemistry, far from setting limits to our understanding of life, will guide it in the right direction." It is no accident that the more firmly psychiatrically inspired ideas take hold of the collective American mind, the more foolishness and injustice they generate. The specifications of the Americans With Disabilities Act (AWDA), a federal law enacted in 1990, is a case in point.

Long ago, American lawmakers allowed psychiatrists to literalize the metaphor of mental illness. Having accepted fictitious mental diseases as facts, politicians could not avoid specifying which of these manufactured maladies were covered, and which were not covered, under the AWDA. They had no trouble doing so, creating a veritable "DSM-Congress," that is, a list of mental diseases accredited by a congressional, rather than a psychiatric, consensus group. Thus, the AWDA covers "claustrophobia, personality problems, and mental retardation, [but does not cover] kleptomania, pyromania, compulsive gambling, and ... transvestism." It is reassuring to know that the Congress of the United States agrees with me that stealing, setting fires, gambling, and cross-dressing are not diseases.

Thus, the various versions of the APA's *Diagnostic and Statistical Manual of Mental Disorders* are not classifications of mental disorders that "patients have," but are rosters of officially accredited psychiatric diagnoses. This is why in psychiatry, unlike in the rest of medicine, members of "consensus groups" and "task forces," appointed by officers of the APA, make and unmake diagnoses, the membership sometimes voting on whether a controversial diagnosis is or is not a disease. For more than a century, psychiatrists constructed diagnoses, pretended that they are diseases, and no one in authority challenged their deceptions. The result is that few people now realize that diagnoses are not diseases.

Diseases are demonstrable anatomical or physiological lesions, that may occur naturally or be caused by human agents. Although diseases may not be recognized or understood, they "exist." People have hypertension and malaria, regardless of whether or not they know it or physicians diagnose it.

Diagnoses are disease names. Because diagnoses are social constructs, they vary from time to time, and from culture to culture. Focal infections, masturbatory insanity, and homosexuality were diagnoses in the past; now they are considered to be diagnostic errors or normal behaviors. In France, physicians diagnose "liver crises"; in Germany, "low blood pressure"; in the United States, "nicotine dependence."

These considerations raise the question: Why do we make diagnoses? There are several reasons: 1) Scientific—to identify the organs or tissues affected and perhaps the cause of the illness; 2) Professional—to enlarge the scope, and thus the power and prestige, of a state-protected medical monopoly and the income of its practitioners; 3) Legal—to justify state-sanctioned coercive interventions outside of the criminal justice system; 4) Political-economic—to justify enacting and enforcing measures aimed at promoting public health and providing funds for research and treatment on projects classified as medical; 5) Personal—to enlist the support of public opinion, the media, and the legal system for bestowing special privileges (and impose special hardships) on persons diagnosed as (mentally) ill.

It is no coincidence that most psychiatric diagnoses are twentieth-century inventions. The aim of the classic, nineteenth-century model of diagnosis was to identify bodily lesions (diseases) and their material causes (etiology). The term "pneumococcal pneumonia," for example, identifies the organ affected, the lungs, and the cause of the illness, infection with the pneumococcus. Pneumococcal pneumonia is an example of a pathology-driven diagnosis.

Diagnoses driven by other motives—such as the desire to coerce the patient or to secure government funding for the treatment of the illness—generate different diagnostic constructions and lead to different conceptions of disease. Today, even diagnoses of (what used to be) strictly medical diseases are no longer principally pathology-driven. Because of third-party funding of hospital costs and physicians' fees, even the diagnoses of persons suffering from *bona fide* illnesses—for example, asthma or arthritis—are distorted by economic considerations. Final diagnoses on the discharge summaries of hospitalized patients are often no longer made by physicians, but by bureaucrats skilled in the ways of Medicare, Medicaid, and private health insurance reimbursement-based partly on what ails the patient, and partly on which medical terms for his ailment and treatment ensure the most generous reimbursement for the services rendered.

As for psychiatry, it ought to be clear that, except for the diagnoses of neurological diseases (treated by neurologists), no psychiatric diagnosis is, or can be, pathology-driven. Instead, all such diagnoses are driven by non-medical, that is, economic, personal, legal, political, or social considerations and incentives. Hence, psychiatric diagnoses point neither to anatomical or physiological lesions, nor to disease-causative agents, but allude to human behaviors and human problems. These problems include not only the plight of the denominated patient, but also the dilemmas with which the patient, relatives, and the psychiatrist must cope and which each tries to exploit.

My critique of psychiatry is two-pronged, partly conceptual, partly moral and political. At the core of my conceptual critique lies the distinction between the literal and metaphorical use of language—with mental illness as a metaphor. At the core of my moral-political critique lies the distinction between relating to grown persons as responsible adults and as irresponsible insane persons (quasi-infants or idiots)—the former possessing free will, the latter lacking this moral attribute because of being "possessed" by mental illness. Instead of addressing these issues, my critics have concentrated on analyzing my motives and defending psychiatric slavery as benefiting the "slaves" and society alike. The reason for this impasse is that psychiatrists regard their own claims as the truths of medical science, and the claims of mental patients as the manifestations of mental diseases; whereas I regard both sets of claims as unwarranted justifications for imposing the claimants' beliefs and behavior on others. Because the secret to unraveling many of the mysteries of psychiatry lies in distinguishing claims from assertions, descriptions, suggestions, or hypotheses, let us briefly examine this concept.

Psychiatrists Have the Power to Accredit Their Claims as Scientific Facts and Rational Treatments

Advancing a claim means seeking, by virtue of authority or right, the recognition of a demand—say, the validity of an assertion (in religion), or entitlement to money damages (in tort litigation). To use my previous example, Muslims, Jews, and

Christians all claim that God created the world in six days and on the seventh He rested. However, each faith names a different day of the week as the day of rest. Similarly, (some so-called) psychotics assert that they hear voices that command them to kill their wives or children; psychiatrists assert that such persons suffer from a brain disease called "schizophrenia," which can be effectively treated with certain chemicals; and I claim that the assertions of psychotics and psychiatrists alike are claims unsubstantiated by evidence. The point, however, is that psychiatrists have the power to accredit their own claims as scientific facts and rational treatments, discredit the claims of mental patients and psychiatric critics as delusions and denials, and enlist the coercive power of the state to impose their views on involuntary "patients."

The difference between a description and a claim is sometimes a matter of context rather than vocabulary. For example, the adjective "schizophrenic" may describe a man who asserts that his wife is trying to poison him (assuming that she is not); but it functions as a claim when, after shooting his wife, the killer's court-appointed lawyer, desperate to "defend" him (perhaps against his nominal client's wishes), claims that the illegal act was caused by schizophrenia and that the killer should therefore be "acquitted" and treated in a mental hospital, rather than punished by imprisonment. Because psychiatrists view mental diseases and their treatments as facts rather than as claims, they reject the possibility that the words "illness" and "treatment" may, as all words, have a literal or metaphorical usage. Although some psychiatrists now concede that hysteria is not a genuine disease, they are loath to acknowledge that it is a metaphorical disease, that is, not a disease at all. Similarly, many psychiatrists acknowledge that psychotherapy—that is, two or more persons listening and talking to one another—is radically unlike surgical and medical treatment. But, again, they do not acknowledge that it is a metaphorical treatment—that is, not a treatment at all.

Psychiatry Is a Branch of the Law and a Secular Religion Rather than a Science or a Therapy

Finally, psychiatrists, who potentially always deal with involuntary patients, delight in the doubly self-serving claim that their patients suffer from brain diseases and that these (psychiatric) brain diseases (unlike others, such as Parkinsonism) render their sufferers incompetent. This claim lets psychiatrists pretend that coercion is a necessary, yet insignificant, element in contemporary psychiatric practice, a claim daily contradicted by reports in the newspapers. Understandably, psychiatrists prefer to occupy themselves with the putative brain diseases of persons called "mental patients" than with the proven social functions of psychiatric diagnoses, hospitals, and treatments.

Lawmakers do not discover prohibited rules of conduct, called crimes, they create them. Killing is not a crime; only unlawful killing is—for example, murder. Similarly, psychiatrists do not discover (mis)behaviors, called mental diseases, they create them. Killing is not a mental disease; only killing defined as due to mental illness is; schizophrenia thus "causes" hetero-homicide (not called "murder") and bipolar illness "causes" auto-homicide (called "suicide").

My point is that psychiatrists, who create diagnoses of mental diseases by giving disease names to personal (mis)conduct, function as legislators, not as scientists. It was this sort of diagnosis making alienists engaged in when they created masturbatory insanity; that Paul Eugen Bleuler engaged in when he created schizophrenia; and that the taskforce committees of the American Psychiatric Association engage in when they construct new psychiatric diagnoses, such as body dysmorphic disorder, and deconstruct old ones, such as homosexuality.

I am not arguing that rule making, such as politicians engage in, is not important. I am merely insisting on the differences between phenomena and rules, science and law, cure and control. Treating the sick and punishing criminals are both necessary for maintaining the social order. Indeed, breakdown in the just enforcement of just laws is far more destructive to the social order than the absence of equitable access to effective medical treatment. The medical profession's traditional social mandate is healing the sick; the criminal justice system's, punishing the lawbreaker; and the psychiatric profession's, confining and controlling the "deviant" (ostensibly as diseased, supposedly for the purpose of treatment). This is why I regard psychiatry as a branch of the law and a secular religion, rather than a science or therapy.

I want to add a brief remark here on the so-called anti-psychiatry movement with which my name is often associated. As detailed elsewhere, I consider the term anti-psychiatry imprudent and the movement it names irresponsible. As a classical liberal, I support the rights of physicians to engage in mutually consenting psychiatric acts with other adults. By the same token, I object to involuntary psychiatric interventions, regardless of how they are justified. Psychiatrists *qua* physicians should never deprive individuals of their lives, liberties, and properties, even if the security of society requires that they engage in such acts. In adopting this view, I follow the example of the great Hungarian physician Ignaz Semmelweis who believed that obstetricians, *qua* physicians, should never infect their patients, even if the advancement of medical education requires that they do so.

I do not deny that involuntary psychiatric interventions might be justified vis-à-vis individuals declared to be legally incompetent, just as involuntary financial or medical interventions are justified under such circumstances. Individuals who are disabled by a stroke or are in a coma cannot discharge their duties or represent their desires. Accordingly, there are procedures for relieving them—with due process of law—of their rights and responsibilities as full-fledged adults. Although the persons entrusted with the task of reclassifying citizens from moral agents to wards of the state might make use of medical information, they should be lay persons (jurors) and judges, not physicians or mental health specialists. Their determination should be viewed as a legal and political procedure, not as a medical or therapeutic intervention.

I have sought to alert the professions as well as the public to the tendency in modern societies—whether capitalist or communist, democratic, or totalitarian—to reclassify deviant conduct as (mental) disease, deviant actor as (psychiatric) patient, and activities aimed at controlling deviants as therapeutic interventions. And I have warned against the dangers of the destruction of self-discipline and criminal sanctions which these practices create—specifically the replacing of penal sanctions with psychiatric coercions rationalized as "hospitalization" and "treatment." To describe the confusion arising from the use of the metaphorical term "mental disease," I have suggested the phrase "the myth of mental illness." For a political order that uses physicians and hospitals in place of policemen and prisons to coerce and confine miscreants and which justifies constraint and compulsion as therapy rather than punishment, I have proposed the name "therapeutic state."

The personal freedom of which the English and American people are justly proud rests on the assumption of a fundamental right to life, liberty, and property. This is why deprivations of life, liberty, and property have traditionally been regarded as punishments (execution, imprisonment, and the imposition of a fine), that is, legal and political acts whose lawful performance is delegated to specific agents of the state and is regulated by due process of law. No physician *qua* medical healer has the right to deprive another of life, liberty, or property. Formerly, when the clergy was allied with the state, a priest had the right to deprive a person of life and liberty. In the seventeenth century, the state began to transfer this role to psychiatrists (alienists or mad-doctors), who eagerly accepted the assignment and have served as state agents authorized to deprive persons of liberty under medical auspices. Now, we are witnessing a clamor for granting physicians the right to kill persons—an ostensibly medical intervention euphemized as "physician-assisted suicide."

It is a truism that the interests of the individual, the family, and the state often conflict. Medicalizing interpersonal conflicts, that is, disagreements among family members, the members of society, and between citizens and the state, threatens to destroy not only respect for persons as responsible moral agents, but also for the state as an arbiter and dispenser of justice. Let us never forget that the state is an organ of coercion with a monopoly on force—for good or ill. The more the state empowers doctors, the more physicians will strengthen the state (by authenticating political preferences as health values), and the more the resulting union of medicine and the state will enfeeble the individual (by depriving him of the right to reject interventions classified as therapeutic). If that is the kind of society we want, that is the kind we shall get—and deserve.

About the Author

Thomas Szasz is professor emeritus of psychiatry at the State University of New York in Syracuse, New York. He is author of The Myth of Mental Illness; Our Right to Drugs: The Case for a Free Market; *and* A Lexicon of Lunacy: Metaphoric Malady, Moral Responsibility, and Psychiatry *(the latter published by Transaction Publishers). His most recent book is* Cruel Compassion: Psychiatric Control of Society's Unwanted.

Note

1 Originally printed in: *Society*, 1 May 1994, Vol. 31, Issue 4, pages 34–39. Reprinted with Permission from Springer-Verlag.

Chapter 24

The Emergence of the UK Critical Psychiatry Network

REFLECTIONS AND THEMES

Pat Bracken, Duncan Double, Suman Fernando, Joanna Moncrieff, Philip Thomas, and Sami Timimi

Summary

The UK Critical Psychiatry Network emerged in the context of ongoing concerns about the limits of a "medical paradigm" for psychiatry and the need to develop alternative ways of working within psychiatry. They carry forward many of the concerns from "antipsychiatry," but many in the group, particularly those interested in postmodern philosophy, have also moved "away from antipsychiatry." They see metaphor as more than an embellishment and as something fundamental to our embodied and encultured nature. Metaphors and cultural myths are not something unique to psychiatry but part of all of our meaning-making activities. That does not mean that anything goes, but it does highlight questions of power in the process of meaning-making around mental difference.

The Critical Psychiatry Network has also increasingly moved beyond earlier critiques of psychiatry because of the way its members have been exposed to the social justice movements of the latter half of the 20th century. These movements include the "colonised people across the globe struggling for freedom … women against patriarchy, the Stonewall riots by gay people in New York against homophobia, and the rise of the civil rights movement in the United States." With this background, critical psychiatrists were deeply sensitized to questions of prejudice and oppression. When the Mad Pride movement arose, they saw similar protests only this time against the dogma of mainstream psychiatry. Critical psychiatrists saw these protests as another understandable social movement. The Critical Psychiatry Network worked to help support the Mad Pride movement's concerns and reform mental health care.

Key themes that the UK group have addressed include the role of postmodern philosophy and social theory in understanding psychiatry, the problem of psychiatric

DOI: 10.4324/9781003148456-28

diagnoses, the increasing use of psychiatric medications, the possibility of new models such as relational psychiatry, and the importance of transcultural issues, race, gender, colonialism, and Eurocentric systems of postempire.

*

Introduction

Psychiatry has always attracted doctors whose interests are broader than human biology, particularly those who are interested in philosophy and politics. When such people start to work in psychiatry, they quickly become aware of the tension that arises from the attempt to blend the complex social issues we refer to as "mental health" problems with a medical framework. Hence the history of psychiatry includes many challenges to the mainstream medical paradigm and initiatives for alternative ways of working that have arisen from within psychiatry itself. The most radical of these was the "antipsychiatry" movement of the 1960s and 1970s which was spearheaded by well-known psychiatrists such as Thomas Szasz and R. D. Laing. However, psychoanalysis, the therapeutic community movement, and the psychobiological approach of leading psychiatrists such as Adolf Meyer, which were all popular and influential in the mid-20th century, also represent alternatives to a narrow biomedical point of view. Though they take different forms and have different emphases, these approaches have in common the recognition of the social and psychological origins of most "mental health" problems and the need for solutions that address these appropriately.

The Critical Psychiatry Network (CPN) first met in 1999 in Bradford, UK, to discuss concern about a range of issues, including changes to the Mental Health Act proposed by the recently elected Labour government, particularly legislation to force psychiatric patients in the community to receive medication against their will. Other concerns were the growing influence of the pharmaceutical industry and biomedical theories of mental illness, and the need to engage positively with the growing voices of critical survivor groups (Thomas & Moncrieff, 1999). To understand more clearly its subsequent work, it's helpful to consider the contexts out of which the group coalesced.

Most of the people who attended the first meeting and became actively involved in the group's work were consultant psychiatrists or senior trainees working in the National Health Service. Some had trained in psychiatry in the 1960s and 1970s, a time when they were encouraged to read the work of Laing and other so-called antipsychiatrists. They did so at a time of political and social upheaval, of colonised people across the globe struggling for freedom from their former colonial powers, women struggling against the patriarchy, the Stonewall riots by gay people in New York against homophobia, and the rise of the civil rights movement in the United States. In the UK, too, psychiatric patients were challenging the power and political authority of psychiatry and its role in their lives. The establishment of the Mental Patients' Union in the early 1970s marked the emergence of an active and critical survivor movement (Spandler, 2006). The evolution of the UK survivor movement is further charted by the Survivors' History Group (see http://studymore.org.uk/MPU.HTM).

Even before CPN came into being, the profession of psychiatry had started to go through profound changes. The publication of the *DSM-III* in 1980 marked the end of the academic domination, at least in the United States, of the profession by psychoanalytic theory and practice, replacing it with the neo-Kraepelinian approach, a new era of "scientific" psychiatry with an emphasis on the diagnosis of psychiatric disorder that was increasingly spoken of in terms of brain disorder. On 18 July 1989, President George Bush Senior signed a decree that the 1990s would be the Decade of the Brain. This promised major developments in understanding the pathology of psychiatric disorder and thus new biological treatments through the new discipline of clinical neuroscience. This marked a major change in the values and priorities of academic departments of psychiatry across the globe. It also strengthened the bonds between the pharmaceutical industry and the profession. Critical psychiatrists were deeply sceptical about these developments, and in 1999, the late Loren Mosher (1999) spoke for many in his letter of resignation from the American Psychiatric Association, in which he expressed his belief that, in reality, he was resigning from the American Psychopharmacological Association.

In the years that followed, members of CPN have contributed a significant body of work, academic papers, blogs, chapters, and books covering a range of issues including postcolonial critiques of psychiatry and mental health, critiques of theories of drug action and the influence of pharma in psychiatry, critiques of diagnosis and the medical model, the origins of critical psychiatry and its relationship to antipsychiatry, and philosophical critiques of psychiatry and mental health practice. These themes are outlined in what follows in this chapter.

In the past, the Network has also been involved in a variety of other activities, including lobbying and demonstrating against government proposals to introduce compulsory treatment in the community and reviewable detention for people with "severe personality disorders," as well as against the influence of the pharmaceutical industry on the profession. For example, in 2002, some members of the Network supported and attended a demonstration organised by Mad Pride and other survivor groups against the influence of pharma on the profession, outside the annual conference of the Royal College of Psychiatrists; and in 2005, members marched with psychiatric survivors on the Kissit demonstrations to protest against the use of compulsory drugging. The Network has also organised a successful series of conferences on contemporary controversies in mental health.

CPN has always been a very informal organisation and, apart from its two cochairs and a secretary, has no "officers." In the years that followed its first meeting, it met biannually to organise a range of activities such as conferences and the writing of academic papers and books covering a wide range of issues. Other important functions of the Network include acting as a "sounding box" for members to share ideas and explore areas for collaboration and as a source of mutual support. The latter has become increasingly important for both junior and senior psychiatrists as health services have become preoccupied with reducing risk, cutting costs, and following guidelines. This can sometimes lead to tensions between services and individual psychiatrists who are trying to prioritise the liberty, independence, and quality of life of their patients. Psychiatry needs to engage with these key issues.

Postpsychiatry

Critical psychiatrists Pat Bracken and Phil Thomas first used the term "postpsychiatry" as the title for a series of articles they wrote for the magazine *Open Mind,* the first of which was published in 1998. This was followed by an article in the *British Medical Journal* (Bracken & Thomas, 2001) and a book (Bracken & Thomas, 2005). Independently, Bradley Lewis (2006) used the term in the title of a book. Sometime later, Bracken and Thomas realised that UK survivor Peter Campbell (1996) had used the term before them when trying to imagine what mental health care would be like without psychiatry.

"Postpsychiatry" was meant to signal a fundamental rethink of how medicine might be involved in the world of mental health. Bracken and Thomas's writing emerged primarily from their clinical work and their realisation that psychiatry would never be an adequate vehicle through which relevant medical insights, strategies, and practices could be brought to bear, in a positive way, on the sort of mental suffering that they encountered in their work. As doctors, they had come to believe that medicine did have a role to play. However, like Peter Campbell, they had also concluded that psychiatry, as a body of assumptions, values, narratives, theories, and priorities, was deeply flawed. Its underlying technical paradigm actually got in the way of good practice. In this way, postpsychiatry was about posing a question: What would a medicine of mental suffering look like if we were able to get beyond the assumptions of psychiatry? Thus, the term postpsychiatry referred to a medical practice that might emerge "after psychiatry."

But there was also a philosophical reference involved. Bracken and Thomas found that they were often of most benefit to people when they deliberately stepped away from psychiatric theories and diagnoses. They wanted to start a discussion about a different form of medical engagement with mental suffering, one that was guided by a sort of "therapeutic doubt" and uncertainty. In this, they wanted to start from a position of "not-knowing," "not-diagnosing," and scepticism towards the dogmas that guided psychiatry under the guise of science. They were influenced by postmodern writers who spoke positively about a move away from metanarratives, away from approaches to knowing that positioned these as foundational. They had come to believe that none of the narratives that had guided psychiatry were adequate in relation to the messy, complicated reality of mental suffering. So, postpsychiatry was also about a questioning of the modernist epistemology that had underpinned psychiatry since its origins in the European Enlightenment.

In addition, they wished to move away from the antipsychiatry of the previous generation. While respectful of the work of Thomas Szasz, they wished to distance themselves from the binary logic that they saw in his writing (Bracken & Thomas, 2010). After their training in medicine and experience of work with diverse communities in different contexts, it was impossible for them not to see the "embodied" and "encultured" nature of all human suffering. It was clear to them that mind and flesh do not inhabit different worlds but exist as one, and all experience of illness (whether it is called physical or mental) is complex. Thinking, feeling, and relating to others are done by the same creature who sleeps, eats, has endocrine problems, and gets old. And the same creature lives its life in the midst of language, culture, and economy. Bracken and Thomas were interested in linguistics, anthropology, and philosophy and had come to believe that states of madness, distress, and dislocation were profoundly "untidy," and that no singular narrative, whether from psychiatry or antipsychiatry, could account for all the suffering that is conventionally called "mental illness." In fact, what they witnessed more than anything was the destructive ways that theories became dogmas and went on to damage and destroy lives.

This is what drew Bracken and Thomas to the work of Foucault, Bauman, and others who might be characterised as "postmodern." They offered a form of scholarship that did not see the contradictions and uncertainties of human reality as irritations that could be eliminated by more science, better science, or more analysis and conceptual clarification. For them, postmodern thought was about facing and accepting the reality that there might not be solutions for all our problems, that there might never be resolutions to all our ethical contradictions nor answers to all the questions we asked of the world.

Crucially, they wanted a form of mental health medicine that worked towards the possibility of meaningful dialogue with the emerging "service-user" movement. They saw that their job as critical psychiatrists was the creation of the conditions wherein genuine dialogue with this movement could take place. The main question for postpsychiatry was: How can we bring biological and medical insights to bear on mental suffering in a way that does not silence, distort, and colonise the understandings that emerge from service users themselves both individually and collectively?

Of course there was no singular answer to this. In their work, Bracken and Thomas have looked for insights from postcolonial scholarship, feminist philosophy, queer theory, mad studies, and critical pedagogy. Gayatri Spivak (1990) argues that educators and scholars who are genuinely trying to get beyond the legacy of colonial forms of knowledge must be engaged in "the unlearning of one's own privilege. So that, not only does one become able to listen to that other constituency, but one learns to speak in such a way that one will be taken seriously by that other constituency" (p. 42). Postpsychiatry represented an attempt to unlearn and to find a way of listening and speaking differently.

Why There Is No Such "Thing" as a Psychiatric Diagnosis

Another important theme for the CPN is the question of psychiatric diagnosis. What do people mean when they talk about mental disorder, mental health, or mental illness? What sort of "thing" is a mental disorder? Where are its boundaries? When does an experience or behaviour become abnormal or disordered or pathological, and who decides, based on what? While the issue of where to place boundaries between the ordinary and not is something medicine often grapples with, when it comes to what we label as "mental health" we have a whole new level of potential confusion, uncertainty, and meanings to get through before we can assert something to be out of the ordinary, abnormal, or disordered. In psychiatry, everything requires interpretation, not just the boundaries (Timimi, 2014, 2020, 2021).

The territory for what we call "symptoms" of a mental disorder is experiences and behaviours that have meanings and that may be interpreted differently by different cultures, different times, and in different settings. This means this is an area of practice where not only are there disagreements and debates about where the boundaries of a condition are, but also we have to take into account the significance and relevance of the diverse meanings that can be attached to these symptoms such that they are seen as symptoms in one interpretive framework but not in another.

Is that patient in front of the doctor who reports intense sadness, difficulty getting to sleep, waking up before 5 o'clock every morning, and a poor appetite suffering from a "depressive disorder" or experiencing understandable heartbreak and grief after the breakup of a long-term relationship a few months back? If one argues both can be true, then of course, culturally speaking the patient may be told she "has" both depression and grief. One (depression), however, cannot be a diagnosis, as it explains nothing but only describes some aspects of the patient's experiences; the other (grief) could be a diagnosis, as it has explanatory pretences. Grief is, in this scenario, being used as an explanation. But we have no access to the patient's inner mental workings; none of us do. With grief, depression, or both, we still do not know what sort of a "thing" we are dealing with. Is it a medical disease in the person's brain, the psychological process of grief, the loss of a social network that she had with that partner, her concern about how this is impacting her son, or the fear of returning to work after a long absence, or is it all of these things? In truth, we don't know anything definitive about what has caused her presentation; neither does she. We can't escape our subjectivity or the patient's, for that matter. We can only guess at the "diagnosis" (proximal explanation).

When it comes to our emotional experiences, we have only embodied experience. We then use words connected with cultural meaning-making systems to attach to that experience. The meaning scaffolding we then use can itself transform our experience of the experience. "You are broken hearted" creates a different scaffold than does "You are depressed" or "You are surviving and recovering from a painful experience," or even "I can see how your suffering has helped you see your life in a transformed way."

In medicine, diagnosis is the process of determining which disease or condition explains a person's symptoms and/or signs. Diagnosis is a system of classification based on cause. Making an accurate diagnosis is a technical skill that enables effective matching of treatment to address specific pathological processes. Pseudo-diagnoses— for example "attention deficit hyperactivity disorder" (ADHD) or "autistic spectrum disorder" (ASD)—cannot explain behaviours or experiences, as there are only symptoms that are descriptions and not explanations (Timimi & McCabe, 2016a, 2016b; Timimi & Timimi, 2015). Even using the word "symptom" is problematic, as in medicine the term usually refers to patients' suffering/experience as a result of an underlying disease process and is therefore associated in our minds with a medical procedure leading to an explanation for the symptom.

We are meaning-seeking creatures and so have used classification systems extensively to classify all manner of things. A diagnostic classification is a classification by explanation, in other words by cause. That's why we say, "My doctor said that the cause of my chest pain was acid reflux, not a heart attack." But psychiatric diagnoses do not explain symptoms. Consider the following example: If we were to ask the question "What is ADHD?" it's not possible to answer that question by reference to a particular known pathological abnormality, as none have been found and therefore there are no tests for ADHD. Instead, to answer the question we will have to provide a description, such as "ADHD is the presence of 'abnormal' levels of poor concentration, hyperactivity, and impulsivity," and so on.

Contrast this with asking the question "What is diabetes?" If a doctor were to answer this question in the same manner by just describing symptoms, such as needing to urinate excessively, thirst, and fatigue, the doctor could be in deep trouble as a medical practitioner, as there are plenty of other conditions that may initially present with these symptoms, and diabetes itself may not present with these symptoms in a recognisable way. In order to answer the question "What is diabetes?" the doctor will have to refer to its pathology involving abnormalities of sugar metabolism, as in "Diabetes is a disease that occurs when blood glucose (sugar) is too high." In most of the rest of medicine, therefore, a diagnosis explains and has some causal connection with the patient's experiences/symptoms. Thus, diagnosis sits in a "technical" explanatory classification framework.

The problem of using a classification like "ADHD" to explain an experience (i.e., as a diagnosis) can be illustrated by asking another set of questions. If a doctor were asked by someone *why* their child is hyperactive and answered that this is *because* they have ADHD, then a legitimate question to ask is "How do you know that this hyperactivity is caused by ADHD?" The only answer they can then give to that question is that they know it's ADHD because they are hyperactive. In other words, if we try to use a classification that can only describe in order to explain, we end up with what philosophically is known as a "tautology." A tautology is a circular thinking trap. A description cannot explain itself. Using ADHD to explain hyperactivity is like saying the pain in my head is caused by a headache or my cough is caused by coughing disorder. In psychiatry what we are calling diagnosis will only describe, it is unable to explain and therefore isn't a diagnosis.

The Myth of the Chemical Cure and Its Implications for Psychiatry

The Critical Psychiatry Network has been particularly concerned about the increasing use of psychiatric medications. Over the past 70 years, drugs have become the main form of treatment for mental health problems. Antidepressants, anxiolytics, and sedatives are widely prescribed by general practitioners for common complaints such as anxiety and depression, and people with more severe mental disorders are invariably treated with at least one sort of psychiatric drug and often several.

The widespread use of psychiatric drugs has contributed to the impression that psychiatric conditions originate in disturbances of biology, which can be reversed using biological means. The use of these drugs is cited as evidence that mental disorders are essentially biological conditions—disorders or diseases of the brain. Yet this conclusion rests on the largely unrecognised assumption that drugs target the underlying biological cause of a particular disorder or its symptoms and that this is the only explanation for their effects. In her work on mechanisms of drug action, Joanna Moncrieff has shown that this assumption does not hold (Moncrieff, 2008).

The conventional view can be referred to as the "disease-centred" model of drug action. This has been adopted from general medicine, where drugs usually do work in this way. Inhaled drugs for asthma, for example, do not treat the cause of the condition but relieve symptoms by reversing the compromising airway obstruction that produces the symptom of wheezing. Psychiatric drugs cannot reasonably be assumed to work in this way, however, because no physical pathology has ever been demonstrated to underpin any type of mental disorder. There is no consistent evidence to link depression with a serotonin abnormality, for example, and it has been proposed that this idea was primarily a marketing technique (Healy, 2015).

Moreover, there is an alternative means by which drugs exert effects in mental disorders, which can be called the "drug-centred" model of drug action (Moncrieff, 2008; Moncrieff & Cohen, 2005). This model highlights that psychiatric drugs alter normal brain functioning in characteristic ways and, by doing so, modify normal mental functions and behaviour. In this sense, they are not fundamentally different from recreational drugs, except that recreational drugs produce alterations that are usually pleasurable, whereas the alterations produced by some psychiatric drugs (e.g., antipsychotics) are usually experienced as unpleasant. The characteristic alterations of mental state and behaviour associated with different classes of psychiatric drugs have been demonstrated in animal and volunteer studies and are reported by patients.

When someone takes a drug with mind- and behaviour-altering properties (whether prescribed or recreational), these changes are superimposed onto the feelings and behaviours that constitute a mental disorder in ways that can explain the apparent "therapeutic" effects of the drugs, as well as some of their unwanted effects. Drugs like benzodiazepines and alcohol, for example, reduce arousal and induce a usually pleasant state of calmness and relaxation. This state temporarily alters one's emotional state and may be experienced as a relief for someone who is intensely anxious, or a brief reprieve for someone who is depressed (commonly referred to as "drowning one's sorrows" in relation to alcohol). Drugs now referred to as "antipsychotics" (previously known as "major tranquilisers") induce a state of "deactivation" characterised by slowing of mental activity and dampening of emotions and motivation (Breggin, 2008). This drug-induced state can reduce the intensity and salience of psychotic symptoms.

It is important that we understand the mode of action of psychiatric drugs correctly because different models of drug action have different implications. The disease-centred model has a bias in favour of drug treatment because it is premised on the assumption that drugs are rectifying an underlying biological abnormality. It has therefore helped drive the medicalisation of behavioural problems and enabled the pharmaceutical industry to capitalise on people's misplaced desire to find a magic bullet for complex emotional and behavioural problems. The drug-centred model, on the other hand, while not discouraging the use of drugs altogether, entails a more transparent and cautious approach. Although it suggests that some drug-induced alterations may be helpful in suppressing some of the distressing emotions or behaviours associated with what we call mental disorders, it also highlights that this is achieved by altering the brain in ways we do not fully understand and whose full consequences we have not properly researched. By doing so, it stresses the potential of drugs to produce dangerous, debilitating, and unpredictable effects.

The drug-centred model presents a fundamental challenge to modern psychiatry. By challenging the disease-centred model, with its idea that psychiatric treatments target underlying diseases or biological symptom-mechanisms in the way that most medical treatments do, the drug-centred model makes it difficult to assimilate the practice of psychiatry into that of medicine. It becomes more difficult to maintain the notion that mental disorders are akin to medical conditions.

If we reject the "medical model" of mental disorders, we are left with the notion that they are a set of human problems, or "ways of being human" (Jenner et al., 1993). The question then becomes, how should we help people whose thoughts or behaviour are causing them distress, and how should society respond to people whose behaviour causes other people distress?

Drug treatment may play a part in both these situations, but the effectiveness and ethics of using chemicals to modify people's thinking and behaviour needs considered debate. Without doubt, drugs that affect the brain can change people's mental state, and some drugs may bring temporary relief through dulling the senses and numbing emotions. We have only to look at the effects of addiction to see the negative side of this, however. Drugs can modify unwanted aggressive and unpredictable behaviour, too, but there needs to be a thorough debate about whether and when it is acceptable to force drugs on someone in the interests of protecting other people's safety or peace of mind.

These are not easy debates to have, and this is one reason for the appeal of the medical approach to understanding and treating mental disorder, because it transforms complex social problems into technical, medical ones. As Thomas Szasz emphasised, the medical model of mental disorder is strategic. The "myth of mental illness" serves the useful function of keeping potentially controversial issues out of the public arena and "permits creation of a therapeutic utopia—a medical fairyland with 'miracle cures' not only for diseases, but for non-diseases as well" (Szasz, 2000).

The future of psychiatry is thus intimately entwined with the future of society as a whole. As long as society needs a myth to keep the peace and manage disorder and discontent, then a system that fosters the idea that mental illness is a brain disease and that treatment is a sophisticated medical process will continue to flourish. In the absence of opportunities for more fulfilling ways of living, some people benefit from the arrangements that the current system offers in the form of the sick role and the chemicals on offer to deaden emotional pain and worry. But many are harmed by the suggestion that they are biologically flawed, that their problems are beyond their control, and that toxic chemicals represent a simple and benign solution for their problems.

From Antipsychiatry to Relational Psychiatry

Another theme important for CPN has been its relationship with antipsychiatry, and critical psychiatry has never hidden its association with antipsychiatry (Double, 2006).

But the term "antipsychiatry" is a complex term. Both R. D. Laing and Thomas Szasz, commonly seen as antipsychiatry's main protagonists, disowned the term. In many ways, antipsychiatry has always been more of a term used by mainstream psychiatry to denigrate criticism that it does not accept. For example, Martin Roth (1973), when he was the first president of the UK Royal College of Psychiatrists, talked about an international movement against psychiatry which he regarded as "anti-medical, anti-therapeutic, anti-institutional and anti-scientific." In this sense, "antipsychiatry" is a label used to marginalise its critics.

Certainly, there were some excesses in antipsychiatry. For example, Laing was taken up by the counterculture of the 1960s and 1970s and, despite his hankering to be reconnected with mainstream psychiatry, he ultimately became more interested in promoting personal growth and authenticity than in changing psychiatry. Szasz's trenchant critique was primarily directed against society's incarceration of people on the basis of the "myth of mental illness." In the end, he wanted to abolish psychiatry, or at least its institutional practices, although he did support and practice an autonomous psychotherapy (despite his dislike of the term "therapy").

Antipsychiatry should not be regarded as merely a negative contribution to psychiatry. Its challenge to the biomedical model of mental illness, in the sense that antipsychiatry did not regard primary mental illness as brain disease, is still valid. It also tended to go further by wanting to abandon the notion of psychopathology altogether. The "anti" element could be said to have more to do with concern about the tendency of psychiatry to objectify people, which can make psychiatry part of the problem rather than necessarily the solution to mental health problems (Jones, 1998).

The term "critical psychiatry" as an alternative to antipsychiatry was probably first used by David Ingleby (1981) in his edited book of the same name. Ingleby moved critical psychiatry on from Szasz's theme of the "myth of mental illness," in the sense that Ingleby, unlike Szasz, accepted that the concept of mental illness is valid. Mental illnesses are seen as meaningful responses to difficult situations. Critical psychiatry argues that psychiatry can be practised without postulating brain pathology as the basis for primary mental illness.

Critical psychiatry is a broad school of thought and tends to be used now as a general term for alternatives to biomedical psychiatry. For example, over recent years, Bonnie Burstow made a case for antipsychiatry (spelt without a hyphen, to distinguish her position from the "anti-psychiatry" of the 1960s and 1970s) seeking the total abolition of institutional psychiatry. At times she used the terms "critical psychiatry" and "antipsychiatry" interchangeably, promoting what she called "anti/critical psychiatry activism" (Burstow, 2019). The critical psychiatry movement includes both reformers and revolutionaries.

Another term that has emerged in CPN circles is "relational psychiatry." The relational psychiatry blog[1] argues that the broader, radical approach of critical psychiatry has outlived its usefulness. For example, debates on Twitter (now called X) can degenerate into arguments about whether mental illness exists and whether mental health problems are somehow different or separate from emotional distress and suffering. Getting too caught up in this argument about whether mental health problems are illnesses could be said to be deflecting attention from the more important task of critiquing mental illness as brain disease.

Critical psychiatry, however it is termed, is not opposed to psychiatry as such and argues for a person-centred shift for practice and research. Moving from a biomedical model of mental illness creates a basis for a more relational practice in psychiatry. In fact, medicine in general, as well as psychiatry, needs to shift from a disease-centred to a more person-centred focus.

Regarding mental illness as equivalent to physical illness does not sufficiently acknowledge the difference between the two. Medicine in general has tried to correct this imbalance over recent years by making its training and practice more patient-centred (Stewart et al., 2003). However, it has not always been very successful in this aim, and arguably medicine still needs to change to be more person-centred. Health services are not always providing the care that people need by treating them holistically. Biomedical progress has been made at a cost and medicine still needs to broaden its approach to illness and disease to include the psychosocial without sacrificing the advantages of biomedicine. Patients and doctors, as far as possible together, shape what should be regarded as illness and how it is treated.

This means that CPN is not completely divorced from the mainstream. In practice, most psychiatrists are not purely biomedical in the sense of simply reducing mental illness to brain disease, or at least some are more biomedical than others. Psychiatrists commonly deflect criticism of the biomedical model by declaring that they are eclectic in their approach, considering psychological and social factors, not just biological ones. Although psychiatrists tend to have no doubt that major mental illness is a disease of the brain, some are inclined to focus solely on this aspect, whereas others want to integrate biological with more psychosocial perspectives. Also, not believing in the biomedical hypothesis of mental illness may not be as unorthodox as it may seem. In fact, there is a long and respectable tradition of thought about the human condition that is far greater than the tendency to reductionism and positivism in general, and in psychiatry in particular. Reductionism can lead to the loss of meaning of human action and a mechanistic psychology may well be impossible to realise in practice.

In mainstream clinical practice, as in CPN, descriptive psychopathology is not studied organically, at the level of neurobiology. History and mental state examination instead produce a formulation of people's problems in terms of differential diagnosis and aetiology. An integrated understanding of mental dysfunction in the context of the whole person, including emotional needs and life issues, forms the basis for all quality clinical practice. It is this foundation that makes psychiatry relational. Marginalising the intentions of critical psychiatry to make practice more relational by labelling it antipsychiatry is, therefore, unhelpful. Its critique has consequences not only for clinical practice but also for psychiatric research, which has become far too focused on presumptive neuroscience.

The contention that primary mental illness should not be reduced to brain disease must not be misunderstood, however. Critical psychiatry is not saying that mind and brain are separate. What it is saying is that minds are enabled by but not reducible to brains. As Adolf Meyer said, "All person disorders must show *through* the brain but not always *in* the brain [his emphasis]" (Double, 2007).

Transcultural Psychiatry and Critical Mental Health

The Critical Psychiatry Network has always been active in questions at the intersection of clinical work and politics. Prior to the 1960s, the notions of culture or "race" were seldom mentioned in connection with clinical work with patients in the UK. But this changed when it became evident, in the 1970s, that psychiatric services were not meeting the needs of immigrants from former British colonies in Asia and the West Indies (Fernando, 1988; MHAC, 1991, 1993) as well as longer-established immigrant groups, such as the Polish (Bavington & Majid, 1982). The discourse on such issues seemed to connect with the notion of "transcultural psychiatry," which was already established at McGill University in Canada and other centres in some European countries. In mid-1976, psychiatrists, clinical psychologists, and social workers working with people of non-European background in the UK formed the Transcultural Psychiatry Society (TCPS), hoping to develop links with similar associations in other parts of Europe and North America. The TCPS held several conferences in the 1980s, including one involving participants from Germany, the Netherlands, Sweden, and France in collaboration with the World Federation for Mental Health on "Mental Health Race and Culture in Europe"; and its members authored several books (Cox, 1982; Fernando, 1988; Fernando & Keating, 2009; Rack, 1982) that attracted much attention, not just in academia but also from official bodies and the general public.

Like CPN, the transcultural psychiatry movement in the UK drew from the work in the 1960s by R. D. Laing and colleagues (Laing, 1960 1961), being critical of the mental health system itself, its political rather than medical or psychological nature. *Sanity, Madness and the Family* (Laing & Esterson, 1970) discussed the "politics of experience"—how human experience, especially that of young people, was structured by power—and pointed to the importance of *context* when experiences are socially constructed into symptoms (for example, of "schizophrenia") such as hearing voices and feelings of passivity or of being controlled by external forces. From a transcultural perspective, much of what psychiatry identifies as "symptoms" of schizophrenia are not really symptoms at all in non-Western cultures but perfectly *natural* experience.

R. D. Laing's work indicated how powerful family systems can be; but "for Black people caught up in the psychiatric system, what is even more powerful is the social-political system … Babylon, the Rastafarian term for oppressive state power" (Cashmore, 1979, as cited in Fernando, 2018, p. 57). An issue frequently cited as being the result of institutional racism is the overrepresentation of Black people diagnosed as suffering from "schizophrenia." In an article in *New Left Review,* R. D. Laing (1964) wrote:

> I do not myself believe that there is any such "condition" as "schizophrenia."
> Yet the label is a social fact. Indeed this label as a social fact is a *political
> event.* This political event, occurring in the civic order of society, imposes
> definitions and consequences on the labelled person.
>
> (p. 64, italics in original)

Fernando (2018) argued that "schizophrenia" is part and parcel of the exercise of power when "white psychiatry" meets Black identity (p. 57). All models of mental illness are predominantly driven by the cultures of the societies in which they develop; and psychiatry itself, being derived in a culturally Western context, is inherently at odds with non-Western ways of thinking about the human condition.

Transcultural psychiatry in the UK initially focused on issues of "culture," but that shifted to issues of "race" (as well as culture), influenced by what patients and clients identified as the basic cause of the problem of high rates of diagnosis of schizophrenia in Black people, suggesting that racism was involved—connecting with social science literature (Centre for Contemporary Studies, 1982; Hall et al., 1978) reporting that what were called "cultural" issues (resulting from the post-war influx to Britain of migrants from ex-colonies) were really about the perceived "racial" identity of these migrants. And the work of Frantz Fanon, translated from the French as *Black Skin, White Masks* (Fanon, 1967a) and *The Wretched of the Earth* (Fanon, 1967b), played an increasing influence on unravelling issues of "race." Increasingly, institutional racism, a term that first appeared in the book *Black Power: The Politics of Liberation in America* (Carmichael & Hamilton, 1967), was blamed for the excessive rates of compulsory treatment of black people coupled with the oppressive nature of the "schizophrenia" label (Fernando, 2003, 2017). As in the civil rights movement in the United States and the struggle of colonised people to shake off European domination, leading to the fall of the major European empires after the end of the Second World War, *liberation* from all Eurocentric systems was talked of, including *critical mental health* (Moodley & Ocampo, 2014), which later encompassed decolonising mental health itself (Wangari-Jones, 2016).

The Future of CPN: Looking Forward

As mentioned in the Introduction above, CPN started in the context of reform of the Mental Health Act (MHA) in England and Wales, which led to the 2007 amendments. Despite CPN's opposition to the introduction of community treatment orders (CTOs), they have now become accepted and are widely used. The MHA in England and Wales is again being reformed (Department of Health & Social Care, 2021), this time to reduce coercion, as detentions continue to rise, rather than focusing on increasing security to manage "risk." But the government proposal is for CTOs to be retained for at least another five years; the impact of the new act on reducing their use will be monitored during this period. This is despite there being research evidence that CTOs do not, in fact, reduce hospital admission compared with previous arrangements (Burns et al., 2013). The Critical Psychiatry Network still believes that the curtailment of individual liberty embodied in CTOs cannot be justified but has not managed to influence government policy.

The issues that brought critical psychiatrists together remain, and indeed, dissent against psychiatry has been magnified and spread by the existence of the internet. People who have been harmed by the imposition of psychiatric diagnosis and taking psychiatric drugs can now find each other more readily and more effectively publicise the harm they have suffered. We live in a contradictory situation in which the majority of the population is now convinced by the biomedical story that moods and emotions arise from chemical aberrations (Pilkington et al., 2013), while a minority denounce psychiatry as a fraud that convinces people they are biologically impaired and prescribes toxic drugs that suppress people's humanity and cause an array of other disabling effects (Berezin, 2016).

The central problem–that psychiatry is a medical specialty that addresses problems that are not essentially medical in nature, or at least not equivalent to other medical conditions–continues to cause tension for psychiatrists, patients, politicians, and the general public. Critical psychiatrists recognise this tension and are prepared to confront its implications and discuss ways in which people can be helped without the use of pseudo-medical diagnoses and potentially harmful biological interventions that modify the brain in ways we do not fully know or understand. With the increasing reach of the pharmaceutical industry and the "psychiatrisation" of more and more aspects of feeling and behaviour (Beeker et al., 2021), this approach is needed more than ever.

Biological psychiatry is deeply entrenched, and it is likely that the wish to find a physical basis for mental illness will never go away completely. A vast research endeavour to uncover the physical causes of mental disorder continues to be generously funded and widely published, despite the fact that it has produced no consistent evidence of a specific biological abnormality in any mental disorder since it started in the 1950s. The strength of the deeply flawed belief that mental disorder can be reduced to abnormal brain activity blinds scientists to the reality of the evidence.

However much CPN may wish for a paradigm shift in psychiatric practice, it may well have to accept that psychiatry will remain a pluralistic, conflictual practice. Psychiatry cannot avoid its history of abusive and inhumane treatment, and these elements have not been eliminated from current practice. Psychiatry does not always make decisions in the best interests of patients, yet it presents itself as though it does, therefore avoiding necessary political and democratic scrutiny. Nonetheless, people still ask for help with their mental health problems, and a critical approach to their management will continue to be required.

Note

1 www.criticalpsychiatry.blogspotcom

References

Bavington, J., & Majid, A. (1982). Psychiatric services for ethnic minority groups. In J. Cox (Ed.), *Transcultural psychiatry* (pp. 87–106). Croom Helm.

Beeker, T., Mills C., Bhugra, D., te Meeman, S., Thoma, S., Heinze, M., & von Peter, S (2021). Psychiatrization of society: A conceptual framework and call for transdisciplinary research. *Front Psychiatry*, *12*, Article 645556. Retrieved June 23, 2021, from https://www.ncbi.nlm.nih.gov/pubmed/34149474

Berezin, R. (2016). *Psychiatric diagnosis is a fraud: The destructive and damaging fiction of biological "diseases."* Mad in America. Retrieved June 23, 2016, from https://www.madinamerica.com/2016/04/psychiatric-diagnosis-is-a-fraud-the-destructive-and-damaging-fiction-of-biological-diseases/

Bracken, P., & Thomas, P. (1998, January/February). A new debate in mental health. *Open Mind—The Mental Health Magazine, 89,* 17.

Bracken, P., & Thomas, P. (2001). Postpsychiatry: A new direction for mental health. *BMJ, 322,* 724–7.

Bracken, P., & Thomas, P. (2005). *Postpsychiatry: Mental health in a postmodern world.* Oxford University Press.

Bracken, P., & Thomas, P. (2010). From Szasz to Foucault: On the role of critical psychiatry. *Philosophy, Psychology and Psychiatry, 17,* 219–228.

Breggin, P. (2008). *Brain-disabling treatments in psychiatry* (Vol. 2). Springer Publishing Company.

Burns, T., Rugkåsa, J., Molodynski, A., et al. (2013). Community treatment orders for patients with psychosis (OCTET): A randomised controlled trial. *Lancet, 381,* 1627–33.

Burstow, B. (2019). From "bed-push" to book activism: Anti/Critical psychiatry activism. In R. Kinna & U. Gordon (Eds.), *Routledge handbook of radical politics.* Routledge.

Campbell, P. (1996). Challenging loss of power. In J. Read & J. Reynolds (Eds.), *Speaking our minds: An anthology* (pp. 56–62). Macmillan, Open University.

Carmichael, S., & Hamilton, C. V. (1967). *Black power: The politics of liberation in America.* Random House.

Cashmore, E. (1979) *Rastaman. The Rastafarian movement in England.* Allen & Unwin.

Centre for Contemporary Cultural Studies (Ed.). (1982). *The empire strikes back. Race and racism in 70s Britain.* Hutchinson.

Cox, J. (Ed.). (1982). *Transcultural psychiatry.* Croom Helm.

Department of Health and Social Care. (2021). *Reforming the mental health act.* www.gov.uk/government/consultations/reforming-the-mental-health-act/reforming-the-mental-health-act

Double, D. B. (Ed.). (2006). *Critical psychiatry: The limits of madness.* Palgrave Macmillan.

Double, D. B. (2007). Adolf Meyer's psychobiology and the challenge for biomedicine. *Philosophy, Psychiatry and Psychology, 14,* 331–339.

Fanon, F. (1967a). *Black skin, white masks.* (C. L. Markman, Trans.). Grove Press. (Original work published 1952)

Fanon, F. (1967b). *The wretched of the earth.* (C. Farrington, Trans.). Penguin Books. (Original work published 1961)

Fernando, S. (1988). *Race and culture in psychiatry.* Croom Helm.

Fernando, S. (2003). *Cultural diversity, mental health and psychiatry. The struggle against racism.* Brunner-Routledge.

Fernando, S. (2017). *Institutional racism and psychiatry and clinical psychology: Race matters in mental health.* Palgrave Macmillan.

Fernando, S. (2018). Moving on from Laing: The politicization of schizophrenia. *Journal of Psychosocial Studies, 11*(1), 50–67.

Fernando, S., & Keating, F. (Eds.). (2009). *Mental health in a multi-ethnic society. A multidisciplinary handbook* (2nd ed.). Routledge.

Hall, S., Critcher, C., Jefferson, T., Clarke, J., & Roberts, B. (1978). *Policing the crisis: Mugging, the state, and law and order.* MacMillan.

Healy, D. (2015). Serotonin and depression. *BMJ, 350,* h1771. https://doi.org/10.1136/bmj.h1771

Ingelby, D. (1981). *Critical psychiatry: The politics of mental health.* Penguin.

Jenner, F. A., Monteiro, A. C. D., Zagalo-Cardoso, J. A., & Cunha-Oliveira, J. A. (1993). *Schizophrenia: A disease or some ways of being human.* Sheffield Academic Press.

Jones, C. (1998). Raising the anti: Jan Foudraine, Ronald Laing and anti-psychiatry. In M. Gijswijt-Hofstra & R. Porter (Eds.), *Cultures of psychiatry and mental health care in postwar Britain and the Netherlands* (pp. 283–92). Wellcome Institute.

Laing, R.D. (1960) *The Divided Self: An Existential Study in Sanity and Madness.* Harmondsworth: Penguin.

Laing, R.D. (1961) *The Self and Others.* London: Tavistock Publications.

Laing, R. D. (1964) 'What is Schizophrenia?', *New Left Review, 28,* 63–9.

Laing, R.D. and Esterson, A. (1970) *Sanity, Madness and the Family.* London: Penguin Books.

Lewis, B. (2006). *Moving beyond Prozac, DSM and the new psychiatry: The birth of postpsychiatry.* University of Michigan Press.

MHAC (Mental Health Act Commission). (1991). *Fourth biennial report 1989–1991.* HMSO Publications.

MHAC (Mental Health Act Commission). (1993). *Fifth biennial report 1991–1993.* HMSO.

Moncrieff, J. (2008). *The myth of the chemical cure: A critique of psychiatric drug treatment.* Palgrave Macmillan.

Moncrieff, J., & Cohen, D. (2005). Rethinking models of psychotropic drug action. *Psychotherapy and Psychosomatics, 74,* 145–153.

Moodley, R., & Ocampo, M. (2014). *Critical psychiatry and mental health: Exploring the work of Suman Fernando in clinical practice.* Routledge, Taylor & Francis Group.

Mosher, L. (1999). *Letter of resignation from the American psychiatric association.* Retrieved November 18, 2020, from https://www.moshersoteria.com/articles/resignation-from-apa/

Pilkington, P. D., Reavley, N. J., & Jorm, A. F. (2013). The Australian public's beliefs about the causes of depression: Associated factors and changes over 16 years. *Journal of Affective Disorders, 150,* 356–362.

Rack, P. (1982). *Race, culture and mental disorder.* Tavistock.

Roth, M. (1973). Psychiatry and its critics. *British Journal of Psychiatry, 122,* 373–8.

Spandler, H. (2006). *Asylum to action: Paddington day hospital, therapeutic communities and beyond.* Jessica-Kingsley. (See particularly chapter 4, The Mental Patients Union, pp. 52–27).

Spivak, G. (1990) *The Post-colonial critic: Interviews, strategies, dialogues.* (S. Harasym, Ed.). Routledge.

Stewart, M., Brown, J. B., Weston, W. W., et al. (2003). *Patient-centred medicine: Transforming the clinical method* (2nd ed.). Radcliffe Medical Press.

Szasz, T. (2000). *Mental disorders are not diseases.* http://www.szasz.com/usatoday.html

Thomas, P., & Moncrieff, J. (1999). *Critical psychiatry.* Retrieved November 16, 2020, from http://www.critpsynet.freeuk.com/healthmatters.htm

Timimi, S. (2014). No more psychiatric labels: Why formal psychiatric diagnostic systems should be abolished. *International Journal of Clinical and Health Psychology, 14,* 208–215.

Timimi, S. (2020). *Insane medicine: How the mental health industry creates damaging treatment traps and how you can escape them.* Kindle Direct Publishing.

Timimi, S. (2021). *A straight talking introduction to children's mental health problems* (2nd ed.). PCCS Books.

Timimi, S., & McCabe, B. (2016a). Autism screening and diagnostic tools. In K. Runswick-Cole, R. Mallet, & S. Timimi (Eds.), *Re-thinking autism: Diagnosis, identity, and equality* (pp. 159–189). Jessica-Kingsley.

Timimi, S., & McCabe, B. (2016b). What have we learned from the science of autism? In K. Runswick-Cole, R. Mallet, & S. Timimi (Eds.), *Re-thinking autism: Diagnosis, identity, and equality* (pp. 30–48). Jessica-Kingsley.

Timimi, S., & Timimi, L. (2015). The social construction of attention deficit hyperactivity disorder (ADHD). In O'Reilly, M. (Ed.), *The Palgrave handbook of child mental health* (pp. 139–157). Palgrave MacMillan.

Wangari-Jones, P. (2016). How to decolonise mental health services. *Open Democracy.* https://www.opendemocracy.net/en/transformation/how-to-decolonise-mental-health-services/

Chapter 25

Crisis Response as a Human Rights Flashpoint

CRITICAL ELEMENTS OF COMMUNITY SUPPORT FOR INDIVIDUALS EXPERIENCING SIGNIFICANT EMOTIONAL DISTRESS[1]

*Peter Stastny, Anne M. Lovell, Julie Hannah, Daniel Goulart,
Alberto Vásquez Encalada, Seana O'Callaghan, and Dainius Pūras*

Summary

Violations of epistemic justice regarding mental difference and mental suffering can easily slide into ethical and human rights abuses—particularly in times of crisis and emergency response. This means that ethical approaches to informed consent and human-rights-based approaches to clinical care are increasingly important in times of crisis. Mental health systems around the world become their most dogmatic, most controlling, and most likely to resort to involuntary hospitalization, mandatory community treatment, and other coercive measures during these times. These coercive measures can be countered by effective human rights approaches. This chapter's authors, made up of a coalition of clinicians, academics, and human rights advocates, summarize their approach to human-rights-based care:

> This paper [chapter] proposes a set of nine critical elements underpinned by human rights principles to support individuals experiencing a serious crisis related to mental health problems or psychosocial disabilities. These elements are distilled from a range of viable alternatives to traditional community mental health approaches and are linked to a normative human rights framework. We argue that crisis response is one of the areas of mental health care where there is a heightened risk that the rights of service recipients may be infringed upon. We further make the case that

DOI: 10.4324/9781003148456-29

the nine critical elements found in advanced mental health care models should be used as building blocks for designing services and systems that promote effective rights-based care and supports.

*

Introduction

Over the last two decades, the United Nations and other organizations have released a number of groundbreaking reports documenting widespread, systemic human rights abuses within mental health systems worldwide.[1] Overall, these documents emphasize the need to seek better health and social outcomes through sustainable means, using a human rights-based approach in keeping with the 2006 United Nations Convention on the Rights of Persons with Disabilities (CRPD) and the right to health framework. These normative standards, along with persistent calls by service users and advocates, have brought attention to the rights of persons with psychosocial disabilities, particularly the right to freedom from coercion in mental health services. They provide the impetus to find suitable practices to transform and modernize mental health care in communities everywhere.

However, the form and substance of rights-based interventions through which mental health service providers, family members, and other engaged citizens might offer support, without resorting to coercive and dehumanizing interventions, remain unclear. While promising non-coercive interventions for persons experiencing serious emotional crises have been piloted in several countries, usually as alternatives to involuntary hospitalization, better evaluation and research is needed to increase their potential for widespread implementation.[2] And although recent publications argue for such rights-based approaches, how to operationalize this evolving framework has yet to be described.[3]

The present paper [chapter] fills this important gap by identifying a set of elements that are likely critical to rights-based support for individuals experiencing serious emotional crises, whether or not they use mental health services. The aim of this paper [chapter] is to help ensure that a rights-based approach to crisis response becomes a distinct and crucial operational component of mental health care. Crisis response is a human rights flashpoint where coercive structures and practices dominate and the human rights threat to individuals is consistently manifest.

The critical elements presented in this paper [chapter] are grounded in the rights-based approach and the right to health. Specifically, they correspond to principles underlying the key normative frameworks enshrined in the CRPD and to the principle of the right to the enjoyment of the highest attainable standard of mental and physical health, which are incorporated into article 12(1) of the International Covenant on Economic, Social and Cultural Rights (ICESCR).[4] We follow the 1946 Constitution of the World Health Organization in defining health as "a state of complete physical, mental and social well-being and not merely the absence of disease or infirmity."[5]

A Quest for Rights-Based Mental Health Systems

Practices with the potential to transform or replace community-based mental health care have been in existence, and many shown to be effective, since the advent of modern community psychiatry in the mid-1960s. Some, such as the Italian and Brazilian experiences, involve large-scale mental health reforms driven by deinstitutionalization and the development of sectorized community mental health services.[6] However, they also include highly innovative, small-scale efforts that have eluded larger systems.[7] These have been spearheaded by former patients or by visionary psychiatrists; many focus on people experiencing psychosis.[8] Most began as alternatives to coercive treatment and enhance personal liberties. Although these initiatives preceded the contemporary human and disability rights discourse by years, they contain critical elements which align with these rights.

A first type of innovation, beginning in the 1970s, involves small, community-based support structures. For example, the Soteria model provides a safe community home, largely non-professional staffing, and minimal medication use as a substantive, non-coercive alternative to acute hospitalization for people experiencing early psychosis.[9] Consumer/survivor/ex-patient groups have established other alternatives to mainstream mental health services for people in crisis.[10] The strongest outgrowth—peer-run respite facilities—provides peer support and non-coercive safe spaces where individuals in crisis can stay for varying periods of time.[11] Some such solidly established initiatives include the Berlin Runaway House (Germany), the Bapu Trust (India), and Western Massachusetts Recovery Learning Community (United States).

A later crisis response paradigm is embodied in the now widespread Open Dialogue model, created in Finland in the 1980s. Instead of an alternative residential setting, Open Dialogue uses systemic network approaches to support individuals in crisis in their homes and communities.[12] Structured conversations between a treatment team, the person in crisis, and members of her social network give equal weight to all viewpoints on the crisis, even those that would elsewhere be dismissed as "psychotic." By engaging persons in crisis with their network members, Open Dialogue attempts to transform the experience of "psychosis" and to destigmatize and empower the person in crisis.[13]

Alternative and "radical" models often show better social and clinical outcomes than "standard care"; others, according to Piers Gooding et al., may contribute to lowering coercive hospitalization.[14] Yet they have failed to spur rights-based, voluntary mental health systems. Instead, involuntary hospitalization, mandatory community treatment, and other coercive measures have risen significantly in Europe and North America, despite consistently poor outcomes.[15] Meanwhile, in the Global South, where mental health care is either lacking or depends almost exclusively on hospitalization, powerful global health actors working to close the "treatment gap" promote interventions focused primarily on medication use, rather than strategies to reduce coercion and safeguard human rights.[16] While advocates critique these neoliberal development strategies, global health proponents argue that only evidence-based practices merit replication.[17] This criterion excludes many rights-based alternatives which are difficult to test through traditional experimental designs.

Yet usual crisis responses (such as police intervention and involuntary hospitalization) are taken for granted without being submitted to the same research standard.

This contradictory situation calls for a wide range of localized innovations that adhere to human rights law while offering workable alternatives to the dominant mental health system.

This paper [chapter] contributes critical elements as guideposts for such efforts. Rather than proposing one paradigm, a competing technology, or total system reform at once, it offers rights-based building blocks that, when endorsed by local stakeholders, can contribute to system reconfiguration of responses to serious mental health crises.

Methodology: Linking Abstract Principles and Practical Responses

To identify critical elements of a rights-based approach to crisis response, we modified Paul Hunt's three-step process for developing a normative framework of human rights principles and values and translating them into practical elements.[18] Whereas Hunt's model moves from the abstract to the practical, we chose to identify already existing practices and confirm their human rights underpinnings.

First, we located the human rights laws and standards that should underpin elements of a rights-based approach (normative framework). Second, we specified a core set of human rights principles and values expressed in this framework. Third, we identified elements of crisis response practices that research shows or that our clinical and advocacy practice suggests are anchored in human rights. Most research to date focuses on whether entire programs, but not specific components, contribute to avoiding hospitalization, and its results are mostly inconclusive. Most studies focus on avoidance of coercion as the outcome, but some studies examine the association of these practices with a subjective sense of empowerment.[19]

The critical elements identified through clinical and advocacy experience are described in the second part of the paper [chapter]. Our practice employs experience-based phenomenological processes to discern what persons in crisis might experience as coercive—a dimension that conventional, positivist evidence-based research may not pick up.[20] Rather than relying on normative criteria based on objective behavioral response, we focus on understanding the singular subjective processes involved in a situation of crisis. This approach better suits the perspective of human rights, especially if social, cultural, and individual differences are to be taken seriously. We selected those elements that seemed aligned with specific human rights principles in the normative framework. The result is a set of nine critical elements that can be operationalized, subjected to research, and embraced as components of rights-based approaches to mental health crises.

Normative Framework

There is no universal definition of a "rights-based approach to health" in general or specific to the mental health context.[21] This paper [chapter] takes a rights-based approach to crisis response to include the full spectrum of civil, political, social, economic, and cultural rights: the rights of the child; the rights to privacy, life, participation, association, non-discrimination, equality, and family; and the prohibition of torture and cruel, inhuman, or degrading treatment or punishment. Health policies, strategies, and programs are to be guided by all these human rights standards and principles and should aim at empowering rights holders and strengthening the capacity of duty bearers. The proposed critical elements emanate from these core normative standards, but they importantly and explicitly foreground the right to the enjoyment of the highest attainable standard of physical and mental health (the right to health) and the specific rights enshrined by the ICESCR, adopted in 1966.

The right to health is recognized in various international and regional human rights treaties and enshrined in the Constitution of the World Health Organization. All states have ratified one or more of these instruments. While the right to health includes both freedoms and entitlements and has been interpreted to encompass both health care and the underlying social and psychosocial determinants of mental and physical health, operationally it has been understood to possess unique elements essential for the effective implementation of a rights-based approach to crisis response.[22]

According to Sofia Gruskin, Dina Bogecho, and Laura Ferguson, a minimal set of operational elements of the right to health includes availability, accessibility, acceptability, and quality (the AAAQ framework), as well as participation, transparency, and accountability.[23] The AAAQ framework finds its legal basis in General Comment 14 of the Committee on Economic, Social and Cultural Rights and is a unique and essential feature of the right to health. How these operational elements of the right to health have been articulated over time both through the CRPD and through the work of authoritative sources, such as the Committee on the Rights of Persons with Disabilities and reports of the United Nations Special Rapporteurs on the right to health and on the rights of persons with disabilities, informs our proposed framework.

The CRPD represents the highest standard of protection for the rights of persons with disabilities. It calls for the full realization of all human rights and fundamental freedoms for all persons with disabilities (actual or perceived), and it outlines specific steps to be taken by state parties to ensure the full and equal enjoyment of these rights.

Emphasizing the universality, indivisibility, and interdependence of human rights, the CRPD effectively contributes to a rights-based approach to crisis response by stressing the principle of non-discrimination and the notion of support in the exercise of rights. Article 12 of the CRPD affirms the legal capacity of all persons with disabilities in all areas of life and acknowledges the role of supported decision-making in exercising legal capacity. Article 14 of the CRPD clarifies that "the existence of a disability shall in no case justify a deprivation of liberty," which the Committee on the Rights of Persons with Disabilities and other bodies and experts have interpreted as an "absolute ban" to involuntary commitment to a mental health facility, including in crisis situations.[24] Furthermore, as underscored by Catalina Devandas, article 25 of the convention reaffirms the right of all persons with disabilities to the enjoyment of the highest attainable standard of health without discrimination, including the right to free and informed consent.[25]

In sum, under the CRPD framework, impairments—whether actual or perceived, or temporary or long standing—cannot be a legitimate ground for the denial or restriction of human rights, particularly in the context of crisis response, which often has been considered as exempted from those very safeguards. The support paradigm of the CRPD calls for non-coercive support responses within and outside the health sector.[26] In doing so, the CRPD questions previous international and regional standards that allow for exceptional circumstances in which the rights of persons with psychosocial disabilities could be restricted in the context of mental health provision.[27] While some CRPD detractors claim that a ban on coercive practices may endanger the right to health of persons with psychosocial disabilities, there is an increasing consensus that the CRPD represents an opportunity to realize a rights-based approach to mental health care.[28]

Key Underlying Principles

The core set of human rights principles and values that underpin the critical elements spring from the need to mitigate the losses of rights described in the ICESCR and CRPD that can occur when individuals experiencing a mental health crisis interact with emergency services and other systems of care. To be diagnosed with a mental illness can be stigmatizing and can result in a loss of social capital for individuals within their communities. In many legal contexts around the world, a diagnosis amounts to being labeled *non compos mentis* and means a loss of the enjoyment of a range of rights under international law. Once this occurs, substitute decision-making takes the place of self-determination. Emergency responders—police, medics, and others—are often empowered to apply force, to medicate without consent, to restrain, and to detain an individual for observation. In the worst such circumstances, individuals experiencing what appears to be a mental health crisis lose not only their rights but also their lives. Most survive the ordeal but, in many countries, they may be detained indefinitely, ostensibly for the safety of the larger community and without the provision of adequate care. In more progressive countries, where deinstitutionalization has advanced, substitute decision-making can remain in force for years, and legally mandated treatment with psychiatric medications as a condition for release from institutional detention or regaining other rights and freedoms is widespread and growing.[29]

The key principles that guide the identification of the critical elements for rights-based mental health care are selected here because they can eliminate substitute decision-making and promote self-determination for individuals within crisis response and systems of mental health support. Without these assurances, crisis situations, whether gradually or rapidly evolving, are likely to result in the immediate and sustained infringement of human rights. Crisis is defined but not limited to a broad range of experiences: sudden or frightening levels of agitation or turmoil; long-term withdrawal and isolation without attention to basic needs, physical health, or safety; suicidal intent; intense interpersonal animosity; expression of extreme fear or beliefs at odds with those of others; elevated mood or behavior; loss of awareness of surroundings; and struggling to plan and use foresight in their actions.

Participation and empowerment. Empowered participation has proved critical in improving care through preserving and bolstering the rights of persons with psychosocial disabilities in countries that have undergone deinstitutionalization, such as the United States, Italy, Portugal, and Brazil, to name some of the best-documented instances. In the United States, empowerment became the central organizing principle among the consumer/survivor/ex-patient movement that emerged from the era of deinstitutionalization and that has improved care for those with the most severe diagnoses, reducing inhumane practices and excessive use of seclusion and restraint. Empowerment and inclusion are proposed by consumer/survivor groups as measures of mental well-being. In our view, empowerment establishes a virtuous cycle of increased freedoms and well-being for those who are diagnosed with mental illnesses. Ideally, all critical elements should either promote or not restrict participation and empowerment.

Equality and non-discrimination. Article 5 of the CRPD upholds a complex substantive model of equality that addresses structural and indirect discrimination, values different layers of identity, and acknowledges intersectional discrimination.[30] Consistent with this strong definition of non-discrimination, the critical elements of mental health programs and systems should "recognize that all persons are equal …, prohibit all discrimination on the basis of disability …, and take all appropriate steps to ensure that reasonable accommodation is provided." Persons with psychosocial disabilities must be supported in exercising rights and should not be restricted in their exercise.

Quality and diversity of care. If the quality of mental health care is deficient, then the right to mental health care is effectively curtailed. Consistent with the principles of non-discrimination and equality, the critical elements should require that programs and systems of mental health care and psychosocial support be of high quality, be at least on par with quality standards for general health care, and demonstrate a record of, or hold reasonable promise of, promoting improved well-being and recovery. The effectiveness of supports should be measurable in ways that are meaningful to the individuals receiving care, and supports should be provided within an organized and accountable network. Because there is no singular recognized cure for any mental health problem, and because both personal and cultural diversity have strong and largely unpredictable effects on mental well-being, a multiplicity of options for care and models of care is essential.

Social inclusion. Social exclusion often lies at the heart of mental health problems and crises and limits the achievability of empowerment while interfering with the basic human need for social connectedness. Therefore, the critical elements must not inhibit and, when applicable, should actively promote social inclusion for and destigmatization of individuals with psychosocial disabilities.

Autonomy and dignity. The principle of autonomy means that individuals can make their own decisions about their lives, with adequate support if required, avoiding substitute decision-making. Respect for autonomy bolsters individuals' rights to choose the types and elements of the care and support they receive and to make decisions about their lives as independently as possible. It must be accounted for within the critical elements of crisis response. Each person should be respected as an individual with the right to autonomy and with the inherent dignity of a free person with equal rights to all others. People with psychosocial disabilities have the right to make decisions that others feel are unwise or with which they disagree.

Critical Rights-Based Elements for Crisis Response

The critical elements of rights-based services for individuals in psychiatric crisis should be underpinned by the five key principles described above. Each of the following nine rights-based critical elements for response to mental health crisis incorporates up to five of these principles (Table 25.1). While no single critical element encompasses all five principles, a human rights-based crisis response integrating more than one element would likely translate all five into concrete practices.

1. Communication and Dialogue

The reality or the belief that it is impossible to be heard and understood is often central to an individual's mental health crisis. Connection to a trusted professional, friend, or "person with experience" can help resolve the immediate situation and avoid coercive consequences. Supportive communication underlies programs ranging from the widely disseminated Friendship Bench, developed in Zimbabwe, to free-standing peer-support techniques.[31] Dialogical encounters, the communication paradigm underlying Open Dialogue and other programs, foster unexpected viewpoints, contradictions, and change. Both paradigms may broaden social capital by reinforcing already available relationships or building new networks around the crisis. The range of dialogical communication can extend from simple one-on-one exchanges to complex engagements in group-formats ("network meetings").

Communication and structured dialogue correspond to three key rights principles. Both facilitate *empowerment*, *autonomy*, and *social inclusion* through listening, gauging the distressed person's tolerance for others present, and involving him or her in deconstructing the situation of crisis. *Social inclusion* is preserved through acceptance of coexisting differences and conflicts, which in turn avoids a collapse of interpersonal relationships. Interventions based on immediate, frequent, and sustained dialogue with people experiencing psychosis have been shown to have better clinical outcomes than usual treatment and to circumvent coercion and overmedication.[32]

2. Presence ("Being With")

Alongside communication, presence—the idea of simply "being with"—responds to the basic human need for authentic human companionship, especially in crisis situations. As a result, it reinforces three rights principles: *participation*, *social inclusion*, and the *autonomy and dignity* of the person in crisis. The art of spending time with a person, without a predetermined objective, has been a key element in pioneering programs for persons experiencing acute psychosis ("altered states"), such as Windhorse, Soteria, Diabasis, and Emanon.[33] Time spent together may occur in a scheduled manner, such as during three-hour "basic attendance" sessions (Windhorse, a crisis support program based on contemplative principles) or 24–78

Table 25.1 Correlation of Critical Elements with Key Underlying Principles

	Participation and empowerment	Equality and non-discrimination	Quality and diversity of care	Social inclusion	Autonomy and dignity
Communication and dialogue	◆			◆	◆
Presence ("being with")	◆			◆	◆
Flexible location		◆		◆	◆
Safe spaces of respite	◆	◆		◆	◆
Continuity			◆		
Peer involvement	◆	◆	◆	◆	◆
Harm reduction				◆	◆
Judicious use of medications			$◆		
Response to basic needs	◆		◆	◆	◆

hour shifts (Soteria) or more spontaneously. Autonomy is preserved through continual renegotiation of the degree of physical closeness and active engagement in a space that protects the safety of the person in crisis. The mere fact of sharing space with someone in extreme distress communicates trust and has been shown to have a sustained calming effect.[34]

3. Flexible Location

Ideally, mental health workers should encounter someone in extreme distress in flexible locations, especially wherever that person happens to be or to feel most comfortable. *Equality, non-discrimination*, and *social inclusion* are preserved through flexibility as opposed to transporting the person to a "special" or stigmatizing place (such as a psychiatric service or institution). *Autonomy and dignity* are assured if the person in crisis invites the worker into his or her home or "personal territory" on the street, or if his or her personal space is safeguarded in shared living spaces.[35]

Mobility, outreach and home visits recognizing flexible location are key components of many community mental health services, including crisis intervention.[36] Ethnographic research has shown that respecting or being welcomed into the spaces occupied by homeless persons in crisis can be conducive to a better understanding and resolution of the situation.[37]

4. Safe Spaces of Respite

Persons in distress may seek safe spaces of "respite" from harmful or traumatizing environments, which may have provoked or could sustain the mental health crisis.[38] Respite spaces can provide around-the-clock support for individuals in crisis, through several-day to two-week stays.[39] Such spaces meet key rights principles of *empowerment, equality and non-discrimination, social inclusion*, and *autonomy and dignity*, as long as decisions to use them are made by the person in crisis or collaboratively.

Respite services involve peer workers, make pantry and cooking facilities continuously accessible, organize group meetings, and allow residents to come and go and pursue outside activities. Overtly illegal acts are not tolerated and can lead to being asked to leave.[40] Trained lay families or friends can also provide relief outside the home. Both types of respite have been shown to have better outcomes than hospitalization and to safeguard human rights.[41] Such rights-based respite approaches must be differentiated from those affiliated with locked or otherwise coercive mental health services.[42]

5. Continuity

Continuity of care remains an elusive goal of mental health services, in spite of widespread consensus regarding its essential role.[43] Continuity of personnel beyond the moment of crisis is almost nonexistent in current systems of care.[44] Critical Time Intervention, peer-bridgers, and Open Dialogue provide continuity by at least one person from the initial encounter through crisis resolution, but they are exceptions to this rule.[45] Such ongoing connection empowers the person and assures *quality and diversity*. In contrast, such typical practices during crisis assessments as "assessment and referral," triage, and other means of handing the person over to another service emphasize technical and managerial solutions rather than the development of emotional bonds. While some respond well to a one-time intervention, the offer of an ongoing relationship provides a powerful tool for persons in crisis to reconstitute their lives, even in the face of fractured connections. Continuity may be especially crucial when the person in crisis is suicidal.

6. Meaningful Peer Involvement

"Experts by experience," also known as peer workers or peer specialists, are trained to use their personal mental health and psychosocial disability experiences to help persons in crisis. While the personal life experiences of anyone who seeks to help others can be used in powerful ways, interventions based on the unique personal experience of extreme mental states and with various treatment responses have been widely embraced. Meaningful peer involvement in crisis situations, alone or with other mental health providers, ideally meets all five key rights principles in our framework.

When peer workers engage and judiciously disclose their personal experiences as they apply to the crisis situation at hand, they support and *empower* the person in crisis in a *non-discriminating* manner that preserves *dignity* and promotes *social inclusion*.[46] To ensure the standard for *quality* that the right to health assumes, peers should be well trained in the subtle and often tacitly acquired skill (for example, Intentional Peer Support). Peer collaboration has been used by some non-peer respites and Open Dialogue teams to generate innovative types of support.[47]

Peer-led services appear to contribute to reducing coercive interventions and the cost of services.[48] In this regard, the extent to which crisis responses require professionalization or can be directly provided by lay or peer practitioners outside medicalized frameworks is an essential question that requires greater attention.[49] To be successful, peer involvement must be meaningful and not be implemented in a tokenistic fashion. In too many instances, peer involvement is encumbered by power imbalances, where peer workers are involved in a superficial manner and have little or no control over crisis responses.[50]

7. Harm Reduction

Harm reduction approaches prioritize access to care by reducing or eliminating behavioral thresholds linked to disturbing, taboo, or even illegal behaviors. This model was pioneered in the domain of substance use services but can be applied to mental health, including for those without substance-related problems. Within the harm reduction paradigm, people are supported in their efforts to eliminate, avoid, or lessen risks associated with mental health problems, such as cutting or other forms of self-harm, unsafe sex, radical isolation, and illicit drug use. In this way, harm reduction assures the principle of *diversity in health care*, through *social inclusion* that respects the *dignity and autonomy* of the person. One can assume that reconceptualizing risk assessment into harm reduction will increase the *quality* of care and its outcomes.

Harm reduction focuses on providing care in a non-stigmatizing manner while tolerating the engagement in risky behavior. Such care is achieved by maintaining a collaborative stance with the person, who may be ashamed and fearful of losing rights due to such behavior, when seeking help. Importantly, harm reduction considerations are different from risk-benefit calculations, since no external assessment of risks or benefits concerning the situation or behavior is involved.[51] In other words, engaging with a broad range of risks in mental health supports is taken as a given, rather than a separate "administrative" layer of concern, which inherently interferes with a host of human rights principles.[52]

Responses to mental health crises that incorporate harm reduction principles may be more acceptable to distressed persons because they destigmatize harmful acts and reduce shame. For example, a person who engages in physical self-harm can be supported by considering less harmful ways instead of provoking categorical interdiction. Still, some situations will require the ongoing presence of another alert human being who may step in to engage the person in a conversation, or even, with permission, to gently prevent them from self-harm by physical contact (for example, through touch, not wrestling).[53]

However, violence against another person should be considered not a psychiatric problem but a likely violation of criminal law. A person in crisis who engages in interpersonal violence may be warned; in addition, the threatened individuals may be protected, and non-discriminatory police intervention may be called on to avert potential harm. Judicial guarantees and safeguards protecting the rights of those accused of a crime should apply in such cases, including the presumption of innocence, the right to a fair trial, and the provision of procedural accommodations.[54]

8. Judicious Use or Avoidance of Psychotropic Medications

Because the distinctions among prescribed psychiatric drugs, over-the-counter remedies, and licit (for example, alcohol) and illicit substances is relatively arbitrary, a harm-reduction approach is applicable to all of them. Meta-analyses suggest that less psychotropic medication is superior to more and that cautious gradual introduction is preferable to an immediate and high-dose prescription. Intermittent use under the person's control is likely less harmful over the short and long term than ongoing "maintenance" administration.[55] However, intermittent use may also increase the risk of harm due to inconsistent effects on receptor sites, an issue beyond the scope of this paper [chapter].[56]

Judicious psychotropic use enhances the *quality and diversity of health care* and ensures the *autonomy and dignity* of the person in crisis. How the person in distress views medication can help determine the most beneficial alternative.[57] Providing medication at the request of the person in crisis—for example, for quick relief of insomnia or intense anxiety—can be an important step in crisis resolution that also protects the person's rights.[58] On the contrary, the forced administration of psychotropic drugs is considered by many to be equivalent to torture and physical abuse.[59] Indiscriminate use of medication can undermine trust; it interferes with optimal, dignified care and frequently ignores the person's preference.

9. Response to Basic Needs

Many, if not most, crises manifested in emotional distress originate in interpersonal problems or environmental stressors (such as poor nutrition; lack of clothing, funds, or access to transportation; housing conditions; and legal problems). Such adversities can push someone from a state of adequate functioning to severe distress.[60] *Empowerment* of the person in distress and *quality and diversity of health care* are promoted when basic needs are addressed immediately. This may involve mobilizing a person's natural support system, collaborating with him or her on problem-solving, and even providing material resources, such as food, clothing, or money, which will yield [the] desired results quickly. Bureaucratic obstacles also often trigger crises, and a competent guide through such mazes (for example, concerning health coverage, financial benefits, or access to essential services) can go a long way. The worldwide Housing First movement advocates for housing without requiring that the person in crisis be in a stable condition.[61]

Practical Application of Critical Rights-Based Elements

Peer-run organizations such as the Western Massachusetts Learning and Recovery Center and Bapu Trust in India incorporate all nine critical elements.[62] Although current mental health systems would be unlikely to accomplish this, it is possible to demonstrate how crisis response can engage the nine critical elements as safeguards of the five key rights principles.

The following example from our work illustrates this possibility in real life. It involves a woman in her forties who was first encountered in the streets when she appeared to be wandering into traffic without paying much attention. When an outreach team pair (peer specialist and social worker) approached her, she seemed intoxicated from alcohol and spoke about scary people who were following her. By listening, without encroaching on her space, the team was able to conclude that the women's fears were outside consensual reality but that she recognized the need to be more careful with street traffic (*communication and dialogue, presence, flexible location, and meaningful peer involvement*).

The same team re-contacted the woman several times on the street and brought her food and warm bedding, which she had requested. She eventually accepted going to a respite space instead of being taken to a psychiatric emergency room (*continuity, respite*, and *basic needs*).

At the respite center, her drinking bothered residents who were trying to stay sober. The respite workers successfully sought a "wet house," which allowed her to drink and supported her in limiting the amount and frequency (*harm reduction*). The outreach team pair continued to spend time with her and support her with nutrition, personal hygiene, and forward planning (*presence* and *continuity*). When the woman complained about medications she had taken in the past, a consultant psychiatrist involved her in a collaborative plan to use medication only as needed which was the least adversely interactive with alcohol (*judicious use of medication*). The team pair helped her apply for long-term supported housing and reconnect with her children.

Accountability

Accountability, one of the most powerful aspects of a rights-based approach, should tie all nine critical elements to a rights-based culture. Accountability is necessary for ensuring that the rights of individuals within a system of care are upheld and that quality of care is preserved.

It is also an essential aspect of how rights-based critical elements can be "rightly" implemented. As such, it requires a system or organization that can embed what is to be accounted for, to assure not only that rights are respected but also that a full range of critical elements, perhaps even beyond those mentioned above, are validly and reliably put into practice as proposed.[63]

In order to succeed in creating a rights-based alternative to coercive standard care, a robust accountability framework should take into account the above critical elements and local law. It should provide means of pressuring existing mental health systems and programs to operationalize alternatives through a plurality of appropriate choices. The adoption of such measures, as well as an effective but not overly onerous approach to ensuring quality of care, must be acceptable to relevant stakeholders, particularly users of mental health services and supports. One example of a tool that can monitor such a process is the World Health Organization's Quality Rights Initiative.[64] Evaluation of crisis response is a crucial component of this accountability framework, and the promotion and upholding of the CRPD standards should be incorporated as outcome measures. Finally, the meaningful and routine inclusion of service users within teams that evaluate, monitor, and report on service implementation and outcomes is an important part of ensuring accountability.

Risks and Limitations

The greatest limitations to establishing supports that uphold human rights for individuals in mental health crisis lie with the vested interests that hold most power within existing mental health systems.[65] The two most prominent are the pharmaceutical industry and the mainstream medical establishment, which is still largely centered around hospital-based services.[66] Half a century ago, antipsychotic medications were heralded by policy makers as miracle cures that would enable those deemed in need of being separated from society to leave psychiatric institutions. The ensuing deinstitutionalization failed largely from lack of adequate community-based alternatives. In the meantime, the efficacy of psychotropic medications has been shown to be equivocal, adverse, even lethal, outcomes (such as dependency, metabolic disease, and suicidality) are not uncommon. Despite this, the pharmaceutical industry and its lobbyists have shaped public policy for decades.[67] Psychiatrists and other mental health professionals are key players in this status quo, and their incentives are skewed toward a focus on short-term evidence of medication effectiveness and away from long-term well-being, recovery, and human rights.[68]

Mainstream critics largely dismiss psychosocial interventions on the grounds that they lack an adequate evidence base. They also argue that implementing such alternatives would put people in crisis and the community around them at risk. Psychosocial interventions, which we argue can preserve rights and improve well-being, are much more complex and difficult to study. Yet their study receives vastly less funding than medication-related research. Researchers should advocate for more funding and develop the evidence base for such alternatives, and civil rights advocates should join forces with them in this effort.

As we have noted, several international developments and reports uniformly decry present conditions and call for a complete revamping of the current mental health system. However, countries, guilds, and mental health systems have yet to take these challenges seriously. Exceptional local efforts to redesign mental health services remain insular and rely on limited funding and practical experience, while broadcasting excellent values and beliefs.

Another important tool that has not been addressed in this paper [chapter] is the availability and promotion of psychiatric advance directives that can be used by persons with psychosocial disabilities in an attempt to influence crisis response in the future.[69] While important to the advocacy movement and to many persons with psychosocial disabilities, of advance directives' the widespread impact on system transformation is still doubtful.[70]

Where Do We Go from Here?

The trajectory within international law clearly bends toward greater freedom and autonomy for people with psychosocial disabilities, although significant barriers to upholding those freedoms and autonomy remain, particularly at a point of crisis when state authorities may intervene. However, since the 1960s, when the era of deinstitutionalization began, a range of alternatives to coercive treatment, especially for those in crisis, have been developed that can show the way toward the realization of rights-based crisis mental health care.

In countries where health systems are less funded and medical professions less powerful than in the Global North, the status quo may resemble the pre-deinstitutionalization era and may be replicating some of the least promising practices in post-colonial settings.[71] Global South nations must rely on cheaper and hence older generic medications, which have high-risk profiles, especially in the short term. As a result, seclusion and restraint, including the chaining of individuals, are frequently used.[72] Implementing the nine critical elements that preserve human rights, for example as part of a comprehensive Open Dialogue approach, requires considerable human interaction by paid staff, and certainly costs more than medication-centered practices.[73] In resource-poor environments, providing training to non-professional lay providers from the community and mental health peers that allows them to assist in preventing coercion and restraint and in implementing basic interventions may help overcome cost barriers.

Based on the characteristics of some of the more promising and prominent alternative models in the literature, we have distilled nine critical elements that incorporate key principles of the right to health. These can provide valuable guideposts for those who are either reforming or developing community mental health supports in an effort to adopt international humanitarian standards of care.

About the Authors

Peter Stastny, MD, is Consulting Psychiatrist at Community Access and the Pratt Institute, New York, USA, and founding member of the International Network towards Alternatives and Recovery.

Julie Hannah is Co-Director of the International Centre on Human Rights and Drug Policy and a member of the Human Rights Centre, University of Essex, UK.

Anne M. Lovell, PhD, is Senior Research Scientist Emerita at INSERM (Institut de Santé et de la Recherche Medicale) at CERMES 3, Villejuif and Paris, France.

Daniel Magalhães Goulart, PhD, is Associate Professor of the Faculty of Education and Health Sciences, University Center of Brasilia, Brazil.

Alberto Vásquez Encalada is Research Coordinator, Office of the United Nations Special Rapporteur on the Rights of Persons with Disabilities, Geneva, Switzerland, and Chair of Sociedad y Discapacidad – SODIS, Lima, Peru.

Seana O'Callaghan is a consultant research scientist in New York, USA.

Dainius Pūras, MD, Clinic of Psychiatry, Vilnius University, Lithuania, is the United Nations Special Rapporteur on the right of everyone to the enjoyment of the highest attainable standard of health.

Note

1 Originally Printed in: *Health and Human Rights Journal*, Vol. 22/1, pp. 105–120. Reprinted with permission.

References

1. N. Drew, M. Funk, S. Tang, et al., "Human rights violations of people with mental health and psychosocial disabilities: An unresolved global crisis," *Lancet* 378/9803 (2011), pp. 1664–1675; European Network of (Ex-) Users and Survivors of Psychiatry, *Submission of the European Network of (Ex-) Users and Survivors of Psychiatry (ENUSP) for the day of general discussion (DGD) on the right of persons with disabilities to live independently and be included in the community, to be held on 19 April 2016* in Geneva. Available at https://www.ohchr.org/Documents/HRBodies/CRPD/ DGD/2016/E uropeanNetworkof_Ex-_Users_and_Survivors_Psychiatry-ENUSP.doc; World Health

Organization, Quality rights, promoting human rights in mental health. Available at https://www.who.int/mental_health/policy/quality_rights/en/; United Nations Working Group on Arbitrary Detention, United Nations basic principles and guidelines on remedies and procedures on the right of anyone deprived of their liberty to bring proceedings before a court, UN Doc. WGAD/CRP.1/2015 (2015); United Nations, Report of the eighth session of the Conference of States Parties to the Convention on the Rights of Persons with Disabilities, UN Doc. CRPD/CSP/2015/5 (2015); C. Devandas, Report of the Special Rapporteur on the rights of persons with disabilities, UN Doc. A/HRC/40/54 (2019).

2. P. Gooding, B. McSherry, C. Roper, and F. Grey, *Alternatives to coercion in mental health settings: A literature review* (Melbourne Social Equity Institute, University of Melbourne, 2018). Available at https://sociale-quity.unimelb.edu.au/__data/assets/pdf_file/0012/2898525/ Alternatives-to-Coercion-Literature-Review-Mel-bourne-Social-Equity-Institute.pdf; S. P. Mann, V. J. Bradley, and B. J. Sahakian, "Human rights-based approaches to mental health: A review of programs," *Health and Human Rights* 18/1 (2016), pp. 263–275.

3. Devandas (2019, see note 1); Parliamentary Assembly of the Council of Europe (see note 1).

4. Convention on the Rights of Persons with Disabilities, G.A. Res. 61/106 (2006) International Covenant on Economic, Social and Cultural Rights, G.A. Res. 2200A (XXI) (1966), art. 12.

5. Convention on the Rights of Persons with Disabilities, G.A. Res. 61/106 (2006) International Covenant on Economic, Social and Cultural Rights, G.A. Res. 2200A (XXI) (1966), art. 12; Constitution of the World Health Organization (1946).

6. D. M. Goulart, *Subjectivity and critical mental health: Lessons from Brazil* (London: Routledge, 2019); A. S. Tarabochia, *Psychiatry, subjectivity, community: Franco Basaglia and Biopolitics* (Oxford: Peter Lang, 2013).

7. L. Mosher and L. Burti, *Community mental health: Principles and practice* (New York: W. W. Norton, 1981).

8. M. W. Cornwall, "Merciful love can relieve the emotional suffering of extreme states," *Journal of Humanistic Psychology* 59/5 (2019), pp. 665–671.

9. L. Mosher, "Soteria and other alternatives to acute psychiatric hospitalization: A personal and professional review," *Journal of Nervous and Mental Disorders* 187/3 (1999), pp. 142–149.

10. P. Stastny and P. Lehmann (eds.), *Alternatives beyond psychiatry* (Berlin: Peter Lehmann Publishing, 2007).

11. L. Ostrow and B. Croft, "Peer respites: A research and practice agenda," *Psychiatric Services* 66/6 (2015), pp. 638–640.

12. J. Seikkula and M. E. Olson, "The open dialogue approach to acute psychosis: Its poetics and micropolitics," *Family Process* 42/3 (2003), pp. 403–418.

13. M. Olson, J. Seikkula, and D. Ziedonis, *The key elements of dialogic practice in Open Dialogue* (Worcester: University of Massachusetts Medical School, 2014); L. P. Kantorski and M. Cardano, "Open Dialogue and the challenges for its implementation: An analysis based on a review of the literature," *Ciência e Saúde Coletiva* 24/1 (2019), pp. 229–246.

14. Gooding et al. (see note 2).

15. A. Turnpenny, G. Petri, A Finn, et al., *Mapping and understanding exclusion: Institutional, coercive and community-based services and practices across Europe: Project report*

(Brussels: Mental Health Europe, 2018); E. Fabris, Tranquil prisons: Chemical incarceration under community treatment orders (Toronto: University of Toronto Press, 2011).

16. D. Pūras and J. Hannah, "Prioritizing rights-based mental health care in the 2030 Agenda," in L. Davidson (ed.), *The Routledge handbook of international development, mental health and wellbeing* (New York: Routledge, 2019); V. Patel, S. Saxena, C. Lund, et al., "The Lancet Commission on Global Mental Health and Sustainable Development," *Lancet* 392/10157 (2018), p. 6; Lancet, *Global mental health 2007*. Available at https://www.thelancet.com/series/ global-mental-health; Lancet, *Global mental health 2011*. Available at https://www.thelancet.com/series/global-mental-health-2011; S. J. Hoffman, L. Sritharan, and A. Tejpar, "Is the UN Convention on the Rights of Persons with Disabilities impacting mental health laws and policies in high-income countries? A case study of implementation in Canada," BMC International Health Human Rights 16/28 (2016).

17. C. Mills, *Decolonizing global mental health: The psychiatrization of the majority world* (London: Routledge, 2014).

18. P. Hunt, "Interpreting the international right to health in a human-rights based approach to health," *Health and Human Rights Journal* 18/2 (2016), pp. 109–126.

19. Gooding et al. (see note 2); Olson (see note 13); Kantorski and Cardano (see note 13); Turnpenny et al. (see note 15).

20. N. K. Denzin and Y. S. Lincoln, *The Sage handbook of qualitative research*, 5th edition (London: Sage, 2018); Tarabochia (see note 6).

21. Hunt (see note 16).

22. Committee on Economic, "Social and cultural rights, general comment no. 14, the right to the highest attainable standard of health," UN Doc. E/C.12/2000/4 (2000); Pūras (2019, see note 1).

23. S. Gruskin, D. Bogecho, and D. Ferguson, "'Rights-based approaches' to health policies and programs: Articulations, ambiguities and assessment," *Journal of Public Health Policy* 31/2 (2010), pp. 138–140.

24. Devandas (2019, see note 1).

25. C. Devandas, "Report of the special rapporteur on the rights of persons with disabilities," UN Doc. A/73/161 (2018), paras. 14–15.

26. Devandas (2019, see note 1), para. 56.

27. Ibid.

28. P. Appelbaum, "Saving the UN convention on the rights of persons with disabilities—from itself," *World Psychiatry* 18/1 (2019), pp. 1–2; M. Scholten and J. Gather, "Adverse consequences of article 12 of the UN Convention on the Rights of Persons with Disabilities for persons with mental disabilities and an alternative way forward," *Journal of Medical Ethics* 44 (2018), pp. 226–233; F. Mahomed, "Establishing good practice in rights-based approaches to mental health in Kenya" (doctoral dissertation, Harvard T.H. Chan School of Public Health, 2019). Available at http://nrs.harvard.edu/urn-3:HUL.InstRepos:40976814; M. Zinkler and S. von Peter, "End coercion in mental health services—Toward a system based on support only," *Laws* 8/3 (2019), p. 19; K. Sugiura, F. Mahomed, S. Saxena, and V. Patel, "An end to coercion: Rights and decision-making in mental health care," *Bulletin of the World Health Organization* 98/1 (2020), pp. 52–58.

29. S. R. Kinsley, L. A. Campbell, and R. O'Reilly, "Compulsory community and involuntary outpatient treatment for people with severe mental disorders," *Cochrane Database of Systematic Reviews* 3 (2017), pp. 1–63.

30. T. Degener, "Disability in a human rights context," *Laws* 5/3 (2016).

31. D. Chibanda, H. A. Weiss, R. Verhey, et al., "Effect of a primary-care based psychological intervention on symptoms of common mental disorders in Zimbabwe: A randomized clinical trial," *JAMA* 316/24 (2016), pp. 2618–2626; R. K. Schutt and E. S. Rogers, "Empowerment and peer support: Structure and process of self-help in a consumer-run center for individuals with mental illness," *Journal of Community Psychology* 37/6 (2009), pp. 697–710.

32. Olson et al. (see note 13).

33. J. Fortuna, "Therapeutic households," *Journal of Contemplative Psychotherapy* 4 (1987), pp. 49–76; Mosher (see note 9); R. Bennett, "The Crisis Home Program of Dane County," in R. Warner (ed), *Alternatives to hospital for acute psychiatric treatment* (Washington, DC: American Psychiatric Press, 1995), pp. 227–236; J. Fortuna, "The Windhorse Program for Recovery," *Journal of Contemplative Psychotherapy* 9 (1994), pp. 73–96.

34. S. Mead and D. Hilton, "Crisis and connection, speaking out," *Psychiatric Rehabilitation Journal* 27/1 (2003), pp. 87–94.

35. E. Goffman, "The interaction order," *American Sociological Review* 48/1 (1983), pp. 1–17.

36. S. M. Murphy, C. B. Irving, C. E. Adams, and M. Waqar, "Crisis intervention for people with severe mental illnesses," *Cochrane Database of Systematic Reviews* 12/5 (2015), pp. 1–89.

37. M. Rowe, *Crossing the border* (Berkeley: University of California Press, 1999).

38. J. Cullberg, S. Levander, R. Holmqvist, et. al., "One-year outcome in first episode psychosis patients in the Swedish Parachute project," *Acta Psychiatrica Scandinavica* 106 (2002), pp. 276–285.

39. B. A. Stroul, "Residential crisis services: A review," *Hospital and Community Psychiatry* 39/10 (1988), pp. 1095–1099; Ostrow and Croft (see note 11).

40. E. E. Bouchery, M. Barna, E. Babalola, et al., "The effectiveness of a peer-staffed crisis respite program as an alternative to hospitalization," *Psychiatric Services* 69/10 (2018), pp. 1069–1074.

41. P. R. Polak and M. W. Kirby, "A model to replace psychiatric hospitals," *Journal of Nervous and Mental Disorders* 162/1 (1976), pp. 13–22; Bennett (see note 33); R. Bellion, "How we invented the Soteria principle," in P. Stastny and P. Lehmann (eds), *Alternatives beyond psychiatry* (Berlin: Peter Lehmann Publishing, 2007); K. Lötscher, H. H. Stassen, et al. "[Community-based crisis home programme: Cost-efficient alternative to psychiatric hospitalization]," *Nervenarzt* 80/7 (2009), pp. 818–826 [in German].

42. M. Heyland, C. Emery, and M. Shatell, "The Living Room, a community crisis respite program offering people in crisis an alternative to emergency departments," *Global Journal of Community Psychology Practice* 4/3 (2013), pp. 1–10.

43. E. F. Torrey, "Continuous treatment teams in the care of the chronic mentally ill," *Hospital and Community Psychiatry* 37/12 (1986), pp. 1243–1247.

44. "New York association of psychiatric rehabilitation services," *Peer Bridger project.* Available at https://www. nyaprs.org/peer-bridger.

45. D. Herman, L. Opler, A. Felix, et al., "A critical time intervention with mentally ill homeless men: Impact on psychiatric symptoms," *Journal of Nervous and Mental Disorders* 188/3 (2000), pp. 135–140.

46. N. Hunter, *Trauma and madness in mental health services* (London: Palgrave and Macmillan, 2018), pp. 201–219.

47. C. Wusinich, D. Lindy, D. Russell, et al., "Experiences of parachute NYC: An integration of open dialogue and intentional peer support," *Community Mental Health Journal* (2020).

48. C. Doughty and S. Tse, "The effectiveness of consumer-led mental health services: An integrative review," *Community Mental Health Journal* 47 (2011), pp. 252–266.

49. Ibid.; M. Chinman, P. George, R. H. Dougherty, et al., "Peer support services for individuals with serious mental illnesses: Assessing the evidence," *Psychiatric Services* 65/4 (2014), pp. 429–441.

50. J. Repper and T. Carter, "A review of the literature on peer support in mental health services," *Journal of Mental Health* 20/4 (2011), pp. 392–411.

51. R. M. Krausz, G. R. Werker, V. Strehlau, and K. Jang, "Applying addictions harm reduction lessons to mental healthcare," *Advances in Dual Diagnosis* 7/2 (2014), pp. 73–79.

52. D. Ougrin, T. Tranah, D. Stahl et al., "Therapeutic interventions for suicide attempts and self-harm in adolescents: Systematic review and meta-analysis," *Journal of the American Academy of Child and Adolescent Psychiatry* 54/2 (2015), pp. 97–107; K. James, I. Samuels, P. Moran, and D. Stewart, "Harm reduction as a strategy for supporting people who self-harm on mental health wards: The views and experiences of practitioners," *Journal of Affective Disorders* 214 (2017), pp. 67–73.

53. Bellion (see note 41).

54. Devandas (2019, see note 1), para. 50.

55. M. I. Herz, W. M. Glazer, M. A. Mostert, et al., "Intermittent vs maintenance medication in schizophernia: Two-year results," *Archives of General Psychiatry* 48/4 (1991), pp. 333–339; P. Stastny, "Taking charge of psychotropic drugs," *Disability Studies Quarterly* 3/2 (1993).

56. V. Aderhold and P. Stastny, "A guide to minimal use of neuroleptics," *Mad in America* (October 2, 2016). Available at https://www.madinamerica.com/2016/10/a-guide-to-mini-mal-use-of-neuroleptics/.

57. T. Van Putten, P. R. May, S. R. Marder, and L. A. Wittmann, "Subjective response to antipsychotic drugs," *Archives of General Psychiatry* 38/2 (1981), pp. 187–190.

58. K. T. Mueser, P. W. Corrigan, D. W. Hilton, et al., "Illness management and recovery: A review of the research," *Psychiatric Services* 53/10 (2002), pp. 1272–1284; Herz et al. (see note 56); J. A. Baker, K. Lovell, and N. Harris, "A best-evidence synthesis review of the administration of psychotropic pro re nata (PRN) medication in in-patient mental health settings," *Journal of Clinical Nursing* 17/9 (2008), pp. 1122–1231; Aderhold and Stastny (see note 56).

59. Office of the United Nations High Commissioner for Human Rights, "UN reports," Available at https://www.ohchr. org/EN/Issues/Disability/Pages/UNStudiesAndRe ports.aspx.

60. M. Rotenberg, A. Tuck, and K. McKenzie, "Psychosocial stressors contributing to emergency psychiatric service utilization in a sample of ethno-culturally diverse clients with psychosis in Toronto," *BMC Psychiatry* 17/234 (2017), pp. 1–7.

61. T. Aubry, G. Nelson, and S. Tsemberis, "Housing First for people with severe mental illness who are homeless: A review of the research and findings from the At Home-Chez Soi Demonstration Project," *Canadian Journal of Psychiatry* 60/11 (2015), pp. 467–474.

62. Western Massachusetts Recovery Learning Community, "RLC articles," Available at https://www.westernmassrlc. org/rlc-articles; C. Mills and B. Davar, "A local critique of global mental health," in S. Grech and K. Soldatic (eds.), *Disability in the Global South: The critical handbook* (Cham: Springer, 2016), pp. 437–451.

63. United Nations, *Rights of persons with disabilities* (New York: United Nations, August 2016), paras. 67–69; Devandas (2019, see note 1), paras. 73–75.

64. World Health Organization, "Quality Rights Initiative (2019)," Available at https://www .who.int/mental_health/policy/quality_rights/en/.

65. Mills (see note 17).

66. D. Ingleby, "How 'evidence-based' is the movement for global mental health?," *Disability and the Global South* 1/2 (2014), pp. 203–226.

67. G. Contino, "The medicalization of health and shared responsibility," *New Bioethics* 22/1 (2016), pp. 45–55.

68. Mills (see note 17).

69. Y. Khazaal, R. Manghi, M. Delahaye, et al., "Psychiatric advance directives, a possible way to overcome coercion and promote empowerment," *Frontiers in Public Health* 2/37 (2014).

70. S. Philip, S. K. Rangarajan, S. Moirangthem, et al., "Advance directives and nominated representatives: A critique," *Indian Journal of Psychiatry* 61/4 (2019), pp. S680–S685.

71. Patel et al. (see note 16); Mills (see note 17).

72. Human Rights Watch, *"Like a death sentence": Abuses against persons with mental disabilities in Ghana* (New York: Human Rights Watch, 2012).

73. S. von Peter, V. Aderhold, L. Cubellis, et al. "Open Dialogue as a human rights-aligned approach." *Frontiers in Psychiatry* 10 (2019), Article 387.

Chapter 26

Sanism

HISTORIES, APPLICATIONS, AND STUDIES SO FAR

Stephanie LeBlanc-Omstead and Jennifer Poole

Summary

Sanism, as LeBlanc-Omstead and Poole explain, "serves as a bedrock for understanding the kind of violence directed at the mad community and the always-present threat to their realization of justice." As a result, "disrupting and dismantling sanism is at the heart of the Mad Studies Project." This chapter works through a historical narrative of the emergence of the term "sanism" and its intersectionality with other forms of prejudice and "isms" that shore up matrices of domination. They also work through some of the multiple uses of the term. For some, such as mad scholar Erick Fabris, sanism is about the very logic of dividing the world into "mad" and "sound." For others, it is about the hierarchy and prejudice that come with that division. One definition that the authors have used for sanism is the "systematic subjugation and a devastating oppression visited on those who have received 'mental health' diagnoses, or who are otherwise perceived to be 'mentally ill.'"

LeBlanc-Omstead and Poole articulate the challenge of sanism as twofold. One is the sanist "epistemic/testimonial smothering" of those who have been negatively impacted by the systems and worldviews of normative psychiatrization. The other is limited understanding and circulation of the term sanism. Mad studies and critical disability studies are contributing to progress in both of these challenges. However, the work so far has been slow and there is still a long way to go. Moreover, the authors point to multiple recent ways that sanism is growing rather than diminishing. They conclude with an invocation of Sins Invalid's understanding of the shared dynamics of oppression: "Our resistance efforts against sanism and toward liberation for mad folx needs to be rooted in the disability justice principle of *collective liberation*."

*

DOI: 10.4324/9781003148456-30

Introduction

This is not the first piece we have written about sanism. We have written as individuals, collaboratively, and collectively; with folx who use, refuse, and push back against the mental health system. We have spent decades thinking, writing, and teaching about sanism because we have experienced its violence firsthand. We have also experienced sanism as a discourse as something that works on and through us, or a set of rules for talking about and doing 'critical mental health' work. In this short chapter, we will do our best to explicate how we have come to understand sanism and how it operates; how we understand scholarship on sanism; how the concept has been taken up or applied in a range of fields; how it is different from, but connected to, stigma; and some of our growing concerns with sanism and its study so far.

We are ever mindful that sanism is operating all day, in every way, in our respective corners of Northern Turtle Island (or what is also known as Canada and the United States). Indeed, as we tried to find the energy to put this piece together, we shared multiple stories of how sanism seems to be growing in its intensity and deployment, as opposed to what we, and many other activists, writers, thinkers, and scholars had always hoped for: that speaking of sanism would reduce sanism, through rendering the once invisible, visible. And yet, despite the speaking, sanism seems to have intensified for many, including those working in the so-called helping professions (ourselves included) and trying to simultaneously navigate systems such as, but not limited to, health, legal, housing, and all of the other systems that serve to discipline, punish, and regulate members of so-called Global North societies.

History

In this next section, we will share how we understand the history of work on/around sanism, always aware of what we do not know. Histories are always precarious and their retelling could always be otherwise. And so, we are deeply mindful of how narratives about sanism may be constructed and fall differently, depending on when, how, and where people are located. For us, we understand sanism as a term that was first coined by American physician and disability rights lawyer, Dr. Morton Birnbaum, whose writing was influenced by his work and conversation with Black legal scholar Florynce Kennedy. Birnbaum's work in the state medical system raised questions for him around what was going on for patients who were housed in residences and various state psychiatric institutions. Following repeated rejection from a number of publishing outlets, Birnbaum (1960) published the article, *The Right to Treatment*, in which he shared observations about what had been witnessed in these institutions and outlined 'sanism.' In a line that could have been written in the present day, Birnbaum (1960) then noted, "Let us continue to improve upon what we are able to do, and not measure success by chemically induced tranquility and the rate at which we discharge patients from our hospitals" (p. 501).

It was in the early 1990s that Dr. Michael Perlin, another disability rights legal scholar, also began writing about sanism. Perlin has since written hundreds of pieces on sanism, how it operates, and where it operates in the legal system. Perlin importantly wrote about the ways sanism (re)produces sanist myths that then operate through society (Perlin, 1992, 1993, 2009, 2013). Perhaps most notable of these, is the sanist myth surrounding the risk of violence, suggesting that persons deemed mad or mentally ill are invariably dangerous (Large & Ryan, 2012). Furthermore, the pervasiveness of sanism, as Perlin has described, makes it so that regular use of words like 'crazy,' 'insane,' or 'psycho' is socially acceptable, and typically regarded as being less violent than other kinds of hate language/speech. We two authors of this chapter have referred to, and are grateful for, Perlin's work, as we have come to understand sanism. Many other folks have deepened and extended the conversation about sanism. Activist Judi Chamberlin, for instance, did not actually use the word sanism but instead used the term *mentalism* to describe a kind of prejudice visited on those who weren't sane (enough). In *On Our Own* (1978) Chamberlin points out that:

> Negative stereotypes of the 'mentally ill' are everywhere and are difficult not to internalize, no matter how sensitive one becomes. This stereotyping has been termed 'sane chauvinism' or 'mentalism' by mental patients' liberation groups. Like sexism, mentalism is built into the language – *sick* and *crazy* are widely used to refer to behaviour of which the speaker disapproves.
>
> (p. 66, emphasis in original)

Chamberlain was an activist first, and a writer who wrote multiple volumes in the years before her passing. We are indebted to and have been molded by this work. We must also revert to the history books to mention the multiple collectives who came together to write against psychiatric sanism and the ways in which sanism divided, disciplined, pathologized, othered, and marginalized thousands of people with various psychiatric diagnoses. If we look to the archives as Geoffrey Reaume has been so particular about, we see that there are multiple groups, including those behind Asylum Magazine, Mad in America (and Canada), and The Icarus Project/Fireweed Collective. It is important that we also acknowledge that many other resistance efforts are not recorded anywhere but are no less vital (Landry, 2021).

For studies on sanism – in addition to work by Perlin, Chamberlain, and Birnbaum – we also look to literature created by Rachel Gorman, Bren LeFrançois, Marina Morrow, Helen Spandler, PhebeAnn Wolframe, Shaindl Diamond, and many more we note below. This collective scholarly archive makes it very clear that the discourse of sanism and about sanism has been with us for 60+ years, but that the practice of othering, and the practice of sanism, is as old as time immemorial. It has shown up in different forms of violence and in various forms of genocide. Indeed, sanism has been known and experienced far longer than its formal study. And despite 60+ years of formal study, of knowledge generation and sharing, not only does sanism continue to thrive, but it has expanded its reach. For instance, sanism is now operating through social media, through professional/disciplinary colleges and licensing, through employment practices, and on university campuses through forced leaves for students and faculty with 'serious mental health issues.'

Sanism Studies

Sanism is defined and described in different ways within and beyond those working toward the Mad Studies project. Rather than focus on the settling of differences between the many ways sanism is understood and languaged (or pinning down one *right* definition of sanism), we work with a diversity of meanings for sanism. Perlin (2008) described sanism as "an irrational prejudice of the same quality and character of other irrational prejudices that cause (and are reflected in) prevailing social attitudes of racism, sexism, homophobia, and ethnic bigotry" (p. 590). Erick Fabris (2011) notes that sanism may be used to refer to, "prejudgement or prejudice against mentally ill people" (p. 9), and he uses it to describe, "the division of persons into 'mad' and 'sound'" (p. ix). Similarly, for Procknow (2017), "Sanism is the perception and 'Othering' of those diagnosed or labeled 'mentally ill' as inferior or abnormal" resulting in "the litany of deprivations, injustices, and inequalities psychiatrized 'Others' within predominately 'sane' cultures face (Didyk, 2016; Diamond, 2013)" (p. 6).

Harrison et al. (2021) draw on Wolframe's (2013) notion of 'sane privilege,' describing sanism as "the societal power structure that privileges normative mood, behavior, and thinking and marginalizes people with mental differences, creating structural oppression of mad and neuro-atypical people" (p. 1). We have previously described sanism as the systematic subjugation and a devastating oppression visited on those who have received 'mental health' diagnoses, or who are otherwise perceived to be 'mentally ill' (LeBlanc & Kinsella, 2016; Poole et al., 2012). Thorneycroft (2020) considers this subjugation and oppression to be the *effect* of sanism, and would prefer to speak of sanism as describing, "the 'ways in which society values certain forms of human consciousness and being over others' (Van Veen et al., 2018, p. 259) –that is, the preference, expectation, and command for the sane mind" (p. 86). Others still have written about different, more context-specific, *kinds* of sanism. Meerai et al. (2016) introduced the notion that sanism "exists on a continuum depending on privilege, and it is always and especially compounded when it is visited on racialized bodies" (p. 20); detailing anti-Black sanism and its relation to white supremacy. Hamer (2011) describes 'state sanism' and 'institutional sanism,' explicating that state sanism orders all citizens into normal and abnormal categories, while institutional sanism assumes that the 'abnormal' are unpredictable and violent. We also take up various forms of sanism in our own work, including but not limited to, 'psy-sanism' (Poole & LeBlanc-Omstead, forthcoming).

Most recently, and as we will elaborate below, we have written about these sanism(s) as contributing to a *settler sanism*. Settler sanism is an expression of white supremacist colonialism and the eugenics project which seeks to destroy and replace with something more compliant, productive, and 'sane' (read: white) (Poole & LeBlanc-Omstead, forthcoming). We can say with confidence that sanism is many things to many different people. Sanism, as it has been taken up to date, is a term used to denote oppression, violence, blatant discrimination, microaggressions, (unequal) power, silencing, Othering, privileging, and division. Sanism – in all of its interpretations – is multi-directional in that it is internalized, externalized, and laterally inflicted.

Applications: Who Is Addressing Sanism, and How?

Law

As we have described above, sanism was first named as such in the legal arena, and particularly by disability rights lawyers, Mortin Birnbaum, Florynce Kennedy, and Michael Perlin. In the time since it was first coined, Perlin has written extensively about sanism, discussing the concept in relation to *pretextuality* (i.e., legal practices sanctioning the use of sanist stereotypes and prejudice, such as testimonial dishonesty and dishonest decision-making) and *therapeutic jurisprudence* (i.e., a 'toolkit' or 'ethics of care,' which encourages lawyers to focus critically on voluntariness, voice, and validation for those they represent). As Parry (2005) explains, "stigma, sanism, and pretextuality combine to make it very difficult for defendants with mental disabilities to be viewed in anything but a negative light when they enter the criminal justice system" (p. 667). Perlin and Lynch (2016) continue to argue that "the [legal] representation of persons with mental disabilities is infected – often, fatally infected – by sanism" (p. 1). Williams (2014), who writes of the legal system's sanist treatment of psychiatrized parents (or those deemed mentally ill), describes sanism as "the last bastion of acceptable prejudice" (p. 3).

Social Work

Over 20 years ago, Wilson and Beresford (2000) quite rightly called out anti-oppressive practice (AOP), which was, at the time, social work's critical theoretical darling. Their critique was that AOP offered a lens into understanding and pushing back on all kinds of oppression and yet had completely overlooked the experience of folx with disabilities including psychiatric survivors, consumers, and other users and refusers of the mental health system. Indeed, since its 'inception,' the late Bonnie Burstow often reminded us that social work had largely overlooked the lived experience and knowledge of mad, psychiatrized, and survivor folx in all of its practice and scholarship, choosing to favor instead a heavily medical and pathologizing approach to so-called 'care' and education (Burstow, 2016).

One of us well remembers their first classroom discussion on sanism at a so-called critical social work program. It was six years after Wilson and Beresford (2000) and decades after Burstow had first raised the alarm in and about social work, but most had never heard of sanism, some argued *for* sanism, citing the so-called 'dangerousness' of their 'clients,' while a handful of students with lived experience of sanism sat in horror and silence. That horror became a project with mad(dened) social work students, illuminating the deep institutional sanism that exists in the profession and its training spaces (Reid & Poole, 2013; Poole et al., 2012). Thankfully, over the last few decades, scholarship on sanism in social work has grown thanks to the leadership of Bren LeFrancois as well as scholars such as Idil Abdillahi, Alise deBie, Chris Chapman, Yaya El-Lahib, Maria Lieggio, Ameil Joseph, Sonia Meerai, Jenna Reid, Jijian Voronka, and so many more. However, so has sanism in social work, as evidenced by increasingly punitive employment and licensing practices that seek to 'gatekeep' and 'protect' the profession from those with lived experience of psychiatric diagnoses (Chapman et al., 2016; Poole et al., 2012). Despite calls for change, studies, and reports (Brown, 2020), the scholarship on sanism in social work has yet to dislodge the deep disciplinary sanism and mental health profiling to which the field continues to hold fast.

Allied Health Professions

The integration of Critical Disability Studies – and (to an even lesser degree) Mad Studies – scholarship into allied health professions education remains limited despite repeated calls for engagement with the critical concepts developed by these fields. Sanism has been named, even afforded a line or two, in discussions of equity and anti-oppression in allied health professions-specific scholarship (e.g., Harrison et al., 2021; Morrow & Hardie, 2014). However, with few exceptions, sanism is seldom taken up in any real depth as a pervasive issue threatening the realization of AOP by allied health professions. In recent years, we have seen pleas from occupational therapy scholars and educators (via written publication, public presentation, and professional seminars) to broaden professional discourse around mental health stigma to include discussion of sanism and the visioning of an anti-sanist praxis (LeBlanc-Omstead & Kinsella, 2019; McCarthy & Doherty, 2019). In a recent special issue of the *American Journal of Occupational Therapy*, Harrison et al. (2021) expressed the hope that sanism (and related concepts) will, "be part of everyday occupational therapy practitioner's awareness" in the not-so-distant future (p. 5).

Higher Education

In the last decade, we have also seen the application of the concept of sanism in thinking about pedagogy and/in higher education. Wolframe (2013) wrote about broadening conversations with her students about anti-oppression to include "saneism" [sic] by way of introducing them to the concept of the "sane privilege backpack" (adapted from Peggy McIntosh's well-known *white privilege knapsack*). Wolframe (2013) describes the sort of unearned privilege that folx deemed or perceived to be 'sane' carry with them and may not be obvious to those who have never lost it. For example, when 'sane' persons seek police assistance or medical attention, their history of 'sanity' will likely not result in their being assaulted, ignored, dismissed, made to wait, or treated as though they are lying, or in receiving diminished quality of care (Wolframe, 2013). Castrodale (2017, 2018) addresses sanism in higher education through their conceptualization of a Mad-positive or Mad-enabling pedagogy. Such pedagogy involves the centering of mad epistemologies or perspectives, pushing back against the dominance of objective/biomedical knowledge in academia. Moving outside of conventional academic spaces, Procknow (2019) recently theorized a 'pedagogy of saneness' related to sane performativity in film, to describe "a process for unpacking how mad-identified viewers come to know who they are, or are not, through renderings of saneness imagined and mapped out cinematically" (p. 15). The area of education perhaps most well-known for addressing sanism is the growing academic field of Mad Studies (LeFrançois et al., 2013).

Mad Studies

The first 'Mad Studies' course was developed and taught by Geoffrey Reaume in 2000. Contrary to popular belief (Burstow, 2016), Reaume taught it first at the University of Toronto (Reaume, 2019) and then found a more supportive home for it at Toronto Metropolitan University (formerly Ryerson) in the School of Disability Studies (also in Toronto). As Reaume (2019) notes, the course drew on history, archives, art, tours of built structures, and multiple other sources of knowledge. Importantly, the term 'Mad' was chosen to get away from the idea that this was a course on the "history of symptomatology" from a medical model perspective (Reaume, 2019, p.31).

For many who now align themselves with the Mad Studies project, sanism serves as a bedrock for understanding the kind of violence directed at the mad community and the always-present threat to their realization of justice. In other words, disrupting and dismantling sanism is at the heart of the Mad Studies project. One of the ways Mad Studies resists sanism is in its centering of the experiential knowledge of those whose lives have collided with the powers of psychiatry, representing a form of ideological opposition to mainstream discourse which privileges 'objective,' 'expert' knowledge of the so-called helping professions (Mellifont, 2019).

Sanism and/or Stigma?

Our thinking, writing, and teaching about (psychiatric) violence and oppression (or sanism) intentionally steers clear of the now ever-popular language of *mental health stigma*. In many cases, and alongside many others, we have urged others to follow suit so that the language of sanism might be elevated to a level of critical importance in our conversations focused on justice, equity, and oppression. Many reasons have been cited for embracing the language of sanism rather than stigma. For Large and Ryan (2012), using the language of sanism makes good sense because "we already understand the pitfalls of other prejudice-based discrimination" and "we know that a propensity to sexism, ageism or racism lies within us all" (p. 1100). Understanding such discrimination or oppression as sanism (as opposed to stigma) then, makes urgent addressing and guarding against sanism as fiercely as one might other systemic oppressions (Large & Ryan, 2012). Others find the language of stigma to be grossly inadequate (Holley et al., 2012) and always too limiting (Thornicroft et al., 2007) in the way that it perpetuates "medical conceptions/language around mental health" and "minimizes the jagged reality of widespread rights abuse and oppression (or sanism) experienced by Mad individuals" (Poole & Jivraj, 2015, p. 201).

Mental health stigma and its studies also tend toward individualizing discourses and responses/interventions, focusing on "the individual being stigmatized and not on the sanist power relations that make stigmatization possible in the first place" (Holley et al., 2012 as cited in Poole & Jivraj, 2015, p. 201). In addition to all these arguments, we also take issue with the fact that stigma does not (necessarily) have a perpetrator per se, but is rather abstract, free-floating, and non-specific. To illustrate, we constantly hear talk (in the media, research, education, mental health campaigns, etc.) about there being a *stigma* surrounding mental health issues (or madness) without any mention of sanism (as systemic oppression). When we stop to consider that we do not typically speak about a *stigma* surrounding gendered or racialized bodies, but instead use the more apt language of sexism and racism or colonialism, we are better able to see *mental health stigma* as problematically 'soft' language, and the importance of a greater embrace of the term sanism. This shift in language acknowledges the discrimination, violence, and oppression experienced by mad persons as systemic, and allows for a greater emphasis on accountability (from ourselves and others).

Stigma studies are not inherently wrong or unnecessary; we need stigma studies. While use of the term sanism is indeed a political decision, we remain open to a myriad of different ways to language and express the harms done to us and others by psy- systems and ideologies. While the language of mental health stigma has obvious limitations – as we have just outlined – we see replacing this language with the term *sanism* as secondary to resisting the silencing or epistemic/testimonial smothering (Dotson, 2011) of those who have been negatively impacted by psychiatrization. In other words, we are not pushing for a monopoly on the language that can be used to name and push back against pathologization and psychiatric oppression.

Where Are We Now?

In our most recent writing on sanism, we continue the work of many before and alongside us – notably, Diamond (2013), Joseph (2015, 2019), Lewis (2019, 2020, 2021), and Sins Invalid (2015) – in disrupting contemporary sanism studies in the form of a (long overdue) acknowledgment of sanism's white supremacist colonial roots (Poole & LeBlanc-Omstead, forthcoming). Drawing inspiration from the ways Lewis (2019, 2021) makes explicit the inseparability of ableism and racism, we reconsidered and disrupted contemporary framings of sanism and anti-sanist resistance efforts, questioning whether these (ever) acknowledge the ways sanism – much like ableism – is conceptually dependent on, and reinforces, racism, colonialism, and patriarchy. The well-documented and theorized white supremacist/racist/colonial foundations of the psy-disciplines have given rise to conceptualizations of 'sanity' that privilege, "European ways of knowing, while also assuming rationality as inherent in some groups based on constructs of 'race,' gender, and class" (Kurchina-Tyson, 2017, p. 3). In its privileging of 'sane' bodyminds (and the oppression of anything Other) – a sanity dependent on "white rationality" (Meerai et al., 2016, p. 24) – sanism is always inherently racist and colonial. As such, "resistance(s) to sanism should fundamentally acknowledge and challenge the colonial legacy of settler psy-sciences and institutions" (Lewis, 2019 as cited in Poole & LeBlanc-Omstead, forthcoming).

Resisting Sanism

For many years, we have operated from the hope/assumption that once the 'invisible' was rendered visible; or the harm and violence of sanism were made known and its insidious operation revealed in our everyday lives (e.g., in our language, policies, education, and practices), that knowledge of this oppression might inspire public outcry and be deemed (at least, socially) unacceptable. However, despite decades (collectively) of naming, resisting, and spreading the word about sanism and the damages it leaves in its wake – often to large audiences of powerful, critical, and well-meaning individuals and organizations – we are left with a sense as we write this piece that sanism is all around us, moving in new and perhaps more insidious ways.

For us in the settler state of Canada, it comes as no surprise that in 2019, a UN report made clear that Canada has failed to live up to its commitments to respect the human rights of people with a psychiatric diagnosis (Devandas-Aguilar, 2019). Since then and during the pandemic, rates of mental distress have skyrocketed as have hospitalizations, suicides, and overdoses, and yet 'treatment' may only be available to those with the resources to access online support via smartphones and computers. Those who were being 'treated' in hospitals report overcrowding, intensified psychiatric assault/abuse, and very poor pandemic protocols (Spencer, 2020). Those who are not 'treated' on an inpatient basis report not just a lack of safe shelter and housing but police harassment and assault (McNally & Dosani, 2021). Additionally, with the passing of Bill C-7 in Canada, it has suddenly become much easier for those labeled with disabilities to 'choose' to end their lives with medical assistance. Disability activists have called the Bill deeply dangerous for mad and disabled people (Disability Filibuster, 2021). All these deeply sanist 'developments' point to what Joseph (2015) names as eugenics; a sanist necropolitics of 'slow death' (Berlant, 2007) meant to rid this world of those who are labeled with a psychiatric diagnosis, disability, or who are perceived to be not sane enough.

So, if naming and speaking about sanism individually is really only the first step toward dismantling it, what else is being done to resist, push back, and disrupt sanism? Many continue to work toward holding Canada accountable to its responsibilities as laid out in the UN Convention on the Rights of Persons with Disabilities. Many continue to work for prisoner's rights, for those held in psychiatric wards, institutions, and by 'community treatment orders,' for those losing or being denied housing, for those being assaulted in 'care' or experiencing psy-sanism at work or in the helping professions. All of this work and more goes on. Additionally, given our understanding that sanism is an expression of white supremacist settler colonial violence, the ongoing movements for Indigenous Sovereignty, Resurgence, Land Back, and water are also vital to resisting the proliferation of sanism(s) we see and feel every day. Colonialism seeks to dehumanize so it can destroy. Sanism is just one way it does that, turning mad or otherwise identified folx into diagnoses, disorders, and 'dangerous' non-humans.

Perhaps our (best) efforts to spread the word or 'raise consciousness' about sanism has in many ways fallen flat because the disappointing reality is that wherever power is at stake, someone stands to benefit from its imbalance. Those carrying around what Wolframe (2013) has called a 'sane privilege backpack' (perhaps unknowingly) may seemingly have very little to gain from resisting sanism individually and/or joining in the Mad fight. So, many of us are able to safely sit in a place of "wilful hermeneutical ignorance," (Pohlhaus, 2012) paying mind only to those social issues that concern us or pose a threat to our comfort.

Summary

The concept of sanism is not new. It is a concept that has been studied and written about for many, many decades in a range of arenas, including disability rights law, across the (so-called) helping professions, in higher education, and the fields of (critical) disability studies and Mad Studies. While public awareness of the term does seem to be growing – albeit only marginally – the effects of sanism in the lives of mad folx seems to have intensified; or are at the very least, not letting up. While some of this may be owing to a lack of agreement over the most appropriate terminology to describe the mistreatment that mad folx continue to face (i.e., mental health stigma versus sanism), perhaps more troubling is the realization that sanism's relentlessness stems from its confluence and inseparability from the other 'isms' that shore up matrices of domination (like the eugenics project and white supremacy). Neglecting to acknowledge this confluence will no doubt be futile. Speaking sanism needs to mean speaking of it as a *settler* sanism; one that is always and inevitably intertwined with and in a mutually beneficial relationship with racism and colonialism. Our resistance efforts against sanism and toward liberation for mad folx need to be rooted in the disability justice principle of *collective liberation* (Sins Invalid, 2015).

References

Berlant, L. (2007). Slow death (sovereignty, obesity, lateral agency). *Critical Inquiry, 33*(4), 754–780.

Birnbaum, M. (1960). The right to treatment. *American Bar Association Journal,* 499–505.

Brown, C. (2020). Critical clinical social work: Theoretical and practical considerations. In C. Brown & J. MacDonald (Eds.), *Critical clinical social work: Counterstorying for social justice* (pp. IX–XXXIX). Canadian Scholars Press.

Burstow, B. (Ed.). (2016). *Psychiatry interrogated: An institutional ethnography anthology.* Springer.

Castrodale, M. A. (2017). Critical disability studies and mad studies: Enabling new pedagogies in practice. *The Canadian Journal for the Study of Adult Education, 29*(1), 49–66.

Castrodale, M. A. (2018). Teaching (with) dis/ability and madness. In M. S. Jeffress (Ed.), *International perspectives on teaching with disability: Overcoming obstacles and enriching lives* (pp. 188–204). Routledge.

Chamberlin, J. (1978). *On our own: Patient-controlled alternatives to the mental health system.* McGraw-Hill Publishing.

Chamberlin, J. (1990). The ex-patients' movement: Where we've been and where we're going. *The Journal of Mind and Behavior, 11*(3–4), 323–336.

Chapman, C., Azevedo, J., Ballen, R., & Poole, J. (2016). A kind of collective freezing-out: How helping professionals' regulatory bodies create "incompetence" and increase distress. In *Psychiatry interrogated* (pp. 41–61). Palgrave Macmillan.

Devandas-Aguilar, C. (2019, April). *End of mission statement by the United Nations special rapporteur on the rights of persons with disabilities.* United Nations Human Rights: Office of the High Commissioner. Retrieved from https://www.ohchr.org/EN/NewsEvents/Pages/DisplayNews.aspx?NewsID=24481&LangID=E.

Diamond, S. (2013). What makes us a community? Reflections on building solidarity in anti-sanist praxis. In B. A. LeFrançois, R. Menzies, & G. Reaume (Eds.), *Mad matters: A critical reader in Canadian mad studies* (pp. 64–78). Canadian Scholars Press.

Didyk, L. A. (2016). *Centering sanism: Stories & visions for mad-positive mental health* [Unpublished Major Research Paper]. Master of Social Work, Ryerson University.

Disability Filibuster (2021, March). *Disabled Canadians and our allies around the world leave it all on the field in the final days of the Bill C7 debate.* Retrieved from https://disabilityfilibuster.ca/

Dotson, K. (2011). Tracking epistemic violence, tracking practices of silencing. *Hypatia, 26*(2), 236–257.

Fabris, E. (2011). *Tranquil prisons: Chemical incarceration under community treatment orders.* University of Toronto Press.

Guterres, J. E. (2018). *Who is enough? An investigation into experiences of exclusion within critical mental health and mad organizing* [Unpublished Major Research Paper]. Master of Social Work, Ryerson University.

Hamer, H. (2011). *Inside the city walls: Mental health service users' journeys towards full citizenship* [Doctoral dissertation, University of Auckland]. ResearchSpace at The University of Auckland. https://researchspace.auckland.ac.nz/handle/2292/11915

Harrison, E. A., Sheth, A. J., Kish, J., VanPuymbrouck, L. H., Heffron, J. L., Lee, D., Mahaffey, L., & The Occupational Therapy and Disability Studies Network. (2021). Guest Editorial – Disability studies and occupational therapy: Renewing the call for change. *American Journal of Occupational Therapy, 75*, 7504170010.

Holley, L. C., Stromwall, L. K., & Bashor, K. H. (2012). Reconceptualizing stigma toward a critical anti-oppression paradigm. *Stigma Research and Action, 2*(2), 51–61.

Joseph, A. (2015). Beyond intersectionalities of identity or interlocking analyses of difference: Confluence and the problematic of "anti"-oppression. *Intersectionalities: A Global Journal of Social Work Analysis, Research, Polity, and Practice, 4*(1), 15–39. https://journals.library.mun.ca/ojs/index.php/IJ/article/view/1407/1226

Joseph, A. (2019). Constituting 'lived experience' discourses in mental health: The ethics of identification/representation and the erasure of intergenerational colonial violence. *Journal of Ethics in Mental Health, 10*(Open Volume), 1–23. https://jemh.ca/issues/v9/documents/JEMH%20Inclusion%20i.pdf

Kurchina-Tyson, A. (2017). *Surveilling 'stigma': Reading mental health literacy as a colonial text* [Master's thesis, Laurentian University]. LU|ZONE|UL. https://zone.biblio.laurentian.ca/handle/10219/2790

Landry, D. (2021, April 28). *"In the business of changing lives": Activist knowledge-practices and the founding of Ontario's consumer/survivor businesses* [Conference panel]. Enacting Disability Justice Panel, presented by Critical Disability Studies Student Association at York University, Toronto, ON, Canada.

Large, M., & Ryan, C. J. (2012). Sanism, stigma and the belief in dangerousness. *Australian & New Zealand Journal of Psychiatry, 46*(11), 1099–1100. https://doi.org/10.1177/0004867412440193.

LeBlanc, S., & Kinsella, E. A. (2016). Toward epistemic justice: A critically reflexive examination of 'sanism' and implications for knowledge generation. *Studies in Social Justice, 10*(1), 59–78. https://doi.org/10.26522/ssj.v10i1.1324

LeBlanc-Omstead, S., & Kinsella, E. A. (2019). Shedding light on a 'hidden prejudice': Considering sanism in occupational therapy. *Occupational Therapy Now, 21*(2), 15–16.

LeFrançois, B., Menzies, R., & Reaume, G. (Eds.). (2013). *Mad matters: A critical reader in Canadian Mad Studies.* Canadian Scholars Press.

Lewis, T. A. (2019, March 5). *Longmore lecture: Context, clarity & grounding.* Talila A. Lewis. https://www.talilalewis.com/blog/longmore-lecture-context-clarity-grounding

Lewis, T. A. (2020, August 17). *Why I don't use "anti-Black ableism" (& language longings).* Talila A. Lewis. https://www.talilalewis.com/blog/archives/08-2020

Lewis, T. A. (2021, January 1). *2021 working definition of ableism.* Talila A. Lewis. https://www.talilalewis.com/blog/january-2021-working-definition-of-ableism

McCarthy, K. & Doherty, B. (2019). Sanism and mad pride: Critical perspectives on mental health. *Occupational Therapy Faculty Conference Presentations, 2.* https://scholar.dominican.edu/occupational-therapy-faculty-conference-presentations/2

Mcnally, D. C., & Dosani, N. (2021, July 26). Violent, militarized park encampment clearings won't end homelessness in Toronto. Here's a human rights approach. *The Toronto Star.*

Meerai, S., Abdillahi, I., & Poole, J.. (2016). An introduction to anti-Black sanism. *Intersectionalities: A Global Journal of Social Work Analysis, Research, Polity, and Practice, 5*(3), 18–35. https://journals.library.mun.ca/ojs/index.php/IJ/article/view/1682

Mellifont, D. (2019). Last Bastion Nevermore! A qualitative exploration of the Australian government's fifth national mental health and suicide prevention plan from the perspective of lessening mental stigma and sanism in the workplace. *Studies in Social Justice, 13*(2), 283–303.

Morrow, M., & Hardie, S. L. (2014). *An intersectional approach to inequity. Creek's occupational therapy and mental health* (5th ed., pp. 188–203). Churchill Livingstone Elsevier.

Parry, J. W. (2005). The death penalty and persons with mental disabilities: A lethal dose of stigma, sanism, fear of violence, and faulty predictions of dangerousness. *Mental & Physical Disability Law Report, 29,* 667.

Perlin, M. L. (1992). On sanism. *SMU Law Review, 46*(2), 373–407. https://scholar.smu.edu/smulr/vol46/iss2/4

Perlin, M. L. (1993). ADA and persons with mental disabilities: Can sanist attitudes be undone. *Journal of Law and Health, 8*(1), 15–45. https://engagedscholarship.csuohio.edu/jlh/vol8/iss1/4/

Perlin, M. L. (2008). 'They're an illusion to me now': Forensic ethics, sanism and pretextuality. In D. Canter, & R. Zukauskiene (Eds.), *Psychology, crime and law: Bridging the gap* (pp. 239–253). Ashgate.

Perlin, M. L. (2009). "Simplify you, classify you": Stigma, stereotypes and civil rights in disability classification systems. *Georgia State University Law Review, 25*(3), 607–639. https://readingroom.law.gsu.edu/gsulr/vol25/iss3/6

Perlin, M. L. (2013). Sanism and the law. *American Medical Association Journal of Ethics, 15*(10), 878–885. https://doi.org/10.1001/virtualmentor.2013.15.10.msoc1-1310

Perlin, M. L., & Lynch, A. J. (2016). Mr. Bad Example: Why lawyers need to embrace therapeutic jurisprudence to root out sanism in the presentation of persons with mental disabilities. *Wyoming Law Review, 16,* 299.

Pohlhaus, G. (2012). Relational knowing and epistemic injustice: Toward a theory of willful hermeneutical ignorance. *Hypatia, 27*(4), 715–735.

Poole, J. & Jivraj, T. (2015). Mental health, mentalism and sanism. In J. D. Wright (Ed.), *International encyclopedia of the social & behavioural sciences* (2nd ed., vol. 15, pp. 200–203). Elsevier.

Poole, J., Jivraj, T., Arslanian, A., Bellows, K., Chiasson, S., Hakimy, H., Pasini, J., & Reid, J. (2012). Sanism, 'mental health', and social work/education: A review and call to action. *Intersectionalities: A Global Journal of Social Work Analysis, Research, Polity, and Practice, 1,* 20–36. https://journals.library.mun.ca/ojs/index.php/IJ/article/view/348

Poole, J., & LeBlanc-Omstead, S. (Forthcoming). *Sanism: Concepts, contestations and consideration.* TBD.

Procknow, G. (2017). Silence or sanism: A review of the dearth of discussions on mental illness in adult education. *New Horizons in Adult Education and Human Resource Development, 29*(2), 4–24. https://doi.org/10.1002/nha3.20175

Procknow, G. (2019). The pedagogy of saneness: Sane-centricity in popular culture as pedagogy. *New Horizons in Adult Education and Human Resource Development, 31*(1), 4–21. https://doi.org/10.1002/nha3.20237

Reaume, G. (2009). *Remembrance of patients past: Life at the Toronto hospital for the insane.* University of Toronto Press.

Reaume, G. (2012). Disability history in Canada: Present work in the field and future prospects. *Canadian Journal of Disability Studies, 1*(1), 35–81. https://doi.org/10.15353/cjds.v1i1.20

Reaume, G. (2019). Creating mad people's history as a university credit course since 2000. *New Horizons in adult education and human resource development, 31*(1), 22–39. https://doi-org.ezproxy.lib.ryerson.ca/10.1002/nha3.20238

Reid, J., & Poole, J. (2013). Mad students in the social work classroom? Notes from the beginnings of an inquiry. *Journal of Progressive Human Services, 24*(3), 209–222.

Sins Invalid. (2015, September 17). *10 principles of disability justice.* https://www.sinsinvalid.org/blog/10-principles-of-disability-justice

Spencer, M. (2020, July). Reporting the COVID crisis at psychiatric hospitals: A missed opportunity. *Mad in America.* Retrieved from https://www.madinamerica.com/2020/07/covid-crisis-psych-hospitals/

Thorneycroft, R. (2020). Crip theory and mad studies: Intersections and points of departure. *Canadian Journal of Disability Studies, 9*(1), 91–121. https://doi.org/10.15353/cjds.v9i1.597

Thornicroft, G., Rose, D., Kassam, A., & Sartorius, N. (2007). Stigma: Ignorance, prejudice or discrimination?. *The British Journal of Psychiatry, 190*(3), 192–193.

Van Veen, C., Ibrahim, M., & Morrow, M. (2018). Dangerous discourses: Masculinity, coercion, and psychiatry. In J. M. Kilty & E. Dej (Eds.), *Containing madness: Gender and 'psy' in institutional contexts* (pp. 241–265). Palgrave Macmillan.

Williams, V. (2014). *'Sanism', a socially acceptable prejudice: Addressing the prejudice associated with mental illness in the legal system.* [Doctoral dissertation, University of

Tasmania]. University of Tasmania Open Access Repository. https://eprints.utas.edu .au/18668/

Wilson, A., & Beresford, P. (2000). 'Anti-oppressive practice': Emancipation or appropriation?. *British Journal of Social Work, 30*(5), 553–573.

Wolframe, P. A. M. (2013). The madwoman in the academy, or, revealing the invisible straightjacket: Theorizing and teaching saneism and sane privilege. *Disability Studies Quarterly, 33*(1). https://dsq-sds.org/article/view/3425/3200

Chapter 27

On Being Insane in Sane Places

BREAKING INTO THE CULT OF THE MENTAL HEALTH INDUSTRY

Noel Hunter

Summary

One of the key paradoxes and conceptual rigidities of the mental health care system is the idea that people are either normal or pathological. This creates a rigid binary that does not do justice to the complexity of people. The mental health professions are largely predicated on the idea that there is a hard line between mental illness and mental wellness and, of course, that the professionals are on the side of wellness. This chapter explores the perspective of a psychologist who went into the field after her experiences as a "seriously mentally ill" patient. That combination, although it makes perfect sense that people might get interested in mental health work because of their own experiences, creates a category problem in rigid binary systems. Hunter discusses topics regarding conformity, silencing, denial, pseudoscience, and ideological blindness. Her goal is, at least momentarily, to bring down the stoic veil of normalcy within the mental health industry.

*

Like many teenage girls of my day, I held a mild obsession with the likes of Marilyn Monroe. She embodied an innocent naivete that somehow also held immense power and idyllic beauty. Posters of her iconic moments adorned my walls, and I would practice her breathy voice and quivering lips while listening endlessly to an album of her songs, which few others even knew existed.

It was not the platinum hair or tight-fitting dresses I was drawn to, however; rather, it was the immense yearning for love and the haunting pain in her eyes that exposed an agony few recognized. I felt an almost indescribable kinship with the woman underneath the caricature, not the sex object everyone else saw. Sadly, Norma Jean Baker, Monroe's real name, grew up with a chronically suicidal and abusive mother, an absent father, and a long history of being passed along and abandoned by

DOI: 10.4324/9781003148456-31

family while being used and objectified by others. Reading about her life and how she managed to overcome such loneliness without anger or cruelty was inspiring. In her films and stories, I discovered one of the few spaces in my life where I felt less alone, perhaps even hopeful. The therapy room, on the other hand, was rarely one of those spaces.

My own mother had a habit, or perhaps a talent, of projecting her internal nightmare onto everyone else, most often her children. Her screams of agony and wishes for death were frequently disowned and proclaimed to be ours. Thus, therapy and the mental health system was part of our life from as early as I can remember. Yet, it was not until my late teens, at the height of my Marilyn obsession, that I was forced to attend individual therapy for myself. It lasted approximately ten minutes.

In that short time, the woman asked almost immediately: "So, I hear that you are a fan of Marilyn Monroe?" To which I somewhat skeptically replied "Yes," hoping that this was an awkward attempt to connect to my wayward Gen X teenage aloofness. Instead, she immediately stated "Why? Because she committed suicide and you will too?" I had never expressed even the slightest suicidal urge in my life.

Not long after, though, my mother would actually die from suicide. I spent many years in and out of mental health services seeking relief and understanding that was not to be found amidst the assumptions, biases, and name-calling that stood in the way. In fact, the biggest lesson I learned was that the harder I sought it, the worse I became. One thing I did accomplish in all those years was racking up a total of ten different diagnoses, a period of experimentation with nine different psychiatric drugs, and the message that I was broken for life. Naturally, as with any good old reaction formation, I decided to pursue a career in the field.

The mental health professions are largely predicated on the idea that there is a hard line between mental illness and mental wellness, with professionals almost always being on the side of wellness. During the first half century of the development of formal psychotherapy, when psychoanalysis was the norm, it was well understood that happiness was not a realistic concept, at least not as a constant, that no lines existed between so-called normal and abnormal, and that the best any of us could hope for was a tolerable level of neuroses (see Freud, 1964).

Suffering and behavioral difficulties existed along a continuum, and trauma, especially in one's childhood, was what led one to creep further along that line. Additionally, during this time, having gone through one's own breakdown and subsequent analysis was seen as an asset, rather than a barrier, to being able to help others do the same. Of course, Sigmund Freud, who first made these ideas popular, veered into theoretical postulations of Oedipal Complexes and psychosexual urges, thereby establishing a chronic pattern within psychiatry of ignoring and dismissing trauma in favor of individual problems and fantasies. Nevertheless, the need for self-analysis and working through one's own neuroses was sacrosanct in becoming a psychoanalyst.

For instance, Carl Jung, one of the most prominent psychoanalysts aside from Freud, notably found himself in the midst of psychosis in his late 30s, describing himself as schizophrenic. Rather than give in to the idea of brain disease and permanent defect, he saw the opportunity in this breakdown to explore the unconscious and greater spiritual meanings in life. He documented much of his journey in what was published in 2009 as *The Red Book*. These experiences became the foundation for his form of psychoanalytic school of thought, still popular in many regions today.

As psychiatry and psychology began flourishing as mainstream professions, however, power dynamics and corruption began to influence many so-called advancements and the directions of change. From the advent of psychiatric drugs to the increased popularity of individual therapies, the mental health professions transformed from those of marginalized doctors overseeing society's rejects to being a central part of society's basic healthcare. In 1980, the *Diagnostic and Statistical Manual* (3rd ed., *DSM-III*; American Psychiatric Association) became a more formalized tool, modeling medical physicians' manuals filled with discrete illnesses, checklists, and medicalized terminology. This was based on consensus factors and politics, rather than actual scientific discoveries of tangible disease processes in the body (e.g., Kawa & Giordano, 2012).

At this same time, Western culture, particularly in the United States, became obsessed with happiness as an ideal that every person should strive for. Most commercials or advertisements promised this elusive state with just one more purchase. Pain and other emotions were nuisances to be erased. And a pill was to be had for everything. This trend continues in the modern day.

Gone was the concept of long-term and in-depth self-reflection and suffering as a means to building wisdom and empathy. Therapists were no longer human beings, but rather cogs in yet another assembly line of capitalist products. For sale were promises of symptom removal, cognitive reprogramming, and relatively quick fixes for life's problems. Hyper-sanity, self-care, and happiness became commodities that only expert clinicians could provide, usually for a hefty price.

A century ago, my experiences of overcoming childhood trauma and emotional breakdown, and the subsequent years of intense self-exploration, analysis, and healing would have been perceived as valuable tools for helping others. My wounds would have been guides toward greater attunement of transference and unconscious motivations and enactments. They would have offered the potential for non-verbal connection and an ability to understand the sometimes un-understandable. Perhaps even more, they might have even been considered spiritual gifts.

Today, however, they are secrets to be kept hidden lest someone find out that I am harboring a dormant life-long illness that could arise at any moment, like the Loch Ness Monster. I am made to be ashamed of what has happened to me and all the work and growth I have done because, according to modern canon, illness is not something that goes away. This is what the ideological medicalization and professionalization of emotional pain and human suffering has done to millions under the guise of objective science. Make no mistake, hard science this is not.

Beware You Might Just Be in a Cult

A cult is roughly defined as a group or movement that adheres to some kind of specific leader or ideology. Regardless of greater rhetoric, the idea that talking to a professional therapist or taking a pill to solve life's troubles is very much an ideology. Further, needing an expensive professional to feel emotionally and spiritually supported is a philosophy culturally based in capitalism. It is quintessentially American to think that one must be highly educated, cost money, and have exclusive expert knowledge for them to be of use in even the most innate and instinctual of activities.

A cult is not just a group that believes in similar ideas, but one where there is punishment if someone questions or defies accepted doctrine. I entered my doctoral studies with a fairly extensive awareness of the research demonstrating a clear link between more severe mental illness diagnoses with chronic childhood trauma (see, for example, Read et al., 2005). Further, there was little solid evidence for theories of genetics or biology playing causal roles in these experiences (e.g., Joseph, 2012; Ross, 2011), and much promise in psychosocial interventions in the process of recovery. These findings and paths of potential development are what made me excited to pursue a clinical degree in the first place. They also are what led me to be threatened with removal from school, training programs, and professionally sanctioned opportunities (see, Hunter, 2015, for a description). Turns out, challenging the status quo in the mental health field is both cause for discipline as well as an additional route for accruing new diagnoses of mental ill-health.

Perhaps an even more disturbing example of this habit of expelling heretics from its ranks is the story of Marcia Angell, former editor-in-chief of the *New England Journal of Medicine*, one of the most respected medical journals in the world. In 2009, she published *The Truth About the Drug Companies: How They Deceive Us and What to Do About It*, a controversial book documenting the problems of corruption within medicine. Upon her apparent devious act of speaking out against the status quo, this once prominent and revered physician was described at large as a conspiracy theorist and subsequently vilified widely by those in power (see Angell's essay, Steinbrook, Kassirer, & Angell, 2015, describing how critics are attacked and ostracized as a norm within medicine).

There is a need for absolute control in cults, and those who stray are marginalized or kicked out of the group altogether. More than anything, however, a cult tends to offer its members all the answers to life, like why bad things happen or why people do bad things. Psychiatry promises those answers in a secular bible called the *DSM*.

Of course, to be able to receive these answers, there are steps to earn such privilege and one is only told enough of what the leaders think they are capable of hearing. Forget about the almost decade of (very expensive) training and professional development years required to be an expert clinician. Or the number of trademarked certificates needed to prove one's worthiness in helping people overcome spiritual and relational pain. Patients themselves can never fully have all the answers, and to receive even some of them they must pay a hefty sum. While anyone can tick off a bunch of yes or no questions online to indicate a diagnosis that is based on a checklist, only the doctor can approve of a checklist of questions he or she expertly conducts. Friends are nice but can never provide support or care that rises to the level of a professional. Yoga, meditation, Tai Chi, and other modalities that have existed for thousands of years to help people in self-exploration and spiritual/emotional healing are seen, at best, as adjuncts to the real help: therapy and/or drugs. Patients must always continue receiving wisdom from their expert for it to be considered genuine.

They are almost never honored for having answers to their own life, especially when they contradict or conflict with the expert's wisdom.

Cult leaders also discourage obtaining information or answers outside of the cult, disparage behaviors or beliefs not accepted within the cult doctrine, and tend to have extensive propaganda and terminology that gives an air of special knowledge. During a particularly difficult period of my life, I decided to seek out therapy to finally address my childhood trauma. During the first intake session, a kindly gentleman asked many questions about my life, including details of my mother's death. What was my experience? What were the smells? He cried. I lost my mind. While still clinging to mere scraps of reality, I decided to decline his invitation to explore the many varied options of brain-altering drugs and instead decided to visit my yoga teacher who was trained in trauma-informed meditation and practice. In reaction to my defiance and apparent lack of insight, I was diagnosed with a new disorder and shunned the next time I tried to revisit the options of therapy at this facility. Reading my records from this time, the diagnosis did, indeed, come as a direct result of my decision to try yoga instead of psychiatry. Imagine getting diagnosed with heart disease because you declined your primary care doctor's advice to take Prozac.

In sum, cults are groups that manipulate and deceive in order to indoctrinate people into a certain belief system that is based on control, obedience, dependency, and conformity.[1] Of course, what really delineates a cult from any other philosophy or religion is how much wider society accepts its ideas. Are the mental health professions a cult any more so than any other ideological group, big or small, in any given community? Maybe, maybe not. But the fact that there could even be the consideration is itself something to be noted. For sure, it is not the objective hardline science it likes to have the image of being.

Pseudoscience as Objective Fact

There are many theories within the mental health professions as to what is normal, why humans act as they do, and what causes people to be *different*. There is the classic idea of the Oedipus conflict and sexual urges as the root of all evil (e.g., Freud, 1887-1902/1950); assertions of the deterioration of the brain and early dementia (dementia praecox, see Kraepelin, 1919); complex notions of split personalities and dissociation (Bleuler, 1950; Fromm-Reichman, 1948; Searles, 1965/1986; Sullivan, 1954); nuanced understandings of complex family dynamics and interpersonal trauma (Schwartz, 1995; Sullivan, 1954); clever taglines like "refrigerator mothers" (see Cohmer, 2014) or "satanic sex cults" (as was popular in the 1980s, see Fraser, 1990; Mulhern, 1994); bold proclamations that a person just thinks all wrong (e.g., cognitive behavioral theories); and, of course, the much-refuted yet ever-popular claim of chemical imbalances. And let us not forget about the once very central eugenics ideals of the basic inferiorities among races and ethnicities that psychology gave "scientific" evidence to support (e.g., Black, 2003).

Whatever the theory of causality, the current paradigm collectively falls under the ruling power of the *DSM*. The vast number of problems with the *DSM* has been detailed elsewhere (e.g., Deacon, 2013; Kinderman, Allsopp, & Cooke, 2017; Owen, 2014, Vanheule, 2017). In general, it is clear that this psychiatry bible lacks validity, and that the categories within do not map onto any objectively identifiable disease process. Yet, somehow these descriptive, loosely defined categories not only have become accepted as factual objective diseases that one "has," but also have come to provide causal explanations for the problems they describe.

This sets up a bullet-proof circular argument for mental health professionals. Imagine that one comes to a doctor saying, "I don't know doc, I just struggle with getting out of bed, I feel down all the time, and I really just hate myself and everyone else around me." Rather than spending time exploring why this might be, the first course of action is to find a label for what is wrong with the patient. The doctor does not want to seem like it is too easy, though, so instead of just saying it is depression outright, he or she says "Well, in order to come up with a differential diagnosis, let me give you this validated questionnaire." No mention is made of the fact that the questionnaire is asking questions based on preconceived biases of what depression is, what emotions are and are not acceptable, and the erroneous assumption that everything people experience is consciously available at the time of answering said questions. This aside, the person answers the questions and meets the minimum threshold for a diagnosis of Major Depressive Disorder. After an hour of exploring many questions and taking tests, the doctor comes back with the obvious: the diagnosis is depression. The patient, momentarily relieved at having a perceived explanation asks, "How do you know for sure?" To which the doctor says "Well, you endorsed certain symptoms that are known to be part of depression." "Ah," says the patient. "So, what causes these symptoms?" to which the doctor confidently replies "Well, depression of course!" In other words, you are sad because sadness causes you to be sad, and no, you cannot self-diagnose yourself as such.

In addition to varied conceptualizations of the problems themselves, there is also a rigid adherence to research designs that are formulated around randomized controlled studies and findings of statistical significance. No hard science utilizes such methods, as they are known to be rife with bias and bare little significance to real-world phenomena. Yet, they provide an air of sophistication and scientific authority. If something cannot be molded into such an experimental design, it is either determined to be unimportant or to not exist at all!

Worse, journals are notoriously biased toward accepting papers that demonstrate statistical significance, adhere to accepted wisdom, and are authored by known researchers, creating an overestimation of the legitimacy of current treatments while ignoring alternatives and negative outcomes (see, for instance, Bowcut et al., 2021; Dal-Re, Bobes, & Cuijpers, 2017; Kuhberger, Fritz, & Scherndl, 2014; Turner, 2013). This sets up a clear cycle of regurgitating the same information while denying access to alternative findings or holes within the current paradigm. Publication and overestimation biases, circular reasoning, cult-like ignorance of alternative findings, and silencing detractors are all fundamental to what makes something a pseudoscience.

Professionals Are Still Humans

There is little that is known for certain about the human mind and brain. There are, however, clear biases and functions that exist for all people, no matter their education,

IQ, or nationality. They are what allow magicians and psychics to astound millions. And they are central to much of what leads such well-intentioned people to do or contribute to illogical or even harmful practices. Even mental health professionals, no matter their claim on superior emotional and mental well-being, succumb to cognitive biases and ideological blindness that can lead to negative attitudes and poor care of vulnerable populations (e.g., Merino, Adams, & Hall, 2018).

The brain is designed first and foremost for efficiency, not rationality. It simply cannot process information without various filters and categorizing functions. Naturally, what gets sorted out tends to be things that a person either finds unimportant, distressing, or challenging to deeply held beliefs or one's ego. Unless one spends a great deal of time in meditation, analysis, or some other deep and ongoing self-reflection, odds are high that these processes largely operate outside of conscious awareness and automatically.

The ability to read the words on this page is due to previous awareness of the representation of the letters and their combinations that the brain can quickly put together in a familiar pattern that is language. These filtration and sorting processes combined with quick retrieval of familiar patterns and experiences are what allows humans to focus on what matters most at any given moment. They also are what lead to typical biases and cognitive errors that can become self-reinforcing over time. The following are just a few of the well-documented biases that tend to be prominent within the mental health professions at both individual and systemic levels (see, for example, Lilienfeld & Lynn, 2014; Snowden, 2003; Yager, Kay, & Kelsay, 2021).

Attributional Biases

In general, attributional biases are made when making judgments and interpretations about others' or one's own behaviors. Attribution theory originated in the 1950s by Fritz Heider and has since been widely studied throughout the social sciences. A number of specific types of attributional errors have been identified in the past 50 plus years, as well as how these biases may lead to certain emotional and behavioral reactions. Fundamental to all biases is the *self-serving* bias which refers to the need to maintain and preserve a positive sense of self (or a positive sense of one's group or family) for purposes of survival. As such, one is inclined to interpret successes as internally caused while negative outcomes are interpreted as due to external factors. Although this bias may not always be present, it most often arises in situations where an attribution is being made against a stranger or a member of the out-group.

At the group level, this same phenomenon is called the *group-serving bias*, wherein one's group is overvalued and any failures are interpreted as due to external factors (such as non-compliant patients or as-yet-to-be-identified illnesses). Considering that most professionals within the mental health fields perceive themselves as part of a group separate from the mentally ill, this broad cognitive error in judgment is likely to rear its ugly head in almost every interaction between professionals and service users.

People, particularly in more individualistic cultures such as the United States, tend to overestimate dispositional or intentional factors in making determinations about others' behaviors, while attributing one's own behaviors to more situational factors.

This *fundamental attribution error* underlies a tendency for mental health professionals, who are inclined to believe themselves to be part of the us, the hyper-sane, and not them, the mentally ill, to interpret their own emotional difficulties as due to their circumstances past and/or present. At the same time, service users, especially those who evoke emotions like anger or helplessness on the part of the clinician, are deemed to have something internally wrong with them that creates their difficulties, whether it is illness or defective personalities or both.

A particularly common form of attributional biases is within the plethora of genetics research that continues to be funded above psychosocial research despite little evidence to continue supporting it and absolutely no clinical utility (Erlandsson & Punzi, 2016; Ioannidis, 2016; Joyner, Paneth, & Ioannidis, 2016; Pickersgill et al., 2013). The *ultimate attribution error* (Pettigrew, 1979) is one wherein a stereotyped group is perceived to behave in problematic ways due to genetics. In other words, when a marginalized group, such as the "mentally ill," behave in ways perceived to be wrong it is because of their genes; however, when positive behaviors are observed, it is often interpreted as being an exception or due to external factors, such as treatment.

Confirmation Biases

Once a set of beliefs about how the world works is formed, the brain filters all new information through this framework. In so doing, it tends to filter out what does not fit with preconceived beliefs, distorts what cannot be filtered out as an interpretation that confirms these beliefs, and/or overestimates supporting evidence for these beliefs in order to support what one already "knows."

Confirmation biases have been documented in areas of diagnoses (e.g., Mendel et al., 2011), treatment evaluation (e.g., Yager, Kay, & Kelsay, 2021), forensic evaluations (e.g., Neal & Grisso, 2014), and policymaking systems within the mental health professions (Lilienfeld & Lynn, 2014). Just like all humans, clinicians see what they want to see, twist reality to fit with their distorted beliefs, and discount disconfirmatory evidence that creates cognitive dissonance. This can become a maddening loop for a patient under the power of a mental health professional wherein the only way one can be heard is if everything is framed in a way that the clinician accepts as truth.

Just-World Theory

The just-world theory (Lerner, 1980) is an oft-cited idea that people have a need to believe that the world is fundamentally good and that bad things only happen to bad people or because it was deserved. The belief in a just-world provides a relief to existential anxieties and fears of not being in control. It allows people to feel generally safe and that there is a sense of justice in the world.

This has been shown to be at the root of victim-blaming (van den Bos & Maas, 2009) and is often associated with adherence to religions or other ideologies (e.g., Hafer and Sutton, 2016). Just-world beliefs can lead to worse therapeutic outcomes and prejudices against people from lower socio-economic classes (e.g., Smith et al., 2011) and blaming of trauma survivors (e.g., Idisis, Ben-David, & Ben-Nachum,

2007). There is no greater support for belief in a just world than to assert that nefarious and mysterious mental illnesses are genetic causes of human suffering rather than face the random acts of cruelty and unfairness rampant throughout all cultures.

Sunk Cost Fallacy

Economics research has demonstrated the tendency for people to continue a behavior or endeavor into which they have already invested significant time, money, and effort. This tendency holds up even when others are the ones who have made the investment (e.g., Olivola, 2018). Perhaps due to an intolerance of cognitive dissonance or an ego-serving refusal to acknowledge that a person is wrong, getting trapped in the cognitive fallacy that one has already gone this far so may as well continue is common. Think of romantic relationships. The longer a couple is together, the harder it becomes to breakup.

Similarly, when one has spent years being indoctrinated into a particular way of thinking and written countless papers and essays on topics accepted as wise and true, while living with a six-figure student loan debt hanging over their head, it becomes quite difficult to admit that one's line of thinking may have been wrong.

Willful Blindness

Although this term originates as a legal term, the concept nonetheless is used to describe the ways in which a person or organization can be blind to the violations of laws and/or humanity that it is either directly causing or complicit to. A proverbial blind eye is turned to the reality of one's actions in order to preserve the ego, avoid conflict, and protect prestige and power. Under the law, this blindness is conceptualized as consciously willful.

In everyday human nature, however, these actions tend to be largely unconscious. Few people are knowingly and consciously lying to themselves in the name of hurting others. Abusive relationships, whether in romance or parental situations, tend to subsist due to willful blindness throughout the family. Most family members are not intentionally hurting each other or wanting children to be hurt. In fact, much abuse is done or allowed to continue in the name of "I'm doing this because I care about you."

Mental health professionals, in particular, tend to pride themselves on their identity as helper. There is a deep need to filter out anything that threatens this identity. Being able to hear and acknowledge the ways in which many mental health practices are not only harmful but a clear and direct violation of human and civil rights[2] is downright impossible for many.

This particularly deleterious cognitive error can be seen at conferences, on social media, in interviews, and more wherein a person presents information regarding some of the harms done within standard mental health and said person is met with personal insults, dismissiveness, claims of inferior education or outright ignorance, and even bullying. It seems these days it is common practice to name-call any critics of the modern mental health paradigm as "anti-psychiatry" and be done with it. As if by donning someone as a heretic proves their ignorance and all evidence he or she may have provided as seen as moot.

In the End There is No Them—Only Us

Much speculation has been had about the specific circumstances of Marilyn Monroe's death. Was it suicide? Did her doctor engage in malpractice? Was there a conspiracy? One thing that is not debated: the mental health professionals around her contributed to rather than mitigated her death. As of 2021, there continue to be commentaries popping up all over the internet and books in bookstores making conjectures as to her "mental illness," almost always concluding that she was a poster child for borderline personality disorder. Scarce is written about the little girl who just wanted a family who loved her and the woman who spent her life trying to fill that hole while dazzling the world. Instead, mental health professionals and all who express their ideas under the umbrella of current mental health ideology have summarily stripped this woman of her beauty, mystery, and mass appeal by boiling her down to a much-maligned label that serves as little more than an epithet. As it was throughout her life, she continues to be dehumanized and objectified, this time in the name of science.

It is hard to acknowledge how much is unknown and uncertain, and how little any of us can control the world around us; to be able to sit with not having answers as to why some children are abused, why some never find love, why some are trapped in poverty while others live a life of gluttony is unbearable to most. Vulnerability in the face of chaos can be overwhelmingly terrifying. But, if we cannot learn to accept ambiguity, uncertainty, and vulnerability even in the most traumatic of situations, what business do we have counseling others on how to live their lives?

Of course, there are many people in the helping professions at all levels who engage in the painstaking work of ongoing self-reflection, looking for alternative explanations and considering conflicting perspectives. Clearly, I myself consider therapy to be something that can be profoundly healing for many. But it is not necessary nor by any means the only way in which one might grow and heal from human suffering.

The proclamations of the system as a whole are to be taken with a grain of salt. The meteoric rise in diagnosable mental illness has run parallel to the rise of the current mental health paradigm. For instance, approximately 17% of Americans are on at least one psychiatric drug (Moore & Mattison, 2017), with a similar number on antidepressants alone in the United Kingdom (a record; "NHS prescribed record number of antidepressants," 2019). Yet, in the last two decades, suicide rates have increased by 35% (Hedegaard, Curtin, & Warner, 2020). It seems that hyper-sanity comes at a steep cost.

Until the mental health professions can start to welcome criticism, explore negative findings, acknowledge biases, and, perhaps more important than anything, recognize that there is no line between mental wellness and illness, then harm will continue to be propagated while understanding, compassion, and empathy become increasingly extinct. We are all human beings struggling in our own ways to cope with a tragic world. It sometimes takes years to really understand how any given individual's behaviors and reactions make perfect sense given the context in which they developed. And none of us has ever nor will we ever have all the answers to life. So, let us stop acting as if we do.

Notes

1 See, for instance, Steven Hassan's *Combating Cult Mind Control: The #1 Best-selling Guide to Protection, Rescue, and Recovery from Destructive Cults*. In his work, Hassan distinguishes between more benign cults that likely exist within our society and we barely notice, versus destructive cults that can result in mass death and ruined lives. His ideas about how to avoid such mind control are a list of the very things that might just get a person kicked out of a mental health program or job, or, as a patient, possibly getting kicked out of therapy or even hospitalized against one's will. These include things like doing your own research, trusting your intuition, asking questions and remaining skeptical, being wary of not being able to get straight answers, asking for proof, fact-checking leaders, and relying on friends and family for support sometimes to the exclusion of group members or leaders.

2 There have been many articles, books, internet posts, magazine articles, TED talks, and more that describe the numerous ways in which standard mental health practices have harmed some (see, for instance, Breggin, 2003; Cohen, 2005; Dillon, 2012; Lacasse & Leo, 2005; Magliano et al., 2013; Whitaker, 2010). There have also been assertions of institutionalized racism, sexism, and discrimination against the LGBTQ community (e.g., Wade, 1993). Further, there is a long history of central ties to the eugenics movement and biases within research that favor White and WEIRD individuals (Western, Educated, Industrialized, Rich, and Democratic; Nielson et al., 2017). Lastly, the United Nations Special Rapporteur on Torture and Other Cruel, Inhuman or Degrading Treatment or Punishment has declared certain practices within Western mental health violations of human rights and has called for substantial systemic change (Mendez, 2013).

References

American Psychiatric Association. (1980). *Diagnostic and statistical manual of mental disorders* (3rd ed.). Washington, D.C.: Author.

Black, E. (2003). *War against the weak: Eugenics and America's campaign to create a master race*. Washington, D. C.: Dialog Press.

Bleuler, E. (1950). *Dementia praecox or the group of schizophrenias*. (J. Zinkin, Trans.). New York: International Universities Press, Inc.

Bowcut, J., Levi, L., Livnah, O., Ross, J. S., Knable, M., Davidson, M., Davis, J. M., & Weiser, M. (2021). Misreporting of results in psychiatry. *Schizophrenia Bulletin*, sbab040, https://doi.org/10.1093/schbul/sbab040

Breggin, P. R. (2003). Psychopharmacology and human values. *Journal of Humanistic Psychology, 43*(2), 34–49.

Cohen, O. (2005). How do we recover? An analysis of psychiatric survivor oral histories. *Journal of Humanistic Psychology, 45*(3), 333–354.

Cohmer, S. (August, 2014). Early infantile autism and the refrigerator mother theory (1943–1970). *Embryo Project Encyclopedia*. ISSN: 1940-5030. http://embryo.asu.edu/handle/10776/8149

Dal-Re, R., Bobes, J., & Cuijpers, P. (2017). Why prudence is needed when interpreting articles reporting clinical trial results in mental health. *Trials, 18*, 143.

Deacon, B. J. (2013). The biomedical model of mental disorder: A critical analysis of its validity, utility, and effects on psychotherapy research. *Clinical Psychology Review, 33*, 846–861.

Dillon, J. (2012). Recovery from "psychosis." In *Experiencing Psychosis*. (J. Geekie, P. Randal, D. Lampshire, & J. Read, Eds.). New York: Routledge.

Erlandsson, S., & Punzi, E. (2016). Challenging the ADHD consensus. *International Journal of Qualitative Studies on Health and Well-being, 11*. doi.org/10.3402/qhw.v11 .31124

Fraser, G. A. (1990). Satanic ritual abuse: A cause of multiple personality disorder. *Journal of Child & Youth Care, Special Issue*, 55–65.

Freud, S. (1887–1902/1950). *The origins of psychoanalysis*. New York: Basic Books.

Freud, S. (1964). *The standard edition of the complete psychological works of Sigmund Freud*. (J. Strachey, Ed.). Macmillan.

Fromm-Reichmann, F. (1948). Notes on the development of treatment of schizophrenics by psychoanalytic therapy. *Psychiatry Journal for the Study of Interpersonal Processes, 11*, 263–273.

Hafer, C. L., & Sutton, R. (2016). Belief in a just world. In *Handbook of Social Justice Theory and Research*. (C. Sabbagh and M. Schmitt, Eds.). New York, NY: Springer.

Hedegaard, H., Curtin, S. C., & Warner, M. (April 2020). Increase in suicide mortality rate in the United States, 1999-2018. *NCHS Data Brief, 362*. Retrieved from https://www .cdc.gov/nchs/data/databriefs/db362-h.pdf

Hunter, N. (2015). Experiences of a "black sheep" in a clinical psychology doctoral program. In *Becoming a clinical psychologist: Personal stories of doctoral training*. (D. Knafo, R. Keisner, & S. Fiammenghi, Eds.). Lanham, MD: Rowman & Littlefield.

Idisis, Y., Ben-David, S., & Ben-Nachum, E. (2007). Attribution of blame to rape victims among therapists and non-therapists. *Behavioral Sciences & the Law, 25*(1), 103–120.

Ioannidis, J. P. A. (2016). Evidence-based medicine has been hijacked: A report to David Sackett. *Journal of Clinical Epidemiology, 73*, 82–86.

Joseph, J. (2012). The "missing heritability" of psychiatric disorders. Elusive genes or non-existent genes? *Applied Developmental Science, 16*(2), 65–83.

Joyner, M. J., Paneth, N., & Ioannidis, J. P. A. (2016). What happens when underperforming big ideas in research become entrenched? *JAMA, 316*(13), 1355–1356.

Kawa, S., & Giordano, J. (2012). A brief historicity of the Diagnostic and Statistical Manual of Mental Disorders: Issues and implications for the future of psychiatric canon and practice. *Philosophy, ethics, and humanities in medicine: PEHM, 7*(2). https://doi.org /10.1186/1747-5341-7-2

Kinderman, P., Allsopp, K., & Cooke, A. (2017). Responses to the publication of the American Psychiatric Association's DSM-5. *Journal of Humanistic Psychology, 57*(6), 625–649.

Kraepelin, E. (1919). *Dementia praecox and paraphrenia*. Chicago, IL: Chicago Medical Book Company.

Kuhberger, A., Fritz, A., & Scherndl, T. (2014). Publication bias in psychology: A diagnosis based on the correlation between effect size and sample size. *PLoS One, 9*(9), e105825.

Lacasse, J. R., & Leo, J. (2005). Serotonin and depression: A disconnect between the advertisements and the scientific literature. *PLoS Medicine, 2*(12), e393.

Lerner, M. J. (1980). The belief in a just world. In *The Belief in a Just World: A Fundamental Delusion*. (M. J. Lerner, Ed.). New York, NY: Springer.

Lilienfeld, S. O., & Lynn, S. J. (2014). Errors/biases in clinical decision making. In *The Encyclopedia of Clinical Psychology*. (R. L. Cautin and S. O. Lilienfeld, Eds.). https://doi.org/10.1002/9781118625392.wbecp567

Magliano, L., Read, J., Sagliocchi, A., Patalano, M., & Oliviero, N. (2013). Effect of diagnostic labeling and causal explanations on medical students' views about treatments for psychosis and the need to share information with service users. *Psychiatry Research*, *210*(2), 402–407.

Mendel, R., Traut-Mattausch, E., Jonas, E., Leucht, S., Kane, J. M., Maino, K., Kissling, W., & Hamann, J. (2011). Confirmation bias: Why psychiatrists stick to wrong preliminary diagnoses. *Psychological Medicine*, *41*(12), 2651–2659.

Mendez, J. E. (February 2013). Report of the Special Rapporteur on Torture and Other Cruel, Inhuman or Degrading Treatment or Punishment. 22nd session of the Human Rights Council, United Nations General Assembly, Agenda Item 3. Retrieved from: http://www.ohchr.org

Merino, Y., Adams, L., & Hall, W. (2018). Implicit bias and mental health professionals: Priorities and directions for research. *Psychiatric Services*, *69*(6), 723–725.

Moore, T. J., & Mattison, D. R. (February 2017). Adult utilization of psychiatric drugs and differences by sex, age, and race [Research Letter]. *JAMA Internal Medicine*, *177*(2), 274–275.

Mulhern, S. (1994). Satanism, ritual abuse, and multiple personality disorder: A sociohistorical perspective. *The International Journal of Clinical and Experimental Hypnosis*, *42*(4), 265–288.

Neal, T. M. S., & Grisso, T. (2014). The cognitive underpinnings of bias in forensic mental health evaluations. *Psychology, Public Policy, and Law*, *20*(2), 200-211.

NHS prescribed record number of antidepressants last year (2019, March 29). *BMJ*, *364*. Retrieved from: https://www.bmj.com/content/364/bmj.l1508.full

Nielson, M., Haun, D., Kartner, J., & Legare, C. H. (2017). The persistent sampling bias in developmental psychology: A call to action. *Journal of Experimental Child Psychology*, *162*, 31–38.

Olivola, C. Y. (2018). The interpersonal sunk-cost effect. *Psychological Science*, *29*(7), 1072–1083.

Owen, M. J. (2014). New approaches to psychiatric diagnostic classification. *Neuron*, *84*(3), 564–571.

Pettigrew, T. F. (1979). The ultimate attribution error: Extending Allport's cognitive analysis of prejudice. *Personality & Social Psychology Bulletin*, *5*, 461–476.

Pickersgill, M., Niewohner, J., Muller, R., Martin, P., & Cunningham-Burley, S. (2013). Mapping the new molecular landscape: Social dimensions of epigenetics. *New Genetics and Society*, *32*(4), 429–447.

Read, J., van Os, J., Morrison, A. P., & Ross, C. A. (2005). Childhood trauma, psychosis, and schizophrenia: A literature review with theoretical and clinical implications. *Acta Psychiatrica Scandinavica*, *114*, 303–318.

Ross, C. (2011). *The great psychiatry scam*. Richardson, TX: Manitou Communications, Inc.

Schwartz, R. C. (1995). *Internal family systems therapy*. New York: Guilford.

Searles, H. F. (1965/1986). *Collected papers on schizophrenia and related subjects.* (Reprint ed.). London: Karnac Books Ltd.

Smith, L., Mao, S., Perkins, S., & Ampuero, M. (2011). The relationship of clients' social class to early therapeutic impressions. *Counseling Psychology Quarterly, 24*(1), 15–27.

Snowden, L. R. (2003). Bias in mental health assessment and intervention: Theory and evidence. *American Journal of Public Health, 93*(2), 239–243.

Steinbrook, R., Kassirer, J. P., & Angell, M. (2015). Justifying conflicts of interest in medical journals: A very bad idea. [Essay]. *British Medical Journal, 350.*

Sullivan, H. S. (1954). *The interpersonal theory of psychiatry.* New York: Norton and Company, Inc.

Turner, E. (2013). Publication bias, with a focus on psychiatry: Causes and solutions. *CNS Drugs, 27*(6), 457–468.

Van den Bos, K., & Maas, M. (2009). On the psychology of the belief in a just world: Exploring experiential and rationalistic paths to victim blaming. *Personality and Social Psychology Bulletin, 35*(12), 1567–1578.

Vanheule, S. (2017). *Psychiatric diagnosis revisited – From DSM to clinical case formulation.* New York: Palgrave Macmillan.

Wade, J. C. (1993). Institutional racism: An analysis of the mental health system. *American Journal of Orthopsychiatry, 63*(4), 536–544.

Whitaker, R. (2010). *Anatomy of an Epidemic: Magic bullets, psychiatric drugs, and the astonishing rise of mental illness in America.* New York: Crown Publishers.

Yager, J., Kay, J., & Kelsay, K. (2021). Clinicians' cognitive and affective biases and the practice of psychotherapy. *The American Journal of Psychotherapy.* Retrieved online: https://doi.org/10.1176/appi.psychotherapy.20200025

Chapter 28

Therapy as a Tool in Dismantling Oppression[1]

Gitika Talwar

Summary

Gitika Talwar's essay, first published in India's Mariwala Health Initiative's *ReFrame III*, draws on her experience working as a therapist and mental health advocate with Bapu Trust in India and with the Cowlitz Tribe in the Seattle, Washington, area of the United States. She argues that a Eurocentric model of mental health is "deficit-based"; its use of allegedly neutral and objective diagnostic labels and methods risks blaming the victim without understanding and acknowledging the reality of oppression. Talwar advocates a "liberation psychology" approach to therapy, which focuses on the individual and their microsystems (e.g., family, friends, work, and school) but can also bring into view larger structures of oppression, exclusion, subordination, and alienation.

The therapist's work, as Talwar sees it, includes not only individual therapy but also working to dismantle oppressive ecosystems. This can involve active collaboration with community-based organizations working toward liberatory/anti-oppressive goals. Talwar argues that the therapist should be open and transparent about this advocacy work. This both/and work requires that the therapist hold together *both* personal work toward self care *and* collective multisystem resistance to oppression. As the therapist balances these different aspects of care, she also recognizes the users (of therapy) as the experts of their experience. Talwar concludes with a quote from Audre Lorde that is well worth repeating: "Caring for myself is not self-indulgence, it is self-preservation, and that is an act of political warfare."

*

Can therapy align with activism to dismantle the influence of oppressive systems, including (but not limited to) racism, casteism, and heteropatriarchy? Could mental health professionals be more vocal within and beyond the clinic about our proliberation and anti-oppressive values in order to become accomplices in the fight for liberation from oppression? This paper [chapter] reflects on how therapy could be a tool to fight oppression by prioritizing "collective multisystemic resistance

DOI: 10.4324/9781003148456-32

and new realities" over "individual Eurocentric symptom reduction" (French et al., 2020).

A Eurocentric model of mental health is deficit-based and uses diagnostic labels to describe a user (client) who, in turn, is expected to be "treated" by an apolitical, value-neutral, and ahistorical therapist. Consistent with the writings and activism of its founder, Latin-American social psychologist Ignacio Martín-Baró,[2] liberation psychology runs counter to the kind of political neutrality typically adopted by mainstream Eurocentric mental health practices (Levine, 2014; Lykes, 2012). Therapists[3] must strive to understand injustice and oppression, and be explicit about their stance against it. When mental health theory meets liberation psychology, therapists attempt to influence the macrosystem, with its incumbent structural inequalities, and devise ways to disrupt its impact. As opposed to adapting to systems because they are typical, we can question systems that are unacceptable. For example, within the framework of feminist therapy, a survivor of domestic violence is supported in seeking a life free from violence. The therapist adopts an explicit position by communicating that violence is unacceptable and responsibility for violence lies with the perpetrator.

A liberation[4] psychology framework acknowledges a multilayered ecosystem. According to Urie Bronfenbrenner (a Russian-American psychologist), who originally proposed this ecological framework in the 1970s, an individual is embedded in a *microsystem* (e.g., family, friends, work, school), a *mesosystem* of relationships within their microsystem (e.g., relationship between family and work), an *exosystem* that indirectly impacts them (e.g., physical environment), and a *macrosystem* of cultural attitudes and ideologies (e.g., casteism or patriarchy). Revisions of the model included a *chronosystem*, which includes lifelong events, historical events, and the like (Bronfenbrenner, 1994). Oppressive ideologies maintain structural inequalities through their influence over the macrosystem and exosystem; for example, anti-Black racism makes the Black community in the U.S. vulnerable to police brutality; casteism among Hindu communities in India, Nepal, and their diaspora can make it harder for people to access education and safe livelihoods; and religious fundamentalism can be used to justify the persecution of religious minorities and the homogenization of neighborhoods.

Mainstream therapy focuses on surviving the trauma of the ecosystem and prioritizes individualistic emotion- and problem-focussed strategies of coping, risking a myopic response to oppression that implicitly blames the victim—for example, failure is a result of not trying hard enough. When the focus of change is limited to the individual's microsystem without acknowledging the reality of oppression, therapy risks becoming a tool for people to adapt to their oppression by either denying the influence of this oppression or disengaging from it (Phillips et al., 2015). Denial and disengagement are reflected in a therapist's silence around oppressive systems that impact the user, particularly avoiding discussion of how the therapist's own privilege or lived experience with oppression impacts the therapeutic relationship. Problem-focussed strategies of coping, such as compensation and empowerment, also prioritize an oppressive system at the cost of those trying to survive it—for example, the Dalit community working doubly hard to get what the Savarna community earns by virtue of unearned caste-privilege

I propose a liberatory therapeutic framework in which therapists collaborate with users to understand how their ecosystem oppresses them and undercuts their sense of agency. Secondly, therapists use a strengths-based lens to celebrate resilience and amplify users' efforts to use their feelings as feedback about needs, which can guide advocating for change while also developing the stamina and self-compassion to prepare for the ongoing process of sociopolitical change. Thus, therapy is embedded in a feedback-informed framework where the therapist and user are two experts who co-create healing by developing a vision for change. The therapist is the mental health expert whereas the user is the expert of their experience. Therapists also invite users to call upon the wisdom anchored in their spirituality, community-held history, and practices. In that sense, the therapist also attempts to undercut the colonizing perspectives embedded in the field of mental health, which is dominated by Euro-American values (e.g. individualism and definitions of "evidence" that reject wisdom passed through non-European or non-American channels).

When therapists actively seek feedback from users about their therapeutic alliance, there is an opportunity to collaboratively create space for healing. Additionally, therapists acknowledge their own role in dismantling an oppressive ecosystem when they vocalize a commitment to liberatory/anti-oppressive values through concrete actions within and beyond the clinic—for example, perhaps an engaged social media or web presence or active collaboration with community-based organizations. Active collaboration with community-based organizations also invites wisdom around the unique mental health needs of the community, the impact of structural inequalities, and/or intergenerational trauma.

In my therapeutic work I also integrate a toolkit for people of color[5] (Adames & Chavez-Duenas, 2017). A line in this toolkit is central to my work: "*The system does not get to determine your worth, dignity and humanity.*" This line is a reminder to create space between one's self-concept and the messages communicated by oppressive systems, thus protecting oneself from internalizing oppressive messages while persevering toward liberation.

Liberatory Framework in Action

A 23-year-old cisgender Sikh-American woman presented with anxiety about failing medical school due to her inability to focus on her studies.[6] During our session she processed how classroom discussions about health disparities had perpetuated racial stereotypes and she felt particularly attuned to the similarity between the racist assumptions made by her classmates and other healthcare professionals. While she experienced rage, her professor and classmates upheld an "objective" (read: devoid of feelings) stance, rendering her mute and making her question whether she could succeed in medical school if "mere class discussions" affected her like this. Validating her rage created a safe space for her to acknowledge the impact of racial microaggressions. I invited her to use her feelings as feedback about her values. She articulated the hope for better discussion about health disparities, and a vision for working toward an equitable healthcare system. We discussed ways she could connect with professionals who shared her vision and could serve as role models. Her rage helped her connect with her values and her vision for the future. Actively celebrating her family's excitement and support around her career goals, she recalled her ancestors who did not have the same oppurtunities she experienced. This offered her a greater sense of meaning and enlarged her perspectives in ways that acknowledged racism but did not center it. Our collaborative therapeutic work is focussed on supporting the steps she takes toward a career in healthcare, ensuring that systems that uphold *White privilege* do not lead her to question her own values and dreams.

Therapy as a Radical Act of Self Care

Emotion-focussed strategies can be used in service of awareness rather than denial and disengagement. A liberatory framework could make therapy more relevant to communities that are silenced by a mental health framework that pathologizes their valid response to oppression. For instance, mindfulness as an emotion-focussed strategy can be used to restore communities fighting oppression by centering their voices in the research and development of mindfulness curriculum (Black, 2017). Correspondingly, privileged communities could use emotion-focussed strategies to build their stamina for listening to the impact of oppression rather than disengaging from it. For instance, Savarna privilege continues to be deeply embedded in the Indian context (including the diaspora) and liberation from the caste system requires Savarnas to respond to feedback with readiness for change rather than denial and disengagement.

On the topic of mindfulness, therapists also need to interrogate the way therapy spaces appropriate ancient practices without regard for the culture and values in which those practices are embedded. A colonial perspective grants cherry-picking of ideas and practices that uphold colonial-capitalist values of productivity and rugged individualism. A decolonizing perspective would honor the spiritual values and wisdom of those practices and explore ways to foster healing, connection and community.

Therapists may also be confronted with the challenge of users who hold privileged identities and who may fear exclusion or judgment by a therapist who names anti-oppressive and decolonial values. This scenario poses an important invitation to the entire mental health practitioner community: How do we co-create healing spaces that address the pain and suffering that is perpetuated by capitalist-colonialist structures? How do we practice compassion and radical acceptance toward ourselves and others while also doing the difficult work of acknowledging privilege and acting in ways that dismantle its harmful effects? How do we use our own lived experience and access (or lack thereof) to power as opportunities to join users in our collective efforts toward liberation?

Therapy must be geared toward thriving alongside fighting oppression. A liberatory framework acknowledges oppression and privilege and ways in which the capitalist-colonialist structures impinge on the freedom of people everywhere.

A liberatory framework also celebrates the joy and legacy of communities that are otherwise viewed purely through a trauma-focussed lens. As Audre Lorde (1988) puts it, "Caring for myself is not self-indulgence, it is self-preservation, and that is an act of political warfare." In the face of ideologies that prioritize the perceptions of the privileged and delegitimize the experiences of the oppressed, entering a therapeutic space that validates and even celebrates liberation is a radical act.

Author Bio

Gitika Talwar, PhD
   Community-Clinical Psychologist and Immigration Advocate.
   Pre-2007: Therapist and mental health advocate with Bapu Trust and a counselor with Aanchal Trust: Support group for lesbian, bisexual, and transgender women.
   Post-2014: Psychologist with Cowlitz Tribe, where she served the urban Native American community in Seattle. She served the student community at the University of Washington-Seattle.

Notes

1 A previous version of this chapter appeared in Reframe (2020), *Beyond Clinical Contexts*, Mariwala Health Initiative, https://mhi.org.in/media/insight_files/ReFrame2020_Beyond_Clinical_Contexts.pdf

2 Ignacio Martín-Baró was a Spanish-born Jesuit priest trained in psychology at the University of Chicago. Through his writings and activism, Martin-Baro devoted his career to making psychology relevant to the community and the individual. During the Salvadoran Civil War, he was killed by the Salvadoran army in November 1989.

3 Martin-Baro explicitly named psychologists; I use this broader term instead, to include a range of disciplines.

4 I strive to use the term "liberation" instead of "anti-oppression" throughout this paper [chapter], analogous to using a strengths-based framework over a deficit-based one.

5 This toolkit is embedded in the sociopolitical context of the United States, where people of color and the Indigenous community experience oppression on the basis of race, gender, immigration status, [and/or] intergenerational trauma. My (evolving) manifesto is further informed by my experiences as a therapist and therapy user and an immigration activist in the United States.

6 To protect confidentiality, this user experience is a fictionalized version of a similar experience.

References

Adames, H. Y., & Chavez- Dueñas, N. Y. (2017). Surviving and resisting hate: A toolkit for people of color. *IC-RACE*. Retrieved April 27, 2020, from https://icrace.files .wordpress.com/2017/09/icrace-toolkit-for-poc.pdf

Black, A. R. (2017). Disrupting systemic whiteness in the mindfulness movement. *Mindful*. Retrieved April 27, 2020, from https://www.mindful.org/disrupting-systemic-whiteness-mindfulness-movement/

Bronfenbrenner, U. (1994). Ecological models of human development. In *International encyclopedia of education* (2nd ed., Vol. 3). Elsevier. Reprinted in Gauvain, M. & Cole, M. (Eds.), Readings on the development of children (2nd ed., 1994, pp. 37–43). Freeman.

French, B. H., Lewis, J. A., Mosley, D. V., Adames, H. Y., Chavez-Duenas, N. Y., Chen, G. A., & Neville, H. A. (2020). Toward a psychological framework of radical healing in communities of color. *The Counseling Psychologist*, *48*(1), 14–46. https://doi.org/10.1177/0011000019843506

Levine, B. E. (2014). Why an assassinated psychologist—Ignored by US psychologists—Is being honored. *Truthout*. https://truthout.org/articles/why-an-assassinated-psychologist-ignored-by-us-psychologists-is-being-honored/

Lorde, A. (1988). *A burst of light and other essays*. Firebrand Books.

Lykes, B (2012). One legacy among many: The Ignacio Martín-Baro fund for mental health and human rights at 21, peace and conflict. *Journal of Peace Psychology*, *18*(1). https://martinbarofund.org/media/readings/

Phillips, N. L., Adams, G., & Salter, P. S. (2015). Beyond adaptation: Decolonizing approaches to coping with oppression. *Journal of Social and Political Psychology*, *3*(1), 365–387. https://doi.org/10.5964/jspp.v3i1.310

Chapter 29

Decolonizing Psychotherapy by Owning Our Madness

Debbie-Ann Chambers

Summary

Chambers asks a key question in this chapter "Is it possible to decolonize oneself?" She answers it through describing her experiences working with the late Frederick Hickling CD, DM, FRCPsych (UK)—an innovative Jamaican transcultural psychiatrist who developed cultural therapies that moved away from individualized clinical models. Hickling found that standard clinical approaches could not effectively challenge the impact of "centuries of White supremacy and colonial oppression, the symptoms of a European psychosis." He developed Psychohistoriographic Cultural Therapy and Dream-A-World Therapy (DAW-CT) for children, which use a team of artists, schoolteachers, and therapists to do cultural process work through theater/art/music/dance sessions.

Chambers found that these group settings were invaluable for "overstanding," a Rastafarian neologism—overcoming and understanding—her own internalized colonization. For Chambers, the process of psychic decolonization was not an individual process, individualism itself being a colonial concept. Chambers found that she had to be in community with others to unbind herself from the "ghosts" of her traditional training, cross boundaries, and decenter herself. In her work with DAW-CT, she was not simply "helping" the marginalized but was joining with a group of people who, through their collective histories and uncovered wisdom, were "formidable knowledge producers and teachers."

*

"Understanding is good
Overstanding is better"

~ Adjani-Okpue Egbe, Artist/Activist

DOI: 10.4324/9781003148456-33

Decolonizing Psychotherapy

There are many things to be said about the need to liberate/decolonize Western psychotherapy. Scholars, including Martin Baro (1994), Friere (1972), Watkins (2015), Hickling (2016, 2020), and others have written about the a-historicity, decontextualization, and disembodiment often rooted in Western theory and practice. They have championed a decolonial praxis which includes developing theories that give preferential option to the economically poor, de-institutionalizing mental health care, accompaniment, negating the negation of racist ideologies, and reclaiming the healing power of indigenous culture so often lost "to the fire that is colonization" (Umebinyuo, 2015, p.). My aim for this chapter, however, is not to advocate for a particular counselling intervention based on the theories and practices of these scholars, though that it is an important task, it is to discuss the messy, destabilizing experience of engaging their decolonial methodologies. I hope to write of encountering the lingering colonialities within as we attempt to do this work. Colonization exists deep within our consciousness (Nandy, 1989) where it lingers and shapes our relationships and processes (Williams, 2016). Efforts to decolonize psychology, then, "require careful attention to the psychic decolonization of its practitioners" (Watkins, 2015, p. 324).

Who am I to take on this task of writing of the messy process of decolonization? I am a Black, "middle-class" Jamaican woman in her early forties who returned home, with social justice tools, after graduate education in North America. Engaging in the work of community mental health in Jamaica, I found myself struggling to use a social justice framework in this former plunder colony. The lessons I have learned and am still learning have raised important questions—Is it possible to decolonize oneself? What does it mean to own our madness in order to face post-colonial reality as the late Professor Frederick Hickling so astutely wrote? Why is it so difficult to shake loose the chains of Western ideology? Why does it matter—to others like me in the Global South and to my colleagues in the Global North that I should raise these questions? I rely heavily on the wisdom of the late Professor Frederick Hickling, Jamaican transcultural psychiatrist. Hickling's central thesis was that the challenge facing descendants of enslaved Africans in the Caribbean is to counter the impact of centuries of White supremacy and colonial oppression, the symptoms of a European psychosis (Hickling, 2016, 2020). We do so by owning our madness, that is, by coming to terms with our collective histories and traumas and recognizing our own negations of our personhood and culture.

The madness I encountered within myself, working in inner-city Jamaica and even now in a post-colonial university setting, is that many parts of me (history, language, and consciousness) were stymied in generations of colonization and this loss has obscured my vision of myself and others and influenced how I approach clinical practice. I have encountered a stubborn tendency to rely on the more traditional (i.e., Western) practices when faced with a lack of resources and institutional pressures, conditions that could otherwise activate a reliance on the decolonial methodologies. I use the term, overstand, a Rastafarian neologism (Pollard, 2000) which means deep, embodied insight, to capture the essence of the work of psychic decolonization as a practitioner of counselling psychology. Rastafarians are a subversive, indigenous religious and cultural group in Jamaica whose modes of speech, dress, religious practice, diet, and so on are a resistance to centuries of White supremacy in Jamaica (Chevannes, 1994).

The Jamaican Context

Jamaica is a Caribbean nation of approximately three million people. Though small, it is has produced some of the world's best-known sport and cultural icons and as such, has a "larger global profile than countries hundreds of times its size" (Patterson, 2019, p. 1). It has even ranked in the top 61 happiest countries in the world (Helliwell, Layard, Sachs, and De Neve, 2020). Contradictorily, Jamaica also has large problems—it is plagued by debt, urban poverty, gross income inequality, and high rates of crime and violence. It is, for example, at the time of this writing, the most murderous country in the Caribbean and Latin America (Harriot & Jones, 2016) with a murder rate of 46.5 per 100,000 people. It is these contradictions that have led noted sociologist, Orlando Patterson, to describe Jamaica as a "confounding island" (Patterson, 2019).

Jamaica's problems with poverty and violence have certainly been shaped by its 500-years history of slavery and colonialism. In her classic poem, "Reporting Back to Queen Isabella," Jamaica's former poet laureate, Lorna Goodison, points to the original violence of colonialism meted out to the indigenous peoples of Jamaica. In the prose, Goodison (2010) has Don Cristobal describe Jamaica as the "fairest isle" with an "overabundance of rivers, food and fat pastures for Spanish horses, men and cattle" and in the most dismissive way also states, "and yes, your majesty there were some people." It is this aspect of colonization that Cesaire (1972) refers to as "thingification"—a reinvention of the colonized as beings less than human, which wreaks enduring spiritual and material havoc in the lives of the colonized.

Jamaica's modern-day issues with violence are also shaped by neo-colonization—the political tribalism (Harriot & Jones, 2016) and economic underdevelopment that arises in its relationship to the economies of the West. Beckford (1999) pointed to Jamaica's plantation economy—a relic of colonialism preserved in neo-colonial trade arrangements—as the main ingredient in its persistent poverty. Patterson (2019) observed that Jamaica's problems with violence can be traced to the period following Jamaica's political independence from Britain in the 1960s when its two political parties began using a system of pork barrel politics to secure votes. This eventually led to the emergence of "garrison" constituencies, communities in which politicians are allied with gang leaders who control communities through violence and who provide much-needed state welfare services. In return for certain levels of immunity, the dons secure votes for the politicians. Thirty to 45 per cent of the capital city's population, mostly Black Jamaicans, live in these inner-city garrisons (Howard, 2005).

Pockets of Resistance

There are often resistance movements to oppressive regimes and ideologies; this is no different in Jamaica's context. The island's history is replete with resistance movements. From the rebellions of enslaved Africans on the island which forced the British to reassess the economic viability of slavery, to the cultural resistance of Rastafari pre- and post-independence. In the book, *Jah Kingdom, Rastafarians, Tanzania and Pan-Africanism in the Age of Decolonization*, Bedasse (2017) notes how the response to Rastafarians in the 1930s from the colonial governance was that they were "riffraff" (p. 20) who were mentally imbalanced; their madness was deemed criminal and as such they were targeted for institutionalization. Bedasse writes:

> Rastafarians saw [Europe's] construction of African inferiority as dialectically related to the construction of European superiority … far from mad, Rastafarians unveiled the insanity of the colonial project's invention of Africa and Africans to serve its own purposes.
>
> (p. 20)

In April of 1963, on Good Friday, the Christian holy day, just months after independence from Britain, Jamaica's first prime minister, Alexander Bustamante, ordered that all Rastafarians be brought in dead or alive, resulting in what is known as Bad Friday; many Rastafarians were murdered by police and several more incarcerated (Hippolyte, 2015). This event highlights the very real danger in advancing anti-colonial discourse and methodology.

Owning Madness: The Messy Process of Decolonization

For this auto-ethnography to make sense, I first need to situate myself in the Jamaican context. I was born and raised in a middle-class Jamaican family, more specifically, I was raised on a sugar estate (former slave estate); my father was the chief accountant and office manager. This meant that while I was surrounded by poverty, I did not experience poverty other than the social help my parents would often give to labourers and I did not accompany those in poverty. This type of cognitive and behavioural distancing from the poor (Lott, 2002) is quite typical in Jamaica. The suburbs of the main city to which I moved in seventh grade, are, for example, often nestled in gated communities safely from the crime of the garrisons.

I moved to New York City for graduate study in 2001. It was during this time that I had life changing contact with the economically poor and the structural violence persons deal with on a daily basis. I worked for two years as a case manager after graduation with the homeless, mentally ill in New York City and so experienced, for the first time, the degradation in navigating a system that did not benefit the people it was intended to serve. These experiences gave rise to an interest in the work of Friere (1972), Martin Baro (1994), and others—scholars who were introduced to me by mentors who saw my interest in social justice. I started to grapple with how I was complicit with an oppressive system in my own country and started to feel a restlessness to return home.

I returned to Jamaica after graduation and began working in the inner-city in a notoriously poor and violent area of Kingston. Within walking distance from the neighbourhood in which I worked, for example, was an infamous "garrison." The Jesuit, a close friend, who pastored a church in the area invited me to facilitate individual and group sessions and to help with the development and evaluation of community programs. On the first few days of working in the neighbourhood, several things were noticeable. There were a plethora of funeral homes—several on one street, one on almost every corner. A middle-aged, single mother whom I saw for individual sessions commented on this one day, saying that death was sold largescale to residents. There was also a lack of garbage collection that caused garbage to be strewn on vacant lots and in gullies and drains. Running water in homes was limited, causing several residents to share outside toilet facilities and standpipes. The heavy presence of soldiers and police in the community gave the community a feeling of being in a war zone. These conditions were indeed traumatogenic, meaning that the "individual and group physical safety, social security and symbolic capacities [were] all simultaneously assaulted" (Layton, Hollander, & Gutwill, 2006, p. 3).

When I began working in the inner-city, it became apparent that I was somehow crossing an age-old boundary, doing something that a well-educated "uptown" Jamaican woman was not do. I was working for people who would "never amount to anything" in the eyes of many Jamaicans. The messages subtly communicated to me by those outside of the context was that I would fail or worse, suffer violence. My own reactions revealed my dis-ease with the boundary crossings. I vividly remember, for example, being embarrassed one day when looking down at my feet and realizing that they were dusty from walking in the neighbourhood and that my shoes were looking well worn. Knowing I had to leave the community to go "uptown" to a meeting later that day left me with anxiety. Would I be seen as unprofessional? Would people know that I appeared this way not because I did not "know better" but because of the circumstances? I was perhaps ironically fearing, like the residents, that I was not amounting to much, that I would fall into an abyss that I could not possibly climb out of.

Other discomforts included the professional boundary crossings so typical in this type of work in the community. My "clients" were people I worked alongside handing out food parcels, people I attended mass with at the local church or hung out with in the shared community spaces. While on the one hand, my studies in social justice validated the need to step outside of the boundaries of Western therapy (Altman, 2010) and my own scholarly writing in graduate school recommended that therapists re-envision their practices in community settings and step outside of traditional paradigms (Smith et al., 2009), on the other hand, doing this work, mostly alone, surfaced anxieties that I was not abiding by the tenants of my profession. I would later call this anxiety, the colonial ghosts of traditional training.

I also struggled with feelings of helplessness and hopelessness. Residents faced a revolving door of crises. One crisis would no sooner be addressed than another crisis would surface. One after the other—housing, assault, hospitalization, death of a loved one, expulsion from a school, or unemployment. Referrals to the local mental health system occasionally added to traumatic experiences. I had the experience once of waiting with an adolescent 12 hours in a psychiatric clinic in rural Jamaica, only to never receive the psychiatric report needed to find the adolescent safe housing. The system seemed hopelessly broken. The attitudes of residents themselves lent to feelings of helplessness. A middle-age Black male of dark skin would unabashedly tell me that he would confide in no one of complexion darker than mine. None of my clinical interventions led to what I deemed insight about his internalized colonization/self-hatred. On days when overwhelmed by my reactions, I questioned my ability to do the work and after only two years I came to the conclusion that I had somehow failed. My immersion in the Jamaican inner-city had strongly confirmed what I had learned in my readings of liberation psychologies, and even what I had written about in professional papers— that is, my psychology had been vastly a-historical and a-contextual. However, applying that insight to the Jamaican inner-city context proved a struggle.

In 2014, I met Professor Frederick W. Hickling. The encounter re-animated my interest in liberation psychologies and raised new questions and hopes for where therapy could go in linking the social-historical to individual and societal behaviour. As a result, I became a member of his clinical research team. Professor Hickling developed Psychohistoriographic Cultural Therapy and Dream-A-World Cultural Therapy (DAW-CT) for children. These cultural therapies are based on ideas of historical analysis to negate historical amnesia and on retrieval of Caribbean cultural expression to negate the historical negation of Afro-Caribbean culture. [The full detailing of these therapies is outside of the scope of the paper, more information can be found in Hickling (2012) and Hickling (2016).]

In the DAW-CT intervention I worked as a cultural therapist with a team of creative artists and schoolteachers; we conducted cultural therapy sessions and art/music/dance sessions with eight- to nine-year-old children in an inner-city primary school. The children, selected by teachers, were those found to have poor academic functioning and/or conduct issues. The group dialogue was dialectical in nature and based on their fantasy of building a new planet on which they could take anything they wanted from this world and leave behind anything they did not want. The children animatedly talked about violence, death, poverty, pollution, and abuse as they fantasized about what they wanted to leave behind. They lent voice to their creative imagination by telling us what they wanted to create and created artistic performances from their insights. These insights were made part of a social discourse when they had a performance to which the Minister of Education was invited.

Working with the children was, as expected, difficult. The behavioural issues were obvious; the school resources were limited. However, the process was transformative. Professor Hickling held a two-hour team meeting each week. During those meetings, a team of artists, psychiatrists, psychologists, and researchers gathered to discuss the interventions' progress, historical events, social issues, and the controlling stereotypes that limited our actions. In those meetings, we would often be charged with shifting gaze from the children's "problems" to owning our madness—the acceptance of deeply colonial messages that caused the system to see the children as bad-behaving things rather than as persons with ontological vocations (Friere, 1972) for freedom. We began to consider that the children, as did we, had a generations-bred culture of resilience that could be activated in the right conditions. Professor Hickling also shared his own early struggle with a system that had deemed him "mad" for siding with the mentally ill incarcerated in the mental hospital, working to de-institutionalize the country's mental health system, and lauding the revolutionary concepts of Rastafarians.

Many more "overstandings," came in interaction with the children. In their natural curiosity, for example, the children would ask me whether I spoke patwah (Jamaican dialect), which high school I went to, or where I lived. These questions had a way of situating me along Jamaica's class hierarchy, and the children, freed in the DAW-CT process from the hierarchical school classroom arrangements, had a way of playfully demanding that I engage them in these discussions. My use of patwah, to the surprise of the children, made me acutely aware of how I engaged local dialect, when and where I spoke it and for what reasons. I experienced myself moving towards more fluency as the weeks rolled on, thus re-engaging, in an embodied way, with aspects of my culture. I was also able to see a definite positive shift in the relationships with the children when I owned my own dispossessed or hidden parts. Of note is that in this space there were no accusations from others about my not fulfilling my potential because of work in the inner-city. The children in this programme, because of their public performances uptown, had garnered much respect in and out of their community.

Engagement with the children, though at times disorienting, surfaced important inner and outer dialogue of who I was as a Jamaican and what cultural aspects of my Jamaican-ness were watered down by a Western education system. My play with the children, which was largely in Jamaican folk music and dance, drumming, and local ring games reignited cultural knowledge and strengths that could not be reignited otherwise. The interaction with the children in this created space also allowed me to view the children's strengths and resilience. This changed, for the better, how I interacted with them. Their poems, which they created themselves with help from the artists, speak to these strengths and resilience. Excerpts are below:

Poem 1.

> Wi want more books
> Wi want more books
> Tell govament seh wi nah
> tun crook
>
> Wi want more books inna we school
> Tell dem we nah tun fool
> Tell everyone we nah tun nuh cruff
> Dats why we waan wi book Dem nuff

Poem 2.

> Yuh see me? I love my family!
> Yuh see me? I love my mommy!

Yuh see me? I love my daddy!
Yuh see me? I never give up yet!
Yuh see me? Ago have success, waan bet?

The poems speak to their desires which were often not seen or taken for granted because they were inner-city children with behaviours deemed as bad or mad in wider society. The poems also speak of their demand to be seen as they were not as the classist, colonized lens deemed them to be. Similar to Hickling's work with patients in the psychiatric hospital in Jamaica, the art forced a re-evaluation of madness/badness.

Re-engaging Institutions

While the Dream-A-World programme catalysed my own psychic decolonization, I must honestly note how maintaining this process was a struggle in my later work in older institutions. What I discovered is that outside of the community of the DAW-CT space and its cultural engagements, I came face to face, once more, with colonial mindsets entrenched in older institutions, even when the mission is well-intentioned. Jamaican poet Kwame Dawes lyrically analyses the situation in his poem, *Ten Imperial Rules*. He writes:

avoid the stench
of reform, it splinters
a simple single sun
into galaxies
a constellation of distracting loyalties.

What I have noticed in myself as I navigate these spaces is an old reliance on the traditional tools of therapy—individual sessions in the office (or virtual space) and working long hours mostly in silos trying to manage the vast needs of a community. The challenge to decolonize has once again become disorienting. However, the lessons are not lost, and the messy struggle continues.

Overstanding

Disorientation

The story of my process highlights several important points. First, disorientation is part and parcel of decolonization. Boulbina (2019) noted that:

we must learn to become disoriented and thereby to become decentered from within ourselves and outside ourselves in order to be able to reach out to regions of humanity long considered backward by European standards

(p. 118)

I was so embedded in the inner-city community that it led to disorientation and decentring; I came into very real contact with parts of me that were disavowed through years of "formal" education. I also crossed cultural boundaries with respect to what is considered appropriate for my social class. In so doing, I crossed the age-old boundaries of class separation in slave practice in the Caribbean where "field slaves" were separated from "house slaves." Perhaps in that decentring, I faced a truth exhorted by Rex Nettleford, Jamaican icon and scholar, that we are all from the cane piece (Ellington, 2010). So, while I initially interpreted my anxieties, helplessness, and questions as failures, they were the decolonizing process at play, an antithesis to the colonial centring of power. Boulbina (2019) further stated:

> Disorientation should therefore not be understood as a failure or absence but as an action … it should not occur by chance but should be sought as a desirable type of perennial indeterminacy.
>
> (p. 122)

The Neo-Colonial Warp

Williams (2016) uses the term, neo-colonial warp, to mean, "a continuation of colonial practices which have become calcified and persistent" (p.2). He further stated that the space, though dysfunctional, is resilient because it is governed by the logic of coloniality, its attractor. While Williams uses this term to speak of the Trinidadian school system and its outmoded hierarchies, curricula, and disciplinary technologies, it could very easily describe my own experience. At times, the warp was outside of me—in institutions, in persons' reactions to my work, and in the culture of the community (such as the comments made to me by my client about skin colour). At other times, the warp seemed to exist within me and the ways in which I fell back on outmoded psychological practices. It also existed in the subtle and not so subtle denigration of culture and ancestral wisdom. My lack of engagement with local dialect in my everyday life was perhaps governed by the logic of coloniality. Erna Brodber, Jamaican sociologist and cultural historian, writes that black scholars have "conned ourselves into believing that true knowledge only exists in white space" (Brodber, 2017, p. 49). Furthermore, the denigration of our local language and cultural sayings results in lacunae in our self-knowledge; it is necessary "to fill this void in order to enact social change" (p. 50). Overstanding this neo-colonial warp and its blockade to filling the void in my own self-knowledge is a significant aspect of my decolonization process.

Community

My narrative strongly speaks to the need for community. Decolonization is not an individual process; it is antithetical to individualism which itself is a colonial concept. Watkins (2015) in referring to accompaniment noted that it is a different social order; it is a concept rooted in interdependency and community well-being, not in an individualistic paradigm. While Watkins speaks of the practitioner accompanying the economically poor and those that the status quo has marginalized, in my experience, the practitioner herself has to be accompanied by others for the psychic decolonization to take place. Professor Hickling and his team created a community around me—of elders and peers. I was the accompanied who:

> [felt] less abandoned and forgotten … In the press of daily struggles [I felt like the accompanied who] feel as though someone has taken the time to listen to their stories, to share the pain and grief they may be feeling, and to lift off their shoulders some of the burdens of the situation.
>
> (p. 329)

In that space, I could then feel secure enough to unbind myself from the "ghosts" of my traditional training to cross boundaries and decentre myself. However, I found that those I walked with in the inner-city were also not simply the accompanied. They formed part of the community; they were not simply the marginalized accompanied I "helped" but in the true sense of community (Dutta, 2018) they were themselves formidable knowledge producers and teachers.

Conclusion

My narrative points to the necessity of entering the messy, disorienting process of decolonization of self. The process, however, is never complete. Colonization is insidious and lingering; its vectors are strong and pull towards the status quo. To participate in this process, then, practitioners have to own their madness. For those who come from histories of colonization, this may mean owning the parts of them labelled mad, uncouth, or uncultured by colonial standards. To not do so is to stymie the power of movements meant to dismantle the logic of coloniality. Freedom, it is said, is a constant struggle. The work can only be done in community, where practitioners are both accompanied and the accompaniers.

Author Acknowledgement

The author would like to acknowledge Dr Nicole D'souza who worked alongside her in the inner-cities of Jamaica and who supported the drafting of this chapter. The author would also like to acknowledge the profound impact of the mentorship of the late Professor Frederick Hickling, Jamaican Transcultural Psychiatrist, on her work.

References

Altman, N. (2010). *The analyst in the inner city: Race, class, and culture through a psychoanalytic lens*. Taylor & Francis.

Beckford, G. L. (1999). *Persistent poverty: Underdevelopment in plantation economies of the third world*. University of West Indies Press.

Bedasse, M. A. (2017). *Jah kingdom: Rastafarians, Tanzania, and Pan-Africanism in the age of decolonization*. UNC Press Books.

Boulbina, S. (2019). Decolonization. *Political Concepts*. https://www.politicalconcepts .org/decolonization-seloua-luste-boulbina/

Brodber, E. (2017). Blackspace and knowledge production. In B. Ndikung (Ed.), *The incantation of the disquieting muse; On divinity, supra-realities or the exorcisement of witchery* (pp. 49–59). The Green Box.

Césaire, A. (1972). *Discourse on Colonialism. 1955* (J. Pinkham, Trans.). Monthly Review Press.

Chevannes, B. (1994). *Rastafari: Roots and ideology*. Syracuse University Press.

Dutta, U. (2018). Decolonizing "community" in community psychology. *American Journal of Community Psychology, 62*(3–4), 272–282.

Ellington, F. (2010, February 14–20). Remembering Prof. *The Sunday Herald*. https:// www.nlj.gov.jm/BN/Nettleford_Rex/bn_nettleford_rm_100.pdf

Freire, P. (1972). *Pedagogy of the oppressed* (M. B. Ramos, Trans.). Penguin Books. (Original work published in 1968).

Goodison, L. (2010). Reporting back to Queen Isabella, Donette Francis, and Sandra Pouchet Paquet. *Small Axe: A Caribbean Journal of Criticism, 14*(2), 179–183.

Hall, S. (1992). The question of cultural identity. In S. Hall, D. Held, & T. McGrew (Eds.), *Modernity and its futures* (pp. 273–325). Sage.

Harriot, A. D., & Jones, M. (2016). *Crime and violence in Jamaica: IDB series on crime and violence in the Caribbean*. Inter-American Development Bank (IDB).

Helliwell, J. F., Layard, R., Sachs, J., & De Neve, J. E. (Eds.) (2020). *World happiness report 2020*. Sustainable Development Solutions Network.

Hickling, F. W. (2012). Psychohistoriography: A post-colonial psychoanalytical and psychotherapeutic model. Jessica Kingsley Publishers.

Hickling, F. W. (2016). *Owning our madness, facing reality in post-colonial Jamaica*. The University of the West Indies: Carimensa.

Hickling, F. W. (2020). Owning our madness: Contributions of Jamaican psychiatry to decolonizing Global Mental Health. *Transcultural Psychiatry, 57*(1), 19–31.

Hickling, F. W., Guzder, J., Robertson-Hickling, H. A., & Walcott, G. W. (2015). Dream-AWorld cultural therapy "scale-up" intervention for school-aged high-risk primary school Jamaican children. *Asia-pacific Psychiatry, 7*(7).

Hippolyte, E. (2015). Bad Friday: Rastafari after coral gardens dir. by Deborah A. Thomas, John L. Jackson Jr. *African Studies Review, 58*(1), 279–281.

Holland, S., Renold, E., Ross, N. J., & Hillman, A. (2010). Power, agency and participatory agendas: A Critical exploration of young people's engagement in participative qualitative research. *Childhood, 17*(3), 360–375.

Howard, D. (2005). Kingston: A Cultural and Literary History. Signal Books.

Layton, L., Hollander, N., & Gutwill, S. (2006). *Psychoanalysis, class and politics*. Routledge.

Lott, B. (2002). Cognitive and behavioral distancing from the poor. *American Psychologist, 57*(2), 100.

Martin-Baro, I. (1994). *Writings for a liberation psychology* (A. Aron & S. Corne, Eds.). Harvard University Press.

Nandy, A. (1989). *Intimate enemy*. Oxford University Press.

Patterson, O. (2019). *The confounding Island: Jamaica and the postcolonial predicament*. Harvard University Press.

Pollard, V. (2000). *Dread Talk: the language of the rastafári*. McGill-Queen's Press-MQUP.

Smith, L., Chambers, D., & Bratini, L. (2009). When oppression is the pathogen: The participatory development of socially just mental health practice. *American Journal of Orthopsychiatry, 79*(2), 159–168.

Umebinyuo, I. (2015). *Homeland. Questions for Ada.* (S. Taaffe & I Umebinyuo, Eds.). Methuen.

Watkins, M. (2015). Psychosocial accompaniment. *Journal of Social and Political Psychology, 3*(1), 324–341.

Williams, H. M. A. (2016). Lingering colonialities as blockades to peace education: School violence in Trinidad. In M. Bajaj & M. Hantzopoulos (Eds.), *Peace education: International perspectives* (pp. 141–156). Bloomsbury.

Williams, H. M. A. (2019). A neocolonial warp of outmoded hierarchies, curricula and disciplinary technologies in Trinidad's educational system. *Critical Studies in Education, 60*(1), 93–112.

Chapter 30

Creating a Cultural Foundation to Contextualize and Integrate Spiritual Emergence

Katrina Michelle

Summary

Sanism intersects with racism, sexism, heteronormism, ageism, childism, ableism, classism, regionalism, and other structures of prejudice, subordination, and inequality. What is less understood is that sanism also intersects with scientism and secularism. These latter isms, scientism and secularism, are fixed—often unthought and unshakable—beliefs that scientific and secular worldviews are superior to other worldviews and represent the progress of civilization and the civilized mind. Unfortunately, these scientific and secular prejudices are common within mental health systems and are baked into the Enlightenment heritage of these systems from their beginnings. As Sigmund Freud put in *Civilization and its Discontents* (1961) with regard to religion and spirituality: "The whole thing is so patently infantile, so foreign to reality, that to anyone with a friendly attitude to humanity it is painful to think that the great majority of mortals will never be able to rise above this view of life" (74). And, even in his strong critique of psychiatry, Thomas Szasz, as we saw in Chapter 23, argued from a similar secularist prejudice against what he called the "theo-mythological foundation" of "religious fiction."

Katrina Michelle's chapter encourages the mental health field to let go of these scientist and secularists prejudices and integrate spiritual emergence into its domains of knowledge and practice. Nearly half of Americans describe having had a mystical experience of some kind. This number has increased dramatically over recent decades, indicating a trend toward the US public's acknowledgment of the role of the mystical and the spiritual in their lives.

Michelle uses the phrase *spiritual emergence* to refer to the developmental process of experiencing mystical or spiritual states. She describes these experiences as evolving over time for a given person and often as arising in times of crisis, need, or introspection. She challenges us to suspend the dominant antispiritual bent of current-day mental health practice in favor of embracing the spiritual as a path of exploration and self-discovery for clients. Michelle further shows how a spirituality-focused stance

DOI: 10.4324/9781003148456-34

has informed her own work and her life. By contextualizing lived experience through the lens of spiritual experience, Michelle forges an intriguing and promising ground on which practitioners might validate and learn from their clients' spiritual selves.

*

Creating a Cultural Foundation to Contextualize and Integrate Spiritual Emergence

When I was in my early twenties, I had a bizarre and immersive spontaneous experience that I could not articulate for many years. Other than the normalized level of stress one expects when riding the subway in New York, the episode had no exceptional precipitating factors, and arrived with neither conscious intention nor substance ingestion. It was as I walked down Lexington Avenue, on Manhattan's Upper East Side, during the course of an ordinary day, that my consciousness was overtaken. In an instant, the known boundaries of my personal identity dissolved and I was swept up into a timeless space of all-encompassing bliss, deep empathy, love, and recognition of my inherent interconnection with the hundreds of New Yorkers bustling around me. Accompanying this was a state of pure and trusted knowing, a revelatory claircognizance that offered a complete and instant recognition of the truths of the multiverse I could not have ever previously imagined. It was profound. It was overwhelming. It far exceeded the parameters of language for me to even begin to try to articulate it. The experience left me stunned, confused, and bewildered. I was absorbed into an infinite space beyond time, yet it was also fleeting, departing as quickly as it arrived, leaving me back in my body moments later to navigate the busy city street. For me, the experience was so awesome and intense that months and even years later, when I would recall it, the visceral memory of it would bring tears to my eyes.

William James (1902) described mystical experiences as having four distinct qualities. He named them to be inherently: (a) ineffable, defying expression so that they can only be understood through direct experience; (b) transient, being of a fleeting nature; (c) noetic, offering a quality of divine knowledge; and (d) passive, in that experiencers cannot control for when they arrive or depart. Reading James' (1902) definition of a mystical experience provided validation to me a decade later when I finally returned to school to study the phenomena. At the time though, as a psychology undergraduate, my rational mind could only interpret this experience through the lens of pathology, the only lens given to us in traditional mental health. A lens which presumes "normal experience" to preclude the mystical. "This must be the first sign of an impending psychotic break," I remember thinking. My grandmother had been diagnosed as schizophrenic and institutionalized. What I had learned in college had led me to believe that my brush with transcendence was actually a disordered genetic predisposition hinting at my fate.

A large-scale survey conducted by Pew Research Center in 2009 (NW et al., 2009) revealed that approximately half of the US public has had a mystical experience. Moreso, this research demonstrates that such experiences have been sharply on the rise since the first such survey in 1962 where only 22% of Americans reported such an experience. Described as a "moment of sudden religious insights or awakening," one in five of those who reported these experiences describe themselves as atheists or agnostics.

Over the past decade, secularized practices such as mindfulness meditation, yoga, breathwork, and psychedelics have become increasingly culturally sanctioned through growing popular interest, mainstream media coverage, and breakthrough scientific research. Yet, because of the dominant material worldview to which our culture subscribes, we have adopted these practices and methodologies distinct from their spiritual foundations. In doing so, we have made them more palatable to a populace hungry for stress reduction, productivity, and resolution for emotional afflictions like depression, burn out, and apathy. We have also given people more opportunities to prime themselves for transpersonal experiences which they have no language or framework to conceptualize.

With the rise of the strictly material worldview and the decline of religious affiliation and participation in spiritual communities, people are placing their trust in mental health professionals for support in making meaning of these extraordinary experiences. Yet, mental health professionals are not trained to be competent in addressing such phenomena, and as a result, often do more harm than good. Erroneous application of disease-model diagnoses that are often followed by psychopharmacological interventions coupled with invalidating and challenging of their clients' experiences often result in additional and complex traumas for those who came seeking solace, support, and guidance from professionals. In order to offer some practical guidelines for helping professionals and experiencers seeking support in this area, I offer an overview of some existing language and frameworks for understanding such experiences.

For the purposes of this chapter, I will define spirituality as the element of our experience that transcends the personal, sensory, material world, allowing for a sense of wonder, awe, and identification with something greater than ourselves. I will use the term "transpersonal" to describe the phenomena associated with the nonlinear states of mystical, spiritual experiences. In order to avoid the stigma associated for some with the word "spiritual," Taylor (2012) advocated for the use of the term "awakening experiences." In my own work, however, I have chosen to use the term "spiritual emergence," as I feel it most closely describes the psychospiritual developmental process of which I understand these phenomena to be a part. The related term, "spiritual emergency," demonstrates that the process of spiritual emergence is not always smooth and is used to describe the elements that can be quite chaotic and disruptive. The terms were first coined by LSD researcher and psychiatrist Stanislav Grof and his late wife Christina Grof (1989), who endured her own spiritual emergency following childbirth.

Researcher Rhea White (Brown, 2000) believed that engaging with one's transpersonal experiences, which she termed exceptional human experiences (EHSs), holds the potential to lead to profound positive transformation that includes an evolution of awareness and an increased sense of meaning in life. She compiled a broad and varied list of examples of these non-ordinary, spontaneous, transcendent experiences. The extensive selection of experiences includes experiences of mediumship, déjà vu, lucid dreaming, faith healing, intuition, kundalini awakening, near-death experiences, noetic experiences, past-life recall, pre-cognition, shamanic experiences, vision quest experiences, unitive experiences, and UFO encounters (Exceptional Human Experiences Network, 2021). These experiences of altered states offer us opportunities to enter into conscious processes of spiritual growth. White highlights the way we choose to engage with such phenomena as key to whether we potentiate or depotentiate the process of awakening (Brown, 2000).

William James (1902) discussed how awakening experiences can be spontaneous and suddenly transformative or of the more gradual and educational variety, being integrated over time as the system learns to hold them. Those who endure the more sudden experiences, without adequate time to understand and integrate them, especially when devoid of a framework of cultural support, may be the ones who find themselves in spiritual emergency. This process can create an array of imbalances, including psychosis, which may not be resolved until one's system has had time to settle into the new state of being and restore itself to equilibrium. In contrast, those who undergo the more educational, subtle progression of spiritual emergence are engaged in a slow and steady process of integration that allows homeostasis to be maintained (Grof & Grof, 1990).

The cognitive dissonance arising from being confronted with transpersonal phenomena for the first time could easily drive someone's memory of the experience into the unconscious, serving as a defense to protect the individual from something so foreign that it threatens to overwhelm the system and potentially lead to decompensation (Brown, 2000). This leads me to wonder about the 50% of the population in the Pew research who did not indicate experiencing transpersonal phenomena. I believe that in fact these transpersonal experiences are commonplace in the range of human experience. Yet, because of the cognitive dissonance at play for all of us, our memory of such events is absorbed by defense mechanisms in order to preserve the structure of the psyche, which may not possess the tools to successfully manage these intense experiences.

Case Study

One person approached me in my private practice several years ago to explore what she had been diagnosed to believe was a bipolar episode of mania. As a woman in her late twenties, she had no history of mental illness and no other precipitating factors. The episode, which consisted of spontaneous, uncontrollable laughter, a persistent state of bliss, and "God connection" for two weeks, was triggered through her graduate studies in spiritual psychology at a prestigious university the previous semester. She and her classmates were engaged in intensive coursework that led them into practical exploration of various spiritual practices. While the intentions of the university were to offer its students a buffet of samplings to add texture to their intellectual studies, what resulted was the activation of latent spiritual energies within my client, and several more of her colleagues. The university had failed to recognize the very real potential for spiritual emergence within its student body. They were immersed in a hodgepodge of introductory spiritual practices through modalities like breathwork, shamanic journeying, energy work, and so on. This institution, dedicated to elevating intellectual study, had failed to consider that the practices they had brought in experts from around the world to deliver could be harmful if not offered within a safe container that was equipped to support the unfolding spiritual energy such practices were established to awaken. Their grand oversight had led my client and others in the program to experience a wide range of transpersonal phenomena which they were ill-equipped to manage. By the time this client had found me a few months later, her episode had subsided and she was left with the scar of a bipolar diagnosis branded on her by an in-network psychiatrist with no education about spiritual emergency.

Our work together was brief, lasting only three months. Together, we reframed her experience as a spiritual emergency and discovered resources to validate her experience and deepen her understanding of the phenomenon. She also greatly benefited from participating in the support group I hosted at the time with others who had endured similar journeys of being misunderstood and pathologized within the mental health system. While our work terminated after a short period, we have kept in touch, and she has not had a similar episode in the five years that have since passed.

Clinical Considerations

While it is clear on many levels that our healthcare system is in need of overhaul, when it comes to sensitively addressing the needs of our clients, we cannot wait for the systemic reform that may well take decades. We can begin by encouraging mental health professionals to become trained in spiritual competencies. Regardless of the personal beliefs of the providers, universalizing our understanding that transpersonal experiences are a part of the normal spectrum of human experience will support all of us in sharing without fear of being shamed and pathologized. By restoring a foundation of trust to the client-therapist relationship in this area, we can support more people in disclosing their experiences, and then as a collective begin to weave a new narrative and begin to create a cultural foundation for spiritual emergence.

A positive step toward normalizing transpersonal experiences within mainstream psychiatry was taken in 1994 when the *Diagnostic and Statistical Manual of Mental Disorders* named a new diagnostic category, V62.89: Religious or Spiritual Problem (Lukoff et al., 2011). The category, updated since its inception for the current version of the manual, the *DSM-5,* can be used when the focus of clinical attention is a religious or spiritual problem. This includes distressing experiences that involve a loss or questioning of faith, problems associated with conversion to a new faith, or questioning of spiritual values that may not necessarily be related to an organized church or religious institution (APA, 2013, p. 725). The original recommendation of the contributors who proposed the category was that it be modified to also include mention of near-death experiences, mystical experiences, psychic experiences, experiences of alien abduction, possession, meditation, and spiritual practice-related experiences (Lukoff et al., 2011). That portion of the recommendation was denied. Nevertheless, the inclusion of this category, which is listed as a supplemental code influencing a client's reason for services, serves to distinguish a spiritual or religious problem as something other than a disease or disorder.

For clinicians who may encounter the client reporting transpersonal experiences, or perhaps as the language becomes more familiar, those self-identifying as going through a spiritual emergence, it is important to keep in mind that the presentation will vary from those who seem joyful to those who are distraught. The process is unique to each individual and a variety of circumstances in one's personal history, such as the presence of traumatic life experiences, quality of one's support system, and openness to experience may all play a role in how they respond. Drawing on your clinical experience, you will be able to assess for safety as you would any client before determining whether the person has adequate supplemental support for the process in which they are engaged.

A common question among mental health providers is around differential diagnosis for spiritual emergence and psychosis. Given the complex and unreliable nature of psychiatric diagnosis, it would be unfair to claim any clear delineations. In considering the nature of spiritual emergency, however, the crisis marks an opportunity for the person to emerge into a state of higher daily functioning, eventually coming to exhibit greatly improved mental health and well-being compared with one's norm prior to the experience (Grof & Grof, 1989; Lukoff, 1985). It is my belief that holding the therapeutic space for the client to positively engage with their process is part of what will determine their outcome to a higher state of daily functioning as opposed to a regressive one.

It is common for people going through the process of spiritual emergence to find themselves so profoundly impacted by an experience that they can no longer continue to function within the same systems, roles, occupations, and relationships that they had prior to the experience (Grof & Grof, 1989). Thus, you may find yourself supporting an individual in reconstructing her life from the ground up, as the consequence of her experiences may lead her to recognize she no longer aligns with the former values that led her to her career, partner, and way of being in the world. As with any significant shift in a person's life, it is best to work with them to make steady and deliberate changes over time rather than making hasty decisions that have long-term impact. Some people I have interviewed have found themselves called to give away millions of dollars when the impulse toward identification with the greater whole of humanity relieves them of their former need for accumulating and hoarding material wealth. You can imagine how one's spouse and children may react to such a person suddenly being moved to such extreme lifestyle changes. In such a situation, it may be easy for our own values to get in the way of how we meet our clients. Maintaining respect for their unique process and reflecting back healthy ways to go about making big changes will best support someone in healthily integrating their experiences.

Conclusion

Not only does our culture not provide us with examples of the latent potentials within our human experience but the systems in which we place our trust seem to encourage us to defer to outer authority and material science when determining the truths by which we live. As a culture, we have largely cut ourselves off from a core part of our nature as inter-connected beings supported by forces that defy the current limits of scientific study, or perhaps more accurately, what science chooses to fund in its research.

Although transpersonal experiences will by nature always be subjective, we can begin to normalize these experiences for individuals by integrating them into the mainstream culture. Just like it has become commonplace to attend a corporate meditation training or take a yoga class at the gym, we are beginning to see the use of psychedelics becoming standard practice within our mental health care system. While there is not necessarily always a precipitating event that leads to a spiritual experience, all of these practices are capable of inducing transpersonal phenomena, awakening us to the process of spiritual emergence or inciting spiritual emergency. As a culture, a responsible stance must include a reverence for the potentials that may arise and having the competency to support people when they do.

Underground psychedelic communities, working with altered states for healing and spiritual growth, have developed an understanding of the importance of supporting each other in integrating these consciousness-shifting experiences after the journeys are complete. It is common these days to find integration circles led by peers, or even therapists, during which people share stories of their experiences while others hold space to receive them without judgment or interpretation. I believe such community groups hold within them immense potential to empower individuals by normalizing their experiences. Beyond that, for those who have had challenging experiences, they can receive ongoing support from others who are more likely to relate.

Psychedelic communities generally have an understanding of the phenomenology of spiritual emergence and spiritual emergency. By creating more shared language and by leaning away from pathological interpretations, we can offer safety for those who find themselves in fear and guide those in need of support to professionals who can delicately hold all interpretations when considering what measures of care would be in the best interest of the person.

Spiritual emergence need not be a lone battle. It takes a community to properly contextualize, support, and integrate it. Creating a cultural foundation for spiritual emergence is not only important for personal development, but also for collective evolution. We are all in relationship to each other all the time. The immense power of the cultural magnet (Wilbur, 2000) shows we can either hold each other down or pull each other up. In order for the evolution of consciousness to occur, every individual must answer the call to spiritual emergence (Teilhard de Chardin, 1959).

Supporting the development of a shared language for and understanding of spiritual emergence matters. Being an uninformed culture is not only inhibiting growth but creating trauma through invalidation and pathologization. Currently, those who experience transpersonal phenomena are a marginalized and underserved population. We must begin to educate our mental health and spiritual professionals and normalize these experiences as a part of the human psycho spiritual developmental process. Together, we may then begin to contribute to a culture committed to embracing the beauty in our shadows and the painful processes that serve as gateways to genuine healing, self-awareness, and evolutionary growth.

www.drkatrinamichelle.com

References

American Psychiatric Association. (1994). *Diagnostic and statistical manual of mental disorders* (4th ed.). Author.

American Psychiatric Association. (2013). *Diagnostic and statistical manual of mental disorders* (5th ed.). Author.

Brown, S. V. (2000). The exceptional human experience process: A preliminary model with exploratory map. *International Journal of Parapsychology*, *11*(2), 69–111.

Exeptional Human Experiences Network. (n.d.). https://www.ehe.org/display/ehe-pagedc08.html?ID=3.

Grof, S., & Grof, C. (1989). *Spiritual emergency: When personal transformation becomes a crisis*. Penguin.

Grof, S., & Grof, C. (1990). *The stormy search for self: A guide for transformational growth through personal crisis*. Penguin.

James, W. (1902). *The varieties of the religious experience*. Longmans Green.

Lukoff, D. (1985). The diagnosis of mystical experiences with psychotic features. *The Journal of Transpersonal Psychology*, *17*(2), 155–181.

Lukoff, D., Lu, F., & Yang, C. P. (2011). DSM-IV religious and spiritual problems. In J. R. Peteet, F. Lu, & W. Narrow (Eds.), *Religious and spiritual issues in psychiatric diagnosis* (pp. 171–198). American Psychiatric Association.

NW, 1615 L. S., Washington, S. 800, & Inquiries, D. 20036 U.-4.-4. | M.-4.-4. | F.-4.-4. | M. (2009, December 9). *Many Americans mix multiple faiths*. Pew Research Center's Religion & Public Life Project. https://www.pewforum.org/2009/12/09/many-americans-mix-multiple-faiths.

Taylor, S. (2012). Spontaneous awakening experiences: Beyond religion and spiritual practice. *Journal of Transpersonal Psychology*, *44*(1), 73–91.

Teilhard de Chardin, P. (1959). *The phenomenon of man*. Harper.

Underhill, E. (1911). *Mysticism*. Dover.

Wilber, K. (2000). *A brief history of everything*. Shambhala.

Chapter 31

The Establishment
and the Mystic

MUSINGS ON RELATIONSHIPS
BETWEEN PSYCHOANALYSIS AND
HUMAN DEVELOPMENT

Marilyn Charles

Summary

Despite Freud's scientific and secular prejudice, there are those in psychoanalysis who have been open to and appreciative of mystical and other nonordinary experiences. Charles builds on her personal and clinical experiences to provide an insightful introduction to these strands in psychoanalysis. She organizes her approach to mystic and other nonordinary experiences through the work of influential British psychoanalyst Wilfred Bion (1897–1979).

Bion suggests that the establishment needs the mystic, and the new idea more broadly, in order to grow, however, at the same time, the establishment is reluctant to change. This creates an uneasy relationship in which growth potentials and mystic insights are resisted and may even be demonized by the group and by the individuals themselves. Bion notes that this happens because of a tendency to move toward safety and the avoidance of dramatic change, which we often experience as catastrophic. This tendency makes it hard for us to navigate changes and shifts of being that take us outside the tamed borders of what has become familiar. But, in contrast to that urge toward safety, individuals and groups also hold the capacity for curiosity, for learning, that invites us to push up against the familiar and to move into new territory. Those who seem compelled to traverse new terrain are often alone in these endeavours and may even feel alien and alienated.

Charles builds on this background to consider ways in which mystical experiences can be supported or undermined (even pathologized) in different therapeutic contexts. She argues for a sensitive therapeutic approach that offers an empathic

DOI: 10.4324/9781003148456-35

and supportive function. This kind of therapeutic resource can help people make meaning from experiences that might otherwise appear catastrophic.

*

When I was in graduate school, I read an article that noted the higher prevalence of what they termed *exceptional people* in families of people diagnosed with schizophrenia. That left me wondering about the capacities that underlie both illness and creativity, a question that has informed many of my explorations into the, at times, fine line between creativity and craziness (see, for example, Charles, 2015; Charles et al., 2011). Psychoanalytic theory, clinical experience, and personal reports suggest—in contrast to biomedical views of psychosis—that people are driven mad by their experience, and that respectful engagement is crucial to well-being, particularly for those such as Van Gogh, for example, whose perspective may be quite idiosyncratic (Charles & Telis, 2009). This latter fact also helps us to understand the plight of inconvenient women incarcerated by their husbands over the years (Charles, 2019). Power imbalances can be very dangerous when the dependent person's truths are not valued.

Humans are born utterly dependent on others for the care and meaning-making that inform identity development. We learn who we are through our relations with others who are both like and unlike ourselves. If caregivers are interested in our particularity, they can help us to better find our way rather than perhaps losing ourselves in our accommodations. But idiosyncrasy can leave us off-balance. Even seemingly small differences can affect our sense of self-in-world. As a left-handed person in a right-handed world, I can recall teachers who tormented me for using scissors incorrectly—turning them upside down so that the blade connected with the paper, which served the purpose but looked quite awkward, I am sure. I also recall my grandmother figuring out how to crochet backwards so that she could teach me the art. I think of her creative resourcefulness and respectful interest with pleasure and gratitude. I try to bring that type of respectful engagement into encounters with those unlike myself, to appreciate *their* gifts, their particularity.

Being somewhat idiosyncratic, myself, I recognize that diagnoses can be more a function of a failure on the part of those using such tools than a reflection of the actual status of the individual being diagnosed. I had an uneasy entry into the world of diagnoses and medical meanings. I could always see something of myself in textbooks and in my patients, which, I think, made me a better clinician but also increased my wariness of the harm that can be done by misunderstanding. That caution invites me to track very carefully the person's story and to be very interested in what they are trying to accomplish and where they encounter obstacles.

Having been born into a family with greater respect for facts than feelings, I yearned for some external validation for the facts I discovered through my feelings. On that journey, I found in Bion a father who, like my own, came from that far remote other side of the brain in which categories and logical reason prevail. Unlike my own father, however, Bion was desperately trying to get to the place where I live, that land of primary, embodied experience that I now think of as the aesthetic realm. Bion's writings helped to combat my father's indictment of me as a "messy kid whose intelligence was wasted" on her. In his writings, we can see him working towards an understanding (he hated that word) of human development that recognized how catastrophic real change can feel. He talked about the eternal choice point between growth and evasion with which we always contend. The realm we term "mystical" or "psychotic" represents one cliff we encounter in our efforts to move towards whatever truths glimmer beyond the knowledge we have received. This cliff becomes a fundamental reckoning point for those drawn by the desire to create meaning, which, according to Milner (1987), wells from "an internal necessity for inner organization, pattern, coherence, the basic need to discover identity in difference without which experience becomes chaos" (p. 84).

Idiosyncrasy and Marginalization

Cultural values affect how particular human qualities will be perceived. Part of what we see in the histories of those noted for idiosyncratic behaviour of whatever sort, is the type of isolation that easily accompanies difference. Marginalization can happen in many forms for many reasons and tends to be experienced as a mark of personal deficit rather than a social problem. Countering that tendency, psychoanalysis helps to contextual character by viewing symptoms in relation to the story being told. This stance seems particularly important with extreme states, for which the possibility of holding meaning is critical. Notably, Lacan speaks of psychosis as a position rather than a disorder, a marginalized position in which speech becomes distorted and it is difficult to hold meanings between people. My clinical experience speaks to the validity of this perspective: it seems clear to me from both the literature and personal and clinical experience that people are driven mad when sense cannot be made from their experience, and that psychotic symptoms tell a story that cannot otherwise be told. Context is everything.

Such difficulties can ensue when there are meanings that cannot be parsed within the family system so that the symptom marks the forbidden meaning in a disguised form. Research shows that in families in which mourning has not been resolved and the sequelae of trauma are carried across generations, inconsistent parenting leaves children vulnerable and dependent (Liotti, 1999; Main & Hess, 1990). Such data invite us to consider ways in which what we term "madness" is a socially constructed phenomenon, driven by the desire to ignore and avoid facing difficult truths, including loss, marginalization, and degradation. When meanings cannot be parsed, it is difficult to learn to make sense of embodied experience, alienating us not only from others but also from ourselves. Difficulties making sense from experience can be also driven by individual characteristics that provide a bad fit between parent and child, making it difficult to translate experience into consensual language.

Disorganized attachment, schizophrenia, and post-traumatic stress disorder are all diagnostic terms, lodged within a system of medical meanings. However, qualities deemed problematic when considered through that lens may, alternatively, be prized by cultures that value those who might be considered extraordinary (Johnson, 1981). The experience of "oneness," for example, can be found in both mystical and psychotic experience (Heriot-Maitland, 2008), an immersion into a primary unity that also typifies the aesthetic moment (Milner, 1987). The profound openness to experience and capacity for absorption integral to creative efforts are also found in psychotic and mystical experience. Studies suggest that *transliminality* may be the link that ties poetic and mystical consciousness together (Ghorbani et al., 2018). "Transliminality" has been defined as "a largely involuntary susceptibility to, and awareness of, large volumes of inwardly generated psychological phenomena of an ideational and affective kind" (Thalbourne & Delin, 1994, p. 25).

Considering commonalities and distinctions between the qualities of experience deemed psychotic or mystical may help us to make sense of ways in which the culture, itself, can either contain and sustain the individual having such experiences or, alternatively, literally alien-ate them in ways that drive them mad. A question undergirding this inquiry is to wonder in what ways the limits in understanding on the part of those who make decisions about such containing or alienating meanings further alienate us all from qualities that have deep and profound social and human value and, therefore, from ourselves and one another. Does our fear of the unknown lead us to founder the developmental efforts and creative capacities of those seekers who might open up different possibilities in whatever field of endeavour might draw them?

Some Clinical Examples

Let us consider a few clinical examples to contextualize our conversations. First, we have a young man who considered himself to be a "mad" painter, able to paint only during frenzied periods in the middle of the night. His painting instructor said that he was not merely a mad painter but rather a gifted artist who had trouble finding his way into painting without the ritual he had developed. The young man, however, felt that there was a forced choice between maintaining his sanity and being able to paint, and so he quit treatment. We can hope that, at some point, he revisited the issue of his psychological and emotional well-being sufficiently to have been able to paint and also build a life.

We can also consider a young woman who was derailed early on in her development. The child of a disturbed mother and a well-intentioned but relatively distant father, the young woman had become sorely distressed in adolescence at encountering erotic feelings that were considered damnable within the tight constraints of her religious community. She had, literally, been driven mad by forces she could neither control nor tolerate. The institutions to which she turned for assistance told her that she was psychotic and treated her accordingly. When I encountered her some years later, she expressed gratitude for having found a mental institution that treated her like a person, saying that this had saved her life. Through her fervent efforts, she was able to come to the limits of what medical treatment could offer and build her own resources through diligent devotion to self-care and personal and spiritual growth. We can wonder what her path might have been if she had been nested within a religious community that valued her idiosyncrasy and truth-seeking and preserved a protective space for her efforts at growth.

A third example is a young man who sought psychoanalytic treatment because he was distressed by difficulties finding his way within the world of people and relationships. Through his readings, he had found the term *schizoid,* and felt that this was a lexicon that recognized his particular difficulties. He, too, worked diligently at personal growth, using many of the strategies employed by the young woman mentioned previously, including reading texts and making diligent efforts in various spiritual practices in the service of truth-seeking. This young man was never diagnosed within the lexicon of medical science or treated from that perspective, leaving him freer to make his own meanings.

We also, of course, have the examples of individuals who have pursued the path of truth-seeking and spiritual growth more actively, and who have been recognized by their various communities as exemplary individuals. We have all likely met such people, who seem to emanate their own peaceful wisdom in ways that can be relieving and soothing to those around them. The working through of our personal demons can take many forms, and there is likely a price for any path. At some level, we are all utterly alone, and yet we are social creatures, dependent upon one another in profound ways.

Social Isolation, Marginalization, and Identity Development

In each of these examples, there was some inner drive, truth, or need in the individual that led the person on an uneasy path. The realm of the unknown presents both allure and fear. Schizophrenia, as a diagnosis, represents a particular conceptualization—and pathologizing—of human experience that formerly was linked with healing and religion (Johnson, 1981; Littlewood & Dein, 2013). Extreme events, such as trance and mystical experiences, have, at times, been held in high esteem, integral to the healing practices within certain social structures, including even within psychiatry itself (Johnson, 1981; Koss-Chioino, 2003).

With sufficient grounding, challenges provide opportunities for growth. Marginalization, however, poses particular difficulties, including increasing the risk of psychosis. Social fragmentation and other socioeconomic factors such as urbanicity, immigration, and socioeconomic level increase marginalization and deplete what have been termed *social capital* (a shared sense of identity based on shared norms, values, trust, and reciprocity) and *community belonging* (linked to physical and emotional attachment to place and persons) (Kirkbride et al., 2007; O'Donohue et al., 2016; Schellenberg et al., 2018). Social stigma is not merely a response to psychosis but is likely implicated in its aetiology (Janssen et al., 2003; Fearon et al., 2006), with social isolation, alienation, and marginalization having profound effects on the developing child and the vulnerable adult (Charles, 2013). Meanings are inevitably contextual, inviting us to consider more carefully links between what has been termed "madness" and mystical or spiritual experience.

The crucial relationships between social capital, community belonging, and identity development demand that environmental factors be taken into account when one is considering how meanings are made from experience. Community belonging is crucial to meaning-making itself. Disruption and social inequalities increase social isolation and impede the positive sense of community belonging so essential to self-worth and self-efficacy (Cantor-Graae & Selten, 2005). These factors also affect the ways in which symptoms are read (Bourque et al., 2011). Studies looking at theory-of-mind deficits highlight the importance of context in terms of how meanings are made, sustained, tested, and refined (Bentall et al., 2009; Kinderman et al., 1998). The presumption of illness makes it difficult to contextualize unusual experiences, make sense of them, and integrate an adaptive understanding.

The social matrix provides the context in which identity develops, at both the familial and the societal levels. Identity development is negotiated in relation to others who may be like and unlike us but who, importantly, sufficiently recognize us as individuals in order that we might locate ourselves in the engagement. In families that have carried the burden of too much trauma to integrate and absorb into the family narrative, the child is left with the impossible task of carrying that knowledge as a stain, a point of darkness the child is haunted by but cannot make sense of. Such knowledge tends to emerge in the form of a symptom that marks those impossible meanings. Legacies of social inequality and discrimination further problematize identity development. Without a secure community network to buffer distress, ongoing stress increases risk (Allardyce & Boydell, 2006) and shame further complicates development (Scheff et al., 2018).

Prevailing social "truths" can be uneasy companions when they demand blindness to other realities. In the gendering of social roles in Western society, for example, basic human values such as empathy and collectivity have been devalued in favour of "objective," rational knowledge in ways that undermine precisely those relationships that might otherwise be reparative. Also undermined is the ability to recognize and respond to the signal functions of affect and other nonverbal meanings so crucial to psychosocial development. Reading emotionality as a problem, without trying to understand the contexts in which symptoms have arisen, amplifies distress and confuses the effects of marginalization with individual attributions regarding "mental illness." This shift from the social to the individual erases precisely those contextual meanings through which individuals might find their way, even under oppressive circumstances—the type of mastery experience that can lead to a stronger identity and more supportive social relationships.

Cultural values affect what can and cannot be seen. We are all prey to the fear of the unknown that results in prejudiced readings of others' worth and behaviour (David, 2011). Along with the demonization of feelings in Western culture, the deprecative labelling of those suffering in our midst invites dangerous "cures" that increase harm rather than relieve suffering (Charles & O'Loughlin, 2013). These types of cultural blind spots not only allow atrocities to occur but also make the sequelae relatively invisible because of internalized negative stances we cannot see (David, 2011). These failures have in common an elision of abjection as a social process that cannot be repaired without attention to the ways in which such meanings become embodied (Fanon, 1952/2008).

Identity is formulated in the moment-by-moment interactions between self and other. Oppressive social forces impede positive self-regard and thereby not only obscure contextual meanings but also invite shame that makes the oppression difficult to recognize, much less fight off. Because identity is formed in the context of early relationships, these difficulties tend to be passed along the generations, becoming even more obscure over time. Psychoanalysis suggests that such meanings become *internalized*, and Tappan (2006) offers the term "appropriated oppression" to explicitly contextualize individual difficulties within the sociocultural context, highlighting the impact of systematic oppression (Banks & Stephens, 2018). Appropriated oppression, if unrecognized, is passed along from parent to child through the dialogical process of identity formation (Fivush et al., 2011).

Jouissance and the Intergenerational Transmission of Trauma

How can we make sense of this oppressive force that drives us towards destruction? Hook (2017) points to a subversive pleasure driving hostility towards difference that persists most strongly at the bodily level. He suggests that such pleasure is not repressed but rather disavowed, allowing a certain satisfaction that can be experienced without having to be recognized. *Jouissance* has to do with an intensity of feeling, characterized by an enjoyment that occurs in the margins, something illicit, that runs counter to what might be seen as acceptable in relation to prevailing norms. "Jouissance then is an enjoyment intermingled with suffering; it is a type of painful arousal poised on the verge of the traumatic; an enjoyment that stretches the subject beyond the bounds of the pleasurable" (p. 607).

Further, Hook suggests that the tendency towards intergroup suspicion, envy, and hatred is not an anomaly but rather is intrinsic to human being, in relation to the sense that others might have the thing one is lacking in the form of a subversive, stolen pleasure. Moving beyond convention represents a break with the social order that inevitably invites reactivity, a relationship that Bion (1977) casts as that of the establishment that needs the mystic in order to grow but fears the change that growth would require. From this perspective, we can think about the paradoxical relationship to the problem of lack pointed to by psychoanalytic conceptions, versus the encounter with lack pointed to in mystical experience. Whereas the former insists that we must face and come to terms with lack, the latter invites us to transcend and transform it.

Ataria (2016) adds to this conversation through his examination of similarities between mystical and traumatic experiences, pointing, in particular, to the encounter with nothingness that stands at the core of each. How we position ourselves in relation to the void is crucial. Vighi (2010) suggests that what is problematic in jouissance is that, when one moves towards an experience of surplus in relation to a void, the void is attributed to an other who is the cause of the lack. Rather than tolerating and thereby transforming the limits of human being through recognition of its ubiquity, one feels demeaned by the idea that something has been taken from us that is enjoyed by others. From that perspective, we can understand why any group that seems to be different will become the focus of not merely suspicion but also a retaliatory and envious hatred (Stavrakis, 1999).

Paradoxically, the guilt we feel for transgression feeds the tenaciousness of our hold on our positions. Psychosis, as something that speaks back to us about what has been closed out of the consensual consciousness and understanding, invites that type of tenacity. The move towards concreteness we find in psychotic speech marks the symbol and also the impossibility of making meaning from it *because* of the denial of the legitimacy of alternative perspectives. Denying alternative truths in this way has been called *epistemic injustice*, the marginalization of the legitimacy of an individuals' experiential truth, as knower of his own experience (Fricker, 2007). Such denial creates a context in which creative thought becomes subversive and even dangerous, conditions that can drive towards madness, against the alternative of internal deadness.

When the social surround misreads one's human value, then survival requires a certain level of isolation and self-protection from the deleterious projections. When essential meanings cannot be told, the holder of such meanings becomes both the symptom-bearer and the historian, telling the story that cannot otherwise be told (Davoine & Gaudillière, 2004). In contrast to ideas about psychosis that presume purely genetic or environmental origins, research points, rather, to a vulnerability model in which intrapersonal and environmental variables play important roles (Zubin & Spring, 1977). Because of what we know about the profound effects of early interpersonal environments on the neurocognitive as well as socio-emotional development of the child, it is important to be able to recognize both environmental vulnerability factors (Shonkoff & Phillips, 2000) and intrapersonal variables that may be linked not only with risk but also with other, more positive outcomes. We will return to this question later.

The Establishment and the Mystic

Recognizing the dysregulating effect of growth and the ways in which we resist whatever invites dysregulation, Bion's (1977) term "catastrophic change" marks the cataclysmic nature of profound psychic growth. He notes that this same tension also exists within groups, such that the *establishment* both needs and resists what he terms variously the *mystic* or the *new idea*. Lacan (1977b, 1977c) locates that tension between the desire for knowledge and the fear of believing in one's own knowing, which keeps us seeking knowledge from others rather than discovering our own. His notion of the *subject who is supposed to know* marks the desire for knowledge that resists learning but rather presumes that the knowledge sought is possessed by another who both keeps it from us and imposes it on us. Each of these theorists, in his own way, points towards the something-more that both entices and persecutes us and, at some level, remains forever out of reach. From this perspective, psychoanalysis takes on the challenge of encountering the unknown without turning away.

It may be precisely at the intersection between psychosis and spiritual experience that we encounter a dichotomy between our discomfort with not knowing and the ethical possibilities inherent in profound growth: catastrophic change. In some sense, we are called forward by the inevitable alterity of the other, the otherness that, in Levinas's (1999) terms, calls to us precisely because it is other. Civilization provides a structure within which we might meet one another—and also face the enormity of the suffering and destruction we encounter—with enough skin/armour to be able to survive. We can think of the cultural *establishment* in terms of the largely *imaginary* (in Lacan's sense) set of presumptions and projections we hold. This reverential scaffolding of cultural meanings and mores tends to imprison us within the confines of our superego-driven, fearful projections, leaving little room for the potentialities that might otherwise inhere.

The current trend in Western neoliberal culture positions religion as a defensive structure, marking the need to distinguish between religion as a societal structure and faith as an aspect of lived experience. The structure and the practice can have strikingly different correlates (Ghorbani et al., 2018). The urge towards the transcendent has been described as a fundamental human need (Fromm, 1950), a *mystical drive* (Ghent, 1990) that I think of, following Bion (1977), as an *aesthetic sensibility*. Gadamer (1975) marks the aesthetic as something inherently and vitally human that disrupts and thereby reveals cultural limits and expectations, inviting an experience of truth that moves beyond the particular, into the universal. This is the territory of Bion's (1977) *truth instinct*, the capacity to move towards either truth or evasion. At this level, development requires a frame through which we can come into finer attunement with an internal sense of truth, integrity, moral authority that is authorized not by an external being but rather by the type of internal sensibility that underlies all creative action.

Gadamer's attempts to locate the aesthetic in relation to truth and method are in line with Bion's definition of passion as a marker of meaning that can also drive us utterly astray. My experience is that those we call psychotic are often mystics who have lost their way, whose passions do not have sufficient context to hold meanings within a relational frame. In these times, when we are wary of spirituality and the structures through which we might meet our mystics with reverence, we tend to drive those seeking truth into the wilderness of the psychiatric establishment. The answers to be found in that realm have little to do with truth-seeking, moving, rather, into the realm of problem-solving. It matters whether we see human suffering as an integral part of living to be understood, worked with, and worked through, or we see such suffering as a mark of aberration to be reduced or eliminated. These are fundamentally different values that orient our efforts in markedly different directions.

Mystical and Psychotic Experience: Distinctions and Commonalities

Given the link between creative and mystical sensibilities (Ghorbani et al., 2018), it seems important to investigate commonalities and distinctions within different types of extreme states. Mystical experience resides in the realm of revelation: absolute, transcendent, and transformational. Its hallmarks are "its internal clarity, power and authority, and depth, as coming-from-elsewhere; its immediate, sudden, non-anticipatable quality such that each experience, each givenness … is experienced as 'overabundant'—suggesting a different kind of presence" (Steinbock, 2012, p. 598). The experience itself can vary, depending on the tenets and spiritual meanings within a particular religious frame. There are no absolute distinctions between mystical and psychotic experiences, rather, the differences lie in the meaning made from the experience (Feliou, 2016) and the impact on the person (Steinbock, 2012).

Without the context of the spiritual frame, a moment of inspiration can be unsettling unless one has some way of grounding oneself in relation to it. Although there can be a regressive feel to such moments, "the inherent rhythmic capacity of the psycho-physical organism can become a source of order that is more stable than reliance on an order imposed either from outside, or by the planning conscious mind" (Milner, 1987, p. 224).

The descriptions of visionary spiritual experiences of religious mystics and individuals diagnosed as psychotic tend to be quite similar (Stifler et al., 1993), distinguished most notably by the contextual meanings that enable the person to make sense of profound and numinous experiences within a consensual framework. Although both experiences involve a discontinuity of normal thought processes, longer lasting and more deleterious in the case of psychosis (Clarke, 2001), the mystical experience "concerns an individual in relationship with transcendent reality and with a community" (Cook, 2004, p. 154). The isolation from the social fabric can result in what Knoblauch (1985) terms an *ego-grasping orientation*, the need to exert control over self and environment, opposing the essential unity or implicit oneness presumed within a spiritual frame.

In Clarke's model, the ego strength of the subject is a critical factor, bringing to mind Jung's distinction between creativity as something into which one dips and psychosis as something into which one falls. From this perspective, sufficient controls are needed to actively explore the deeper recesses of mind and spirit without becoming lost or overwhelmed. Such protective scaffolding can come from the presumptions held in common with those around us as well as our own faith in ourselves.

Religiosity and spiritual experience have been pathologized by psychiatry. Through that lens, what might be termed numinous, mystical, or visionary spiritual moments become delusions and hallucinations (Baldacchino, 2016). In the absence of "clear dividing lines between veridical perceptions and hallucinations" (Collert et al., 2012, p. 85), the defining characteristic that distinguishes between ideology and psychopathology "is the sociocultural distance between the ideas and beliefs of the person holding them and his social reference group," most particularly, whatever group has the power to ordain meanings (Vardy & Kaplan, 2008, p. 478).

Psychopathology, then, may best be understood not in relation to the actual symptom but rather in terms of the social isolation that "isolates its bearer and renders him a deviant in his group by impeding his communication with the group members" (Vardy & Kaplan, 2008, p. 479). Much as in Bion's depiction of the relationship between the establishment and the mystic, visionary experiences may best be viewed not as purely personal but rather as relevant to all members of a community, offering "vicarious benefits to many as it informs and inspires their own experiences of human life" (Cook, 2004, p. 154). From that perspective, pathologizing such experiences distances us from potential learning about our own humanity.

We can see that the most important distinction between psychotic and mystical states lies not in the form or content but rather in the context in which the event occurs. Spiritual practice provides a framework through which to make sense of and integrate experiences that might otherwise prove destabilizing. The ability to return to a consensual framework and relate to the subjectivity of others and to one's own needs for self-care is crucial (Brett, 2003). Spiritual practice affords a way of recognizing links between the transcendent vision and the mundane world it relates to, such that the vision enriches our perception of our world and does not entirely isolate us from the social surround. In contrast, contends Brett, in psychosis, the investment is in preserving meaning by isolating it from the world from which it is drawn, which further isolates the individual. Artistic efforts can be seen as one means for preserving and sharing the meanings intuited in moments of creative inspiration.

Metaphors and Meaning

Similar to Brett's perspective (2003), the crucial dividing line for Lacan (1997) has to do not with reality but with the firmness of the conviction and the possibility of reflection. Psychotic speech becomes metonymic: there is no as-if, but rather *like* becomes *same*. Metaphor, in contrast, allows meanings to multiply, which requires not only semantic associative capacities but also an appreciation of other mental states that includes the possibility of an interchange between two separate minds (Ribolsi et al., 2015). Trauma can force meaning out of experience, making it difficult to make such connective links. The symptoms, then, mark the meanings that cannot be spoken, driving us towards madness if we cannot bridge the gaps (Davoine & Gaudillière, 2004). Trauma speaks in its own tongue, requiring what Felman (1995) calls *the witness,* to reinstate what has been omitted back into communal experience.

The de-realization of meaning can be seen as a refusal or inability to distinguish between the vision and the context in which it occurred (McGhee, 2003). In contrast:

> the Buddhist practitioner undergoes a transformation of their worldview, but they come to see the world differently, or more fully, or more adequately; they do not see a different world. The psychotic person falls into a state of delusion; the spiritual practitioner falls out of delusion.
>
> (p. 345)

Sufficient grounding is required in order to learn from the extreme experience rather than have reality collapse into an incomprehensible and untenable unity.

Psychosis and spiritual experience each seem to be nested in the primary process realm of experience, which functions at the level of metaphor, an aesthetic dimension in which "it is an inner harmony between the finite and infinite that fills the symbol with meaning" (Gadamer, 1975, p. 70). At that juncture, we are closer to the profound truths that are potentially transformative but entail a surrender to the unknown, transforming our relationship to both fear and possibility. For Gadamer, "the absolute moment in which a spectator stands is at once self-forgetfulness and reconciliation with the self. That which detaches from everything also gives him back the whole of his being" (p. 113); "the transformation is a transformation into the true" (p. 101).

This type of transformation is part of an intrinsic and evolving need for transcendence:

basic to a human being's ritual and aesthetic needs for a pervasive quality which we call the *numinous*: the aura of a hallowed presence. The numinous assures us, ever again, of *separateness transcended* and yet also of *distinctness confirmed,* and thus of the very basic sense of "I."

(Erikson, 1982, p. 12, italics in original)

A relationship to the sacred that *points beyond itself* (Tillich, 1957), this is the terrain of what psychoanalysts call the *third* perspective, which pulls us out of symbiotic or dyadic agreements in ways that allow space for creative engagement, the type of *play* that forms the bedrock of the universe of creative, aesthetic, and transcendent experience (Gadamer, 1975; Winnicott, 1971).

Psychoanalysis, as an enterprise that moves towards integration of primary and secondary process, provides a useful vertex through which to consider what may arise out of self-other experience but also transcend and transform it. This move towards transcendence is also the realm of aesthetic and religious ecstatic experience, informed by the primary process, through which familiar forms and patterns of experience resonate in ways that are profound and experience-near (Loewald, 1978). The encounter with such primary truths can be both tantalizing and terrifying, marked by patterns of emergent symbols that bring us into the realm of myth and metaphor. Symbols are not merely static but rather emergent functions that make it possible to recognize the multiple and potential meanings underlying what we had thought was merely "reality" (Milner, 1987). Because of their transformative potential, symbols "enable us to play with aspects of experience that are not accessible to conscious thought, including whatever might be too terrifying if it were to be perceived as too 'real'" (Charles, 2005, p. 487).

Psychoanalytic field theories invite respect for the possibilities afforded by a being-with-another that opens up rather than closes down possibilities. There is the inherent rhythmic capacity that Milner (1987) refers to in her expositions of the aesthetic sensibilities underlying creative activity. This creative area of transitional space has been described by Kristeva (1986a) as the *chora,* an underlying rhythmic, energetic patterning of experience upon which our becoming rests. Similar to Milner's recognition of the need to temporarily give up "the discriminating ego which stands apart and tries to see things objectively and rationally and without emotional colouring" (p. 97), Kristeva contrasts a *logic of identification* that locates itself within the dominant discourse of the society, with a *dynamic of signs.* The latter refuses linear temporality in favour of an aesthetic, spiritual discourse that calls to us directly, Milner's psycho-physical rhythms through which patterned meanings are recognized.

Although we tend to rely on verbal language to forge bonds with one another, words can be at odds with other ways of making meaning that are more driven by affect or "the infinitesimal significations with the relationships with the nature of their own bodies" (Kristeva, 1986b, p. 199). The allegiance to that type of internal truth marks a crucial ethical injunction that we also see in Bion and Lacan, who place a personal ethics—Bion's *truth instinct* (Grotstein, 2004; originally described in terms of *passion* in Bion, 1977) or Lacan's (1992) *desire of the subject*—at the heart of profound intrapsychic development.

Highlighting the importance of a more affectively engaged way of knowing, Kristeva (1982, 1986c) traces a path of embodied development that must come through the personal feelings that arise from facing the limit, not through the pillars of received knowledge. This leads, she suggests:

> to the active research, still rare, undoubtedly hesitant but always dissident, being carried out by women in the human sciences; particularly those attempts, in the wake of contemporary art, to break the code, to shatter language, to find a discourse closer to the body and emotions, to the unnamable repressed by the social contract.
>
> (1986c, p. 200)

In this way, Kristeva invites us to break through the constrictions of the social world that can become a "sacrificial contract" (p. 200). Kristeva's position here is similar to that of Lacan (1977b), who writes, "The function of language is not to inform but to evoke" (p. 86). Language speaks and hides in relation to our ambivalent desire to know and to be known, and yet, inevitably, we reveal ourselves: "The symptom *is* metaphor whether one likes it or not, as desire *is* metonymy" (Lacan, 1977a, p. 175).

And yet, as our investigations into differences between psychotic and spiritual experience show us, in the search for meaning—and for safety—we also must seek answers from without in order to anchor and organize our experience. For Campbell (1988), the position of the shaman, whose wisdom comes from direct experience, marks the allure of and aversion to direct knowledge. As the character who uses externally sanctioned authority to invite recognition of internal truths, the shaman serves a function similar to that of the psychoanalyst, a potential also present in the position of the mystic and the psychotic. Those who speak from beyond consensual knowledge are both desired and feared but also potentially form a bridge between internal and external truths in relation to one's own authenticity. Human development depends upon the external vantage point that helps to contain and organize our experience, but always in relation to our emergent capacity to make our own meanings in line with an internal sense of truth.

Epiphanic visionary experiences—including the psychotic and the mystical—can be seen as grounded in the types of deep truths embodied in Kristeva's *chora*, a rhythmic articulation rather than a disposition, "a nonexpressive totality formed by the drives and their stases in a motility that is as full of movement as it is regulated" (1986a, p. 93). "Nourishing and maternal" (p. 94), the chora is organized through an *ordering* rather than according to a law. Following Klein (1930/1975), Kristeva marks the transition from the concreteness of metonymic meanings towards symbol usage: "The kinetic functional stage of the *semiotic* precedes the establishment of the sign," (p. 95), she says. In this way, in line with Bion's truth instinct, Kristeva posits an embodied organizational framework that structures human meaning-making.

This framework allows for the surrender found in visionary experience, the type of absorption Gadamer (1975) describes in relation to the aesthetic moment. The paradoxical need for surrender in order to move beyond a point of impasse is also at the core of Lacan's (1977b) ideas about the need to break through the confines of the Imaginary—the transference relationship—into something authentic and engaged that both demands and makes possible a different level of truth-telling. That juncture can provide a terrible rupture between self and context when transgenerational trauma has impeded knowing. For example, I have been working with a young man who has a fierce desire to divest of the "upholstery" with which most people cover over the truths that feel too raw, too bare to disclose. His family tries to reach out to him but their words become barriers to the closeness each both longs for and occludes. Paul becomes the mystic who speaks truth in his particular haiku form, unupholstered and seemingly obscure, yet cutting to the core as best he can, trying desperately to find something real in relationship.

Aesthetics and Humanism

Focusing our investigation on the all-too-human quest for greater knowledge and self-development brings us in line with Gadamer's (1975) positioning of ethics within a tradition of self-cultivation that has its roots in mediaeval mysticism. That framework endorses cultivating one's innate natural capacities towards a transformative self-revelation that is embedded within "the ancient mystical tradition, according to which man carries in his soul the image of God after whom he is fashioned and must cultivate in himself" (p. 12). This view is very much in the spirit of Winnicott's (1971) *becoming*, which presumes the centrality of history in meaning, including the interpenetration of person, world, and experience. For Gadamer, "to seek one's own in the alien, to become at home in it, is the basic movement of spirit, whose being is only return to itself from what is other" (p. 15).

   In line with Bion's (1967) injunction to eschew memory or desire, Gadamer advocates for a forgetting that affords the possibility "of total renewal, the capacity to see everything with fresh eyes, so that what is long familiar combines with the new into a many levelled unity" (p. 16). Gadamer (1975) also recognizes, much as we find in Lacan (1978), the importance of the angle from which an idea or event is approached, saying: "To pass over something does not mean to avert the gaze from something, but to watch it in such a way that rather than knock against it, one slips by it" (p. 17). This passage highlights the importance of the witness who can follow respectfully the movements of the person trying to find their own way in their own journey, enabling us also to be respectful of the bumps and bruises so that we might, together, build a navigational map that is in relation to the person's own experience.

Aesthetics and the Sublime

Mysticism and creative inspiration can each bring us into the realm of the sublime, a region of human experience that presumes a universal aesthetic principle. I think that what Freud terms libido may be best understood in terms of a drive towards the aesthetic that is profoundly embodied and affective—sensual rather than sexual, informed by the rhythmic patterns alluded to by Milner and Kristeva. Bion (1977) highlights this aesthetic dimension of experience, in which *passion* is a marker of the emotional truth of meanings revealed through the senses, and myth is a way of organizing the elements and marking patterns. This is the territory Freud (1900) refers to as primary process, and Matte-Blanco (1975) further explicates in his descriptions of symmetrical logic, the condensed and displaced, timeless, and affectively laden symbolic logic of dreams. Recognizing the essential patterns of experience helps us to accept the complexity—and move further into it—rather than foreclose on it.

These patterns hold meanings that call to us from the unconscious, formulating sensibilities we can grasp if we are sufficiently open. The artist, the mystic, and the psychotic are each, in their own way, in the position of primary knower, a position that can be precarious but also can be seen as an attempt to constitute oneself as knower. As subjects in their own right, they lay claim to the legitimacy and importance of their own particular perspectives rather than placing the other—illegitimately— in the place of the primary knower and thus using the other to subvert their own unique becoming.

Conclusion

The uneasy relationship between the establishment and the truth-seeker, and the ease with which lack of recognition can undermine one's sense of truth, are important to consider when making judgements about extreme states and the people who experience them. We have seen that ego integrity can be a crucial factor in enabling an individual to tolerate and learn from visionary experiences. Beyond one's own initial experience, support from a respectful community can be crucial to ongoing stability and meaning-making. Just as culture can provide a means and language through which extreme experiences can be valued, sustained, and learned from within a particular community of belief, so, too, the culture can provide just the opposite. Fear can be a powerful force, invited by readings of visionary experience as madness. In this regard, the clinician potentially serves a useful stabilizing function by helping to make meaning from experiences that may initially appear psychotic from the perspective of Western medicine or of the family that restricts itself in relation to the unformulated trauma. Our caution may be most important in relation to experiences we do not fully understand, and the realm of the sacred by definition defies rational understanding:

> A perceptive diagnostician needs to be something of an anthropologist in being able to connect the diagnostic structures of sanity with models of sanctity if only to be able to provide a better treatment that does not itself perversely disavow the experience of the Real with our patients.
>
> (Baldacchino, 2016, p. 408)

These considerations invite us, as we sit with those who find themselves situated outside consensual culture, to try to hear the call of truth and enter as empathically as we can into resonance with their experience. From that place, we are in a better position to find the links between their words and experience and our own, and to have a sense of where the difficulties arise for them. It is difficult to witness the depth of suffering; yet, in such respectful engagement, the person who has become lost may find themselves and begin to locate themselves in relation to the life story that could not previously be formulated. Identity is built within the context of contextual meanings built in respectful, intimate engagement with one another. Human development depends on those unique individuals who reach out into the darkness and help us all move beyond the places where convention limits our growth. Rather than fearing that we might mistake craziness for creativity, perhaps we would do better to cherish idiosyncrasy where we find it and try to assist those we encounter in getting their bearings and finding their way—also, in the process, learning and recognizing that each person has gifts and stories to share.

References

Allardyce, J., & Boydell, J. (2006). Review: The wider social environment and schizophrenia. *Schizophrenia Bulletin*, *32*(4), 592–598.

Ataria, Y. (2016). Traumatic and mystical experiences: The dark nights of the soul. *Journal of Humanistic Psychology*, *56*(4), 331–356.

Baldacchino, J. P. (2016). Visions or hallucinations? Lacan on mysticism and psychosis reconsidered: The case of St. George of Malta. *British Journal of Psychotherapy*, *32*(3), 392–414.

Banks, K. H., & Stephens, J. (2018). Reframing internalized racial oppression and charting a way forward. *Social Issues and Policy Review*, *12*(1), 91–111.

Bentall, R. P., Rowse, G., Shryane, N., Kinderman, P., Howard, R., Blackwood, N., Moore, R., & Corcoran, R. (2009). The cognitive and affective structure of paranoid delusions: A transdiagnostic investigation of patients with schizophrenia spectrum disorders and depression. *Archives of General Psychiatry*, *66*(3), 236–247.

Bion, W. R. (1967). Notes on memory and desire. *Psychoanalytic Review*, *2*, 272–273.

Bion, W. R. (1977). *Seven servants*. Heinemann.

Bourque, F., van der Ven, E., & Mala, A. (2011). A meta-analysis of the risk for psychotic disorders among first- and second-generation immigrants. *Psychological Medicine*, *41*, 897–910.

Brett, C. (2003). Psychotic and mystical states of being: Connections and distinctions. *Philosophy, Psychiatry, and Psychology*, *9*(4), 321–341.

Campbell, J. (1988). *The power of myth*. Viking Press.

Cantor-Graae, E., & Selten, J. P. (2005). Schizophrenia and migration: A meta-analysis and review. *American Journal of Psychiatry*, *162*, 12–4.

Charles, M. (2005). Patterns: Basic units of emotional memory. *Psychoanalytic Inquiry*, *25*(4), 484–505.

Charles, M. (2013). Bullying and social exclusion: Links to severe psychopathology. In M. O'Loughlin (Ed.), *Working with children's emotional lives: Psychodynamic perspectives on children and schools* (pp. 207–226). Jason Aronson.

Charles, M. (2015). *Psychoanalysis and literature: The stories we live*. Rowman & Littlefield.

Charles, M. (2019). Women and madness in context. In M. H. Brown & M. Charles (Eds.), *Women & psychosis: Multidisciplinary perspectives* (pp. 11–35). Rowman & Littlefield.

Charles, M., Clemence, J., & Biel, S. (2011). Psychosis and creativity: Managing cognitive complexity on unstructured tasks. In L. DellaPietra (Ed.), *Perspectives on creativity* (Vol. 2, pp. 107–122). Cambridge Scholars Publishing.

Charles, M., & O'Loughlin, M. (2013) The complex subject of psychosis. *Psychoanalysis, Culture, and Society, 17*(4), 410–421.

Charles, M., & Telis, K. (2009). Pattern as inspiration and mode of communication in the works of Van Gogh. *American Journal of Psychoanalysis, 69*, 238–262.

Clarke, I. (2001). Psychosis and spirituality: The discontinuity model. In I. Clarke (Ed.), *Psychosis and spirituality: Exploring the new frontier* (pp. 129–142). Hoboken, NJ: Wiley.

Cook, C. C. H. (2004). Psychiatry and mysticism. *Mental Health, Religion & Culture, 7*(2), 149–163.

Collert, D., Dudley, R., & Mosimann, U. P. (2012). Visual hallucinations. In J. D. Blom & I. E. C. Sommer (Eds.), *Hallucinations: Research and practice*. Springer.

David, M. F. (2011). *Internal racism: A psychoanalytic approach to race and difference.* Palgrave Macmillan.

Davoine, F., & Gaudillière J. M. (2004). *History beyond trauma: Whereof one cannot speak, thereof one cannot stay silent* (S. Fairfield, Trans.). Other Press.

Erikson, E. (1982). *The life cycle completed.* W. W. Norton.

Fanon, F. (2008). *Black skin, white masks* (R. Philcox, Trans.). Grove Press. (Original work published 1952)

Fearon, P., Kirkbride, J. B., Morgan, C., Dazzan, P., Morgan, K., Lloyd, T., Hutchinson, G., Tarrant, J., Fung, W. L. A., Holloway, J., Mallett, R., Harrison, G., Leff, J., Jones, P. B., & Murray, R. M. (2006). Incidence of schizophrenia and other psychoses in ethnic minority groups: Results from the MRC AESOP study. *Psychological Medicine, 36*, 1541–1550.

Feliou, G. (2016). Saturated phenomena and their relationship to 'extreme experiences': A phenomenological comparison between mystical experiences and psychotic and depressive experiences based on Jean-Luc Marion's philosophy. *Existential Analysis, 27*(1), 121–136.

Felman, S. (1995). Education and crisis, or the vicissitudes of teaching. In C. Caruth (Ed.), *Trauma: Explorations in memory* (pp. 13–60). Johns Hopkins University Press.

Fivush, R., Habermas, T., Waters, T. E. A., & Zaman, W. (2011). The making of autobiographical memory: Intersections of culture, narratives, and identity. *International Journal of Psychology, 46*, 321–345.

Fricker, M. (2007). *Epistemic injustice: Power and the ethics of knowing.* Oxford University Press.

Fromm, E. (1950). *Psychoanalysis and religion.* Yale University Press.

Freud, S. (1900). The Interpretation of Dreams. *Standard Edition*, 4 & 5. London: Hogarth Press, 1971.

Gadamer, H. G. (1975). *Truth and method.* Continuum.

Ghent, E. (1990). Masochism, submission, surrender: Masochism as a perversion of surrender. *Contemporary Psychoanalysis, 26*, 108–136.

Ghorbani, N., Ebrahimi, F., Watson, P. J., & Chen, Z. J. (2018). Poets and transliminality: Relationships with mystical experience and religious commitment in Iran. *Psychology of Religion and Spirituality.* http://dx.doi.org/10.1037/rel0000174

Grotstein, J. S. (2004). The seventh servant: The implications of a truth drive in Bion's theory of 'O'. *International Journal of Psychoanalysis, 85*, 1081–1101.

Heriot-Maitland, C. P. (2008). Mysticism and madness: Different aspects of the same human experience? *Mental Health, Religion & Culture, 11*(3), 301–325.

Hook, D. (2017). What is enjoyment as a political factor? *Political Psychology*, *38*(4), 605–620.

Janssen, I., Hanssen, M., Bak, M., Bijl, R. V., de Graaf, R., Vollebergh, W., McKenzie, K., & Van Os, J. (2003). Discrimination and delusional ideation. *British Journal of Psychiatry*, *182*, 71–76.

Johnson, C. L. (1981). Psychoanalysis, shamanism and cultural phenomena. *Journal of the American Academy of Psychoanalysis*, *9*(2), 311–318.

Kinderman, P., Dunbar, R., & Bentall, R. P. (1998). Theory-of-mind deficits and causal attributions. *British Journal of Psychology*, *89*, 191–204.

Kirkbride, J. B., Morgan, C., Fearon, P., Dazzan, P., Murray, R. M., & Jones, P. B. (2007). Neighbourhood-level effects on psychoses: Re-examining the role of context. *Psychological Medicine*, *37*, 1413–1425.

Klein, M. (1975). The importance of symbol-formation in the development of the ego. In *Love, guilt and reparation and other works 1921–1945* (pp. 219–232). Hogarth Press. (Original work published 1930)

Knoblauch, D. L. (1985). Applying Taoist thought to counseling and psychotherapy. *American Mental Health Counselors Association Journal*, *7*, 52–63.

Koss-Chioino, J. D. (2003). Jung, spirits and madness: Lessons for cultural psychiatry. *Transcultural Psychiatry*, *40*(2), 164–180.

Kristeva, J. (1982). *Powers of horror: An essay on abjection.* (L. S. Roudiez, Trans.). Columbia University Press.

Kristeva, J. (1986a). Revolution in poetic language. In T. Moi (Ed.), L. S. Roudiez & S. Hand (Trans.), *The Kristeva reader* (pp. 89–136). Columbia University Press.

Kristeva, J. (1986b). Stabat mater. In T. Moi (Ed.), L. S. Roudiez & S. Hand (Trans.), *The Kristeva reader* (pp. 160–186). Columbia University Press.

Kristeva, J. (1986c). Women's time. In T. Moi (Ed.), L. S. Roudiez & S. Hand (Trans.), *The Kristeva reader* (pp. 187–213). Columbia University Press.

Lacan, J. (1977a). The agency of the letter in the unconscious or reason since Freud. In A. Sheridan (Trans.), *Écrits* (pp. 146–178). W. W. Norton.

Lacan, J. (1977b). The function and field of speech and language in psychoanalysis. In A. Sheridan (Trans.), *Écrits* (pp. 30–113). W. W. Norton.

Lacan, J. (1977c). The subversion of the subject and the dialectic of desire in the Freudian unconscious. In A. Sheridan (Trans.), *Écrits* (pp. 292–325). W. W. Norton.

Lacan, J. (1978). *The four fundamentals of psychoanalysis* (J. A. Miller, Ed.; A. Sheridan, Trans.). W. W. Norton.

Lacan, J. (1992). *The ethics of psychoanalysis* (J. A. Miller, Ed.; D. Porter, Trans.). W. W. Norton.

Lacan, J. (1997). *The seminar of Jacques Lacan III: The psychoses. 1955–1956.* W. W. Norton.

Levinas, E. (1999). *Alterity and transcendence* (M. B. Smith, Trans.). Columbia University Press.

Liotti, G. (1999). Disorganization of attachment as a model for understanding dissociative psychopathology. In J. Solomon & C. George (Eds.), *Attachment disorganization.* Guilford Press.

Littlewood, R., & Dein, S. (2013). Did Christianity lead to schizophrenia? Psychosis, psychology, and self-reference. *Transcultural Psychiatry*, *50*(3), 397–420.

Loewald, H. (1978). Primary process, secondary process, and language. In *Papers on Psychoanalysis* (pp. 178–206). Yale University Press, 1980.

Main, M., & Hesse, E. (1990). Parent's unresolved traumatic experiences are related to infant disorganized/disoriented attachment status: Is frightened and/or frightening parental behavior the linking mechanism? In M. Greenberg, D. Cicchetti, & E. M. Cummings (Eds.), *Attachment in the preschool years: Theory, research, and intervention* (pp. 161–182). University of Chicago Press.

Matte-Blanco, I. (1975). *The unconscious as infinite sets: An essay in bi-logic.* Duckworth.

McGhee, M. (2003). Mysticism and psychosis: Descriptions and distinctions. *Philosophy, Psychiatry, and Psychology, 9*(4), 343–347.

Milner, M. (1987). *The suppressed madness of sane men: Forty-four years of exploring psychoanalysis.* Tavistock.

O'Donoghue, B., Lyne, J. P., Renwick, L., Madigan, K., Staines, A., O'Callaghan, E., & Clarke, M. (2016). Neighbourhood characteristics and the incidence of first-episode psychosis and duration of untreated psychosis, *Psychological Medicine, 46,* 1367–1378.

Ribolsi, M. R., Feyaerts, J. & Vanheule, S. (2015). Metaphor in psychosis: On the possible convergence of Lacanian theory and neuro-scientific research. *Frontiers in Psychology, 6,* 664. https://doi.org/10.3389/fpsyg.2015.00664

Scheff, T., Daniel, G. R., & Sterphone, J. (2018, March–April). Shame and a theory of war and violence. *Aggression and Violent Behavior, 39,* 109–115.

Schellenberg, G., Lu, C., Schimmele, C., & Hou, F. (2018). The correlates of self-assessed community belonging in Canada: Social capital, neighbourhood characteristics, and rootedness. *Social Indicators Research, 140*(2), 597–618.

Shonkoff, J. P., & Phillips, D. (Eds.). (2000). *From neurons to neighborhoods: The science of early childhood development.* Committee on Integrating the Science of Early Childhood Development. National Academy Press.

Stavrakakis, Y. (1999). *Lacan and the political.* Routledge.

Steinbock, A. J. (2012). *Evidence in the phenomenology of religious experience.* Retrieved July 19, 2019, from www.academia.edu

Stifler, K., Greer, J., Sneck, W., & Dovenmuehle, R. (1993). An empirical investigation of the discriminability of reported mystical experiences among religious contemplatives, psychotic inpatients, and normal adults. *Journal for the Scientific Study of Religion, 32*(4), 366–372.

Tappan, M. B. (2006). Reframing internalized oppression and internalized domination: From the psychological to the sociocultural. *Teachers College Record, 108,* 2115–2144.

Thalbourne, M. A., & Delin, P. S. (1994). A common thread underlying belief in the paranormal, creative personality, mystical experience and psychopathology. *Journal of Parapsychology, 58,* 3038.

Tillich, P. (1957). *The dynamics of faith.* Harper & Row.

Vardy, M. M., & Kaplan, B. M. (2008). Christ/Messiah delusions revisited: Toward an anthropological definition of religious delusions. *Psychoanalytic Review, 95*(3), 473–487.

Vighi, F. (2010). *On Žižek's dialectics.* Continuum.

Winnicott, D. W. (1971). *Playing and reality.* Routledge.

Zubin, J., & Spring, B. (1977). Vulnerability: A new view of schizophrenia. *Journal of Abnormal Psychology, 86*(2), 103–126.

Chapter 32

Rethinking Psychiatry with Mad Studies

Bradley Lewis

Summary

This chapter starts with an articulation of the current world of US psychiatry and then imagines how this world might shift through a mad studies perspective. For insight into contemporary psychiatry, the author looks at two recent textbooks published by the American Psychiatric Association. He also considers the "virtual education center" sponsored by Sunovion Pharmaceuticals, the maker of Latuda—a medication approved for treatment of clinical depression. The education center is dedicated to mental health providers and contains material from key opinion leaders in US psychiatry. A close read of this material highlights many of the sanist worldviews and problematic logics at the heart of contemporary US psychiatry.

Mad studies assistance, as the author sees it, helps mental health work move beyond sanist logics and opens clinical work in three critical and affirmative ways: (a) taking the diversity of people's perspectives seriously; (b) nurturing mad-positive models of mental difference; and (c) joining narrative medicine to adopt a narrative hermeneutics paradigm for clinical psychiatric work.

Contemporary US psychiatry and mad studies are worlds apart in many ways, but nonetheless there are concrete steps that mental health workers can make to help build a more mad-positive mental health community and a more mad-positive world.

*

Those of us who do clinical work and are also mad studies advocates are left with a critical question: How can mad studies help reimagine clinical work? I focus my consideration of this question on US psychiatry, where my clinical work is located. US psychiatry has a range of issues unique to itself, but, at the same time, these issues overlap in important ways with mental health care more broadly. I start with an articulation of contemporary US psychiatry and then imagine psychiatry transforming through mad studies assistance. Mad studies brings three critical and affirmative standpoints to clinical psychiatry: (a) taking the diversity of people's perspectives seriously; (b) nurturing mad-positive models of mental difference; and (c) joining narrative medicine to adopt a narrative hermeneutics paradigm for clinical psychiatric work.

DOI: 10.4324/9781003148456-36

Contemporary US Psychiatry

To get a window into contemporary US psychiatry, I turn to two recent textbooks of psychiatry published by the field's leading organization—the American Psychiatric Association (APA). These textbooks do not represent the entire field of US psychiatry or even individual practitioners in all their density, complexity, and contradiction, but they do provide useful examples of how a major institution of psychiatry, the APA, understands and represents itself. The two texts, *The American Psychiatric Association Publishing Textbook of Psychiatry* (2019) and *Introductory Textbook of Psychiatry* (2021), dive quickly into the details of psychiatric diagnosis and treatment with little to no discussion of broad philosophical questions or paradigm choices the field has made.

The qualifying label "biopsychiatry," which is often used in mad studies literature to describe contemporary US psychiatry, continues to fit well with the definitions, conceptual models, and paradigm choices these texts articulate and recommend. *The Introductory Textbook of Psychiatry* (ITP), for example, tells us that "the primary purposes of psychiatry as a discipline within medicine are to define and recognize illnesses, to identify methods for treating them, and ultimately to develop methods for discovering their causes and implementing preventive measures" (Black & Andreasen, 2021, preface). The textbook explains:

> The study of psychiatry, the branch of medicine devoted to the study of mental illnesses, is therefore a discipline dedicated to the investigation of abnormalities in brain function manifested in diseases that afflict individuals in interesting and important ways. The clinical appearance of these abnormalities may be obvious and severe, as in the case of schizophrenia, or subtle and mild, as in the case of an adjustment disorder.
>
> (Introduction)

The biopsychiatry center of this psychiatric self-identification shows up with ITP's emphasis on "mental illnesses" understood as "aberrations" and "abnormalities in brain function manifested in diseases." For biopsychiatrists, abnormalities in brain function cause mental illness and the goal of diagnostic psychiatry is to identify these abnormalities, from the most severe all the way to seemingly situational states like "adjustment disorder." ITP articulates the goal of biopsychiatry as advancing "clinically and scientifically" to the point that "specific treatments for particular disorders or groups of symptoms" are possible (Introduction). This does not always mean biomedical treatments, but when ITP gives treatment examples, medications are in the foreground.

The American Psychiatric Association Publishing Textbook of Psychiatry (APATP) is similar except that it calls the paradigm of psychiatry it prefers "precision psychiatry." APATP uses this term to describe an emerging approach to psychiatry that seems even more aggressively centered on biomedical science and diagnostic logics than the one promoted by ITP (Roberts, Hales, & Yudofsky, 2019). Precision psychiatry, for editors of APATP, "captures the prowess of the present and the promise of the future," and chapter 28, devoted to precision psychiatry (Williams, Ball, & Kircos, 2019) explains why:

A revolution is under way in psychiatry. We are witnessing the emergence of precision medicine for psychiatry: "precision psychiatry." Precision psychiatry is an integrative approach, one that pulls together the scientific foundations of the discipline and recent technological advances and directs them toward closing the gap between discovery and clinical translation.

The chapter goes on to explain:

The goals of precision psychiatry are threefold: precise classification (i.e., a specific understanding of the pathophysiology of each individual patient—what has gone wrong?), precise treatment planning (i.e., tailoring treatment plans in a personalized manner—how can we fix what has gone wrong?), and precise prevention (i.e., targeted and tailored prevention strategies—how can we keep things from going wrong?).

But, despite the excitement and the new name, "precision psychiatry" is still basically biopsychiatry since, as APATP emphasizes, the "primary focus is on the organ of dysfunction in psychiatry: the brain," and, as such, the primary treatments of interest are biomedical.

For additional insight into how the paradigm of biopsychiatry is practiced, taught, and researched, I turn now to the pop-up advertisement for Latuda that appeared on my computer when I looked up the APA textbooks in my university library. Latuda is an "antipsychotic medication" sold by Sunovion Pharmaceuticals and approved by the FDA in 2010 for the treatment of "schizophrenia." In 2013, Latuda was given approval for treatment of "depressive episodes" combined with "bipolar I disorder." When I follow the pop-up advert to the Latuda website section devoted to clinicians, I find treatment recommendations very similar to those in the APA textbooks (Sunovion ProFile, n.d.) The Sunoivon-sponsored Latuda website shows us a seemingly happy family—a smiling and engaged mother, father, daughter, and family dog—having a picnic in an urban park (see Figure 32.1). The website text tells clinicians that "Latuda may help your patients suffering from depressive symptoms

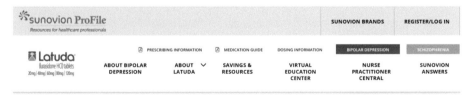

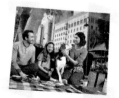

LATUDA may help your patients suffering from depressive symptoms get to where they want to be

Figure 32.1 Sunovion ProFile, Latuda.

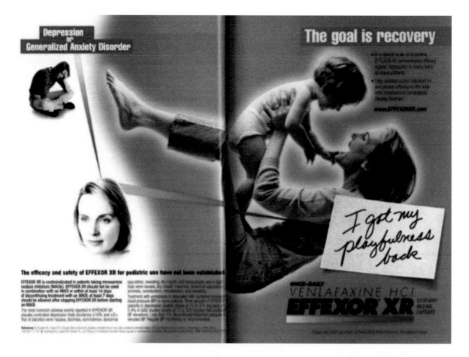

Figure 32.2 Effexor XR, 2001.

get where they want to be." This suggests that one or more of the family members had a depressive episode in the past, took Latuda, and are now where they want to be—happy, engaged, enjoying a picnic. The image is placed in a larger notebook of "cases" implying that, after taking Latuda, people become normal and "grateful for small things."

The Latuda website works from the same perspective as an older antidepressant ad for Effexor (see Figure 32.2). The Effexor ad shows a woman looking straight at the reader, who is presumably a psychiatrist since the ad is published in a psychiatric journal. The woman in the ad is likely being interviewed by a biopsychiatrist who interprets signs and symptoms for either depressive episodes or generalized anxiety symptoms (portrayed in the black-and-white image at the top left). The psychiatrist prescribes Effexor and the woman becomes happy and engaged with her young child: "I got my playfulness back."

The APA textbooks follow the same approach as the adverts. ITP (chapter 6) tells us that, once a diagnosis has been made, "several medications are available to treat depression" and that they "work by altering levels of various neurotransmitters at crucial nerve terminals in the central nervous system." ITP recommends that "treatment should begin with an SSRI because agents in this medication class are well tolerated and safe in overdose" and goes on to outline a treatment course, the use of additional or "augmenting" medication if the first medication is not effective, and recommendations for various other medication complications. The expectation is that "most patients will improve relatively quickly, even within the first 1–2 weeks after starting medication, although full response will take longer." In the same chapter, ITP tells us that the medications have similar effectiveness and that, when treated, "65%–70% of persons … will improve markedly." This means that persons will lose their sadness and lack of interest and become happy (or at least not sad) and engaged in their lives like the people in the ads.

After detailing medication treatments, ITP includes a section on "other treatments"—making clear that anything besides biological treatments is "other." For example, supportive psychotherapy shows up in this section, not so much as a treatment but as a way to help people cope with having a psychiatric disorder.

> Experiencing an episode of mood disorder is often a major blow to the patient's confidence and self-esteem. Consequently, most patients could benefit from supportive psychotherapy in addition to whatever medications are prescribed. … Work, school performance, and interpersonal relationships all can be impaired because of a mood disorder. It is important to help patients assess these problems and recognize that the *illness is responsible*—rather than feeling that they themselves are responsible—and to instill confidence that they can now begin to restore and repair whatever injuries have occurred as a consequence of their episode of mood disorder. (chapter 6, italics added)

We can get a further sense of how the biopsychiatry model plays out in the clinical encounter by going to the "virtual education center" of the Latuda website.[1]

The virtual education center contains "hypothetical case" presentations, mock interviews, and psychiatric education lectures from key opinion leaders in biopsychiatry, including Stephen Stahl, MD, PhD; David Sheehan, MD; Rakesh Jain MD, MPH; Roger McIntyre MD, FRCPC; and Kiki Chang, MD. All these experts have distinguished academic careers in psychiatric research, education, and practice, and all are active consultants and advisers to the pharmaceutical industry, including in this situation, Sunovion, the maker of Latuda.

The case of "Katie" presented by Dr. Chang is perhaps the most informative for our purposes since Katie is new to psychiatry and is being diagnosed for the first time (Figure 32.3). Katie is a 15-year-old young woman who is being brought to a psychotherapist by her mother. Katie's mother is concerned because Katie is not doing well in school:

> Mother: Katie's having a really hard time with 10th grade. September was bad. October it was worse. I can't get her out of bed in the morning, and she's starting to miss a lot of school. When she does go, she calls me wanting to come home early. Sometimes she gets in bed right after soccer practice without eating her dinner. That's not normal, is it?

The therapist shares the mother's perspective: "Katie, is that accurate? It sounds like your Mom is worried about you." Katie's mother adds that Katie is "even thinking about quitting the soccer team. And she *loves* soccer!" Also, her grades are bad and

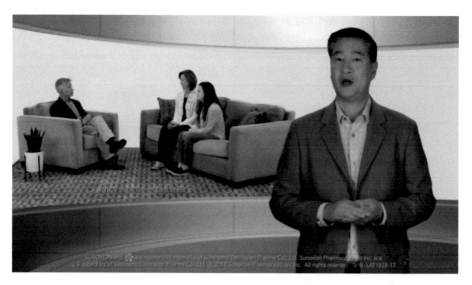

Figure 32.3 Kiki Chang, MD, presenting "Hypothetical Case" (Latuda Website).

"two teachers say she is very quiet, and she doesn't talk in class. They said she sits in the back row with her head down on her desk." The therapist asks with some alarm and disbelief: "Katie, is that true? You don't participate in class?"

Dr. Chang, in his educational commentary, explains that making a diagnosis can be difficult in patients like this. He adds that therapists, when confronted with these situations, will often refer patients to a psychiatrist like him for a consultation. He further explains that, in a case like Katie's, if he sees "persistent depressive symptoms in a child or adolescent, and [doesn't] detect any history of mania," he will likely diagnose "major depressive disorder and prescribe an antidepressant." He also adds, however, that even he might be mistaken, the diagnosis is tricky, and this might well be a "typical first step in the journey of a child who [will later be] diagnosed with bipolar depression."

But, when we listen to Katie's voice, even from within this promotional copy, we start to see a deep problem with biopsychiatry—the way it navigates difference. Katie, for her part, does not see her situation as a "disorder." She sees the problem coming from the institution of "school," and she says so unambiguously: "I can't stand school." She singles out high school in particular: "High school is so useless. I wish it was over already." And she argues that the school system overall "is a waste!" Her understanding of the situation, in other words, is not that she has an internal problem like clinical depression or bipolar depression, but that the external environment of school is deeply problematic. For Katie, something is rotten in the institution of school. Accordingly, she is not interested in college, and she does not care about her grades in high school. She is tired and worn out, doesn't want to go to school anymore, doesn't feel like trying or participating, and is just holding out, wishing "it was over already." Nothing about being in school makes her happy. On top of that, she feels forced to play soccer, which she does not like although she has had to pretend that she does. And, because of her difference from others (who presumably do like the institution of school), she is mistreated by the other students and finds that "no one likes me."

This deep difference of perspective means that Katie, her mother, her teachers, the therapist, and Dr. Chang end up at an impasse. They have diametrically opposite perspectives on the situation. Katie sees the problem as mostly coming from external factors, and everyone else (or so it seems) believes that the problem is coming from individual diagnostic factors within Katie. And not only do they have different perspectives, none of the psychiatrists—Dr. Stahl, Sheehan, Jain, McIntyre, or Chang—and indeed none of the psychiatrists trained according to the APA textbooks, have a way of navigating this conflict and difference beyond a logic that the psychiatrists are right and anyone who disagrees is wrong. This is because for biopsychiatrists mental difference is organized around the scientifically "true," and therefore difficult to dispute, "abnormalities in brain function." The emerging form of biopsychiatry, precision psychiatry, pushes this truth of abnormal brain function even further, to the point of an absolute and ideally indisputable "precise classification (i.e., a specific understanding of the pathophysiology of each individual patient—what has gone wrong?)." The consequence of this way of looking at things is that differences of opinion with scientific "truth" can be seen only as at best "false" and at worst "pathological."

When psychiatrists understand different perspectives as either true or false, normal or pathological, patients who have "false" perspectives must be reeducated so they see the "true" perspective of the clinicians. If reeducation does not work, clinicians can pathologize the disagreement as a symptom of mental illness. Clients disagree because they are "out of touch with reality"; they have "lack of insight," or "anosognosia"—the neurological inability of someone with mental illness to perceive his or her illness. This is something of an unarguable tautology because to be a "patient," to be "mentally ill," would be to be out of touch with reality in some way.

Mad Studies Assistance

The notion that people who come to clinical care, or are brought there, are "out of touch with reality" and/or are pathological easily slides into a core problem of biopsychiatry: sanism—the structural devaluing of people, their contributions, perspectives, feelings, and goals based on a logic of truth versus pathology. It is precisely here where mad studies can help. Rather than trying to navigate differences of perspective that emerge in clinics through a sanist logic of right/true/sane versus wrong/false/insane, psychiatry can open up its perspective in three ways. *First*, it can take people seriously by being curious about and inclusive of additional, non-normative, perspectives. *Second*, it can rethink pathological models like biopsychiatry in relationship with mad-positive models of mental difference. And *third*, it can adjust its logic of truth by moving outside the dominant paradigms toward more inclusive fourth-force approaches to mental difference.

Taking People and Different Perspectives Seriously

To take Katie seriously would be to treat her with respect and dignity and as someone whose insights are worthy of careful consideration. It would mean treating her as one would want oneself to be treated. It would mean, at its most basic, taking her perspective—that there is something rotten in the institution of school—seriously. And that would require being curious about this perspective, doing comparative research with other people who share it, and working to understand how that perspective makes sense.

One of the most interesting comparisons that the biopsychiatrists could make would be with work done by their own colleagues at the National Academy of Medicine (NAM). The academy has become concerned because an epidemic of difficulties similar to Katie's is happening to physicians, medical students, and health care workers in the institution of medicine. The statistics outlined by NAM are alarming: physicians have a 50% burnout rate and a 39% rate of depression, nurses have a 23%–31% rate of emotional exhaustion and a 24% rate of PTSD, and physicians die by suicide each year at a rate two times the national average (National Academy of Medicine, 2019).

Unlike Katie's mother and her therapist, however, NAM did not turn to biopsychiatry for consultation. Instead, NAM put together a committee of peers in an "action collaborative" to assess the situation, develop a conceptual model for what was happening, and make recommendations (Brigham et al., 2018). The committee was made up of medical educators, nurses, pharmacists, medical physicians, and medical board specialists. No psychiatrists seem to have been invited, or if they were, they all declined to participate or perhaps left because they did not like the findings.

The first thing that stands out about the action collaborative conclusions is that they did not understand the problems their colleagues were having as clinical depression. Rather, they saw the problem in nonpathological terms of burnout, well-being, and resilience. For "burnout," they used a definition that could easily fit Katie's situation as well: "a syndrome characterized by emotional exhaustion, depersonalization (i.e., cynicism), and loss of work fulfillment" (p. 2). The collaborative found that most research on burnout includes "both individual (e.g., internal) and external (e.g., environmental and organizational) resources and demands" (p. 3). The second thing that stands out is that, just as with Katie's perspective, the literature on burnout "suggests that external factors carry more weight" and that "external factors in systems and culture often have a larger effect … in well-being than individual factors do" (pp. 3, 5).

The NAM collaborative brought all of this together to come up with their own model of well-being and resilience that includes both "external" and "individual" factors (see Figure 32.4). The external factors make up the larger part, and they include sociocultural factors, regulatory and business factors, organizational factors, and education/practice factors. The individual factors include health care role, personal factors, and skills and abilities. For NAM, in no uncertain terms, improvement in the institution of medicine is required to reduce clinician burnout. This means changing the external problems, reimagining the health care role, helping

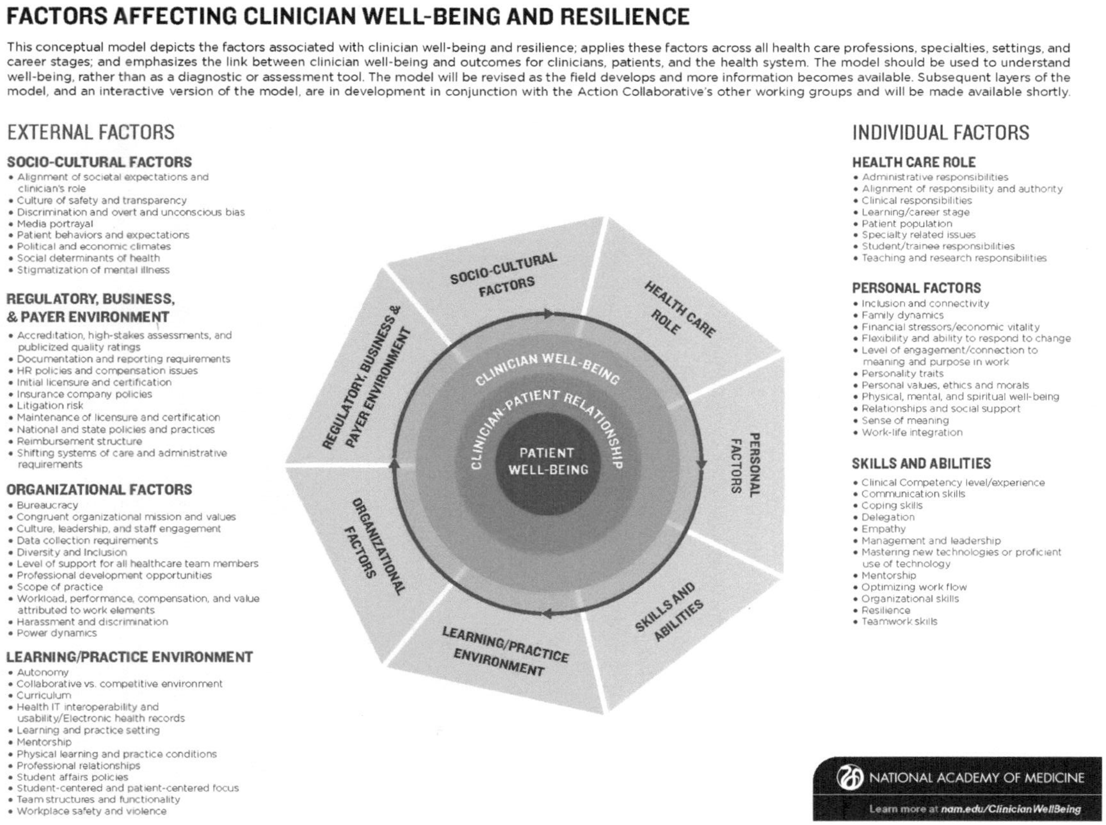

FACTORS AFFECTING CLINICIAN WELL-BEING AND RESILIENCE

This conceptual model depicts the factors associated with clinician well-being and resilience, applies these factors across all health care professions, specialties, settings, and career stages; and emphasizes the link between clinician well-being and outcomes for clinicians, patients, and the health system. The model should be used to understand well-being, rather than as a diagnostic or assessment tool. The model will be revised as the field develops and more information becomes available. Subsequent layers of the model, and an interactive version of the model, are in development in conjunction with the Action Collaborative's other working groups and will be made available shortly.

EXTERNAL FACTORS

SOCIO-CULTURAL FACTORS
- Alignment of societal expectations and clinician's role
- Culture of safety and transparency
- Discrimination and overt and unconscious bias
- Media portrayal
- Patient behaviors and expectations
- Political and economic climates
- Social determinants of health
- Stigmatization of mental illness

REGULATORY, BUSINESS, & PAYER ENVIRONMENT
- Accreditation, high-stakes assessments, and publicized quality ratings
- Documentation and reporting requirements
- HR policies and compensation issues
- Initial licensure and certification
- Insurance company policies
- Litigation risk
- Maintenance of licensure and certification
- National and state policies and practices
- Reimbursement structure
- Shifting systems of care and administrative requirements

ORGANIZATIONAL FACTORS
- Bureaucracy
- Congruent organizational mission and values
- Culture, leadership, and staff engagement
- Data collection requirements
- Diversity and inclusion
- Level of support for all healthcare team members
- Professional development opportunities
- Scope of practice
- Workload, performance, compensation, and value attributed to work elements
- Harassment and discrimination
- Power dynamics

LEARNING/PRACTICE ENVIRONMENT
- Autonomy
- Collaborative vs. competitive environment
- Curriculum
- Health IT interoperability and usability/Electronic health records
- Learning and practice setting
- Mentorship
- Physical learning and practice conditions
- Professional relationships
- Student affairs policies
- Student-centered and patient-centered focus
- Team structures and functionality
- Workplace safety and violence

INDIVIDUAL FACTORS

HEALTH CARE ROLE
- Administrative responsibilities
- Alignment of responsibility and authority
- Clinical responsibilities
- Learning/career stage
- Patient population
- Specialty related issues
- Student/trainee responsibilities
- Teaching and research responsibilities

PERSONAL FACTORS
- Inclusion and connectivity
- Family dynamics
- Financial stressors/economic vitality
- Flexibility and ability to respond to change
- Level of engagement/connection to meaning and purpose in work
- Personality traits
- Personal values, ethics and morals
- Physical, mental and spiritual well-being
- Relationships and social support
- Sense of meaning
- Work-life integration

SKILLS AND ABILITIES
- Clinical Competency level/experience
- Communication skills
- Coping skills
- Delegation
- Empathy
- Management and leadership
- Mastering new technologies or proficient use of technology
- Mentorship
- Optimizing work flow
- Organizational skills
- Resilience
- Teamwork skills

NATIONAL ACADEMY OF MEDICINE

Learn more at *nam.edu/ClinicianWellBeing*

Diagram labels (hexagonal model): PERSONAL FACTORS · HEALTH CARE ROLE · SKILLS AND ABILITIES · SOCIO-CULTURAL FACTORS · LEARNING/PRACTICE ENVIRONMENT · REGULATORY, BUSINESS & PAYER ENVIRONMENT · ORGANIZATIONAL FACTORS · CLINICIAN WELL-BEING · CLINICIAN-PATIENT RELATIONSHIP · PATIENT WELL-BEING

Figure 32.4 Factors affecting clinician well-being and resilience.
Source: Brigham, T., C. Barden, A. L. Dopp, A. Hengerer, J. Kaplan, B. Malone, C. Martin, M. McHugh, and L. M. Nora. 2018. A journey to construct an all-encompassing conceptual model of factors affecting clinician well-being and resilience. *NAM Perspectives*. Discussion Paper, National Academy of Medicine. https://doi.org/10.31478/201801b. Reproduced with permission from the National Academy of Sciences, Courtesy of the National Academies Press, Washington, DC.

clinicians achieve personal goals, and expanding education to include personal and interpersonal well-being skills and abilities.

Another place where Katie's clinicians could get comparative perspectives with regard to the institution of school is the internet database Mad in America, where people critical of sanist approaches to mental difference publish blogs, articles, music, visual art, and videos. The Mad in America database shows a wealth of perspectives similar to Katie's on the institution of school. In other words, with just a little curiosity, we can see that Katie is not alone. A Yale Child Study Center survey, for example, found that "nearly 75% of the [high-school] students" they studied self-reported negative feelings about school (Belli, 2020). Mad in America covers a wide range of external issues contributing to these negative feelings. There are deep problems with student isolation and lack of social connection (Cathcart, 2019), limited and problematic parental engagement (Cathcart, 2021), complex social and emotional consequences of school bullying and violence (Cathcart, 2020), outdated and problematic approaches to school counseling (Cathcart, 2018; Peters, 2017), and superficial mental health screening programs that are covers for a "pharmaceutical invasion" of schools (Cook, 2019; Davidow, 2016), as well as a dire need for more and better social and emotional learning programs in schools (Troeger, 2017).

One Mad in America blogger, Michael Corrigan, EdD, in 2014, contextualized student problems by looking at the way school systems overvalued standardized testing.

> The fact that we spend far more billions of dollars on standardized testing than apparently everything else combined, is evidence that our kids' safety and helping each student prepare for the test of life is far less important than preparing them for a life of tests.

We have created a system, Corrigan argues, where standardized test scores are "more important than providing the basic human needs" that are "first and foremost in order to even pursue enlightenment." In a nutshell, Corrigan concludes we must reverse our educational values: "What SHOULD be *the* #1 priority of our schools? KIDS! Not test scores! They deserve nothing less."

But, as Katie explains, it is not easy to be hopeful because high-school problems are intertwined with college problems and larger cultural problems. Alexandra Robbins (2019), writing in the *Atlantic Monthly*, finds that "one in five college students reports having had suicidal thoughts over the past year." A college counselor Robbins interviews describes:

> a remarkable increase in the number of kids who are just falling apart, checking out, harming themselves and medicating themselves. There are more suicide attempts, students cutting themselves, more hospitalizations, more cases of anorexia and bulimia, every year. And there is every sign that this will continue to rise, unabated, into the foreseeable future.

Robbins understands this phenomenon as coming from a larger "overachiever culture" that has caused "drastic changes in schools and homes prioritizing prestige, high-stakes testing, and accountability at the cost of families and schools." One Illinois high-school senior she interviews, sounding very much like Katie, puts it this way: "Many students view life as 'a conveyor belt' making monotonous scheduled stops 'at high school, college, graduate school, a job, more jobs, some promotions, and then you die.'"

In one last example of the way that Katie is "not alone," Mad in America blogger Douglas Bloch, a survivor of depression and now a teacher, author, and coach, develops related concerns for society at large. Bloch (2014) argues that we are living in an "age of melancholy." It is not just in our high schools, colleges, and medical institutions that people are having problems; we must face the fact that "society" can "become depressed." We live in a time when "evidence … from a study of 9,500 adults … found that people born near the end of the 20th century were three times more likely to develop depression than those born earlier." Bloch puts the blame on materialist culture, which leaves us cut off and disconnected from what matters: we are disconnected from our feelings, from one another, from a sense of time, from a sense of mortality, from the earth, from curiosity, creativity, and wonder, and from our spirit. For Bloch:

> We can no longer afford to view depression solely as a problem of the individual. The health of the society and the health of its individuals are inextricably linked. To end the worldwide epidemic of depression, we must combine individual psychological therapies with new social and economic systems that respect the earth and more fairly distribute the worlds resources. Such models already exist. What we need is the political will to implement them. If we can do so, we will be able to create a more equitable culture that optimizes the mental and emotional health of each of its citizens.

In short, Bloch and all of these Mad in America perspectives are telling us what Katie is telling us and what second-wave feminism told us years ago: the personal is political. And Katie is hardly the only one who feels this. When people, like Katie, come to the clinic with these concerns, we should take them seriously—not simply pathologize them.

Mad-Positive Models of Mental Difference

Even if the personal is political, that fact does not make it less personal. Individuals who are sensitive to social/political problems and who have feelings similar to those of Katie or Bloch or the Illinois high-school senior must find their way as individuals. How might Katie, or others with Katie's perspective, navigate these social problems and concerns. This is the second place where curiosity about the mad studies perspective can be helpful for psychiatry. How have people with lived experience of mental difference narrated and navigated the world in ways that reduce suffering and burnout and increase joy and human flowering?

A key way that mad studies has found to do so is through embracing mad-positive, or generative, models of psychic difference (Castrodale, 2019; Wilson, 2008, p. 69). These models are counterintuitive since mad-positive models—such as political, creative/expressive, and spiritual models—go against the grain of most clinical models. Unlike pathological models, mad-positive models frame psychic difference as *something positive rather than something negative*. From a mad-positive perspective, psychic difference from the norm is something to value, to be proud of, to channel, and even to celebrate (Lewis, 2017). This perspective is in sharp contrast to common clinical models, including the biopsychiatry but also psychoanalytic, cognitive-behavioral, interpersonal, and family models—all of which explain psychic difference in terms of pathology and dysfunction. Mental difference, from these pathological models, is something to be diminished, dampened, shocked, and even surgically removed.

Mad-positive models, by contrast, are generative. They organize psychic difference and psychic suffering around positive valuations of *sensitivity* and *yearning*. Common pathological approaches tell people to lessen their sensitivities and yearning through various medication or psychotherapy interventions. The cultural-stereotype refrains from pathological models—"stop being so sensitive," "grow up," "take your meds," "see your shrink"—all ask us to dampen our sensitivities and our yearnings. But when we move to mad-positive models, we turn the kaleidoscope 180 degrees the other way. Sensitivity and yearning become generative states to appreciate, an advantage rather than a disadvantage.

To see how this works, we can start with the social/political model that Katie uses. As we saw above, Katie is deeply sensitive to the social and political problems of the institution she is most directly exposed to—high school. If one uses a social/political model, it does not make sense to say that Katie is "out of touch with reality." Our Mad in America research shows us that many people share Katie's politics and many are more radical than Katie. But, at the same time, these perspectives are not "normal." Katie's mother, therapist, doctors, and possibly teachers seem to have none of these school concerns. Indeed, most people—who by being in the majority become the "normal" people—are not focused on the social/political problems of school. So when we say that Katie is sensitive, more sensitive than "normal," we are saying that she has a more subtle barometer or Geiger counter for these problems than do most "normal people."

At the time of her interview, Katie does not seem to have a developed political understanding of her experience or to be yearning for political change. "Yearning," as I am using it here, is described by bell hooks (2015) as a "common passion" and "sentiment" of longing for change that many suffering from social/political problems feel (p. 12). The particular social/political problems may be different, but the underlying longing and passion for change is shared across these political differences. As hooks puts it, "the shared space and feeling of 'yearning' opens up the possibility of common ground where all these differences might meet and engage one another" (p. 13).

Martin Luther King (1997) says it beautifully:

> Psychologists have a word which is probably used more frequently than any other word in modern psychology. It is the word "maladjusted." This word is the ringing cry of the new child psychology. Well, there are some

things in our social system to which I am proud to be maladjusted and to which I suggest that we ought to be maladjusted.

I never intend to adjust myself to the viciousness of lynch-mobs. I never intend to become adjusted to the evils of segregation and discrimination. I never intend to adjust myself to the tragic inequalities of an economic system which takes necessities from the masses to give luxuries to the classes. I never intend to become adjusted to the madness of militarism and the self-defeating method of physical violence.

History still has a choice place for those who have the moral courage to be maladjusted. The salvation of the world lies in the hands of the maladjusted.

(pp. 285–6)

From this social/political perspective, Katie's psychological difference from the norm, her maladjustment, is not a pathology. It is a sensitivity that might someday become a political yearning and might well be channeled into political activism or engaged research or creative work to help reverse the social suffering being caused by our current school system. In this way, using a generative social/political model rather than a pathological model, we can say that Katie's sensitivity is a valuable maladjustment. Only through maladjustment do we have hope of changing deep political problems.

Similarly, from the perspective of an artistic/creative model, we can see that a "sensitive artist" is nearly always a good thing. And, likewise, from a spiritual perspective, we admire a spiritual person's sensitive yearning for higher levels of consciousness and mystical experience. From a political perspective, we want revolutionaries like Mahatma Ghandi and Martin Luther King to be sensitive to political oppression and to help us be less prone to injustice, inequality, and political dysfunction. Similarly, we do not want our artists or our spiritual seekers to dampen their sensitivity or put their yearnings in a quiet room. We need our artists to help make the world more beautiful and more creatively rich, and we need our spiritual seekers to help keep us more in touch with spiritual values and spiritual depth.

There is nothing abstract about these possibilities for generative models. The pages of mad studies personal essays and memoirs, such as *We've been Too Patient: Voices from Radical Mental Health* (Green & Ubozoh, 2019); *Searching for a Rose Garden: Challenging Psychiatry, Fostering Mad Studies* (Russo & Sweeney, 2016); and *Outside Mental Health: Voices and Visions of Madness* (Hall, 2016), are full of testimonies for the value of mad-positive models of mental difference. As so many have shown, political, creative, and spiritual sensitiveness and yearnings can all be crucial catalysts that help transform not only people but also cultures and subcultures. All of these sensitivities and yearnings allow people to access generative realms of being that many "normal" people can never reach.

Mad-positive models also help people find community, connection, and friendship. Mental difference from the norm, by definition, can leave a person feeling isolated, disconnected, and abnormal. All of the generative models involve helping people find connections. When one uses a political, artistic, or spiritual model, one almost always shifts communities. One goes from a normal community—usually not that interested in politics, the arts, or spirituality—to a community that is very interested in these concerns. Even organizing around mental difference itself, coming together with other mad studies people and the larger disability studies community, all of whom are concerned about normal approaches to mental difference, can be a source of shift from isolation to community. In Katie's case, as we saw, a big part of the difficulty around her feelings about high school was that she felt "nobody likes her" and that she "lets everyone down."

The mad pride group formerly known as the *Icarus Project* understood this so well that the group spearheaded a key part of their organizing around consciousness-raising groups. In their workbook, *Friends Make the Best Medicine*, they outline how isolating mental difference can be and how much a shift in community can yield a shift in the way one feels:

> We have other people's language in our heads and on our tongues. Words like "disorder" and "disease" offer us one set of metaphors for understanding the way it feels to experience our lives through our particularly volatile minds and souls, but it is such a limited view. ... It controls how we feel about ourselves and whether we connect with other people. ... We need to start talking and networking—finding common ground and common language with the other people around us. We need to get together in groups and find language for our stories that make sense to us and leave us feeling good about ourselves. Unlearn social conditioning about what it means to be 'sick' and 'healthy'. We need to reclaim our dreams and scheme up ways to make them happen. We need to share everything we've figured out about how to be a human being. We need to love ourselves as we are.
>
> (Icarus Project, 2013, p. 4)

From this perspective, if Katie's school had a mad studies community, she could reduce her isolation and disconnection from the norm immediately. No treatment required.

Peter Tyrer, a British community psychiatrist, although not a mad studies scholar, used related insights to introduce a model of therapy he calls "nidotherapy." The term "nido" comes from the Latin word *nidus*, or "nest" (Tyrer, 2019). Tyrer argues that the metaphor of a nest can help us understand human cultural embeddedness. Using this metaphor as a guide, someone using a nidotherapy approach looks to see if a person's presenting difficulties have more to do with his or her cultural location—his or her "nest"—than with the particular person.

> The aim is to help the individual take up an acceptable role again, not to correct a biochemical disturbance, exorcize an unresolved conflict or recondition behavior. In many instances it will be realized quickly that the person being seen for help is not really unwell at all and is just in the wrong place at the wrong time.
>
> (Tyrer & Steinberg, 2005, p. 110).

Interestingly, a nidotherapy approach can allow mad-positive approaches to at least partially enter the clinical world. Nidotherapy, like mad-positive approaches, is not focused on changing the person unless that is something the person wants.

Nidotherapy and mad-positive approaches work with the person to locate the cultural environment where he or she best fits. Tyrer finds that "once the changes are made, the state of patient-hood is no more" (Tyrer & Steinberg, 2005 p. 111). What nidotherapy does not do, however, and what mad-positive approaches would do, is help build additional cultural spaces where yearning and sensitivity are valued and channeled.

Joining Narrative Medicine and Adopting a Narrative Hermeneutics Paradigm

A third way that mad studies can be of assistance to US psychiatry is by helping psychiatry shift its underlying paradigm. Taking people seriously, appreciating different perspectives, and engaging in the values of mad-positive models get to the heart of mad studies concerns to center "the perspectives and goals of those who have experienced madness, mental difference, altered mental states, mental suffering, and those who have felt harmed by psychiatric or psychological treatments" (Fletcher, 2025). This centering is also at the heart of the disability studies rallying cry "Nothing about us without us," and it is central to the call for epistemic justice in psychiatry and mental health care through the reduction of sanism. In the example of Katie, the treatment team's dismissal of her perspective is part of an effort to help Katie without Katie's input. Far from meeting the larger social goal of "nothing about us without us," it is, at the individual level, everything about Katie without Katie. Individual psychiatrists and therapists can avoid this kind of testimonial injustice by taking a shift to more inclusive paradigms.

Psychotherapy education author Jones-Smith (2016), in her book *Theories of Counseling and Psychotherapy*, calls the many inclusive paradigms that have emerged in psychotherapy the "fourth force" in mental health care. These fourth-force paradigms emerge after psychoanalytic, cognitive-behavioral, and existential humanistic paradigms (the first three "forces") in psychotherapy. Jones-Smith groups these fourth-force paradigms under the heading "social constructivism and postmodernism," and they include multicultural, transcultural, feminist, lesbian and gay, solution-focused, and narrative therapies (p. 373). We can also include "open dialogue," which has been a favorite in mad studies, in fourth-force approaches as well (Seikkula and Arnkil). A common ground across these fourth-force perspectives is that all these paradigms approach difference with care and subtlety and a recognition of the human aspects of meaning-making. Rather than "expert knows best," or in Katie's case, "everything about Katie without Katie," these fourth-force approaches demonstrate much more appreciation of a range of different perspectives and possibilities and are much less likely to cause the kind of epistemic injustice seen in Katie's situation.

Scholars of epistemic injustice call this range of worldviews "epistemic pluralism," which, as Fricker (2000) puts it, "acknowledges the existence of many different perspectives on a shared world" (p. 159; see also Allen, 2017, p. 193; Medina, 2011, p. 26). Epistemic pluralism is essential to epistemic justice because tolerating a diversity of perspectives requires accepting pluralism. Unfortunately, biopsychiatry, unlike these fourth-force paradigms, does not lend itself to appreciation and understanding of this range of different perspectives. Instead, biopsychiatry usually supports a hidden pedagogy of *one, and only one, true world*. This hidden pedagogy creates the opposite of epistemic pluralism: epistemic dogmatism and injustice (Kidd, Medina, & Pohlhaus, 2017). One way out of this hidden pedagogy is to adopt a version of what Fricker (2000) calls "perspectival realism" (p. 159). Different perspectives and different zeitgeists organize the real in different ways. There is a "real" world, but at the same time, it is multifaceted enough to allow different interpretations and different ways of life.

As Jones-Smith book makes clear, there are many forth-force philosophical and conceptual routes to Fricker's "perspectival realism." But for US psychiatry today, I would argue for narrative hermeneutics as an ideal route to the kind of epistemic pluralism needed for epistemic justice in psychiatry. This is primarily a strategic move, since narrative hermeneutics, unlike like Jones-Smith's "fourth-force" approaches, has already entered medicine. Narrative hermeneutics is the basic paradigm for "narrative medicine," a rapidly emerging new paradigm for medical work and therefore psychiatric work (Brockmeier & Meretoja, 2014; Charon et al., 2016; Lewis, 2011; Spencer, 2021). Narrative hermeneutics approaches to medicine and psychiatry are particularly adept at tending to the epistemological aspects, as well as the ontological and ethical aspects, of meaning-making (Lewis, 2011, forthcoming). Narrative hermeneutics develops an epistemology of perspectival pluralism, an ontology of pluridimesional ways of life, and an ethics that takes seriously questions of who gets to decide how to approach meaning-making and which meaning to live (Freeman, 2017, 2020; Meretoja, 2014, 2017). Psychiatrists can develop this narrative hermeneutics perspective by joining with their colleagues in narrative medicine to move beyond epistemic dogmatism and injustice (Charon et al., 2016).

Narrative medicine and narrative hermeneutics can help psychiatry achieve perspectival realism and epistemic pluralism through a deep understanding that psychiatric knowledge and psychiatric truth always involve questions of interpretation and meaning-making (Lewis, 2011, Forthcoming). Narrative hermeneutics, like philosophical hermeneutics, sees humans as meaning-making creatures, or as Charles Taylor (1985) so memorably put it, "self-interpreting animals"—we are constituted by the way we interpret ourselves and our worlds (p. 96). This builds on Hans-George Gadamer's (1970) foundational insight that interpretation is not

> an isolated activity of human beings but a basic structure of our experience of life. We are always taking something as something. That is the givenness of our world orientation, and we cannot reduce it to anything simpler or more immediate.
>
> (p. 87)

Narrative hermeneutics adds to philosophical hermeneutics by layering in narrative meaning-making as part of the larger process of human meaning-making (Brockmeier & Meretoja, 2014; Freeman, 2017; Ricouer, 1991, 1992). This narrative addition, as narrative medicine has found, is particularly relevant for interpreting ideas of self, identity, and difference and for how we tell the stories of our lives (Lewis, 2011, 2017). From this perspective, an ideal paradigm shift for psychiatry is for psychiatrists to see the discipline as a form of philosophical and narrative hermeneutics and to join with their colleagues in narrative medicine to work out what this means for clinical research, education, and practice.

Importantly, narrative hermeneutics would not jettison psychiatric science—just as narrative medicine has not had to jettison medical science. Katie's psychiatrists and even the precision psychiatrists would still be able to use clinical science to add to psychiatric knowledge. But, and this is critical, this science would no longer be able to trump other ways of knowing and other perspectives as happened in the Katie interview. Psychiatric science would become an interpretation, one that works through the methods of science, but an interpretation nonetheless. This interpretation would not be totalitarian; it would be pluralistic. It would be open to alternative interpretations and alternative approaches. It would do this not only at the "testimonial" level but also at the "hermeneutic" level of reorganizing the field to bring in a diverse array of research topics and practice approaches beyond the ones that dominate today. These topics and approaches would include those pivotal to mad studies, such as the role of social determinants, the role of art and creativity, the role of spirituality, the role of friendships and community, and the role of the deep prejudice of sanism, just to name a few.

Conclusion

It is important to understand that to practice mental health care is to be part of a contentious domain. The US psychiatrists who write the APA textbooks know this because for many years they have walked through a wall of protest and dissent outside the APA convention (Figure 32.5). These protesters are trying hard to be heard by giving interviews, by calmly explaining, by yelling, by making jokes, by artistic work, by creating posters, by creating videos, by writing readers, and by organizing to create alternatives. They are voicing the very concerns Katie might have if she were there: "Nothing about us without us," "Bet your ass we are paranoid," "Mental health is driving me crazy," "Label jars, not people," "Housing, not Haldol," "Psychiatry is outdated science," and, perhaps most important, "Another world is possible."

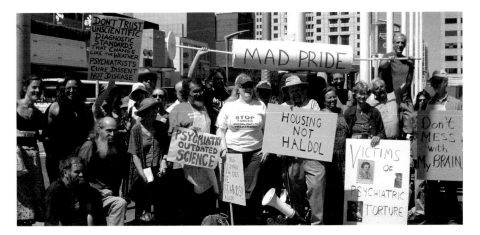

Figure 32.5 Protest of the American Psychiatric Association, 2009.
Source: Mindfreedom International.

Psychiatry must take these protesters seriously, and it must engage with the larger mad studies community trying to understand and develop these concerns.

Unfortunately, US psychiatry, as the APA textbooks make clear, is going the other way. Rather than take these voices and concerns seriously, normative US psychiatry is trying to quiet dissent and force compliance by pushing toward more rigorous biomedical frames, more aggressive biotech surveillance, more insistence on biomarkers, and more use of "precision" rhetoric. As it did with Katie's psychiatrist, this approach will put APA psychiatry in coalition with big pharma and the biotech industry more than with their clients, large sections of the general public, their own colleagues who have different perspectives, and the mad studies and disability studies communities.

The way forward in this situation is for US psychiatry to change its approach. But there is little sign that this will happen soon. Short of a revolution, clinicians practicing in the belly of the current paradigm can use mad studies assistance to form interdisciplinary and transdisciplinary alignments and coalitions with emerging mad studies, disability studies, and narrative medicine programs, texts, events, and communities. This book is an ideal example of that possibility and what it brings to an understanding of US psychiatry.

In addition, clinicians working in dominant paradigms can bring mad studies perspectives to their current therapeutic work through a position that China Mills (2014) calls "sly normality." Taking people's perspectives seriously, engaging with mad-positive models of mental difference, and adopting a narrative hermeneutics framework for understanding, when done well, can be a form of "passing" in mainstream settings. These mad studies approaches can pass as quality, "person-centered," or "narratively competent" clinical work while at the same time being deeply subversive to dominant paradigms. Clinicians using mad studies sly normality can serve, even in the most dogmatic clinical settings, as underground railroads to alternatives beyond the mainstream for those people who are unhappy with the dominant options. In Katie's example, a psychiatrist using these "sly normality" tactics and mad studies perspectives would allow for much greater epistemic justice in the work.

In the spirit of these very live options and possibilities, even in the midst of US psychiatry's current retrenchment in the other direction, let me conclude with an invitation. If you are a clinician concerned, as many clinicians are, with where mental health care is going, and if any or all of these mad studies perspectives make sense to you, let me formally welcome you to the mad studies community! Whether you are on the sly or ready to come out and join in the protest, your voices and your shoulders to the wheel are much appreciated!

Note

1 https://www.sunovionprofile.com/latuda-bpd/virtual-education-center, accessed 2/12/22.

References

Allen, A. (2017). Power/knowledge/resistance: Foucault and epistemic injustice. In I. J. Kidd, J. Medina, & G. Pohlhas (Eds.), *The Routledge handbook of epistemic injustice* (pp. 187–194). Routledge.

Belli, B. (2020, January 30). National survey: Students' feelings about high school are mostly negative. *Mad in America.* https://www.madinamerica.com/2020/02/national-survey-students-feelings-about-high-school-mostly-negative/

Black, D., & Andreasen, N. (2021). *Introductory textbook of psychiatry* (7th ed.). American Psychiatric Press. https://doi-org.proxy.library.nyu.edu/10.1176/appi.books.9781615373758

Bloch, D. (2014, June 30). Living in an age of melancholy: When society becomes depressed. *Mad in America.* https://www.madinamerica.com/2014/06/living-age-melancholy-society-becomes-depressed/

Brigham, T., Barden, C., Dopp, A. L., Hengerer, A., Kaplan, J., Malone, B., Martin, C., McHugh, M., & Nora, L. M. (2018). A journey to construct an all-encompassing conceptual model of factors affecting clinician well-being and resilience. *NAM Perspectives.* Discussion Paper, National Academy of Medicine. https://doi.org/10.31478/201801b

Brockmeier, J., & Meretoja, H. (2014). Understanding narrative hermeneutics. *Storyworlds, 6*(2), 1–27.

Castrodale, M. (2019). Mad studies and mad-positive music. *New Horizons in Adult Education and Human Resource Development, 31*(1):40–58.

Cathcart, S. (2018, May 30). Time for a paradigm shift in school psychology interventions. *Mad in America.* https://www.madinamerica.com/2018/05/time-paradigm-shift-school-psychology-interventions/

Cathcart, S. (2019, September 25). How social dynamics at school impact teen suicide. *Mad in America.* https://www.madinamerica.com/2019/09/social-dynamics-school-impact-teen-suicide/

Cathcart, S. (2020, November 16). Bystander training to prevent bullying improves student mental health. *Mad in America.* https://www.madinamerica.com/2020/11/bystander-training-prevent-bullying-improves-student-mental-health/

Cathcart, S. (2021, January 7). Parent engagement in student achievement and how schools can help. *Mad in America.* https://www.madinamerica.com/2021/01/parent-engagement-student-achievement-schools-can-help/

Charon, R., DasGupta, S., Hermann, N., Irvine, C., Marcus, E. R., Colsn, E. R., Spencer, D., & Spiegel, M. (2016). *Principles and practices of narrative medicine.* Oxford University Press.

Cook, J. A. (2019, March 1). How "Mental Health Awareness" exploits schoolchildren. *Mad in America.* https://www.madinamerica.com/2019/03/mental-healthcare-in-schools/

Corrigan, M. (2014, May 28). What should be the #1 prioirity of our schools? *Mad in America.* https://www.madinamerica.com/2014/05/1-priority-schools/

Davidow, S. (2016, January 16). Middle school invasion: When the pharmaceutical companies come to town. *Mad in America.* https://www.madinamerica.com/2016/01/middle-school-invasion-when-the-pharmaceutical-companies-come-to-town/

Effexor XR. (2001). *Archives of General Psychiatry, 58*(4), 368–69.

Fletcher, E. (2025). Theoretical considerations in mad studies. In J. Russel, A. Ali, & B. Lewis (Eds.), *Mad studies reader*. Routledge.

Freeman, M. (2017). Narrative hermeneutics. In J. Martin, J. Sugarman, & K. Slaney (Eds.), *The Wiley handbook of theoretical and philosophical psychology* (pp 234–247). Wiley Blackwell.

Freeman, M. (2020). Psychology as literature: Narrative knowing and the project of psychological humanities. In J. Sugarman & J. Martin (Eds), *A humanities approach to the psychology of personhood*. Routledge. https://doi-org.proxy.library.nyu.edu/10.4324/9780429323416

Fricker, M. (2000). Feminism in epistemology: Pluralism without postmodernism. In M. Fricker & J. Hornsby (Eds.), *The Cambridge companion to feminism in philosophy* (pp. 146–165). Cambridge University Press.

Gadamer, H. (1970). *On the scope and function of hermeneutical reflection* (G. B. Hess & R. E. Palmer, Trans.). Continuum.

Green, L. D., & Ubozoh, K. (Eds.). (2019). *We've been too patient: Voices from radical mental health*. North Atlantic Books.

Hall, W. (Ed.). (2016). *Outside mental health: Voices and visions of madness*. Madness Radio.

hooks, b. (2015). *Yearning: Race, gender and cultural politics*. Routledge.

Icarus Project. (2013). *Friends make the best medicine* (2nd ed.). Icarus Project.

Jones-Smith, E. (2016). *Theories of counseling and psychotherapy: An integrative approach* (2nd ed.). Sage.

Kidd, J., Medina, J., & Pohlhaus, G. (Eds.). (2017). *The Routledge handbook of epistemic injustice*. Routledge.

King, M. L. (1997). The 'New Negro' of the South: Behind the montgomery story. In C. Carson, S. Burns, S. Carson, D. Powell, & P. Holloran (Eds.), *The papers of Martin Luther King, Jr.: Volume 3. Birth of a new age* (pp. 280–286). University of California Press.

Lewis, B. (2011). *Narrative psychiatry: How stories can shape clinical practice*. Johns Hopkins University Press.

Lewis, B. (2017). A deep ethics for mental difference and disability: The 'case' of Vincent van Gogh. *Medical Humanities, 43*, 172–176.

Lewis, B. (Forthcoming). Psychiatric truth and narrative hermeneutics. In H. Meretoja & M. Freeman (Eds.), *The use and abuse of stories: New directions in narrative hermeneutics*. Oxford University Press.

Mad in America. (2021, August 3). Retrieved August 3, 2021 from https://www.madinamerica.com/

Medina, J. (2011). Toward a Foucaultian epistemology of resistance: Counter-memory, epistemic friction, and *guerrilla* pluralism. *Foucault Studies, 12*, 9–35.

Meretoja, H. (2014). Narrative and human existence: Ontology, epistemology, and ethics. *New Literary History, 45*(1), 89–109.

Meretoja, H. (2017). *The ethics of storytelling: Narrative hermeneutics, history and the possible*. Oxford University Press.

Mills, C. (2014). Sly normality: Between quiescence and revolt. In B. Burstow, B. A. LeFrançois, & S. Diamond (Eds.), *Psychiatry disrupted: Theorizing resistance and crafting the (r)evolution* (pp. 208–224). McGill-Queen's University Press.

Mindfreedom International. (n.d.). https://mindfreedom.org/

National Academy of Medicine. (2019). *Action collaborative on clinician well-being and resilience.* https://nam.edu/initiatives/clinician-resilience-and-well-being/

Peters, S. (2017, June 7). Humanistic counseling effective in schools, study finds. *Mad in America.* https://www.madinamerica.com/2017/06/humanistic-counseling -effective-schools-study-finds/

Ricoeur, P. (1991). Life in quest of narrative. In D. Wood (Ed.), *On Paul Ricoeur: Narrative and interpretation.* Routledge.

Ricoeur, P. (1992). *Oneself as another.* University of Chicago Press.

Robbins, A. (2019, March 15). Kids are the victims of the elite-college obsession. *Mad in America.* https://www.madinamerica.com/2019/03/kids-victims-elite-college -obsession/

Roberts, L., Hales, R., & Yudofsky, S.. (2019). *The American psychiatric association publishing textbook of psychiatry* (7th ed.). The American Psychiatric Press. https:// doi-org.proxy.library.nyu.edu/10.1176/appi.books.9781615372980

Russo, J., & Sweeney, A. (Eds.). (2016). *Searching for a rose garden: Challenging psychiatry, fostering mad studies.* PCCS Books.

Seikkula, J., & Arnkil, T. E. (2006). *Dialogical meetings in social networks.* Karnac Books.

Sunovion ProFile. (n.d.). *Latuda.* https://www.sunovionprofile.com/latuda-bpd/

Spencer. D. (2021). *Metagnosis: Revelatory narratives of health and identity.* Oxford University Press.

Taylor, C. (1985). *Human agency and language: Philosophical papers I.* Cambridge University Press.

Troeger, R. (2017, September 27). Study investigates long-term effects of social and emotional learning programs. *Mad in America.* https://www.madinamerica.com /2017/09/study-investigates-long-term-effects-social-emotional-learning-programs/

Tyrer, P. (2019). Nidotherapy: A cost-effective systematic environmental intervention. *World Psychiatry, 18*(2), 144–45.

Tyrer, P., & Steinberg, P. (2005). *Models for mental disorder* (4th ed.). John Wiley and Sons.

Williams, L., Ball, T., & Kircos, C. (2019). Precision psychiatry. In L. Roberts, R. Hales, & S. Yudofsky (Eds.), *The American psychiatric association publishing textbook of psychiatry,.* The American Psychiatric Press. https://doi-org.proxy.library.nyu.edu /10.1176/appi.books.9781615372980

Wilson, E. (2008). *Against happiness: In praise of melancholy.* Farrar, Straus and Giroux.

Part IV. Daring Activists

DOI: 10.4324/9781003148456-37

MAD ACTIVISTS ARE PART OF A social movement that has gone by many names: "mad liberation," "antipsychiatry," "mental patients' liberation," "psychiatric survivor," "ex-patient," "ex-inmate," "mental health consumer," "c/s/x" (short for consumer/survivor/ex-patient), "neurodiversity," "radical mental health," "mad resistance," "mad pride," and simply "the movement." The variety of terms for what can be seen as a single movement speaks to the common ground and the diversity of concerns, perspectives, and histories of the people involved in mad activism. To understand this social movement, it helps to think through both the commonalities and the diversities.

The key common-ground issues are the social toxins we have been discussing through the reader—sanism, epistemic injustice, and structural inequality—and the way these can create harmful experiences and abuses for those who engage with mental health systems. These mental health systems are vast, and while not everyone has a bad experience, many mad activists (including ourselves) have had direct experiences with the oppressive and pernicious aspects of the system (Morrison, 2006). Many of us are drawn to mad activism when we or someone among our family or close relations has been diagnosed and/or treated by the system and that experience has made things worse rather than better. Whatever problems first brought us to the mental health system—either of our own volition or through the insistence, manipulation, or force of others—mental health care left us with additional problems caused by the system itself. In other words, we found the mental health system wounding to our being or to someone we cared about. We realized we were not alone in these often alienating and oppressive systems, and we became "activated" to change the system.

Mental health care, despite its manifest efforts to be beneficial, can be wounding in multiple ways: physically, psychologically, spiritually, socially, and politically, just to name a few. Physically, medical-model treatments for mental difference are often aggressive (compared with more holistic approaches) and have multiple side effects. The life expectancy for people diagnosed with mental illness is 20% lower than for the general population—a significant part of this has to do with iatrogenic side effects of psychiatric medications (Thornicroft, 2011). Mental health treatments are also physically damaging; they overlap with incarceration in various ways—what Ben-Moshe (2020) calls "carceral ableism"—which can easily turn punitive and violent, resulting in a range of bodily harms. Psychologically, the mental health system can be wounding, alienating, and deskilling through multiple processes associated with diagnostic labels that harbor sanist and pathological hierarchies. These hierarchies can be dehumanizing, at times changing our self-definition to someone who is "mentally ill, dysfunctional, broken, or crazy." Spiritually, the mental health system's persistent secular stance risks neglecting and pathologizing people's spiritual and existential frames of meaning, which are vital to their wellbeing. Socially, those who have been through the mental health system are more likely to experience social isolation, alienation, discrimination, and abuse.

Politically, mental health and interconnected systems divert attention from problems of social justice, community development, structural violence, and inequity. By labeling mental difference and distress as individual deficiencies, they make invisible the institutional abuse enacted by these systems, furthering distress and suffering. Understanding how these interconnected systems can perpetuate harm requires us to adopt a social and political imagination that moves beyond mental health systems isolated from other systems. We have to see how the mental health system fits with Katheryn Pauly Morgan's outer squares of the medical industrial complex and the larger politics of technocracy, patriarchy, structural alliances, and political economy (Figure P.2 in Critical Scholars). Disability activist Mia Mingus also provides a helpful visualization of these larger links in her article 'The Medical Industrial Complex' in her blog *Leaving Evidence*.[1]

As we discussed in the Introduction to Part II (Critical Scholars), we have found Naomi Klein's (2007) concept of "disaster capitalism" helpful in this domain. By disaster capitalism, we mean the way mental health systems contribute to social/political causes of mental distress and debility while at the same time profiting from and distracting us from these systems (by blaming biological or cognitive variables). In short, mental health systems risk blaming the victims and profiting from them at the same time. Mad activism associated with the Occupy movement provides a good example of activists who are making this political connection. Here is how they put it in their handbook, *Mindful Occupation: Rising Up Without Burning Out* (2012):

> It's easy to see connections between radical mental health and the Occupy movement. After all, both movements are challenging the objectification of persons and nature at large. In the radical mental health movement, we raise our voice against the mainstream mental health system in which our complex experiences are objectified into labels that fit cookie-cutter understandings of mental health. In the Occupy movement, we raise our voice against the corporate-centered

culture where our lives are treated as objects whose purpose is to bring financial gain to corporations.

(p. 19)

Activists within the disability justice movement have also laid the groundwork for an intersectional movement that combats and contextualizes madness and sanism within a broader critique of systems that treat certain body-minds as more dysfunctional and disposable than others. Combating ableism on all fronts requires that we understand

> no body stands outside the consequences of injustice and inequality. … What our bodies require in order to thrive, is what the world requires. If there is a map to get there, it can be found in the atlas of our skin and bone and blood, in the tracks of neurotransmitters and antibodies.
> (Morales, 2013)

The disability justice framework moves beyond a "rights-based" model that invisibilizes the roots of inequity, toward an end to ableism and sanism in all its manifestations in and through the forces of colonialism, white supremacy, capitalism, and heteropatriarchy (Berne, 2020). Speaking to the intersectionality required of disability justice and related movements, Patty Berne writes in *Skin, Tooth, and Bone: The Basis of Movement is Our People, A Disability Justice Primer* (2020), "We are in a global system that is incompatible with life. There is no way to stop a single gear in motion—we must dismantle this machine."

The frequently used rallying cries for mad pride activism also help us see the common ground of the movement. These rallying cries overlap with those from other social movements such as the women's movement, disability rights movement, and social justice movements: "The personal is political," "Nothing about us without us," and "Another world is possible." Some are specific to mad pride, such as "You bet your ass we are paranoid" chanted over a large paper hypodermic needle.

Perhaps the most important and most counterintuitive rallying cry is "mad pride" itself. Within a normative system, mental difference and distress is an illness. There is nothing, as one critic puts it, to be "proud" about:

> Mental illness is an illness, just as cancer is an illness; and people die from both. … Mental illness is not an identity. Nor is it something I wish to celebrate. … Mental illness is ruthless, indiscriminate and destructive.
> (Allan, 2006)

The problem with this perspective is threefold. First, it declares dogmatically that there is one truth of mental difference and that "truth" tells us that our difference "is an illness." This "truth" leaves out all the epistemic justice issues of who gets to decide, for whom, and through what forms of participation. Second, this dogmatic pathologization loses sight of a notion of pride that is deeply tied to the goal of reclaiming the very ground of equal citizenship. As French protesters have highlighted, "We are, above all, citizens here. There are no patients, no users, just people and citizens who want to shout out loud: 'We exist, with our differences.'

That is what Mad Pride is about" (quoted in Haigh, 2016, p. 202). Third, dogmatic pathologization reinforces sanist prejudice and leaves out the many ways that mental difference and mental suffering can have positive value.

For mad pride activists, to be outside the norm can be seen as a "gift"–particularly if our sensitivities and our thin skins give us access to understandings that we and others need. Sensitivity to beauty, the sublime, and aesthetic value, as we discussed in the Innovative Artists section, can be a good thing, a gift rather than a pathology. Similarly, sensitivity to political injustice and sensitivity to spiritual depth can be a good thing. We want our artists, our political leaders, and our spiritual seekers to be sensitive and to yearn for another world–in short, to feel and know aspects of the world outside the norm. This mad-positive openness to and pride in the value of sensitivity and yearning does not mean romanticizing mental difference and/or distress. As Sascha DuBrul explains in Chapter 34, the activist group the Icarus Project often used the compound term "dangerous/gift" to highlight the values of difference and at the same time the difficulties and challenges of difference in a normative world.

In addition to these many common grounds, there is also considerable diversity and, at times, tensions within the mad pride movement. Historically, the most prominent voices within the movement have been made up of White, middle-class folks from the Global North whose analysis of oppression within the mental health system failed to acknowledge, let alone center, the experiences of Blacks, Indigenous survivors, or movement organizers from the Global South. This mirrored in some ways the treatments, models, and frameworks from the Global North that have been historically privileged despite biomedical psychiatry having far-reaching impacts worldwide as a colonial project of social control. The inequity within the movement itself, mirroring the wider culture of colonialism, White supremacy, and racism, has sidelined intersectional experiences of oppression such as ableism, homophobia, racism, ethnocentrism, sexism, and more. International and intersectional movement collaboration has been crucial to finding a polyphony of answers to questions of inequity, drawing on creative works of prison abolition, environmental justice, disability justice, trans liberation, and many other liberatory movements. Because many people who are harmed by the mental health system either find their way there by way of, or get funneled into, carceral, medical, educational, or other institutions, the resistance to these systems also can't be siloed from the lens and experiences of people suffering multiple systemic injustices.

We can see these differences and tensions in the mad pride movement as falling out along multiple lines of continuation. Here are some of the most common:

- For some, the goal is to reform the mental health system. For others, the goal is to vastly shrink or do away with mental health systems.
- For some, the goal is to remove all notions of bodily or neurological causation of mental difference and to focus solely on psycho-social-political-aesthetic-spiritual differences. For others, the goal is to see biological and neurological difference as the result of trauma from these other issues, or as simply as human neurodiversity, not pathology.

- For some, the focus is more single-issue-oriented around mental difference and sanism. For others, the focus is much more intersectional to highlight the many overlapping prejudices, discriminations, and subordinations between sanism and racism, sexism, homophobia, classism, colonialism, ableism, and so on.
- For some, the focus is on larger social and political structures of inequality and subordination—the outer squares of Morgan's medicalized hegemony or Mingus' medical industrial complex—which often push people into mental distress and suffering. For others, the focus is much more on the inner circles of mental health systems and the power dynamics between mental health knowledge systems and mental health providers.
- For some, the focus is local or national. For others, the focus is global and international.
- For some, the goal is the creation of separatist groups—for example, groups composed of only clinicians or groups without clinicians at all. For others, the goal is the creation of hybrid groups with participants from multiple locations.
- For some, the goal is critique of mental health systems. For others, the goal is to build new possibilities outside the system for reskilling ourselves and for providing mutual aid in times of need.

Mad studies approaches to mad activism, as we see them, take seriously all these differences and tensions as well as the many common grounds between activists and activist groups. From a mad studies perspective, understanding both the diversity and the commonality of the mad movement provides leverage for coalition as well as separatist tactics and strategies. The goal for all, as we see it, is a less sanist world, more epistemic justice around mental difference, and a world with less structured violence, inequality, and debilitation. The route to these goals can vary in different times, for different people, and for different projects. At large, the following chapters highlight our collective and diverse visions for a less exclusionary, more just, and more democratic future. Nothing about us without us. Indeed, nothing without us.

Note

1 Mia Mingus' website link: https://leavingevidence.wordpress.com/2015/02/06/medical-industrial-complex-visual/

References

Allan, C. (2006, September 26). Misplaced pride. *The Guardian*. https://www.theguardian.com/commentisfree/2006/sep/27/society.socialcare

Ben-Moshe, L. (2020). *Decarcerating disability: Deinstitutionalization and prison abolition*. University of Minnesota Press.

Berne, P. (2020, June 16). What is disability justice? *Sins Invalid*. https://www.sinsinvalid.org/news-1/2020/6/16/what-is-disability-justice

Haigh, S. (2016). "Mad Pride France": Disability, mental distress, and citizenship. *Journal of Literary & Cultural Disability Studies, 10*(2), 191–206.

Klein, N. (2007). *The shock doctrine: The rise of disaster capitalism.* Metropolitan Books / Henry Holt.

Morales, A. L. (2013). *Kindling: Writings on the body.* Palabrera Press.

Morrison, L. (2006). A matter of definition: Acknowledging consumer/survivor experiences through narrative. *Radical Psychology, 5.* http://www.radpsynet.org/journal/vol5/Morrison.html

Occupy Mental Health Project. (2012). *Mindful occupation: Rising up without burning out.* https://mindfuloccupation.org/files/booklet/mindful_occupation_singles_latest.pdf

Thornicroft, G. (2011). Physical health disparities and mental illness: The scandal of premature mortality. *The British Journal of Psychiatry, 199,* 441–442.

Chapter 33

The Ex-Patients' Movement

WHERE WE'VE BEEN AND WHERE WE'RE GOING[1]

Judi Chamberlin

Summary

Judi Chamberlin (1944–2010) is an icon in the movement for social justice around mental health and mental difference. Her work, and the work of mad pride activism more broadly, can be understood in the context of her personal experiences. For Chamberlin, as for the women's movement more broadly, the personal is political. Chamberlin's personal story began when she was 21 years old, and when she went to her medical doctor because of feelings of deep depression.

> After a while, he [the doctor] suggested I sign myself into a hospital because I was just not functioning, I was so depressed. And I just thought, "Oh a hospital's a place where you get help." And you know, I'd been in hospitals for surgery and things like that, and didn't think of it as having anything to do with your fundamental rights. So I just said, "OK, I'll try it."
>
> (Hall, 2006)

Very quickly Chamberlin found out that even though she had signed in "on a voluntary basis," she was confined against her will. "You can't leave when you want to leave, which was absolutely shocking to me." She found the whole experience traumatic, making her situation more difficult than it was before. This has been a common ground of so many in the mad pride movement, mental health "help" ended up making things worse. When Chambers eventually did get out, she started working with other former patients in the Boston area to change the system. The group called themselves the Mental Patients Liberation Front.

David Oaks, founder of Mindfreedom International (another beacon for mad pride activism in the US), describes Chamberlin's early work:

DOI: 10.4324/9781003148456-38

> When I arrived at this storefront in Cambridge, Mass. [1976], I was a
> senior Harvard student, had been locked up five times, so I was referred
> by Harvard to volunteer there. ... I walked in, and it was a little radical
> ragtag group, Mental Patients Liberation Front. And Judi was right in
> the thick of folks, just really warm, community organizer. One thing
> she immediately helped teach a lot of people was basic 101 about mental
> health liberation: That we're equal; that we have rights.
>
> (Shapiro, 2010)

Chamberlin went on to write *On Our Own: Patient Controlled Alternatives to the Mental
Health System* (1979), which became an inspiration and manifesto for other people
going through similar experiences. Her book first coined the term "mentalism,"
which Chamberlin continues to use in the chapter printed here: "'Mentalism' and
'sane chauvinism' [are] a set of assumptions" that people diagnosed with mental
illness are "incompetent, unable to do things for themselves, constantly in need
of supervision and assistance, unpredictable, likely to be violent or irrational or
so forth." Chamberlin found it doubly tragic that not only did the general public
hold these "crippling stereotypes," but these stereotypes often became forms of
"internalized oppression" for the victims themselves.

Robert Whitaker, the author of *Mad in America* (2001) and publisher of madinamerica
.com, describes Chamberlin as "incredibly fierce. ... She knew her mind, she spoke
her mind, and she didn't worry if she offended people who were listening" (Shapiro,
2010). Chamberlin was irreverent, "brilliant," plus a "joy to be around." She was also
"incredibly brave," because "it obviously takes a lot of bravery to confront a society
that's had a different belief before." Chamberlin followed in the footsteps of "Black
pride" to reclaim "mad" as something that was human and valuable in a problematic
world: "She changed it from ... a pejorative word." She said to the world, "We are
worthy individuals, and our minds our worthy, and they're to be respected."

In 1990, when Chamberlin wrote this article, she was working for the Ruby
Rogers Advocacy and Drop-In Center in Cambridge, Massachusetts. That center
no longer exists, but for a comparable contemporary advocacy see the Wildflower
Alliance[2] and the work of Caroline Mazel-Carlton (Berger, 2022).

Here is how Chamberlin introduced the article printed here:

> The mental patients' liberation movement, which started in the
> early 1970s, is a political movement comprised of people who have
> experienced psychiatric treatment and hospitalization. Its two main
> goals are developing self-help alternatives to medically-based psychiatric
> treatment and securing full citizenship rights for people labeled "mentally
> ill." The movement questions the medical model of "mental illness," and
> insists that people who have been labeled as "mentally ill" speak on their
> own behalf and not be represented by others who claim to speak "for"
> them. The movement has developed its own philosophy, and operates
> a variety of self-help and mutual support programs in which ex-patients
> themselves control the services that are offered. Despite obstacles, the
> movement continues to grow and develop.

*

A complete history of the mental patients' liberation movement is still to be written. Like other liberation struggles of oppressed people, the activism of former psychiatric patients has been frequently ignored or discredited. Only when a group begins to emerge from subjugation can it begin to reclaim its own history. This process has been most fully developed in the black movement and the women's movement; it is in a less developed stage in the gay movement and the disability movement (of which the ex-patients' movement may be considered a part).

The "madman," as defined by others, is part of society's cultural heritage. Whether "madness" is explained by religious authorities (as demonic possession for example), by secular authorities (as disturbance of the public order), or by medical authorities (as "mental illness"), the mad themselves have remained largely voiceless. The movement of people who call themselves variously, ex patients, psychiatric inmates, and psychiatric survivors is an attempt to give voice to individuals who have been assumed to be irrational – to be "out of their minds."

The ex-patients' movement began approximately in 1970 but we can trace its history back to many earlier former patients, in the late nineteenth and early twentieth centuries, who wrote stories of their mental hospital experiences and who attempted to change laws and public policies concerning the "insane." Thus, in 1868, Mrs. Elizabeth Packard published the first of several books and pamphlets in which she detailed her forced commitment by her husband in the Jacksonville (Illinois) Insane Asylum. She also founded the Anti-Insane Asylum Society, which apparently never became a viable organization (Dain, 1989). Similarly, in Massachusetts at about the same opinion Elizabeth Stone, also committed by her husband, tried to rally public opinion to the cause of stopping the unjust incarceration of the "insane."

In the early part of this century, Clifford Beers, a wealthy young businessman, experienced several episodes of confused thinking and agitation which caused him to be placed in a mental hospital. Following his recovery, Beers (1953) wrote a book, *A Mind that Found Itself*, which went through numerous editions and which led to the formation of the influential National Committee on Mental Hygiene (later the National Association for Mental Health) Dain (1989) states that

> Beers was outspoken about abuse of mental patients and passionate in defending their rights and damning psychiatrists for tolerating mistreatment of patients. But he eventually toned down his hostility to psychiatry as it became obvious that for his reform movement to gain the support he sought at the highest levels of society it would have to include leading psychiatrists. Although he envisioned that eventually former mental patients and their families would be recruited into the movement, the public's persistent prejudice against mentally disturbed people and Beers' own doubts and inclinations, plus pressures from psychiatrists, drew him away from this goal.
>
> (pp.9–10)

Dain also notes, in passing, the formation of the Alleged Lunatics' Friend Society in 1845 by former patients in England. On the whole, however, this early history is obscure, and the development of modern ex-patient groups in the United States at the beginning of the 1970s occurred primarily without any knowledge of these historical roots.

Although the terms have often been used interchangeable, "mental patients' liberation" (or "psychiatric inmates' liberation") anti-psychiatry are not the same thing. "Anti-psychiatry" is largely an intellectual exercise of academics and dissident mental health professionals. There has been little attempt within anti-psychiatry to reach out to struggling ex-patients or to include their perspective. The focus in this paper is on ex-patient (or ex-inmate) groups I identify the major principles that have guided the development of the ex-patients' movement, sketch the recent history of this movement, describe its major goals and accomplishments, and discuss the challenges facing it in this decade.

Stigma and discrimination still make it difficult for people to identify themselves as ex-mental patients if they could otherwise pass as "normal," reinforcing public perceptions that the "bag lady" and the homeless drifter are representative of all former patients. Like the exemplary black persons of a generation or two ago – who were held to be "a credit to their race" and, by definition, atypical of black people generally – so the former mental patient who is successfully managing his or her life is widely seen as the exception that proves the rule.

Guiding Principles of the Movement

Exclusion of Non-Patients

In the United States, former patients have found that they work best when they exclude mental health professionals (and other non-patients) from their organizations (Chamberlin, 1987). There are several reasons why the movement has grown in this direction – a direction which began to develop in the early 1970s, influenced by the black, women's and gay liberation movements. Among the major organizing principles of these movements were self-definition and self-determination. Black people felt that white people could not truly understand their experiences; women felt similarly about men; homosexuals similarly about heterosexuals. As these groups evolved, they moved from defining themselves to setting their own priorities. To mental patients who began to organize, these principles seemed equally valid. Their own perceptions about "mental illness" were diametrically opposed to those of the general public, and even more so to those of mental health professionals. It seemed sensible, therefore, not to let non-patients into ex-patient organizations or to permit them to dictate an organization's goals.

There were also practical reasons for excluding non-patients. Those groups that did not exclude non-patients from membership almost always quickly dropped their liberation aspects and became reformist. In addition, such groups rapidly moved away from ex-patient control, with the tiny minority of non-patient members taking on leadership roles and setting future goals and directions. These experiences served as powerful examples to newly-forming ex-patient organizations that mixed membership was indeed destructive.

In attempting to solve these organizational problems, group members began to recognize a pattern they referred to as "mentalism" and "sane chauvinism," a set of assumptions which most people seemed to hold about mental patients: that they were incompetent, unable to do things for themselves, constantly in need of supervision and assistance, unpredictable, likely to be violent or irrational, and so forth. Not only did the general public express mentalist ideas; so did ex-patients themselves. These crippling stereotypes became recognized as a form of internalized oppression. The struggle against internalized oppression and mentalism generally was seen as best accomplished in groups composed exclusively of patients, the process of consciousness-raising (borrowed from the women's movement).

Consciousness-Raising

The consciousness-raising process is one in which people share and examine their own experiences to learn about the contexts in which their lives are embedded. As used by the women's movement, consciousness-raising helped women to understand that matters of sexuality, marriage, divorce, job discrimination, roles, and so forth were not individual, personal problems but were instead indicators of society's systematic oppression of women. Similarly, as mental patients began to share their life stories, it became clear that distinct patterns of oppression existed and that our problems and difficulties were not solely internal and personal, as we had been told they were. The consciousness-raising process may be hampered by the presence of those who do not share common experiences (e.g., as women or as mental patients). As the necessity for consciousness-raising became more evident, it provided still another reason for limiting group members.

Consciousness-raising is an ongoing process, with people and groups constantly recognizing deeper levels of oppression. Within an ex-patient group various activities often lead to further consciousness-raising experiences. For example, a group may approach a local newspaper or television reporter to write a story about the group's work or to give its viewpoint on a current mental health issue. If the group's representatives are treated respectfully and their opinions listened to, no consciousness-raising issues arises. If, however, the reporter is unwilling to listen to the group's representatives or seems to disbelieve them or makes comments about their mental status, it can become an occasion for further consciousness-raising. Whereas, before the advent of the patients' liberation movement, the group might have altered its strategy or even disbanded after such a discouraging incident, armed with the knowledge that they have run into systematic discrimination they can decide how to proceed. They may complain to the reporter's superior. They may raise questions about discrimination against mental patients. Because of consciousness-raising, they will have a clear idea of what they are facing.

Historical Development of the Movement

Like many new developments in the United States, mental patients' liberation groups began primarily on the east and west coast and then spread inland. Among the earliest groups were the Insane Liberation Front in Portland, Oregon (founded in 1970), the Mental Project in New York City, the Mental Patients' Liberation Front in Boston (both founded in 1971), and the Network Against Psychiatric Assault in San Francisco (founded in 1972). Local groups took a long time to establish ongoing communications, because they were not funded and membership consisted mostly of low income individuals. The development of two major means of communication, the annual Conference on Human Rights and Psychiatric Oppression, and the San Francisco-based publication, *Madness Network News*, helped the movement to grow. Interestingly, both the Conference and *Madness Network News* began as mixed groups but later were operated and controlled solely by ex-patients (see below).

The first Conference on Human Rights and Psychiatric Oppression was held in 1973 at the University of Detroit, jointly sponsored by a sympathetic (non-patient) psychology professor and the New York City-based Mental Patients' Liberation Project (MPLP). Approximately fifty people from across the United States (and Canadian representatives) met for several days to discuss the developing philosophy and goals of mental patients' liberation. The leadership role of ex-patients was acknowledged; for example, the original name proposed by the sponsoring professor for the conference ("The Rights of the Mentally Disabled") was roundly rejected as stigmatizing. Although no plan was made in Detroit to continue the conference, the practice later developed of designating an attending group to sponsor the next year's conference. The conference became limited to patients and ex-patients only in 1976. Conferences were held annually through 1985 (see below for later developments).

Madness Network News began as a San Francisco-area newsletter in 1972 and gradually evolved into a newspaper format covering the ex-patients' movement in North America as well as worldwide. *Madness Network News'* original core group included both self-styled "radical" mental health professional and ex-patients, but within a few years a major struggle ensued and the paper was published solely by ex-patients. There were also struggles between women, and men ex-patients resulting in special women's issues edited by all-women, all-ex-patient staffs. *Madness Network News* existed solely on subscription income, which was sufficient to cover printing and mailing cost, but did not allow for salaries. For many years this publication was the voice of the American ex-patients' movement, a journal which published personal experiences, creative writing, art, political theory, and factual reporting, all from the ex-patient point of view. Madness Network News ceased publication in 1986.

The heart of the movement, however, continued to be the individual local group. Although some groups existed for only short period, the overall number of groups continued to grow. Most groups were started by a small number of people coalescing out of a shared anger and a sense that through organization they could bring about change. Groups were independent, loosely linked through *Madness Network News* and the annual Conference. Each group developed its own ideologies, terminology, style and goals. Groups were known by an astonishing variety of names, from the straightforward (Mental Patients' Alliance; Network Against Psychiatric Assault) to the euphemistic (Project Acceptance; Reclamation, Inc.). Some groups were organized as traditional hierarchies with officer and held formal meetings while other groups moved toward more egalitarian structures with shared decision-making and no formal leadership. Groups were united by certain rules and principles: mental health terminology was considered suspect; attitudes that limited opportunities for mental patients were to be discouraged and changed; and members' feelings – particular feelings of anger toward the mental health system – were considered real and legitimate, not "symptoms of illness."

The activities of various groups included organizing support groups, advocating for hospitalized patients, lobbying for changes in laws, public speaking publishing newsletters, developing creative and artistic ways of dealing with the mental patient experience, etc. The two primary thrusts were advocacy and self-help alternatives to the psychiatric system, as it quickly became clear to each group that its own membership's needs largely fell into these two areas.

Different groups developed different terminologies to describe themselves and their work. "Ex-patient" was a controversial term because it appeared to embrace the medical model; *Madness Network News* promoted the use of "ex-psychiatric inmate," which became widespread. Other groups referred to themselves as "clients," "consumers," or "psychiatric survivors." Differences in terminology stressed differing emphases and priorities' clearly the individuals labeling themselves "inmates" or "survivors" took the more militant stance.

Because most groups existed with little or no outside funding they were limited in their accomplishments. The question of funding generated numerous controversies, as did the question of reimbursement for organizational labor. Even if the group decided it had no objection in principle to receiving outside funding, obtaining such funding was difficult. Potential funding sources tended to look askance on ex-patient groups – especially groups that rejected psychiatric ideology and terminology. Moreover, foundations which funded community organizing efforts did not view ex-patient groups as falling within their purview. Finally, state departments of mental health were seldom approached because of their role in running the very institutions in which group members had been oppressed. And those mental health departments that were approached were highly skeptical of the ability of ex-patient groups to run their own projects.

Gradually, however, inroads were made. Members of ex-patient groups demanded involvement in the various forums from which they were excluded – conferences, legislative hearings, board, committees and the like Although at first in only the most token numbers, ex-patients were slowly invited to take part in such forums. Often groups had to insist on being invited, however.

Once involved in such meetings, ex-patients could move in two different tactical directions: cooperation or confrontation. Clearly, much was said in these forums which directly contradicted the movement's developing ideology. While most such meetings featured a reliance on psychiatric terminology and diagnosis, and on the assumption that patients existed in a lifetime dependency relationship, the patients' movement stood in opposition to the medical model and in support of self-reliance and self-determination. Although ex-patients' objections to such mentalist assumptions were often used as a reason to exclude ex-patients from future meetings, it is to the movement's credit that the ex-patients did speak up and object to much of what was being said Frequently-heard objections from professional participants were that the ex-patients "polarized the discussion" or were "disruptive." Professionals sometimes chose to work with non-movement identified ex-patients who were much more likely to be compliant. For example, the most publicly visible post to go to an ex-patient in the 1970s — as one of the twenty-member President's Commission on Mental Health — went to a woman who had never worked with an ex-patient group but who had written about her patienthood experience in professional journals.

However, from this forum, as from others, the movement refused to be excluded. Movement activists packed many of the Commission's public hearings, testifying eloquently about the harmfulness of the psychiatric treatments they had experienced while pleading for enforcement of patients' rights and funding of patient-run alternatives to traditional treatment. The Commission's final report acknowledged the role of alternative treatments, stating that many of the latter "are wary of being classified as mental health services, convinced that such a classification entails a medical perspective and implies authoritarian relationships and derogatory labeling" ("Report," 1978, p. 14). The report went on to note that "groups composed of individuals with mental or emotional problems are in existence or are being formed all over the United States" (pp. 14-15).

The movement also demanded its inclusion in a series of conferences organized by the Community Support Program (CSP), a small division of the National Institute of Mental Health (NIMH). CSP, which began in the late 1970s, focused on providing assistance to programs in community settings. However, in the movement's view, these programs often perpetuated many of the worst features of institutionalization, including labeling, forced drugging, and paternalistic control. The participation of ex-patients in CSP conferences (even though the movement activists were vastly outnumbered by mental health professionals) forced CSP to acknowledge the importance of funding patient-run programs as a part of community support. Such recommendations would not have been made — indeed, would not even have been considered — without the tenacity of movement activists who insisted on being heard.

Participation in professionally-sponsored conferences and meetings produced an additional unintended benefit. It enabled ex-patients to meet each other and learn from one another. Such contacts, especially by people from different geographical areas, were previously difficult but later became a source of inspiration and support during the exercise of an otherwise thankless task — to present the patient viewpoint to audiences that were often indifferent or even hostile toward that view.

Self-Help and Empowerment

Gradually, the movement began to put some of its principles into action in the operation of self-help programs as alternatives to professional treatment. Although the Mental Patients' Association (MP A) in Vancouver, Canada, began operating its drop-in center and residences within months of its founding in 1971, the first such projects did not appear in the United States until the late 1970s, largely because funding was unavailable.

Programs that developed out of the ex-patients' movement tend to be skeptical about the value of the mental health system and traditional psychiatric treatment

(Chamberlin et al., 1989). Members usually gravitate to these groups because they have had negative experiences in the system. Often, members are angry, and their anger is seen by the group as a healthy reaction to their experiences of abuse by the mental health system. At the same time, members, despite their distrust of the system, may simultaneously be involved in professionally-run programs. Members of user-run services are free to combine their participation in self-help groups with professionally-run services, in whatever proportion and combination each member determines.

Through successes experienced in self-help groups, members are enabled to take a stronger role in advocating for their own needs within the larger mental health system. Empowerment means that members have a voice in mental health matters generally – they reject the role of passive service recipient. Group members found themselves moving naturally into the role of advocate, representing the needs of clients on panels, boards, and committees. This may require accommodation on the part of other groups and group members such as administrators, policy makers, legislators, and family members, who typically have listened to everyone but the client about client needs.

Self-help groups do not exist in a vacuum. Even a group that sees itself as totally separate from the mental health system will, of necessity, have some interactions with it, while groups that have been aided or brought into existence by mental health professionals will need to devise their own ways of making themselves autonomous from the larger system. By taking on a role other than that of the passive, needy client, self-help group members can change the systems with which they interact, as these systems adjust to respond to clients in their new roles as advocates and service providers.

Self-help is a concept, not a single program model. The concept is a means by which people become empowered and begin to think of themselves as competent individuals as they present themselves in new ways to the world By its very nature, self-help combats stigma, because the negative images of mental patients ultimately must give way to the reality of clients managing their own lives and their own programs. The successes of self-help groups have been striking. Groups are handling annual budgets that may be in the hundreds of thousands of dollars; producing newsletters, books, and pamphlets; educating other clients and professionals about group work; influencing legislation and public policy; publicizing and advocating on their own behalf in the media; and, in general, challenging stereotypes and creating new realities. At the same time, individual group members may still be battling the particular manifestations that led to their being psychiatrically labeled in the first place. Self-help is not a miracle nor a cure-all, but it is a powerful confirmation that people, despite problems and disabilities, can achieve more than others (or they themselves) may have ever thought possible.

Advocacy

Self-help is one of two co-equal aspects of the ex-patients' movement; the other is advocacy, or working for political change. Unlike groups such as Recovery Inc.

or Schizophrenics Anonymous, patient liberation groups tend to address problems that go beyond the individual. The basic principle of the movement is that all laws and practices which induce discrimination toward individuals who have been labeled "mentally ill" need to be changed, so that a psychiatric diagnosis has no more impact on a person's citizenship rights and responsibilities than does a diagnosis of diabetes or heart disease. To that end, all commitment laws, forced treatment laws, insanity defenses, and other similar practices should be abolished.

Ending involuntary treatment is a long-term goal of the patients' liberation movement. Meanwhile, movement activists work to improve conditions of people subjected to forced treatment, and to see that their existing rights are respected, keeping in mind that these are interim steps within a basically unjust system.

Existing laws have the power to compel people to receive treatment for mental illness. This almost never occurs in the case of physical illness, except in the rare instances when courts overrule parent who refuse medical treatment for a child. The courts in these instances assume the *parents patriate* role, acting in lieu of parents in what the court defines as the child's best interest. When a person of whatever age is ordered by a court to undergo psychiatric treatment, this same *parens patriae* power comes into effect. This connection between the legal and medical systems places the mental patients at a disadvantage that is not faced by patients with physical illnesses.

In addition to the *parens patriae* doctrine, which assumes that a mentally ill individual is incapable of determining his or her own best interest, an additional doctrine, the police power of the state, is used to justify the involuntary confinement of individuals labeled mentally ill. This doctrine is based on the assumption that mentally ill people are dangerous and may do harm to themselves or to others if they are not confined. The belief in the dangerousness of the mentally ill is firmly rooted in our culture. It is especially promoted by the mass media, which frequently run stories in which crimes of violence are attributed to mental illness. If the alleged criminal has been previously hospitalized, the fact is prominently mentioned; if not, frequently a police officer or other authority figure will be quoted to the effect that the accused is "a mental case" or "a nut." In addition, unsolved crimes are often similarly attributed. Both the *parens patriae* power and the police power relate to the stereotyped view of the prospective patient – that he or she is sick, unpredictable, dangerous, unable to care for himself or herself, and unable to judge his or her own best interest.

The movement's advocacy has focused on the right of the individual not to be a patient, rather than on mere procedural safeguards before involuntary treatment can be instituted. A major lawsuit testing this right was field by seven patients at Boston State Hospital in 1975, many of whom had been members of a patients' rights group that met weekly in the hospital with the aid of the Mental Patients' Liberation Front. The suit, originally known as Rogers v. Macht, was called, in later stages, *Roger v. Okin and Rogers v. Commissioner of Mental Health* (1982). It established a limited right-to-refuse-treatment (i.e., psychiatric drugs) for Massachusetts patients.

Since *Rogers v. Commissioner*, right-to-refuse-treatment cases have been decided in a number of states, including New York (*Rivers v. Katz*, 1986) and California (*Reise v. St. Mary's Hospital*, 1987), and the right has been established administratively in some other states. While the movement first greeted these decisions as victories, it has become clear that, in practice, these reforms do little to change the power relationship between patients and psychiatrist Each procedure (varying from state to state) provides one or more methods to override the patient's decision to refuse drug; and whether the procedure is administrative or judicial, the end result is that most drug-refusing patients whose cases are heard are forced, ultimately, to take the drugs, despite the ostensible right to refuse them (Appelbaum, 1988). Many movement activists have become discouraged and no longer believe that the courts will help people avoid involuntary patienthood through the mechanism of the right to refuse treatment.

Many individuals in the ex-patients' movement first encountered a critique of the mental health system – a critique which confirmed their feelings – in the works of Thomas Szasz. In such books as *The Myth of Mental Illness* (1961) and *The Manufacture of Madness* (1970), in a career spanning more than thirty years, Szasz has always spoken powerfully about the essential wrongness of forced psychiatric treatment, and the fallacy of defining social and behavioral problems as illnesses. In a recent paper, Szasz (1989) provides a devastating critique of the mental patients' "rights" movement, which has been guided largely by lawyers and non-patients.

> Rallying to the battle cry of "civil rights for mental patients," professional civil libertarians special-interest-mongering attorneys, and the relatives of mental patients joined conventional psychiatrists demanding rights for mental patients – *qua* mental patients. The result has been a perverse sort of affirmative action program: since mental patient are ill, they have a right to treatment; since many are homeless, they have a right to housing; and so it goes, generating even a special right to reject treatment (a right every non-mental patient has *without* special dispensation). In short, the phrase "rights of mental patients" has meant everything but according persons called "mental patients" the same rights (and duties) as are accorded all adults *qua* citizens or persons,
>
> (p.19)

The National Association of Psychiatric Survivors (NAPS), founded in 1985 as the National Alliance of Mental Patients, promotes the same ideals Szasz espouses. The first item in its *Goals and Philosophy Statement* reads:

> To promote the human and civil rights of people in and out of psychiatric treatment situations, with special attention to their absolute right to freedom of choice. To work towards the end of involuntary psychiatric intervention, including civil commitment and forced procedures such as electroshock, psychosurgery, forced drugging, restraint and seclusion, holding that such intervention against one's will is not a form of treatment, but a violation of liberty and the right to control one's own body and mind. We emphasize freedom of choice for people wanting to receive psychiatric services through true informed consent to treatment which includes the right to refuse any unwanted treatment We will also work to assure the rights of all people who have been psychiatrically labeled including but not limited to people in halfway houses, day treatment,

residential facilities, vocational rehabilitation, nursing homes, psycho-social rehabilitation clubs as well as psychiatric institutions.

(NAPS, no date, p. 1)

This is the essence of "mental patients' " liberation. NAPS was formed specifically to counter the trend toward reformist "consumerism," which developed as the psychiatric establishment began to fund ex-patient self-help. Ironically, the same developments which led to the movement's growth and to the operation of increasing numbers of ex-patient-run alternative programs, also weakened the radical voices within the movement and promoted the views of far more cooperative "consumers." The very term "consumer" implies an equality of power which simply does not exist; mental health "consumers" are still subject to involuntary commitment and treatment, and the defining of their experience by others.

It is not surprising that once the Community Support Program at NIMH began funding "consumer" conferences, the International Conference on Human Rights and Psychiatric Oppression disbanded. The first CSP-funded conference, "Alternatives '85" was held in Baltimore in June 1985; the last International Conference in Burlington, Vermont, in August of that year. The dissolution was aided by a group of "consumers" who may have seen the liberation perspective as a threat. At the same time, some extreme radicals opposed any form of organization as oppressive, believing that a totally decentralized and unstructured movement could accomplish its goals.

Madness Network News disintegrated the next year. Its all-volunteer staff became exhausted by the effort of putting out the newspaper with no found but member subscriptions, and they were succeeded by a very small group of extreme radicals who published only one issue-critical of anyone attempting to develop organizational structure or sources of funding for movement activities. The paper then ceased publication, leaving a gap in movement communication that went unfilled for several years. Although Dendron, a newsletter published by the Clearinghouse on Human Rights and Psychiatry in Eugene, Oregon, began publishing shortly there after, only recently has it become as visible within the movement as had been *Madness Network News*.

Where the Movement Stands Now

At present, many groups exist that claim to speak "for" patients, that is, to be patients' advocates. Even the American Psychiatric Association claims this role, as does the National Alliance for the Mentally III (NAMI), a group primarily composed of relatives of patients, which enthusiastically embraces the medical model and promotes the expansion of involuntary commitment and the lifetime control of people labeled "mentally ill." However, a basic liberation principle is that people *must* speak for themselves.

Former patients recognize numerous currents of opinion within their community (which, after all, numbers in the millions). There are groups whose members promote the illness metaphor (e.g., National Depressive and Manic-Depressive Association); groups whose members promote self-help in conjunction with treatment for illness (e.g., Recovery, Inc.); groups whose members see themselves as consumers (e.g., the National Mental Health Consumers Association); and groups whose members see themselves as liberationists (e.g., National Association of Psychiatric Survivors). However, it is safe to say that by far the largest number of patients and ex-patients are those who identify with *none* of these organizations – indeed most patients and ex-patients have probably never even heard of these groups.

The movement continues to face formidable obstacles. The psychiatric/medical model of "mental illness" is widely accepted by the general public. Indeed, new psychiatric "illnesses" are being "discovered" all the time and psychiatry now claims that social deviants – from rapists to repetitive gamblers – are suffering from a variety of newly defined "mental illnesses Psychiatry is entrenched, as well, in the courts, the prisons, the school, and all major institutions of society.

At the same time, there are many hopeful signs for the movement. The ex-patients' movement is developing alliances with the physically disabled, with the poor, and with ex-patients in other countries. Physically disabled people have organized their own self-help programs, using the model of independent living. According to the principles of independent living, any person – no matter how physically disabled he or she may be – can live independently if provided with the proper supports. Such supports must be individualized – a person may need special equipment, personal care attendants, modified transportation vehicles, and so forth. The particular mix of supports is determined by the individual, in consultation with an independent living specialist (who is also a physically disabled person). As the disability rights movement has grown, it has become a powerful force for legal change as well. For more than ten years, this movement has lobbied in favor of the Americans with Disabilities Act, the so-called civil rights bill for the disabled. The bill was signed into law on July 26, 1990. Although the ex-patients' movement entered that struggle late, the final version of the Act does include persons with "psychiatric disabilities" under its protections.

Linkages of the ex-patients' movement with the impoverished include efforts at affordable housing, campaigns for universal medical insurance, and involvement in the Rainbow Coalition. It has proved extremely useful for ex-patient activists to become involved in these activities – not only do ex-patients require the services being advocated but demystification in the eyes of one's allies can serve an invaluable purpose. When labeled as "mentally" ill" – a nameless, faceless person – the "mental patient" may be seen as the enemy; as a co-worker and a colleague, facing the same problems and struggling for the same solutions, the ex-patient becomes an individual: knowable and understandable.

The growing internationalization of the ex-patients' movement is another sign of the movement's growth and strength. As groups exchange newsletters, and attend meetings and conferences, a shared ideology is developing. Although the lack of a solidifying terminology continues to be troubling, such variety does not necessarily indicate wide variations in viewpoints and activities. Whether group members call themselves clients, consumers, ex-patients, users, or psychiatric survivors, groups throughout the world are united by the goals of self-determination and full citizenship rights for their members.

It is true that the vast majority of former patients remain unorganized, but this challenge is being met. As groups become more visible, they recruit more members. This occurs because ex-patient groups speak to a truth of the patienthood experience: that people's anger and frustration are real and valid, and that only by speaking out can individuals who have been harmed by the entrenched power of psychiatry mount a challenge against it.

Notes

1 Originally published in *The Journal of Mind and Behavior*, Summer and Autumn, 1990, Vol. 11, No. ¾ by the Institute of Mind and Behavior, inc. Reprinted with permission.
2 The Wildflower Alliance Website can be accessed here: https://wildfloweralliance.org/

References

Appelbaum, D. (1988). The right to refuse treatment with antipsychotic drugs: Retrospect and prospect. *American Journal of Psychiatry*, 145, 413–419.

Beers, C. (1953). *A mind that found itself.* Garden City, NY: Doubleday.

Chamberlin, J. (1979). *On our own: Patient-controlled alternatives to the mental health system.* New York: McGraw-Hill.

Chamberlin, J. (1987). The case for separatism. In I. Barker and E. Peck (Eds.), *Power in strange places* (pp. 24–26). London, England: Good Practices in Mental Health.

Chamberlin, J., Rogers, J.A., and Sneed, C.S. (1989). Consumers, families, and community support systems. *Psychosocial Rehabilitation Journal*, 12, 93–106.

Dain, N. (1989). Critics and dissenters: Reflections on 'anti-psychiatry' in the United States. *Journal of the History of the Behavioral Sciences*, 25, 3–25.

National Association of Psychiatric Survivors. (No date). *Goals and philosophy statement.* Unpublished manuscript.

Report to the President for the President's Commission on Mental Health. (1978). *Volume I.* Washington, DC: United States Government Printing Office.

Riese v. St. Mary's Hospital, 209 Cal. App. 3rd, 1303, 1987.

Rivers v. Katz, 67 N.Y., 2nd, 485, 1986.

Rogers v. Commissioner of Mental Health, 390 Mass. 498, 1982.

Szasz, T. (1961). *The myth of mental illness.* New York: Hoeber-Harper.

Szasz, T. (1970). *The manufacture of madness.* New York: Dell.

Szasz, T. (1989, July). The myth of the rights of mental patients. *Liberty*, pp. 19–26.

Editor's References

Berger, D. (2022, May 17). Doctors gave her antipsychotics. She decided to live with her voices. *The New York Times.*

Hall, W. (Host). (2006). *Madness radio.* https://www.madnessradio.net/madness-radio -judi-chamberlin-psychiatric-survivor-movement/

Shapiro, J. (Host). (2010, January 19). Advocate for people with mental illness dies. Morning edition. *NPR.* https://www.npr.org/templates/story/story.php?storyId =122706192

Chapter 34

The Icarus Project

A COUNTER NARRATIVE FOR PSYCHIC DIVERSITY[1]

Sascha Altman DuBrul

Summary

The Icarus Project (2002–2020) took its name from the ancient Greek myth of Icarus, who famously uses wings fashioned from wax and feathers to escape imprisonment. But, alas, Icarus flies too close to the sun, his wings melt, and he tumbles into the sea. The myth works in the context of mental diversity to provide an alternative to overly pathological and romantic approaches to mental difference. Icarus's wings allow him to see and know and do things beyond the norm, but they also come with risks and challenges. Icarus's wings are comparable to the kinds of difference that are often labeled and pathologized as "mental illness." In the language of the Icarus Project, these differences can often be better understood as "dangerous gifts." They provide opportunities outside the norm, but they can also be challenging, especially in a world structured by sanist prejudice. The Icarus Project has an archive of their materials available (https://icarusprojectarchive.org/). Some participants took on new leadership and changed its name to the Fireweed Collective in 2020. The Fireweed Collective (https://fireweedcollective.org/) uses a healing justice lens to continue the work of disrupting the harms of the mental health system and fostering education and mutual aid. Some Icarus Project participants have also been active in forming the Institute for the Development of Human Arts (IDHA), which offers transformative mental health education and community development (https://www.idha-nyc.org/).

This chapter by one of the Icarus Project's cofounders, Sascha DuBrul, was first written in 2014. It gives the background of the Icarus Project's emergence and early history. Here is the abstract DuBrul provided for the article when it was first published:

> Over the past 12 years, I've had the good fortune of collaborating with others to create a project which challenges and complicates the dominant biopsychiatric model of mental illness. The Icarus Project,

DOI: 10.4324/9781003148456-39

founded in 2002, not only critiqued the terms and practices central to the biopsychiatric model, it also inspired a new language and a new community for people struggling with mental health issues in the 21st century. The Icarus Project believes that humans are meaning makers, that meaning is created through developing intrapersonal and interpersonal narratives, and that these narratives are important sites of creativity, struggle, and growth. The Icarus counter narrative and the community it fostered has been invaluable for people around the world dealing with psychic diversity—particularly for people alienated by mainstream approaches. But, despite the numbers of people who have been inspired by this approach, the historical background of the Icarus Project is hard to find. It exists primarily in oral history, newspaper articles, unpublished or self-published Icarus documents, and in internet discussion forums. As the co-founder of the Icarus Project, I use this article to make my understanding of that history and its key documents more widely available.

*

Emergence of the Icarus Project

In September of 2002, I wrote an article for the *San Francisco Bay Guardian* that was read by thousands of people entitled "The Bipolar World" (DuBrul). It was about my personal struggles in the mental health system, the biopsychiatric model that dominates it, and my desire for a new way of looking at my diagnosis of "bipolar disorder." I was 27 years old and had been writing stories and articles for years within my insular community of punks and anarchists, but this was the first time that my words had made it into a more mainstream publication. It was also the most personal article I had ever written with details about dramatic hospitalizations, psychotic delusions, and struggles with suicidal depression.

I wrote about how at times I felt like the entire universe was crawling under my skin, and yet at other times, I felt as though I had been given a divine mission to save the world. Then I wrote about how the medications I was taking actually seemed to be helping me, but how distrustful I was of the medical model. I was concerned with how closely it seemed to be tied to the capitalist system and with how confusing and alienating the whole situation left me feeling. I ended the story by saying:

> But I feel so alienated sometimes, even by the language I find coming out of my mouth or that I type out on the computer screen. Words like "disorder," "disease," and "dysfunction" just seem so very hollow and crude. I feel like I'm speaking a foreign and clinical language that is useful for navigating my way though the current system but doesn't translate into my own internal vocabulary, where things are so much more fluid and complex...
>
> In the end, what it comes down to for me is that I desperately feel the need to connect with other folks like myself so I can validate my experiences and not feel so damn alone in the world, so I can pass along the

lessons I've learned to help make it easier for other people struggling like myself. By my nature and the way I was raised, I don't trust mainstream medicine or corporate culture, but the fact that I'm sitting here writing this essay right now is proof that their drugs are helping me. And I'm looking for others out there with similar experiences.

Our society still seems to be in the early stages of the dialogue where you're either "for" or "against" the mental health system. Like either you swallow the antidepressant ads on television as modern-day gospel and start giving your dog Prozac, or you're convinced we're living in Brave New World and all the psych drugs are just part of a big conspiracy to keep us from being self-reliant and realizing our true potential. I think it's really about time we start carving some more of the middle ground with stories from outside the mainstream and creating a new language for ourselves that reflects all the complexity and brilliance that we hold inside.

(DuBrul, Sascha Altman 2002)

Within 2 days of the article going to print, my inbox was filled with email from people who had read the story and related somehow to my words. I never would have imagined that my story would have resonated with so many others from different communities and lifestyles, and it was an incredibly empowering feeling. For the first time in my life, I learned the important lesson that when you are brave enough to tell your own story, other people often feel compelled to tell you their story as well. I learned about the liberatory power of speaking our personal truths and about the power of personal narratives to challenge the power of the dominant narrative.

One of the people who initially wrote to me with a particularly compelling story was a person named Jacks McNamara. We began corresponding over email, met shortly thereafter, and within the span of an evening and a morning decided to create a place for people like us who had been through the mental health system and were diagnosed with bipolar disorder to tell their stories. We started with a website, calling it the Icarus Project. Shortly after meeting, we wrote an initial vision statement:

> As the ancient Greek myth is told, the young boy Icarus and his inventor father Daedalus were imprisoned in a maze on an island and trying to escape. Daedalus was crafty and made them both pairs of wings built carefully out of wax and feathers, but warned Icarus not to fly too close to the blazing sun or his wings would fall to pieces. Icarus, being young and foolish, was so intoxicated with his new ability to fly that he soared too high, the delicate wings melted and burned, and he fell into the deep blue ocean and drowned. For countless generations, the story of Icarus' wings has served to remind us that we are humans rather than gods, and that sometimes the most incredible of gifts can also be the most dangerous.
>
> The Icarus Project was created in the beginning of the 21st century by a group of people diagnosed in the contemporary language as Bipolar or Manic-Depressive. Defining ourselves outside convention we see our condition as a dangerous gift to be cultivated and taken care of rather than as a disease or disorder needing to be 'cured.' With this double edged blessing we have the ability to fly to places of great vision and creativity, but like the boy Icarus, we also have the potential to

fly dangerously close to the sun—into realms of delusion and psychosis—and crash in a blaze of fire and confusion. At our heights we may find ourselves capable of creating music, art, words, and inventions which touch people's souls and change the course of history. At our depths we may end up alienated and alone, incarcerated in psychiatric institutions, or dead by our own hands.

Despite these risks, we recognize the intertwined threads of madness and creativity as tools of inspiration and hope in this repressed and damaged society. We understand that we are members of a group that has been misunderstood and persecuted throughout history, but has also been responsible for some of its most brilliant creations. And we are proud.

While many of us use mood-stabilizing drugs like Lithium to regulate and dampen the extremes of our manias and the hopeless depths of our depressions, others among us have learned how to control the mercurial nature of our moods through diet, exercise, and spiritual focus. Many of us make use of non-Western practices such as Chinese medicine, Yoga, and meditation. Often we find that we can handle ourselves better when we channel our tremendous energy into creation: some of us paint murals and write books, some of us convert diesel cars to run on vegetable oil and make gardens that are nourished with the waste water from our showers. In our own ways we're all struggling to create full and independent lives for ourselves where the ultimate goal is not just to survive, but to thrive. Despite the effort necessary just to stay balanced and grounded, we intend to make the world we live on better, more beautiful, and way more interesting.

The Icarus Project Website is a place for people struggling with Manic-Depression outside the mainstream to connect and build an alternative support network. We hope to learn from each others' mistakes and victories, stories and art, and create a new culture and language that resonates with our actual experiences of this "disorder" rather than trying to fit our lives into the reductionist framework offered by the current mental health establishment. We would like this site to become a place that helps people like us feel less alienated, and allows us, both as individuals and as a community, to tap into the true potential that lies between brilliance and madness.

(The Icarus Project 2002)

Thus, very early on in our work together, Jacks and I developed a counter narrative to the dominant biopsychiatric narrative. We spoke clearly of our desire not for a reduction of stigma or a cure for our disease but for a new culture and language of mental health. We considered the mainstream narrative to be a reductionist framework offered by the current mental health establishment, and we emphasized our desire to step outside that framework and into new territory.

We talked about our biodiesel cars and graywater systems, which represented our countercultural values and alternative knowledge; our stories about painting murals and writing books highlighted the role art and creativity would play in shaping our work. Our narrative, which recognized both lithium and yoga as equally valid means to handling our sensitivities, opened up a much needed space in the dialog about self-care and mental health. We recognized the intertwined threads of madness and creativity as tools of inspiration and hope in a repressed and damaged society. We linked madness and creativity, speaking of them as "tools of inspiration." Even more powerfully, we flipped the script and pointed our fingers back at the society in which we were raised. Furthermore, we expressed an understanding that we are members of a group that has been misunderstood and persecuted throughout history but that has also been responsible for some of its most brilliant creations. It was a powerful beginning.

Narrative Strands of Our New Story

Before going further with the Icarus Story, let me step back to provide some context. Our response to the label "bipolar" was not a "normal" response, which is why the Icarus Project brought a new perspective to psychic diversity. To create this perspective, we drew inspiration from many social movements and subcultural communities that came before us. So even though our response was unusual, it did not arise in a vacuum. In creating the Icarus Project, we wove together the ideas and practices in these movements to imagine a powerful new counter narrative to the dominant mental health narrative that went beyond a questioning of the language around "bipolar" and critiqued the system itself. A review of our cultural, social, and political roots places our work in a larger context and adds to the richness and depth of the Icarus Project as a whole. It also articulates the world views and ways of life from which Icarus emerged. These worldviews are not in the mainstream, they are not "normal," but they have a long history of solidarity behind them. Although there are surely more, I have identified eight social, political, cultural, and ecological movements that most notably inspired the Icarus Project. Some of these movements were very conscious to us, some were just part of the cultural background in which we lived.

Anarchism

For nearly three centuries, anarchists were at the forefront of contending undemocratic, unaccountable forms of power. From the Spanish Civil War to the 1960s counterculture, anarchist ideas and actions have played an important role in political and social movements (Marshall 2010). Since the end of the Cold War in 1989, there has been a resurgence in anarchist organizing, most notably during the protests against the World Trade Organization in the streets of Seattle 1999 (Graeber 2002). Many early Icarus participants identified with the anarchist political tradition and its emphasis on prefigurative political ideals, mutual aid, and direct action. Our original organizing vision was based on Food Not Bombs (Butler and McHenry 2002), an anarchist project which began as part of the anti-nuclear movement and is a type of direct action and mutual aid: acquiring free food, cooking it as a group, and serving it in a public place.

Anti-Psychiatry

Though we did not fully understand it in the early days, we were walking in the footsteps of a large body of knowledge and thought from the 1960s, grouped under the category of *Anti-Psychiatry* (Cooper 1967). Anti-psychiatry is a term used to refer to a configuration of groups and theoretical constructs that question the fundamental assumptions and practices of psychiatry, such as its claim that it achieves universal, scientific objectivity. In the United States, the body of ideas known as anti-psychiatry were passed down and put into practice in what became known as the Psychiatric Survivors Movement by organizations such as Mindfreedom International based in Eugene, Oregon (Glasser 2008). While the Icarus Project had much in common with this project, we tended to have a more nuanced relationship to psychiatric medications than many in the survivor movement. Also, we were younger than most in the survivor movement and had never experienced long-term hospitalizations or institutionalization. That set us apart and made us more appealing to many of our generation who had emergency room and short-term hospital run-ins with the psychiatric establishment typical of today.

Permaculture/Sustainable Ecology

From the beginning, the vision and spirit of the Icarus Project drew a great deal of inspiration from the worlds of sustainable agriculture and the body of knowledge collectively referred to as *Permaculture* (Mollison 1997). Within the first months of its formation, both Jacks and I were working on Community Supported Agriculture (CSA) farms, understanding that our sensitivities (labeled by society as "bipolar disorder") could be kept in check by keeping close to the earth and prioritizing the cultivation of food in a community context. Both an economic farming model and an international movement, CSA re-prioritizes the relationship between farmers, the food that they grow and the families that consume their products. Icarus has always had a culture that prioritizes and celebrates food. Many of the most powerful metaphors in the Icarus Project are drawn from ecology and sustainable agriculture: from roots and seeds to the comparison of monoculture fields with monocultures of the mind.

Permaculture refers to a set of principles for developing sustainable human systems by mimicking systems that occur in nature (Mollison 1997). Among the useful ideas in permaculture are: using and valuing diversity, using small and slow solutions; integrating rather than segregating, understanding the important relationship between the wild and the cultivated, understanding that the problem holds the keys to the solution, catching and storing energy, and stepping back to observe patterns in nature and society. Like the Icarus Project, Permaculture has gone from a set of ideas and principles gathered from a diverse group of people and places to an action oriented international signifier for a thriving movement.

LGBTQ Movement

The Lesbian/Gay/Bisexual/Transgender/Queer (LGTBQ) movement is large and diverse; within it there is an incredible amount of outsider and resistance stories that have inspired the work of the Icarus Project. The watershed event for both the radical and mainstream LGBTQ community was the 1969 Stonewall riots in New York City where, for the first time, an LGBTQ community publicly reacted militantly in the face of oppression in a way that was widely reported. Until 1973 homosexuality was on the American Psychiatric Association's official list of mental disorders. (Bayer

1987). In the 1980s, an organization called ACTUP (AIDS Coalition to Unleash Power) coordinated an incredibly successful campaign to raise awareness about government complicity in the AIDS crisis and build a successful movement based around direct action activist culture and queer identity (Shepard and Hayduk 2002). Icarus has drawn a lot of inspiration from the success of the radical portions of the Queer Pride movement.

What we have in common is the focus on personal politics, looking at a marginalized identity and reclaiming it as a point of pride. Icarus members' common shouts of "mad pride" (Glasser 2008) have much in common with the loud and vibrant articulation of gay pride or queer pride. It helps that many of the early (and contemporary) Icarus organizers identify as some shade of queer. At the heart of our connection is the utilization of pride around an oppressed identity to inspire political action and the understanding that when we stop being afraid of being exposed for a shamed identity, there is nothing that can stop us.

Harm Reduction

The harm reduction movement is centered in the experiences of drug users, sex workers, people involved in street economies, and criminalized communities. There are many ways to frame the war on drugs in the United States and many ideological angles from which to view it; one angle is that it has been a massive and successful propaganda exercise to demonize drug users and destabilize Black and brown communities. Drug users are first criminalized for using outlawed substances, and then, as a result of how they must obtain drugs, forced to engage in additional criminal behavior in order to maintain their habits and addictions. Thus, a drug user becomes a deviant - a transgressor who is incompetent and selfish, destined for jails, institutions or death. The message is that drug users do not care about their own health, the health of their friends or colleagues and certainly not the greater public health. The harm reduction movement challenges these ideas.

At the core of the harm reduction movement is the belief that everyone has the right to determine the circumstances of his or her own life, including care (Inciardi and Harrison 2000). This principle is also at the core of the Icarus Project. Early in our visioning, we embraced the complexities of our individual members' relationship to psychiatric medications, use of recreational substances, life style choices and outsider identities. One of our first website forums was titled "Give Me Lithium or Give Me Meth," and it was a place to share stories about members relationships to illegal drugs. The Icarus Project embraced the spirit of the harm reduction movement in its publishing of the *Harm Reduction Guide to Coming Off Psychiatric Drugs* (Hall 2007), which gathered the best information and valuable lessons we could find about reducing and coming off of psychiatric medication.

Global Justice Movement

From the beginning, the Icarus Project viewed itself in terms of a larger political context, as one part of a struggle for mutual liberation. The Global Justice Movement describes the loose collection of individuals and groups—often referred to as a movement of movements— placing a significant emphasis on transnational solidarity uniting activists in the global South and global North. Usually traced historically to the Zapatista Uprising in Chiapas, Mexico on January 1, 1994, the Global Justice Movement is an anti-capitalist movement that weaves together the struggles of many movements, including an emphasis on grassroots organizing, popular education, and strong critique of capitalism (Notes from Nowhere 2003). Our original web designer was from Indymedia, one of the key online activist networks in the early part of the 21st century and a hub of the Global Justice Movement. Not long after we published our first book, *Navigating the Space Between Brilliance and Madness*, we learned that it was being read widely in the Zapatista activist community of San Cristobal de las Casas, Chiapas, Mexico.

Counterculture

In 1968, Theodore Roszak coined the term "counterculture" to refer to the intersection of Vietnam War protesters, dropouts, and rebels of various stripes who had an effect on the larger dominant culture (1968). In the 1960s, the counterculture was strong in numbers and cultural influence. Today, many of the most powerful ideas have either been co-opted in the service of capitalism or marginalized. Countercultural ideas are transmitted through music and art, and they offer creative ways of disseminating ideas, connecting with allies and realizing goals. The following is a brief mention of some of the countercultures that have inspired the Icarus Project via their ideologies, practices, approaches and goals.

The *Beat Generation* is a term used to describe a group of American post-WWII writers who came to prominence in the 1950s, as well as the cultural phenomena that they both documented and inspired (Charters 2003). Central elements of Beat culture included experimentation with drugs and alternative forms of sexuality, an interest in Eastern religion, a rejection of materialism, and the idealizing of exuberant means of expression and being (Charters 2003). *Howl*, written by Allen Ginsburg in 1956, chronicles the repressive culture of America in the 1950s. It reads as a transmission from an earlier time in a language that has clearly influenced the nature of our modern slang-filled English. *Howl* was dedicated to Carl Solomon, whom Ginsburg befriended in a Rockland County psychiatric hospital. The following excerpt captures an aspect of the Beat culture that has influenced the Icarus Project in major ways: "I'm with you in Rockland/where there are twenty-five thousand mad comrades all together singing the final stanzas of the Internationale…" (Ginsburg 1956, 18) The weaving together of madness and the history of leftist politics is familiar. The words are not mainstream but are transmissions from the underground to the underground—now in the mainstream for everyone to see.

Jack Kerouac was the archetypal beat writer – the explorer of the open roads of America. One of the most famous quotes from his influential book *On the Road* articulates the feeling of the Beats and their relationship to the "mad":

> The only people for me are the mad ones, the ones who are mad to live, mad to talk, mad to be saved, desirous of everything at the same time, the ones who never yawn or say a commonplace thing, but burn, burn, burn, like fabulous yellow roman candles exploding like spiders across the stars

and in the middle you see the blue centerlight pop and everybody goes "Awww!"

(1957, 21)

We consciously resurrected this Beat language in the Icarus Project, referring affectionately to one another as "mad ones," the nod to earlier times and cultures that contributed to the artistic foundation of our project.

Punk Rock

As one of the founders of the Icarus Project, I can safely say that the culture of punk rock held a critical and important role in our project's tone and vision. Emerging in the 1970s in London and New York before spreading to cities over the globe, punk rock was initially a reaction to the sterile conformity of commercial rock and roll and disco culture. It inspired a lot of creative protest music during the Reagan and Thatcher era of the 1980s. An emphasis on questioning authority, rebellious distrust of government, and an anti-materialistic DIY (Do It Yourself) ethic. The British version of punk had direct influences from the Situationists, a clever revolutionary student movement from the 1960s in Paris (Marcus 1989). The Situationists were proto-punks, inspired by the ideas of breaking down barriers imposed by modern capitalist society and creating "situations" where new visions might emerge. Woven into the ideology of punk is an understanding that society is sick and that acting crazy is totally natural. Growing up immersed in the punk scene in New York in the 1990s, I learned how to be proud of sometimes feeling crazy and, if anything, learned to revel in it while celebrating difference and nonconformity.

The story of punk, and of countercultures generally, are useful in explaining an important aspect of the cultural vision and strategy of the Icarus Project. In 1994, punk went through a revival in the mainstream with the rise in popularity of bands like Nirvana and Green Day. I watched the subculture in which I had been immersed suddenly become currency for mass culture with both positive and negative results. One positive result was that more people had the opportunity to be exposed to the alternative political and social messages by which punk rock music is characterized. On the negative side, capitalist consumer culture's process of marketing a product required that many of the themes of social change be toned down or altogether removed from the music (Frank 1997). As a result, the counternarrative associated with punk rock culture was somewhat diluted. For Icarus, this history meant that important cultural work can start in the underground, but at the same time, this work can easily become co-opted.

Navigating the Space between Brilliance and Madness

Pulling these many strands together, the Icarus Project initially focused on the identity narratives of bipolar disorder, and much of our language was geared towards radical political activists. But it quickly became clear that our message was reaching people outside of the counterculture from which we were born. Shortly after the website went live in November 2002, I embarked on a cross-country tour in a beat-up 1982

Toyota pickup truck, facilitating workshops in community spaces and collective house kitchens. I had never organized mental health discussions, but I had facilitated a lot of meetings and taught permaculture and seed saving workshops. I was used to public speaking and creating space for dialog, but nothing like this. I started with a basic set of questions which evolved into some incredible discussions.

An example of the way in which we used our words to carve out a space in the psychic architecture of the community around us is illustrated in the following passage, an excerpt from the original flier used to advertise the meetings and gatherings of the Icarus Project.

Walking the Edge of Insanity

Navigating the World of Mental Health as a Radical in the 21st Century

> As creative folks skeptical of the conventional social system, what does it mean within our extended community for someone to be "mentally ill" or struggling with traditional labels such as "clinical depression," "bipolar disorder," or "schizophrenia?" How helpful is the modern psychiatric paradigm that revolves around medicine and mental disorders and how much of it is really just a function of powerful pharmaceutical corporations, public funding cuts, and a society that equates productivity with health? Are there other frameworks for understanding what it means to be "crazy?" Are there alternative ways to heal? How do we begin the process?
>
> Chances are pretty high that if you're reading this, you or someone you care about has been grappling with these questions for years. Come join an open discussion and learn more about The Icarus Project, a radical support network by and for people struggling with the dangerous gifts commonly labeled as mental illnesses. The Icarus Project envisions a new culture and language that resonates with our actual experiences rather than trying to fit our lives into a conventional framework. By joining together as individuals and as a community, we hope to create space where the intertwined threads of madness and creativity can inspire hope and transformation in a repressed and damaged world.
>
> (The Icarus Project 2006)

The following season, Jacks and I were both apprenticing on organic farms, she in California and me in the Hudson Valley of New York. The Icarus Project website was up and running, and a virtual community began to evolve around the discussion forums. We were attracting interesting people, creating discussion forums with names like "Alternate Dimensions or Psychotic Delusions" and "Experiencing Madness and Extreme States." There was no place else where people who used psych meds and people who did not, people who identified with diagnostic categories and people who did not, could all talk with each other and share stories. Because of the outreach in the anarchist and activist community, there was a high percentage of creative people with a radical political analysis. And with the (seeming) anonymity of the Internet, people felt comfortable being honest and sharing intimate stories about their lives. Our website served as a refuge for a diverse group of people who were learning the ways in which new narratives could be woven about their lives.

After a generous and serendipitous donation (from a wealthy woman whose daughter was diagnosed with bipolar disorder) in the winter of 2003, Jacks and I reunited and spent two intense months compiling the writings of people on the website with our own writings into a book that we self-published under the title: *Navigating the Space Between Brilliance and Madness – A Reader and Roadmap of Bipolar World*. Here is a passage from the introduction:

> The two people putting together this reader you hold in your hands have been diagnosed with "Bipolar Disorder," the most recent medical language for what was once known as Manic Depression. It is considered a disease of the mind. The statistics are that 6 million people in the United States have some form of the disorder, and that 1 out of 5 people left untreated will eventually kill themselves. But this "illness" is more than a bunch of statistics, or a set of symptoms. For those of us who live with this awkward label, the phenomenon it describes is something fluid and hard to pin down, yet none of us can escape its effects on our lives. We share common patterns and eerily common stories, some devastating and some inspiring—and so few of them have actually been mapped…
>
> In this little book we've assembled an atlas of maps, back and forth through the subconscious and consciousness, from hospital waiting rooms to collective house kitchens, from the desert to the supermarket. The pages we are giving to you chart some of the underground tunnels beneath the mainstream medical model of treatment, tunnels carved by brave and visionary people before us, and tunnels we're helping to carve ourselves with our friends. They go beyond three dimensions. They are maps made up of ideas and stories and examples from many people's lives. They are maps of our souls as well as the world outside. Some of these maps will help you to navigate through the existing architecture of the mental health establishment; some of them might help you figure out for yourself where you stand in relation to the larger ecosystem of the earth and the people who inhabit it.

After this publication, The Icarus Project grew in earnest. Our website became increasingly well know; our book was in its third printing; and we had completed three incredibly successful tours. Our Icarus discourse of dangerous gifts was becoming audible among the larger community around us, despite our subcultural backgrounds and unorthodox messages, we were onto something that people found compelling. We had tapped into a desperate need for a more creative look at mental health and wellness. The biopsychiatric model, though incredibly profitable for some, left many of us out in the cold as far as understanding our mental health issues and how they related to the rest of the world.

Through contacts in the non-profit funding world, Jacks and I met with Anthony Wood, Executive Director of the Ittleson Foundation, and talked over ideas for a proposal to partner with an older, more established organization in New York named Fountain House to do outreach on college campuses. A radical mental health organization when it was founded in the 1940s, Fountain House became the parent of an international network of mental health Clubhouses (the International Center for Clubhouse Development.) Like most mental health agencies, Fountain House uses the traditional language of mental illness, but also, like most mental health agencies, they were desperate for ideas that could attract young people. Below is a section from our proposal to the Ittleson Foundation:

> Community support is a vitally important part of the healing process no matter what form of treatment an individual chooses. While there are numerous conventional support structures available for adults, family members, and those who are comfortable with the medical model of mental illness, there are very few peer-based support structures created by and for young and creative populations. Most of the support structures currently available in this country have been established by institutions, mental health professionals, and large bureaucratic organizations like NAMI, the National Alliance for the Mentally Ill. While these groups have indubitably helped thousands of people suffering from mental illness, they have also alienated countless individuals who do not identify with the conventional paradigm of the "mental health consumer." The majority of our members have indicated that they did not consider any of the participants in traditional support groups to be their peers, and subsequently felt even more alone in their struggles to understand the extremes of their experience.
>
> Traditional support organizations frequently speak in terms of "psychiatric disability," "disease," and "eradicating mental illness" (the first objective in NAMI's mission statement). The members of The Icarus Project, by contrast, have consistently expressed that our project – with its unique conception of mental illness as a potential gift of great vision, creativity, and compassion that must be harnessed and respected, as well as an incredible hardship – is one of the only places where they can find meaningful support from true peers. The archetype of the mythical Icarus, who uses the gift of wings to fly to places of incredible beauty but crashes after recklessly flying too close to the sun, has proven a much more resonant metaphor for our members' extremes of experience than the paradigm of disease.
>
> (The Icarus Project 2004).

The day we found out we had received the grant from Ittleson, we were hanging the first Icarus Project art show at a radical community center/art gallery on the Lower East Side of New York known as ABC No Rio. It was surreal; not only were they giving us $80,000 to work on our dream project, but we had also stepped suddenly into a world of legitimacy to which we never expected to gain access. Within 6 months of receiving the grant, we recruited a handful of amazing organizers, collectivized our organization, and revised our mission and vision statements to reflect our evolving political and social analysis. In short, this was the statement, not just of a non-profit, but of an aspiring movement:

Icarus Project Mission Statement (2005)

Our Mission

The Icarus Project envisions a new culture and language that resonates with our actual experiences of 'mental illness' rather than trying to fit our lives into a conventional framework. We are a network of people living with and/or affected by experiences that are often diagnosed and labeled as psychiatric conditions. We believe these experiences are dangerous gifts needing cultivation and care, rather than diseases or disorders. By joining together as individuals and as a community, the intertwined threads of madness, creativity, and collaboration can inspire hope and transformation in an oppressive and damaged world. Participation in The Icarus Project helps us overcome alienation and tap into the true potential that lies between brilliance and madness.

Our Vision

Together, we seek new space and freedom for extreme states of consciousness. We support alternatives to the medical model and acknowledge the traumatic legacy of psychiatric abuse. We recognize that we all live in a crazy world, and believe that sensitivities, visions, and inspirations are not necessarily symptoms of illness. Sometimes breakdown can be the entrance to breakthrough. We call for more options in understanding and treating emotional distress, and we advocate for everyone, regardless of income, to have access to these choices. We respect diversity and embrace harm-reduction and self-determination in treatment decisions. Everyone is welcome, whether they support the use of psychiatric drugs or not, and whether they identify with diagnostic categories or not. To ensure we remain honest and untamed, we do not accept funding from pharmaceutical companies. We invite anyone who shares the Icarus vision and principles to join us, and choose "The Icarus Project" or any other name for the independent efforts that inspire them.

Our Principles

Beyond the medical model *While we respect whatever treatment decisions people make, we challenge standard definitions of psychic difference as essentially diseased, disordered, broken, faulty, and existing within the bounds of DSM-IV diagnosis. We are exploring unknown territory and don't steer by the default maps outlined by docs and pharma companies. We're making new maps.*

Educating ourselves about alternatives *A lot of what the media, medical establishment, and institutions tell us about "mental illness," psych drugs, and how we have to live our lives is just not true. We educate ourselves and each other. We question what we hear on TV and read in doctor's office brochures. We explore holistic and spiritual approaches to handling our extreme states of consciousness. We learn as much as we can about any medical treatments, and encourage each other to make informed choices. Icarus is a sanctuary for people thinking outside the mainstream and creating their own definitions of health and wellness.*

Balancing wellness and action *Icarus is a place for supporting each other in practicing real self-care. This includes but is not limited to: making sure we don't neglect our personal basics like food, rest, exercise, and community; encouraging each other to commit to the amount of work we can actually do, and not push ourselves past our limits; and challenging ourselves to find daily routines and projects that help us live out our dreams and have enough structure to get by.*

Access *We don't need more alternatives that only rich people can afford. All Icarus gatherings follow the policy that 'no one is turned away for lack of funds.' We work to create options and choices that are available to all.*

Non judgment and respect for diversity *We welcome people who support psych drugs and people who do not, as well as people who use diagnostic labels and people who do not identify with those terms. We do not exclude people on the basis*

*of politics, lifestyle choice, diagnostic history, recreational drug use, "criminal"
behavior, or other outsider identities. We all have a lot to learn from each other, so
we respect each others' choices. While the current social system and medical model
have the tendency to divide us, we want our understanding of and experiences with
madness to unite us.*

*Non-hierarchy and anti-oppression Local groups need to be anti-
authoritarian, inclusive, and working against racism/classism/sexism/
homophobia and other oppressions. As a radical mental health support network,
our affiliated groups create safe and challenging spaces where oppressive behavior
is not tolerated.*

*Nonviolence We believe that we will bring about lasting change in the world
through dialogue, compassionate listening, mutual aid, and grassroots networks
of support. We hope these approaches contribute to forming viable alternatives to
the current system of government, bureaucracy, domination, and corporate culture.*

*Transparency We believe in public access to information about how we are
making decisions, spending money, distributing responsibility, and otherwise
delegating the work of organizing together.*

(The Icarus Project 2005)

These are revolutionary words and acknowledge our relationship to history and
our debt to the movements and cultural workers that have come before us. These
words put us outside all the other organizations working in our field, affirming to
everyone our radical stance in the true meaning of radical: from the roots to the
extremes. No one else in the field of mental health was talking about non-hierarchy
and transparency in this way. We were bringing the radical narratives and models
into the door of the mainstream.

Later that year we created a collective document which we called *Friends Make the
Best Medicine: A Guide to Creating Community Mental Health Support Networks* that people
around the world download from our website and use as a guide for starting local
Icarus Project support groups. Here is part of the introduction.

Underground Roots and Magic Spells

Visions for Resisting Monoculture and Building Community

*You can see it all from the highway: enormous monocrops of identical corn plants
that reach for miles bordered by an endless sea of strip malls, parking lots, and
tract housing. You can see it on our kitchen counters and in our classrooms: the
same can of soda on the table in Cairo and Kentucky, the same definitions of
"progress" and "freedom" in textbooks around the world. Monoculture — the practice
of replicating a single plant, product or idea over a huge area— is about the most
unstable, unsustainable, unimaginative form of organization that exists, but in
the short term it keeps the system running smoothly and keeps the power in the
hands of a small number of people. In the logic of our modern world, whether
it's in the farmer's field or in the high school classroom, diversity is inefficient
and hard to manage. Powerful people figured out awhile time ago that it's a
lot easier to control things if everyone's eating the same foods, listening to the
same music, reading the same books, watching the same TV shows, and speaking*

the same language. This is what we call the monocult, and while everyone is supposedly more and more connected by this new "global culture," we're more and more isolated from each other. Things feel more and more empty, and so many of us end up lonely and rootless, wondering why everything feels so wrong.

Out in the wild things are very different. In old forests everything is connected, from the moss and lichens to the ferns and brambles to the birds and beetles. In our human minds we separate all the parts of the forest into separate pieces when a lot of the time it can be more helpful to view the forest as one giant organism with separate parts all working together. The trees of a forest intertwine their roots and actually communicate with each other underground. You see it most visibly along ravines and creek beds where a cut-away hillside reveals totally asymmetrical tangle of roots that no scientist could ever have imagined or planned out with all his laws of physics. Something in that tangle explains how those trees can lean out at all kinds of gravity-defying angles and hang their necks into the strongest winds and still survive, bending but not breaking, adapting with unpredictable curves and angles to the way the world breathes and shines and rains and burns. Concrete can't do that. There are a lot of lessons to be learned from the way life evolves and gets stronger in the wild. Something about the living architecture of chaos and time, multi-tiered forests and microscopic algae, outlasts any of the straight lines and square institutions we're told to believe in.

We believe that people do not belong in grids and boxes of rootless lonely monocultures. Humans are adaptable creatures, and while a lot of people learn to adapt, some of us can't handle the modern world no matter how many psych drugs or years of school or behavior modification programs we've been put through. Any realistic model of mental health has to begin by accepting that there is no standard model for a mind and that none of us are single units designed for convenience and efficiency. No matter how alienated you are by the world around you, no matter how out of step or depressed and disconnected you might feel: you are not alone. Your life is supported by the lives of countless other beings, from the microbes in your eyelashes to the men who paved your street. The world is so much more complicated and beautiful than it appears on the surface.

There are so many of us out here who feel the world with thin skin and heavy hearts, who get called crazy because we're too full of fire and pain, who know that other worlds exist and aren't comfortable in this version of reality. We've been busting up out of sidewalks and blooming all kind of misfit flowers for as long as people have been walking on this Earth. So many of us have access to secret layers of consciousness you could think of us like dandelion roots that gather minerals from hidden layers of the soil that other plants don't reach. If we're lucky we share them with everyone on the surface–because we feel things stronger than the other people around us, a lot of us have visions about how things could be different, why they need to be different, and it's painful to keep them silent. Sometimes we get called sick and sometimes we get called sacred, but no matter how they name us we are a vital part of making this planet whole.

It's time we connect our underground roots and tell our buried stories, grow up strong and scatter our visions all over the patches of scarred and damaged soil in a society that is so desperately in need of change.

(The Icarus Project 2006)

With this statement, we attempted to define ourselves in opposition to the cold logic of the DSM-IV. The same way that monoculture corn fields are horrible for the environment but profit a few, the monocultures of the mind are a disaster to our planet, our communities and personal lives. The Icarus vision, a weaving of multiple counternarratives, throws the cold DSM narrative on its head and grows a new world with the broken pieces.

A Dandelion Conclusion

Biopsychiatry remains the dominant narrative of mental health despite the fact that it has faced tremendous resistance. Indeed, over the same years that the Icarus Project developed, biopsychiatry has become the focus of widespread critique (Whittaker 2011; Tamini and Cohen 2008; Lane 2007; Morrison 2005). New approaches to mental health focus on stories and narratives echoing many of Icarus Project perspectives and emerging from a variety of sources (Stastny and Lehman, 2007). Yet, despite widespread critique and alternatives, biopsychiatry remains the invisible common sense on our television screens and in our medical culture. It is the overwhelming option that is available to us when we and our loved ones are in distress, and it is the language in our mouths when we try to talk about our most intimate struggles with our minds. Biopsychiatry is the mainstream that we all drink from and, for many of us, the story that keeps us feeling trapped in psychic boxes like we are sick and diseased, rootless and alone.

In the preceding pages I have shared with you the attempts of my community to actively and creatively counter the biopsychiatric narrative and way of life. Early on in our struggle, we came up with a metaphorical symbol, an image that carries a story which best conveys our resilience in the long battle to redefine how our culture understands mental health. This is the symbol of dandelion roots and their relationship to soil.

It is a rule of nature that the ground does not stay bare for very long. Wherever soil has been disturbed, there are always seeds that come along which grow into plants with roots and leaves that cover the bare soil, providing homes for all kinds of creatures and enriching the earth through their cycles of life and death. These plants are called pioneer plants because they lay the groundwork for the inevitable successions that follow. Many of the most common pioneer plants are the ones we are trained to see as weeds, plants like the dandelion whose strong taproot extends far below the depleted topsoil to the deep layers of subsoil that hold hidden minerals underground. The dandelion pulls these minerals up and incorporates them into its leaves and flowers; when it dies all the nutrients that were locked underground join the upper layers of soil, making them available to the next generation of plants growing in the soil.

We have learned, in the Icarus Project, to see the dandelion–this wild and unpredictable plant that reaches into the fertile darkness of underground places–as a symbol for our work. Many of the ideas from the Icarus Project are taken from the cultural and political underground, from important stories and wisdom that are not so easy to find in the topsoil of mainstream culture. Many of our visions for the future emerge from the depths of our own experiences as the mad ones whose roots reach down into the darkness but whose voices open up into the light.

Pioneer plants tend to create thousands of tiny seeds that are lightweight, sometimes with fine hairs that act like parachutes, keeping them afloat in the wind and preventing them from succumbing too quickly to gravity. We see the Icarus Project setting seed and releasing messages from hidden worlds that just might travel far and wide and colonize patches of damaged soil all over the planet, slowly transforming old stories into new, laying the groundwork for inevitable changes. In this spirit, the dandelion serves as an organic metaphor for our strategy and our vigilant hope going into the future.

Note

1 Originally printed in the *Journal of Medical Humanities,* vol. 35, pp. 257–271 (2014). Reprinted with permission.

References

Bayer, Ronald. 1987. *Homosexuality and American Psychiatry: The Politics of Diagnosis.* Princeton: Princeton University Press.

Butler, C. T. and McHenry, Keith. 2002. *Food Not Bombs.* Berkeley, CA: Sharp Press.

Charters, Ann. 2003. *The Portable Beat Reader.* Berkeley, CA: Penguin Classics.

Cooper, David. 1967. *Psychiatry and Anti-Psychiatry.* London: Tavistock Publications.

DuBrul, Sascha Altman. 2002. "The Bipolar World." *San Francisco Bay Guardian,* September 25. http://theicarusproject.net/articles/the-bipolar-world.

DuBrul, Sascha Altman and McNamara, J. 2003. *Navigating the Space Between Brilliance and Madness.* New York: The Icarus Project. Accessed November 30, 2012. http://theicarusproject.net/files/navigating_the_space.pdf.

Frank, T. 1997. *The Conquest of Cool: Business Culture, Counterculture, and the Rise of Hip Consumerism.* Chicago: University of Chicago Press.

Ginsburg, Allen. 1956. *Howl.* San Francisco, CA: City Lights Books.

Glaser, Gabrielle. 2008 "'Mad Pride' Fights a Stigma." *The New York Times,* May 11. Accessed June 12, 2012. http://www.nytimes.com/2008/05/11/fashion/11madpride.html?pagewanted=all.

Graeber, David. 2002. "The New Anarchist." *New Left Review* 13,61–73.

Hall, Will. 2007. *Harm Reduction Guide to Coming Off Psychiatric Drugs.* New York: The Icarus Project.

Inciardi, James A. and Harrison, Lana D. 2000. *Harm Reduction: National and International Perspectives.* Los Angeles: SAGE Publications.

Kerouac, Jack. 1957. *On The Road.* San Francisco, CA: City Lights Books.

Lane, Christopher. 2007. *Shyness: How Normal Behavior Became a Sickness.* New Haven: Yale University Press.

Lewis, Bradley. 2006. *Moving Beyond Prozac, DSM, and the New Psychiatry: The Birth of Post-Psychiatry.* Ann Arbor: University of Michigan Press.

Marcus, Greil. 1989. *Lipstick Traces: A Secret History of the Twentieth Century.* Boston: Harvard University Press.

Marshall, Peter. 2010. *Demanding the Impossible: A History of Anarchism.* Oakland: PM Press.

Mollison, Bill. 1997. *Permaculture: A Designer's Manual.* Tasmania, Australia: Tagari Publications.

Moncrieff, Joanna. 2008. "Neoliberalism and Biopsychiatry: A Marriage of Convenience." In *Liberatory Psychiatry: Philosophy, Politics, and Mental Health*, edited by Carl I. Cohen and Sami Timimi, 235–255. Cambridge: Cambridge University Press.

Morrison, Linda. 2005. *Talking Back to Psychiatry: The Psychiatric Consumer/Survivor/Ex-Patient Movement.* London: Routledge.

Notes from Nowhere, ed. 2003. *We Are Everywhere: The Irresistible Rise of Global Anti-Capitalism.* New York: Verso.

Roszak, Theodore. 1968. *The Making of a Counter Culture: Reflections on the Technocratic Society and Its Youthful Opposition.* Garden City, NY: Doubleday & Company

Stastny, Peter and Lehman, Peter. 2007. *Alternatives Beyond Psychiatry.* Berlin: Peter Lehman Publishing.

Shepard, Benjamin and Hayduk, Ronald. 2002. *From ACT UP to the WTO: Urban Protest and Community Building in the Era of Globalization.* New York: Verso.

Tamini, S. and Cohen, C., eds. 2008. *Liberatory Psychiatry.* Cambridge: Cambridge University Press.

The Icarus Project. 2002. "Original Origins and Purpose Statement." Accessed July 8, 2014. http://www.theicarusproject.net/icarus-organizational/origins-andpurpose.

The Icarus Project. 2004. "Grant Proposal to the Ittleson Foundation." Accessed November 30, 2012. http://www.coactivate.org/projects/icarusproject/grant-proposals-and-grant-reports.

The Icarus Project. 2005. "Mission Statement." Accessed November 30, 2012. http://theicarusproject.net/about-us/icarus-project-mission-statement.

The Icarus Project. 2006. "Friends Make the Best Medicine." Accessed November 30, 2012. http://www.theicarusproject.net/icarus-downloads/friends-make-the-best-medicine.

Whitaker, R. 2011. *Anatomy of An Epidemic: Magic Bullets, Psychiatric Drugs, and the Astonishing Rise of Mental Illness in America.* New York: Random House.

Chapter 35

Ending Coercion[1]

Alberto Vásquez Encalada

Summary

Vásquez Encalada crucially helps us distinguish between "hard coercion," or the explicit force, violence, and intrusion often legitimized and normalized through mental health law, and "soft coercion," a perhaps even more insidious form of deception, pressure, manipulation, and gaslighting that can destroy the possibility of making informed decisions. While the former has received quite a bit of attention in human rights advocacy, the latter can seem fundamental to psychiatry in a way that may lead us to wonder whether "mental health services based on human rights is not an oxymoron."

Vásquez Encalada analysis is rooted in his experience as a survivor, citing moments when he may have voluntarily and consensually received mental health treatment, but like so many, solely due to the fact that he was not offered any other options, nor could he previously imagine anything different. Taking the reader through the profound collaborative work of the United Nations Committee for the Rights of Persons with Disabilities, Vásquez Encalada gives us hope and reminds us that while ending coercion is the beginning of the process, we must keep our vision for systemic transformation and liberation as our true north.

*

Point of Departure

Fifteen years ago, back in 2005, I started working at the Peruvian Congress. I was 24 years old, with long hair and very little desire to wear a suit. At that point in my life, I was facing a breakdown. I spent my days in profound and inescapable sadness. I hated my career, had few real friends, and felt like my life was sinking, plagued by insomnia, migraines, and a precocious array of disappointments.

My office was run by a left-wing congressman, Javier Diez Canseco. A natural leader committed to progressive battles, Javier was also a person with a disability. For this reason, he promoted the creation of a multiparty commission for disability studies, dedicated to analysing the situation of this group and preparing legislative

DOI: 10.4324/9781003148456-40

proposals that would enable the full exercise of their rights. Back then, I did not know anything about disability, and my true motivation for working in that commission was to avoid working in a law firm.

Shortly after joining the commission, I had my first "official" crisis. So many years of fear and anguish drove me to collapse one morning in the middle of a family breakfast. That same day I had my first appointment with a psychologist, and, in the following weeks, the number of my diagnoses and prescriptions snowballed.

An Irish colleague once shared that psychiatry had saved his life and, at the same time, taken away his will to live. I do not know if I would say the same. Indeed, for a couple of years, I did not feel anything. Neither sadness nor joy—nothing. I lived doped, drowsy. While everything I did was voluntary and my treatment taken with my consent—and for a long time, I felt grateful—the truth is that I had no alternative. It was either that or go back to the hell I had experienced before. Nothing else was on offer, nor could I imagine anything different.

A Totalitarian Threat

In mid-2006, I left Congress and joined the Ombudsperson's Office, where one of my work areas was monitoring mental health establishments. One of the first things I learned while visiting these mental health facilities was that coercion is a universal reality—something I confirmed later, visiting psychiatric hospitals in other countries as part of my work at the Office of the United Nations Special Rapporteur on the rights of persons with disabilities.

On one hand, there is *hard* coercion: that of force, confinement, and intrusion—intrusion through injections, drugs, and loss of control and self. It is undoubtedly the darkest side of psychiatry. Around the world, almost without exception, mental health systems exert physical and psychological coercion on people daily, including institutionalisation, involuntary commitment, community treatment orders, forced medication, electroconvulsive therapy, sterilisation, isolation, physical and pharmacological restraints, and conversion therapies, among other practices that diminish the dignity, autonomy, and integrity of people. Contrary to what the psychiatric *establishment* claims, these practices are not exceptional but are on the rise (Frances, 2012; Sashidharan, Mezzina, & Puras, 2019).

Hard coercion is made legal in many countries through mental health legislation. Mental health laws may seem like a good idea until you take the trouble to read them. There is a promise of greater access to services and protection of human rights, but the reality is that all mental health laws in the world, without exception, place limitations on the human rights of service users. Through mental health laws, coercion is legitimised and normalised.

It is difficult to understand how *hard* coercion has its place in care and treatment. The mere possibility of using force to compel a person to follow a "treatment" denatures the notion of care. Further, it invalidates the possibility of making a free and informed decision. Even where force is not explicit, the threat overshadows the relationship between the doctor and the individual, creating a marked power asymmetry. Indeed, the evidence tells us that people may voluntarily consent to internment or treatment just to avoid the humiliation and stigma of forced intervention (Szmuckler, 2015). Like a totalitarian regime, power is concentrated in the system and takes away personhood, independence, and individuality—basically any departure from the norm and status quo.

On the other hand, there is also *soft* coercion, that of family and societal pressure and the lack of alternatives. Some authors refer to it as informal coercion (Pelto-Piri, Kjellin, & Hylén, 2019). There are different forms of *soft* coercion: deception (*strategic dishonesty*); authoritarian or disciplinary styles, which verticalise the doctor-user relationship; family pressure and manipulation, including the threat of cutting off connections and gaslighting; and social pressure in general, which pushes people to stay within the bounds of so-called normality.

The lack of alternatives to the biomedical model of mental health should also be considered a form of *soft* coercion in the sense that it represents another form of deception and propaganda. As the United Nations Special Rapporteur on the Right to Health reminded us, the biomedical discourse has the monopoly on most mental health systems, inculcating that mental health problems are biologically based and medication is the best, if not only, course of action (Puras, 2017). Under this mainstream discourse, buttressed by the media and biased evidence, it is difficult, if not impossible, to make an informed decision.

It could be argued that *hard* coercion, that of literal force, is far more pernicious and has more profound effects than *soft* coercion, including trauma, psychological damage, injury, and even death (Kersting, Hirsch, & Steinert, 2019). But *soft* coercion entrenches the totalitarian model: the denial of human diversity, the loss of the actual possibility of making informed decisions, and the reduction of an individual's value to their function within the economic and social system.

A New Hope

Adopted in 2006, the United Nations Convention on the Rights of Persons with Disabilities brought us hope for change, for a humanity in which difference is accepted and diversity is valued (United Nations International Convention on the Rights of Persons with Disabilities, 2006). Drafted with the active participation of the disability movements, including many users and survivors of psychiatry from different parts of the world, the Convention reminds us of the universality of human rights: all persons with disabilities must enjoy all human rights and fundamental freedoms on equal terms with others. Differences, actual or perceived, cannot be a valid reason for the limitation of rights.

The Convention also represents a paradigm shift in the way disability is understood and addressed. Building on the social model, the Convention conceptualises disability as the result of the interaction between a person with disabilities and the attitudinal and environmental barriers the person faces in exercising rights. That is, disability is not intrinsic to the individual but is the result of the lack of opportunities to participate in social life.

To reflect this understanding, the expert body in charge of its monitoring, the United Nations Committee on the Rights of Persons with Disabilities, uses the term "persons with psychosocial disabilities" (United Nations Committee on the Rights of Persons with Disabilities, 2014). This term seeks to recognise all people who experience discrimination and social barriers based on a mental health diagnosis or subjective distress regardless of how they self-identify. Furthermore, it aims to reflect a social rather than medical approach to mental health experiences, focusing on attitudinal and environmental barriers individuals face that impede their participation and inclusion.

This new human rights model of disability is based on principles such as dignity and personal autonomy, equality and non-discrimination, intersectionality, and the recognition of disability as part of human diversity. It questions the status quo and offers alternative responses to traditional institutions. The Committee has pointed out on several occasions that the Convention prohibits coercive measures in mental health systems because they are contrary to the right to equal recognition of legal capacity, personal liberty and security, personal integrity, and the right to health and the prohibition of torture and ill-treatment (United Nations Committee on the Rights of Persons with Disabilities, 2014).

Article 12 of the Convention recognises that persons with disabilities enjoy legal capacity in all aspects of life on an equal basis with others. Thus, contrary to most civil codes and mental health laws that make "exceptional" limitation of the exercise of rights legal for this population, the Convention upholds the individual's right to make legally binding decisions, such as entering into contracts, voting, and consenting to or rejecting medical treatment. In addition, the Convention recognises that people with disabilities have the right to support for the exercise of their legal capacity, and therein lies the paradigm shift embodied by the Convention: recognising and valuing the interdependence of the human experience (United Nations Committee on the Rights of Persons with Disabilities, 2015).

Article 14 of the Convention expressly prohibits the deprivation of liberty on the grounds of disability. The Committee has clarified that this prohibition extends to cases in which deprivation of liberty is based on additional criteria such as the need for treatment or the consideration that the person poses a risk to self or others (United Nations Committee on the Rights of Persons with Disabilities, 2015). As such, the involuntary admission of a person to a mental health facility contravenes the right to liberty and security of the person and the principle of free and informed consent (art. 25, lit. d). Furthermore, when detention involves involuntary treatment and the forced administration of medication, this practice also violates the right to personal security and integrity (art. 17), as well as protection against torture and ill-treatment (art. 15).

In this sense, the Convention represents an unequivocal international mandate to respect, protect, and fulfil all the rights of all persons with disabilities and, along these lines, to transform existing health systems to eliminate all forms of coercion. This is the opinion not only of the Committee on the Rights of Persons with Disabilities but also of various human rights mechanisms and experts and agencies of the United Nations, including the World Health Organization (United Nations

High Commissioner for Human Rights, 2017; United Nations Committee on the Rights of Persons with Disabilities, 2015; Puras, 2020; Working Group on Arbitrary Detention, 2015; World Health Organization, 2019b). One hundred eighty-three states and the European Union have ratified the Convention and thereby assumed the obligation to comply with these standards and take all necessary legislative, policy, and other measures to give effect to the rights therein. This includes a duty to review their mental health laws.

Human Rights–Based Mental Health Services: An Oxymoron?

Based on the past and present human rights violations in mental health systems, many may wonder whether talking about mental health services based on human rights is not an oxymoron—a combination of two words of opposite meaning. For example, in a very sharp article, Jasna Russo and Stephanie Wooley (2020) contemplate whether there can be such a thing as "human psychiatry."

The main concern of these authors is how mental health systems are appropriating the discourse of the Convention and human rights and, in this process, denaturing it (*Berlin Manifesto*, 2019; Appelbaum, 2019). Indeed, in recent years, under pressure from the United Nations human rights system, initiatives and publications have emerged from psychiatry that take the Convention as their starting point, particularly the mandate to guarantee access to support for decision-making, but in many cases are empty of content. This process of co-opting critical instances is not new, and much has been written about denaturing the recovery approach or peer support spaces (Madrid & Castillo Parada, 2018).

In this sense, I agree with Russo and Wooley (2020) that the implementation of the Convention cannot be seen as another mental health reform. Instead, this treaty is a call to transform the social and political structures that sustain the discrimination and marginalisation faced by persons with psychosocial disabilities, which, among other things, legitimise the actions of psychiatry. As Transforming Communities for Inclusion (TCI), a global organisation of persons with psychosocial disabilities, predominantly from Asia and the Pacific, points out, responses framed by the medical model that restrict freedom, choice, and opportunity have failed (TCI Asia Pacific, 2018). The reforms of mental health systems, although necessary, cannot be considered sufficient to implement our rights. The inclusion of people with psychosocial disabilities implies a paradigm shift at many levels: from the medical model to the social model; from "mental disorder" to disability or psychosocial diversity; from "mental health" to inclusive development; from institutionalisation to life in the community; and from "treatment" to support systems (TCI Asia Pacific, 2018). Along the same lines, the Latin American Network of Psychosocial Diversity (2019), in its Lima Declaration, called for constructing a new paradigm that accepts "psychosocial diversity" as a fact and principle derived from human diversity and recognises us as experts by experience.

Therefore, to talk about mental health and human rights (without falling into an oxymoron), it is not enough to incorporate elements of the Convention as part of another mental health reform process. It requires systemic transformation to overhaul the starting points and approaches. Ending coercion is an urgent but insufficient step. It is essential to reassess and reposition the role of the right to health and mental health systems. It is necessary to turn our gaze towards the social factors that determine subjective distress and the exclusion of our difference: discrimination, violence, institutionalisation, poverty, and social exclusion in general. In the health sector, this may be called addressing the social determinants of mental health. In the Mad movement, we call it achieving social justice and human rights.

Furthermore, alternatives need to be built inside and outside the system: peer groups, spaces for respite or rest, open dialogue, safe spaces to talk about suicide, and the like (Gooding et al., 2018). The leadership and direct experiences of people with psychosocial disabilities in the design and implementation of these alternatives is essential to achieve this. As Tina Minkowitz and others have noted, mental health crises would evolve better with proper peer support and support services, and further demedicalising these processes will help (Minkowitz, 2019; Stastny et al., 2020).

Coercion in Mental Health: A False Necessary Evil

To convince, arguments from authority are not enough. Although the Convention prohibits coercion, the truth is that a good part of the population and the majority of policymakers and service providers believe that coercion is a necessary evil. This conviction is not spontaneous but the legacy of a system that is more than 300 years old. And although fundamental rights cannot be subject to the majority's discretion, advancing legislation and policies is essential to dismantling these false premises.

The truth is that coercion is ineffective on its terms, and there is limited evidence to support its effectiveness (Gooding, 2017). The first argument favouring coercion is that it protects and saves lives, whether that of one person or those of third parties. Common sense would lead us to think that this is true, since one of the most used criteria for using coercive measures is the risk to oneself or others. The problem is that there is no evidence to support this claim.

On one hand, it is extremely difficult, if not impossible, to predict who represents a risk to third parties, given the low rate of violence among people with psychosocial disabilities (Mossman, 2009). The evidence tells us, on the contrary, that there is a widespread bias of dangerousness associated with psychosocial disability that is prevalent in the general population, including service providers (Stuber et al., 2014). On the other hand, there are no reliable methods to determine who will commit suicide. Although risk factors have been identified, there is no way to predict suicide before the act itself (Pokorny, 1983; Kessler et al., 2020). Instead, some authors warn that coercion can increase the risk of suicide because many people who require help do not go to services or choose not to reveal their suicidal thoughts for fear of coercive measures (Jordan & McNeil, 2019).

A second argument is that coercion facilitates access to mental health services. That has been the central argument for expanding community (involuntary) treatment orders in many countries (Bertolín Guillén, 2011). However, several studies have shown that such measures have not achieved their objective of fulfilling greater adherence to treatment and reducing hospitalisation rates or producing better clinical and social outcomes (Rugkåsa, 2016). Likewise, in a general way, various publications have pointed out that coercion affects the therapeutic bond and, in this way, prevents the recovery process (World Health Organization, 2019a).

A third argument is that the use of coercion is an exceptional measure to be used when there are no alternatives. As we have said before, coercion is on the rise and there is little unusual about it. But more important, there have been several "alternatives" to coercive measures inside and outside mental health systems for many years, from Open Dialogue in Finland and other countries to mutual support groups in Kenya (Open Dialogue, 2022; USP-K, 2018). These services and interventions, although not perfect, have proven effective in ensuring rights-based responses even in crises (Gooding et al, 2018). Therefore, it should come as no surprise that many of these services have been designed and led by people with psychosocial disabilities.

Although this does not pretend to be a legal article, it is worth affirming that the fact that the coercive measures are neither suitable nor necessary to achieve the presumably legitimate purposes that it pursues should lead us to the conclusion that such actions do not comply with the criteria of the test of reasonableness of restrictions to human rights.

Point of No Return

Almost 15 years have passed from those days I spent as an advisor to the Disability Studies Commission in the Peruvian Congress. So much has changed in my life, and much has changed the debate on mental health and human rights. It seems unbelievable, but my first mental health assignment on that commission was to write a mental health bill—a Mad in charge of dreaming the future of mental health of the country. I confess that I failed that time: I could not imagine anything different. Or I had no real chance to do it.

Today, I write these lines from a different experience and identity, from the conviction that we can imagine another system to provide support and respond to the actual problems that cause distress.

There is no turning back.

Note

1 *This chapter was originally written in Spanish for Juan Carlos Cea Madrid (ed.), *Sin locxs no hay revolución. Activismo en primera persona desde América Latina*, Locooperativa, 2021, In press.

References

Appelbaum, P. (2019). Saving the UN convention on the rights of persons with disabilities—from itself. *Editorial WPA, 18*(1).

Berlin Manifesto for a Humane Psychiatry. (2019). http://berliner-manifest.de/english

Bertolín Guillén, J. M. (2011). Community treatment orders: Bioethical basis. *European Journal of Psychiatry*, *25*(3), 134–143. https://dx.doi.org/10.4321/S0213–61632011000300003

Frances, A. (2012, August 8). A clinical reality check. *Cato Unbound*. https://www.cato-unbound.org/2012/08/08/allen-frances/clinical-reality-check

Gooding, P. (2017). *A new era for mental health law and policy: Supported decision-making and the UN convention on the rights of persons with disabilities* (pp. 88–96). Cambridge University Press.

Gooding, P., McSherry, B., Roper, C., & Grey, F. (2018). *Alternatives to coercion in mental health settings: A literature review*. Melbourne Social Equity Institute. https://socialequity.unimelb.edu.au/news/latest/alternatives-to-coercion

Jordan, J. T., & McNiel, D. E. (2019). Perceived coercion during admission into psychiatric hospitalization increases risk of suicide attempts after discharge. *Suicide and Life-Threatening Behavior*. https://doi.org/10.1111/sltb.12560

Kersting, X., Hirsch, S., & Steinert, T. (2019). Physical harm and death in the context of coercive measures in psychiatric patients: A systematic review. *Frontiers in Psychiatry*, *10*, 400. https://doi.org/10.3389/fpsyt.2019.00400

Kessler, R. C., Bossarte, R. M., Luedtke, A., Zaslovsky A. M., & Zubizarreta J. R. (2020). Suicide prediction models: A critical review of recent research with recommendations for the way forward. *Mol Psychiatry*, *25*, 168–179. https://doi.org/10.1038/s41380-019-0531-0

Latin American Network of Psychosocial Diversity (Redesfera Latinoamericana de la Diversidad Psicosocial). (2019). Locura Latina, Declaración de Lima. In J. C. Madrid (Ed.), *Por el derecho a la locura. La reinvención de la salud mental en América Latina* (2nd ed.).

Madrid, J. C., & Castillo Parada, T. (2018). Locura y neoliberalismo. El lugar de la antipsiquiatría en la salud mental contemporánea. *Política y Sociedad*, *55*(2).

Minkowitz,Tina. (2019). *Positive policy to replace forced psychiatry, based on CRPD*. https://www.academia.edu/39229717/Positive_policy_to_replace_forced_psychiatry_based_on_CRPD

Mossman, D. (2009). The imperfection of protection through detection and intervention lessons from three decades of research on the psychiatric assessment of violence risk. *Journal of Legal Medicine*, *30*, 109–140. https://doi.org/10.1080/01947640802694635

Open Dialogue. (2022). *An international community*. http://open-dialogue.net/

Pelto-Piri, V., Kjellin, L., Hylén, U., Valenti, E., & Priebe S. (2019). Different forms of informal coercion in psychiatry: A qualitative study. *BMC Res Notes*, *12*, 787. https://doi.org/10.1186/s13104-019-4823-x

Pokorny, A. D. (1983). Prediction of suicide in psychiatric patients: Report of a prospective study. *Arch Gen Psychiatry*, *40*(3), 249–257. https://doi.org/10.1001/archpsyc.1983.01790030019002

Puras, D. (2017). *Report of the special rapporteur on the right of everyone to the enjoyment of the highest attainable standard of physical and mental health* (A/HRC/35/21). United Nations Digital Library.

Puras, D. (2020). *Report of the special rapporteur on the right of everyone to the enjoyment of the highest attainable standard of physical and mental health* (A/HRC/44/48). United Nations Digital Library.

Rugkåsa, J. (2016). Effectiveness of community treatment orders: The international evidence. *Revue canadienne de psychiatrie*, *61*(1), 15–24. https://doi.org/10.1177/0706743715620415

Russo, J., & Wooley, S. (2020). The implementation of the convention on the rights of persons with disabilities: More than just another reform of psychiatry. *Health and Human Rights Journal*, *22*(1). https://www.hhrjournal.org/2020/06/the-implementation-of-the-convention-on-the-rights-of-persons-with-disabilities-more-than-just-another-reform-of-psychiatry/

Sashidharan, S. P., Mezzina, R., & Puras, D. (2019). Reducing coercion in mental healthcare. *Epidemiology and Psychiatric Sciences*, *28*(6), 605–612. https://doi.org/10.1017/S2045796019000350

Stastny, P., Lovell, A., Hannah, J., Goulart, D., Vásquez, A., O'Callaghan, S., & Puras, D. (2020). Crisis response as a human rights flashpoint: Critical elements of community support for individuals experiencing significant emotional distress. *Health and Human Rights Journal*, *22*(1). https://www.hhrjournal.org/2020/06/crisis-response-as-a-human-rights-flashpoint-critical-elements-of-community-support-for-individuals-experiencing-significant-emotional-distress/

Stuber, J. P., Rocha, A., Christian, A., & Link, B.G. (2014). Conceptions of mental illness: Attitudes of mental health professionals and the general public. *Psychiatric Services*, *65*(4), 490–497.

Szmukler, G. (2015). Compulsion and "coercion" in mental health care. *World Psychiatry: Official Journal of the World Psychiatric Association (WPA)*, *14*(3), 259–261.

Transforming Communities for Inclusion—Asia Pacific (TCI Asia Pacific). (2018). *Bali declaration*. https://www.tci-asia.org/bali-declaration/

United Nations Committee on the Rights of Persons with Disabilities. (2014). *General comment No. 1, Article 12: Equal recognition before the law* (CRPD/C/GC/1). United Nations Committee on the Rights of Persons with Disabilities.

United Nations Committee on the Rights of Persons with Disabilities. (2015). *Guidelines on the right to liberty and security of persons with disabilities* (A/72/55, Annex). United Nations Committee on the Rights of Persons with Disabilities.

United Nations High Commissioner for Human Rights. (2017). *Mental health and human rights* (A/HRC/34/32). United Nations High Commissioner for Human Rights.

United Nations International Convention on the Rights of Persons with Disabilities. (2006). *In force since 3 May 2008*. Ratified by 184 States Parties.

Users and Survivors of Psychiatry in Kenya (USP-K). (2018). *The role of peer support in exercising legal capacity*. http://www.uspkenya.org/wp-content/uploads/2018/01/Role-of-Peer-Support-in-Exercising-Legal-Capacity.pdf

Working Group on Arbitrary Detention. (2015). *United Nations basic principles and guidelines on remedies and procedures on the right of anyone deprived of their liberty to bring proceedings before a court* (A/HRC/30/37). Working Group on Arbitrary Detention.

World Health Organization. (2019a). *Freedom from coercion, violence and abuse*. WHO QualityRights Core Training: Mental Health and Social Services, Course Guide. https://apps.who.int/iris/bitstream/handle/10665/329582/9789241516730-eng.pdf

World Health Organization. (2019b). *QualityRights materials for training, guidance, and transformation*. https://www.who.int/publications/i/item/who-qualityrights-guidance-and-training-tools

Chapter 36

Language Games Used to Construct Autism as Pathology[1]

Nick Chown

Summary

Nick Chown's work as an autism advocate, mentor, researcher, and trainer has been enriched and inspired by his scholarship on the philosopher Ludwig Wittgenstein. This chapter uses Wittgenstein's philosophy to highlight "neurotypical language games" that problematically shape the very language of "autism" and "non-autism." These language games underlie almost all research funding and publication, and they contain one-sided assumptions that autism is a "bad thing" and that the cure of autism is a "good thing." This perspective results in research almost exclusively devoted to the "cause" and "treatment" of this bad thing, heavily focused on questions of "genetics, neuroscience, and the search for a cure."

Chown advocates for a "macroethics" approach to this research. Macroethics, as opposed to microethics, questions whether research devoted to eradicating autism and other categories of neurodivergence should be undertaken at all. This is particularly true when autism self-advocates argue that autism is a "neurological difference associated with societal oppression," an argument that is consistent with those of many disability studies scholars.

For Chown, crude good/bad perspectives about autism and non-autism have been so insinuated into our language games we have trouble doing justice to the complexities involved. He does not argue that we should ignore "the challenges faced by some autistic people, and their carers." But we should also not ignore the ways that neurotypical language games and their eradication-oriented research protocols are causing equally deep challenges.

*

Ludwig Wittgenstein counselled against the bewitchment of our intelligence by means of our language, by which he meant that we risk misunderstanding something as a result of failing to notice logical errors in language used to describe it. Some scholars believe that autistic thinking is more individualistic and less likely to be stuck in the rut of conventionality. So, an autistically neurodivergent perspective on language use is

DOI: 10.4324/9781003148456-41

valuable in identifying the bewitchment of intelligence that concerned Wittgenstein. I also argue that a failure of neurotypical society to appreciate that societal language games are, by definition, *neurotypical* language games has adverse consequences for autistic people because of the inevitability of cultural biases favouring neurotypicality. The philosopher Sandy Grant has written that

> as long as there is language it will bewitch us, we will face the temptation to misunderstand. And there is no vantage point outside it. There is no escape from language-games then, but we can forge a kind of freedom from within them.[2]

Might it be possible for an autistic person to escape a neurotypical language game – and all language games *are* neurotypical – and observe it from an external vantage point?

Wittgenstein introduced the concept of language games. Various of his ideas – including the language game concept – are relevant to an understanding of autism. A language game is the language associated with a particular activity that gives the activity its meaning. For example, the job interview is an activity where language is used in special ways. When an interviewer asks an interviewee to talk about their weaknesses, both parties should know that the response has to demonstrate self-awareness on the part of the interviewee; to provide a detailed description and analysis of weak points would be to misunderstand this particular language game. It is my view that the term 'language game' does not do full justice to Wittgenstein's intention because it implies a sole focus on language rather than the social interaction of which language is a part (albeit a very important part). Szasz refers to the 'game-playing model of human behavior' (Szasz, 2010, p. 250) and to the importance of 'rules'[3] in human social interactional gameplaying. I believe this is what language games are about.

While neurotypical language relating to autism inevitably reflects neurotypical perspectives on autism, societal understandings of autism will benefit from autistic perspectives that reflect the lived experience of autism. For instance, many autistic people consider that the monotropism theory of autism – developed by neurodivergent scholars – describes what it is like to be autistic better than any other theory (Murray, Lesser, & Lawson, 2005). And the double empathy hypothesis (Milton, 2012) – which draws attention to the bi-directional nature of the difficulty autistic and non-autistic people often have understanding each other – was also developed by a neurodivergent scholar. In addition to the language game concept, I draw attention to Wittgenstein's counsel against bewitchment of our intelligence through misuse of language. On occasions, and perhaps due to the subtlety of language, we draw conclusions that appear sound but that on investigation are found to be illogical. For example, the concept of the broader autism phenotype – which is thoroughly embedded in medical understandings of autism – is based on the illogical assumption that a cluster of traits used to screen for autism, and that any human being may present with, are somehow 'autistic traits' indicative of a subclinical presentation of autism in the general population known as the broader autism phenotype (Chown, 2019). This chapter begins a Wittgensteinian analysis of aspects of societal language use to demonstrate the value of a neurodivergent perspective in the identification of researcher misunderstandings of aspects of autism with the potential to influence ethical consideration of research to cure/prevent autism adversely.

First, it will be demonstrated that a failure to appreciate that societal language games are *neurotypical* language games can have adverse consequences where autism is concerned because of the inevitability of cultural biases in favour of neurotypicality. Second, it will be demonstrated that misuse of language can give rise to false beliefs about autism that may become embedded as received opinion in language games. In the first situation, the value of 'missing' neurodivergent perspectives will be shown directly. In the second situation it is contended that more individualistic (and possibly also more logical) thinking styles in autism may enable identification by autistic scholars of language misuse, that might otherwise remain hidden, as the thought processes of autistic people are less likely be influenced by pre-existing conceptual frameworks.

A substantial amount of autism research and its associated funding and publicity is focused on genetics, neuroscience, and the search for a cure (Pellicano, Dinsmore, & Charman, 2014). Although there has been considerable discussion of ethical matters in the autism research literature, most of this discussion refers to what one might call 'micro' ethical subjects such as informed consent and anonymisation. These subjects are important but of no relevance to an investigation of the ethics of research to eradicate autism. This is because discussion of 'micro' ethical subjects presupposes that the research being undertaken is research that is ethically valid. I describe a fundamental issue, such as whether a particular type of research should be undertaken at all, as a 'macro' ethical subject. Researchers rarely, if ever, discuss their justification for undertaking their study. There has been very little discussion of the ethics of autism cure/prevention in the literature (Bovell, 2015). Virginia Bovell's work is one of only two thesis-length discussions of this subject. She notes that there has been very little attempt to define the terms 'cure' and 'prevention' in relation to autism. Pursuance of a cure for autism has been problematised on ethical grounds by only a limited number of scholars. For instance, Majia Holmer Nadesan has written of the 'latent dangers lurking in a geneticization of autism devoid of environmental mediation' as well as the 'potential for ... prenatal testing potentially ushering in a new eugenics' (Nadesan, 2013, p. 137).

Wittgenstein's view of moral justifications is summed up well in the following quotation:

> Nothing we can do can be defended absolutely and finally. But only by reference to something else that is not questioned. I.e. no reason can be given why you should act (or should have acted) *like this,* except that by doing so you bring about such and such a situation, which again has to be an aim you accept. '
>
> (Wittgenstein, 1984, p. 16, author's italics)

If, like me, you believe him to be correct that there are no categorical imperatives or deity-given moral compasses, and therefore no absolute and final justification for what one does (and doesn't do), you will also agree with me that those who advocate eradicating autism must accept its eradication as a justifiable aim per se. This is presumably because in their view it is a disorder, and disorders are, by definition, harmful, and thus at odds with living a good life. It seems that most of those who would eradicate autism if they could, undertake their research on the basis of an aim they accept as a 'given', or at least without being willing to be transparent about their justification. Pellicano and Stears (2011) tell us that scientists defend the spending of the vast majority of autism research funds on research into genetics and neuroscience on the basis that: (1) identifying children at risk for autism before they show signs of autism will enable much earlier intervention than is currently the case, and (2) there will be medical benefits to improve the health of autistic individuals. If, indeed, these are the main defences used to justify such research, they appear disingenuous. This is due to the apparent focus on benefiting autistics being in clear contrast to the emphasis on seeking a cure for autism – sometimes expressed as 'prevention' – of funding bodies such as the National Alliance for Autism Research, Cure Autism Now, and Autism Speaks. Bovell (2015, p. 49) writes that 'sometimes the purpose of [autism] investigations falls short of any kind of articulated explanation beyond a "knowledge for knowledge's sake" perspective' which holds that 'potential benefits are somehow self-evident' (ibid., p. 50). She concludes that much autism research is based on autism being a 'bad thing' and cure a 'good thing'.

Where scientists justify research with the potential (if not the specific aim) of eradicating autism or other categories of neurodivergence, on a simple belief in the importance of seeking a cure for diseases and mental disorders, the issue is that it is not at all clear that these categories *are* mental disorders or are *always* mental disorders. Many autistic self-advocates and others have put forward a case that autism is neurological difference coupled with societal oppression as understood by the social models. While the language game associated with the 'cure' of diseases and disorders is uniformly positive, as indeed it should be, the inclusion of a phenomenon within the diagnostic manuals giving legitimacy to the search for a cure, is a matter for both political and scientific debate (Kapp, 2020). This can lead to the inclusion of diagnoses in the manuals that are categorically *not* diseases or disorders, with all the adverse consequences of such bad decision-making. One only has to consider the situation regarding gays and lesbians to appreciate that inclusion of a so-called disorder in a diagnostic manual can be problematic. Certain sexual orientations were included in the Diagnostic and Statistical Manual of Mental Disorders until as recently as 1987 and it was another three years before the World Health Organization removed the same orientations from their International Classification of Diseases (ICD-10). Debates about sexuality then shifted from psychiatry into the moral and political spheres as institutions could no longer justify discrimination against gay and lesbian people on the basis of (supposedly) scientific arguments used to pathologise them. Drescher (2015, p. 572) writes that

> Most importantly, in medicine, psychiatry, and other mental health professions, removing the diagnosis ['homosexuality'] from the DSM led to an important shift from asking questions about 'what causes homosexuality?' and 'how can we treat it?' to focusing instead on the health and mental health needs of LGBT patient populations.

Neurodiversity advocates would like to see similar developments in relation to autism. While many advocates support the search for a cure for conditions co-occurring with autism (co-morbidities) such as anxiety, gastrointestinal disorders, sleep disorders, and epilepsy (ibid.), that is because – unlike autism itself – they do not regard these as being core to the very nature of their being.

There have only been a limited number of investigations into the ethics of eradicating autism to date (e.g. Anderson, 2013; Barnbaum, 2008; Barnes & McCabe, 2012; Bovell, 2015; Chapman, 2019; Pellicano & Stears, 2011; Walsh, 2010). These authors all take an anti-discriminatory, anti-eradication stance except for Barnes and McCabe,[4] whose work is an investigation of the issue of choice (whether a cure should be made available for those who want one), and Barnbaum who writes that there is 'something intrinsically limiting in an autistic life' and appears to support the eradication of autism (Barnbaum, 2008, p. 154).[5] Anderson considers autism to be a valid identity and possibly even to have given rise to a culture. Walsh has challenged those who would prevent disability coming into the world, pointing out that preventing Asperger's would of necessity mean that the exceptional abilities associated with it would be lost to society. Liz Pellicano and Marc Stears set out an ethical objection to cure and prevention of autism but, importantly, one that only applies in the context of *living individuals.* Robert Chapman challenges the assumption underlying the dominant view of autism that it is inherently at odds with the ability to lead a good life. He concludes that there is no 'decisive reason to think that being autistic, in and of itself, is at odds with either thriving or personhood' (Chapman, 2018, p. 1). Bovell considers that research to cure/prevent autism is ethically indefensible. After unpacking the issues surrounding the ethics of curing/preventing autism she concludes that 'reference to prevention and/or cure as a desirable *general* goal[6] is neither clinically/scientifically coherent nor morally legitimate' (Bovell, 2015, p. 364, author's italics). Her point that 'To talk in approving terms about prevention and cure implies that a world where there are no more autistic people would be a better world' (ibid., p. 364) is the thinking that lay behind the call for scientists engaged in research to cure and/or prevent autism to justify the ethical validity of their work (Chown & Leatherland, 2018).[7]

As already stated, the fundamental point here is the vexed question as to what autism is; is it a mental disorder or disease or a natural human difference? Bovell calls this the 'analogy challenge' as both positive analogies and negative analogies have been drawn in relation to autism. There is no definitive answer to this question as yet. Many autistic scholars believe that no researcher should ever assume that it is appropriate to seek to destroy any aspect of humanity without societal acceptance of the justification for their work, an acceptance that must be based on the most thorough of investigations and debates because the very survival of a category of people depends upon it. My aim here is to indicate how a Wittgensteinian grammatical perspective can uncover hidden instances of language bewitchment of relevance to the undertaking of autism cure/prevention research. The relevance arises from the risk of misleading our attempts to understand what autism is. This can lead to situations where issues become separated from concerns about their morality. Baumann refers to such separation as 'adiaphorisation' which he defines as 'stratagems of placing, intentionally or by default, certain acts and/or omitted acts regarding certain categories of humans *outside* the moral-immoral axis – that is, outside the "universe of moral obligations" and outside the realm of phenomena subject to moral evaluation' (Bauman & Donskis, 2013, p. 40, author's italics). He says that exemption of adiaphoric acts from ethical consideration due to social consent enables those acts to be committed without those involved facing any moral stigma or needing to worry their consciences about them. Scholars' failure to discuss the ethics of their research, and society's failure to call scholars to account for their failure, is adiaphorisation. The ethics of autism research must be brought into the 'universe of moral obligations'. Wittgenstein argued that certain aspects of language use can bewitch our intelligence. This chapter discusses examples of language misuse giving rise to false beliefs about autism.

Wittgensteinian Grammatical Investigation of Autism Language

By taking steps to avoid language games 'bewitching our intelligence' we will be in a better position to see concepts for what they really are, not what they appear to be when language clouds the understanding. A Wittgensteinian grammatical investigation[8] involves an exploration of a language game and the rules governing it, not an investigation of language structure. His primary focus was on the confusions that misuse of words can cause. This chapter discusses examples of language confusion that impact upon debates relating to the ethics of autism because they give rise to false beliefs about autism: neurotypical[9] language games;[10] illogical language moves; and confusing language.

Neurotypical Language Games

Milton's double empathy hypothesis argues that communication difficulties between neurotypical and autistic people are bi-directional in nature. Hughes (2019, personal communication) refers to such difficulties as reciprocal misunderstandings. If arguing that misunderstandings on the part of autistic people arise from a cognitive defect associated with autism, it could be argued on the basis of double empathy that the difficulties neurotypical people have understanding autistic people are due to a cognitive defect in neurotypicality. Alternatively, the difficulties autistic and neurotypical people have in communicating with each other could be due to society's language games being neurotypical language games based on neurotypical understandings of autism.

First, let us consider an issue arising from a medical language game taken from Bovell (2015, p. 280). She writes that 'engaging with the community of people who are most affected and able to reflect on [intervention practices] is likely to be essential, given the sorry history of autism having been drastically misunderstood by "outsiders" in the past'. Examples of misunderstandings include autism being caused by poor mothering (Kanner/Bettelheim); autism involving social isolation (Kanner); autism only affecting children (Kanner); autistic people being intellectually disabled; autistic individuals being unable to feel or express emotions; all autistic people lacking empathy and/or theory of mind. There are many more myths and misunderstandings, and they have probably all been perpetuated by non-autistic scholars who have just as much difficulty empathising with autistic people as vice versa[11] (Chown, 2014; Milton, 2012). Milton and Bracher (2013) argue that the absence of autistic voices from work to generate knowledge about autism results in both epistemological and ethical problems as non-autistic people cannot have lived experience of being autistic. Unless and until medical language games of autism are allowed to develop with contributions from autistic scholars, they will remain prone to perpetuating misunderstandings about autism that impact theory and practice.

Let us now consider a cultural language game. Sarah Pripas-Kapit (2020, p. 25) writes that while

> authors such as Temple Grandin and Donna Williams introduced mainstream audiences to the concept of autistic people narrating their own experiences, their works still relied on ableist ideas about autism promoted by non-autistic scientific 'experts' and parents. They positioned autism as a tragedy.

She points out that Sinclair (1993), who had a thorough understanding of parental perspectives on autism, challenged the assumption that autism is always tragic and that parental grief for the 'loss' of the expected child is the inevitable result of autism. The 'autism as tragedy' trope is an example of a cultural perspective on autism inextricably linked with neurotypicality,[12] and with which most autistic self-advocates would disagree. Parents of autistic children have contributed to the development of the neurodiversity movement, and some autistic individuals agree with the tragedy trope, so it is wrong to speak of necessarily opposed neurotypical and autistic attitudes. However, with cultural attitudes towards autism having developed in a neurotypical society where cure and prevention discourses are prominent, the language games of autism have inevitably developed in accordance with neurotypical society's cultural biases. Autistic self-advocates and the developing autistic online culture are effecting some change to this situation but unless and until autistic viewpoints are accepted as valid this cultural bias will continue.[13]

Illogical Language Moves

It is argued that those who believe in the existence of a broader autism phenotype (BAP) are led astray by misuse of language (Chown, 2019). Human traits indicative of autism are included in a screening cluster for a good reason – that there is a strong indication of autism if an individual has the cluster traits – but scholars then generally make the unjustified leap into thinking that having some of the cluster traits implies the existence of a broader autism phenotype of individuals who do not justify a diagnosis of autism but have a sufficient number of its features to be ... what? The BAP concept appears so nebulous that it is difficult to devise a suitable descriptor for people supposedly in this category other than 'member of the BAP', which says nothing. How many of the criteria in an autism screening cluster would a person need to qualify for membership of a BAP rather than them being undeniably non-autistic, and what would the cut-off point be for actually being autistic? Including certain traits in a diagnostic cluster for autism does not mean that individuals with some, but not all, of these traits are in a 'somewhat, but not fully, autistic' category.

Those who believe this have been bewitched by the hidden transition from 'human trait associated with autism' to an 'autistic trait' that implies a degree of autism,[14] whatever this may mean. Human beings can present with any combination of human traits. So human traits in a diagnostic cluster for autism may be seen in non-autistic people. This does not imply that these individuals are not autistic enough to justify a diagnosis of autism, whatever this may mean. It is simply that they have some of the human traits used to diagnose autism because at present we have no better means of diagnosing autism than by using (a cluster of) behavioural criteria (ibid.).

Confusing Language

Here again, let's consider two examples. First, there is an example of the reification of a piece of confusing language in autism that Bovell has discussed. She points to the crucial distinction between treating a co-morbidity and treating autism itself, writing that 'in the treatment vs acceptance debate, much of the defence of the pro-treatment group rested on their emphasis on co-morbidities that could/should be treated, and their rejection of the idea that painful co-morbidities should be 'accepted' rather than challenged' (2015, p. 275). As mentioned earlier, this position would be accepted by most autistic advocates. Pro-treatment groups usually call for treatment of associated health needs, not autism itself. But 'treating autism' is a far handier descriptor than, say, 'treating medical conditions associated with autism'. In other words, what began life as a headline-grabbing form of words designed to attract attention, can become something it was never intended to be, that is, a statement that autism *itself* should be treated. Of course, 'treating autism' may mean exactly that in some cases; my point is that it sends a wrong message when it does not mean what it says.

The second example is also sourced from Bovell and is an example of how crude language can oversimplify debate by concealing its underlying complexity. In relation to the impact of the problematic aspects of autism on families, such as sleep deprivation and challenging behaviour,[15] she stresses that

> Given the heterogeneity of autism, and indeed of families, there are multiple different narratives in which problems … either do not feature, or feature only at a particular point in time, and which in any case are perceived as being compensated for by some of the benefits that an autistic family member will bring.[16]
>
> (Ibid., p. 288)

She refers to the crude 'disabled vs non-disabled' debates relating to autism that serve to conceal the complexity resulting from such heterogeneity. In the same way that I have drawn attention to the complexities between NT and autistic perspectives on autism, scholars should avoid crude binaries that cannot reflect the heterogeneity of attitudes to autism.

Conclusions

Overcoming 'an instance of moral blindness – when one comes to see the moral salience of something one did not see before' – requires moral perception (Wisnewski,

2007, p. 123). Baumann (in Baumann & Donskis, 2013) refers to situations where issues become separated from concerns about their morality, which enables acts to be committed without those involved facing any moral stigma or needing to worry their consciences about them. It is my contention that the failure of most scholars working towards the cure/prevention of autism to openly discuss the ethics of their research, and the failure of society to call these scholars to account, is an example of both the separation Baumann refers to and a failure of moral perception. University ethics committees should cover the macro issue of whether or not curing/preventing autism is morally acceptable as well as the usual micro issues. Society should insist on full debates about *all* ethical issues relating to autism research.

No valid case has yet been made that the health of the social body requires the amputation of the autistic parts of the body (cf. Bauman & Donskis, 2013). Work to remove autism from the social body should not proceed in the dark space of a moral vacuum; such a fundamental issue must be brought out into the clear light of day. To ensure ethical matters in autism research are given the attention they are due, I recommend that:

1   all autism research projects should undertake an ethical impact assessment (EIA) for consideration by the university's ethics committee;
2   university ethics committees should make these impact assessments, and their deliberations on them, publicly available.

These recommendations are in line with the approach taken to ethical matters by the Human Brain Project (HBP) which 'Recognizing that its research may raise various ethical ... issues has made the identification, examination, and management of those issues a top priority' (Salles et al., 2019, p. 380). The issues referred to include the values that inform, and the *ethical permissibility* of, research.

Virginia Bovell (2015, p. 86) writes that 'a crude perspective on autism, either as something that is bad and should be eliminated, or as something that is good that should be celebrated, does not do justice to the complexity of human experience'. The challenges faced by some autistic people, and their carers, must not be ignored. But we should also reflect on the fact that non-autistic individuals can pose serious challenges. In the same way that I have no qualms in saying out loud that the apparently non-autistic Donald Trump presents a clear and present danger to civilised society, I consider the campaigner Greta Thunberg[17] – who has spoken[18] of the autistic strengths that she believes have enabled her to take on a climate change activist leadership role at a young age – to be a wonderful asset to society.

Acknowledgements

My thanks to Hanna Bertilsdotter Rosqvist, Robert Chapman, and Anna Stenning for their valuable input, and to Virginia Bovell whose work was a major influence.

Notes

1 Originally printed in *Neurodiversity Studies*, edited by Hanna Bertilsdotter Rosqvist, Nick Chown and Anna Stenning, and published by Routledge. Reprinted with permission.

2 https://aeon.co/ideas/how-playing-wittgensteinian-language-games-can-set-us-free

3 Rules of social interactional game-playing are not codified like the rules of cricket or chess. They are subtle, complex, and generally learned via osmosis during the formative years.

4 Barnes and McCabe (2011, p. 268) ask their readers to 'reflect on whether the world is better with or without a cure [for autism]' which suggests that the incidence of autism also concerns them.

5 One of few statements in Barnbaum's book that suggests she may not support the full eradication of autism is her reference to certain studies that 'locate — a moral sense in persons with autism' (Barnbaum, 2008, p. 111). This quotation is of particular interest to me because she appears to recognise that the ability to recognise moral questions is not a matter of neurotype.

6 It is a general goal as she reserves the right for a mother to have the final decision on whether or not to give birth.

7 The *Autonomy* journal has published the letter under Julia Leatherland's sole name.

8 Wittgenstein did not use the term 'grammar' in accordance with its dictionary definition. His definition of this term refers to the rules that govern word usage. He wrote that 'grammar … has somewhat the same relation to the language as … the rules of a game have to the game' (PG, I, 23).

9 I use the term 'neurotypicality' simply to draw a distinction between majority cognition and autism.

10 Wittgenstein intended the language game concept 'to bring into prominence the fact that the speaking of language is part of an activity' (PI 23) which gives language its meaning.

11 The bi-directional difficulty in understanding was named 'double empathy' by Damian Milton.

12 Some parents are involved in the neurodiversity movement and some autistic individuals support the search for a cure for autism. But the 'autism as tragedy' trope *is* a neurotypical concept.

13 One reason for this is that many autistic people do not disclose their autism because of the stigma still associated with autism and the risk of damaging their professional careers.

14 The DSM-5 has introduced the concept of the severity of autism. The extent of the autism-friendliness of an environment influences the apparent severity of autism presentation.

15 Sleep deprivation and challenging behaviour are not restricted to autistic children.

16 As was pointed out to me by Joanna Baker-Rogers, these benefits (which can apply in the case of children with many different labels) include the love they inspire in their family, friends, and carers.

17 I do NOT argue that autistic people are only 'acceptable' to society if they have social utility.

18 https.7/edition.cnn.com/videos/tv/2019/02/01/amanpour-greta-thunberg.cnn

References

Anderson, J. L. (2013). A Dash of autism. In J. L. Anderson & S. Cushing (Eds.), *The philosophy of autism* (pp. 109–142). Plymouth: Rowman & Littlefield.

Barnbaum, D. R. (2008). *The ethics of autism: Among them but not of them*. Bloomington, IN: Indiana University Press.

Barnes, R. E., & McCabe, H. (2012). Should we welcome a cure for autism? A survey of the arguments. *Medicine, Health Care and Philosophy, 15*(3), 255–269.

Bauman, Z., & Donskis, L. (2013). *Moral blindness: The loss of sensitivity in liquid modernity*. Cambridge, UK: Polity Press.

Bovell, V. (2015). *Is the prevention and/or cure of autism a morally legitimate quest?* (Unpublished doctoral dissertation). University of Oxford.

Chapman, R. (2018). *Autism, neurodiversity, and the good life: On the very possibility of autistic thriving* (Unpublished doctoral dissertation). University of Essex.

Chapman, R. (2019). Neurodiversity theory and its discontents: Autism, schizophrenia, and the social model of disability. In R. Bluhm (Ed.), *The Bloomsbury companion to philosophy of psychiatry* (pp. 371–390). London: Bloomsbury Academic.

Chown, N. (2014). More on the ontological status of autism and double empathy. *Disability & Society, 29*(10), 1672–1676.

Chown, N. (2019). Are the 'autistic traits' and 'broader autism phenotype' concepts real or mythical? *Autism Policy and Practice, 2*(1), 46–63.

Chown, N., & Leatherland, J. (2018). An open letter to Professor David Mandell, Editor-in-Cliief, 'Autism' in response to the editorial 'A new era in autism'. *Autonomy, 1*(5). Available at: www.larry-arnold.net/Autonomy/index.php/autonomy/article/view/CO1/html

Drescher, J. (2015). Out of DSM: Depathologizing homosexuality. *Behavioral Sciences, 5*(4), 565–575.

Hughes, L. (2019). Personal communication to the author.

Kapp, S. K. (Ed.). (2020). *Autistic community and the neurodiversity movement: Stories from the frontline*. London: Palgrave Macmillan.

Milton, D. E. (2012). On the ontological status of autism: The 'double empathy problem'. *Disability & Society, 27*(6), 883–887.

Milton, D. E., & Bracher, M. (2013). Autistics speak but are they heard? *Medical Sociology Online, 7*(2), 61–69.

Murray, D., Lesser, M., & Lawson, W. (2005). Attention, monotropism and the diagnostic criteria for autism. *Autism, 9*(2), 139–156.

Nadesan, M. (2013). Autism and genetics profit, risk, and bare life. In J. Davidson & M. Orsini (Eds.), *Worlds of autism: Across the spectrum of neurological difference* (pp. 117–142). Minneapolis, MN: University of Minnesota Press.

Pellicano, E., Dinsmore, A., & Charman, T. (2014). What should autism research focus upon? Community views and priorities from the United Kingdom. *Autism, 18*(7), 756–770.

Pellicano, E., & Stears, M. (2011). Bridging autism, science and society: Moving toward an ethically informed approach to autism research. *Autism Research, 4*(4), 271–282.

Pripas-Kapit, S. (2020). Historicizing Jim Sinclair's 'Don't mourn for us': A cultural and intellectual history of neurodiversity's first manifesto. In S. K. Kapp (Ed.), *Autistic community and the neurodiversity movement*. London: Palgrave Macmillan.

Salles, A., Bjaalie, J.G., Evers, K., Farisco, M., Fothergill, B. T., Guerrero, M., ... & Walter, H. (2019). The human brain project: Responsible brain research for the benefit of society. *Neuron, 101*(3), 380–384.

Sinclair, J. (1993). Don't Mourn for Us. *Our Voice, 1*(3). Retrieved December 2019, from www.autreat.com/dont_mourn.html

Szasz, T. (2010). *The myth of mental illness: Foundation of a theory of personal conduct*. New York: Harper Perennial.

Walsh, P. (2010). Asperger syndrome and the supposed obligation not to bring disabled lives into the world. *Journal of Medical Ethics, 36*(9), 521–524.

Wisnewski, J. J. (2007). *Wittgenstein and ethical inquiry: A defense of ethics as clarification*. London: Continuum.

Wittgenstein, L. (1984). *Culture and value*. Chicago, IL: University of Chicago Press.

Wittgenstein, L. (2005). *Philosophical grammar*. Berkeley: University of California Press.

Wittgenstein, L. (2009). *Philosophical investigations*. Hoboken, NJ: John Wiley & Sons.

Chapter 37

The Black Wisdom Collective

Kelechi Ubozoh

Summary

In this chapter we hear from three Black women who are leaders in the movement for mental health treatment alternatives: Celia Brown, Vanessa Jackson, and Keris Jän Myrick. They weave lessons from history and lived experience to show the complex and nuanced intersections between race, community, and healing. They emphasize the power of the Black community as a source of restorative practice and the widespread community-based efforts to build culturally relevant treatment practices ranging from consciousness-raising, to self-help skills, to creating alternative drop-in centers for consumers and survivors. They discuss the need to learn from intersecting activist efforts in order to build a cohesive mad pride movement that deliberately honors and incorporates Black practitioners, activists, and survivors. Their personal stories illustrate the ways individuals heal while holding collective and ancestral grief within their meaning-making of personal narrative.

The Mad Movement can thrive as a responsive and culturally nuanced force if it recognizes that lived mental health experiences necessarily intersect with race, ethnicity, class, and migration histories. This chapter shows the power of Black healing, as well as the power of historical reclamation and activism as means to restore wellness within communities that have faced brutality and racism in the mental health system.

*

Author's Note

On December 11, 2022, one of the movement leaders interviewed for the following piece, Celia Elise Brown, became an ancestor. She joined a lineage of Black ancestors in the Mad Movement to whom our future is greatly indebted. I am grateful to Celia for her generous spirit and the opportunity to capture some of her wisdom in the development of this collective work. Messages from her family, dearest friends, and colleagues are included at the end of this chapter in her memory.

DOI: 10.4324/9781003148456-42

The Collective

Race, identity, community, and perception: a tangled web of words that merge at the intersection of being Black and 'mad' and which follow me into every interaction, presentation, and written word. Watching the ongoing graphic Black deaths at the hands of law enforcement while enduring performative activism instilled the urgency of grounding my work in the Black community as a restorative practice.

In 2020, I started holding healing spaces for Black people all over the world. Later, I embarked on an oral history research project to capture the voices of Black leaders in the Mad Movement.

I must admit, I first felt shame. Shame that I did not know the stories of these Black ancestors who fought cross-movement, who shared identity and complexity of being Black and Mad and missing from various conversations. The names I started to learn are ones that have largely been erased from our history. And as I was learning from our contemporaries in this Movement, I was weaving together their stories with those of our ancestors. The contribution of this chapter is, I hope, also part of an active reclamation of the voices of our ancestors who have been erased. I would like to name some of them here, because their contributions guided this work.

This work pays homage to Ben Riley, who at the young age of 19 led what was called a five hour 'inmate riot' of 80 Black people in the Rusky State Hospital in Texas in 1955. The list of demands included an end to beatings of psychiatric prisoners, better counseling, organized exercise periods, and the same rights as white psychiatric prisoners like food, showering, and freedom of movement.

We are indebted to Lois Curtis, who bravely advocated for her right to independence while in psychiatric incarceration. Her persistence in seeking a life in community led to the Olmstead Decision in 1999, which created the first legal framework in the U.S. for the right of people with disabilities to live their lives with the highest degree of community integration possible.

We are grateful for the wisdom of Malidoma Patrice Somé whose 1995 book *Of Water and Spirit* initiated a global and ongoing conversation about the colonialist exporting of American psychiatric values and the importance of healing through an Indigenous African lens. This conversation was part of a cross-cultural invitation to reframe mental illness, as Somé urged to witness mental illness as 'the birth of a healer.'

We honor Cookie Gant, an African American lesbian and disabled psychiatric survivor, artist, and photographer who was a founder of MindFreedom International's coalition, served on that Board for many years, and co-founded MindFreedom Michigan.

We uplift the work of Darnell Levingston and DeWitt Buckingham, the founders of Black Men Speak in California. They brought their lived experience and vulnerability to their tireless efforts to support Black Men in processing pain and trauma as well as to addressing substance use and its impact on their peers.

Their stories, and the stories of countless other beloved Black ancestors who experienced harm or death within the psychiatric system, weave together the pain and hope of our shared history. We honor the many more who have powered our movement without spotlight, recognition, and whose names we may not know. May their memories live on in their words and in our work.

The Black Wisdom Collective is a contribution to our living history. This discussion engages three contemporary Black Movement leaders who weave lessons and history through their personal narratives, wisdom through their experiences navigating racism in the Mad Movement, and considerations for the future of Black liberation.

Background on the Black Movement Leaders

Celia Brown is a nationally recognized psychiatric survivor and longtime advocate for people with psychiatric disabilities. Celia started her activism work in 1986 when she met leaders in the consumer/survivor/ex-patient movement like Judi Chamberlin and Howie T. Harp. Celia was instrumental in developing the first Peer Specialist civil service title in the country and was one of the first Peer Specialists in New York State. Celia served as the President of MindFreedom International, which also positioned her as the main representative to the United Nations. Celia is also the founder of Surviving Race: The Intersection of Injustice, Disability and Human Rights and the International Network Toward Alternatives and Recovery (INTAR). She served as the position of Regional Advocacy Specialist for the Office of Consumer Affairs at the NYC Field Office, New York State Office of Mental Health.

Vanessa Jackson is an activist, Soul Doula, and the author of *In Our Own Voice: African-American Stories of Oppression, Survival and Recovery in Mental Health Systems* and *Separate and Unequal: The Legacy of Racially Segregated Psychiatric Hospitals*, monographs on the history of African American psychiatric experiences. After nearly two decades of working in mental health and social services as a licensed clinical social worker, Vanessa had a nervous 'breakthrough' where she began to rethink her beliefs and practice regarding mental health and emotional wellbeing. She spent years researching African American psychiatric history and worked with ex-patients, consumers, and staff of segregated asylums. Vanessa is a nationally recognized speaker on mental health issues with a focus on culturally conscious therapy and therapy with marginalized populations. As the owner of Healing Circles, Inc. based in Atlanta, she provides politically conscious and clinically sound counseling and healing workshops and supports activists in creating healthy and balanced lives.

Keris Jän Myrick is a national and internationally known mental health advocate with over 15 years of experience in mental health services innovations, transformation, and peer workforce development. She is recognized for her innovative and inclusive approach to mental health reform and the public disclosure of her personal story. She serves on the board of Disability Rights California (DRC) and previously served on the Board of the National Association of Peer Specialists (N.A.P.S.). She previously held positions as the Chief of Peer and Allied Health Professions for the Los Angeles County Department of Mental Health, the Director of the Office of Consumer Affairs for the Center for Mental Health Services (CMHS) of the United States Health and Human Services' Substance Abuse and Mental Health Services Administration (SAMHSA), and President and CEO of Project Return Peer Support Network, a Los Angeles-based, peer-run nonprofit. Keris currently works as the Vice President of Partnerships at Inseparable, a national policy organization and is the creator and host of the podcast, Unapologetically Black Unicorns, which examines mental health and racial justice.

These leaders weren't interviewed together, but their words were brought together to form a story. These unfiltered stories challenge us to take action, do our own work, and do our collective work. They speak for themselves.

How did you come into the movement? What were your first experiences like?

Celia: I have been in the movement for over 20 years, and I have to tell you that before I found the Movement, I was just not really doing well. I was in and out of the hospital. I knew that there was something different than . . . the treatment I was receiving. But I didn't have anybody or an exposure of a new way of thinking about my treatment and my life. Because back in the 80s, when I was in the hospital, the thinking was you had a chemical imbalance. . . And because you have a perceived diagnosis, you could be in the hospital for the rest of your life and get unwanted treatments without informed consent for the rest of your life. So, that was the thinking then. One of the things that I needed to do when I was in the hospital is say, you know, do I have this disorder that they say I have? Or who am I as a person? How does it differ?

When I was in this residential treatment housing center, I was considered quote 'high functioning.' So, they decided to have me, and another peer go to Troy, New York, near Albany, to this conference called 'Self Help Vision.' And this is back in 1986, I believe. When I got there, I met people who actually were in the movement at that time, because they started to be in the movement around the late 60s and 70s. So, I met Judi Chamberlin, I met Joe Rogers, I met Howie the Harp, I met Ed Knight, who's somebody who promoted self-help skills throughout New York State. And we were just sort of having a session and doing a lot of consciousness-raising that we're in control of our own lives, and that we can make our own treatment decisions. And that was a radical thing to be thinking; that someone who's labeled with a mental illness can actually decide what it is they want for their lives, that just wasn't heard of. So, they were saying that they were creating alternatives, like drop-in centers for people who were consumers, survivors, ex-patients . . . giving support to their fellow ex-patients and survivors, and consumers. That was unheard of. Only the medical profession was supposed to be giving you all this treatment, and support, like psychiatrists and social workers, nurses. It really could never be us. You know?

So, I was so intrigued. And I went up to Judi Chamberlin and I said, 'who's allowing you to do this?' And she said, 'no one, we're just doing it because we're free. We're liberated.' . .. And a light grew in me, and I said, 'Oh, my God, I'm free.' I got other people who are like minded. . .. I found them.

So, I went back to the Bronx, and I developed a support group, with the residents and staff there. And you can imagine what happened; here, I'm trying to empower people and give support and help with what their rights are, that kind of thing.

Yeah, [laughs], and so that was disbanded. But what happened is that I found some other like minded people in the Bronx . . . and we developed the Interexpressive support group and we would meet outside of the residence and just supported each other. Support is so important, to know that someone validates your experience. And if you are thinking one thing about yourself, but you have a system saying, 'oh no that's not you, you're schizophrenia, you're bipolar, that's who you are, you're nobody else.' I was somebody's daughter, sister, you know, I'm a woman. I'm a Black woman. I'm not the diagnosis. I know that some people identify with a label, it supports them. . . I think everybody should have their own choice, whether I agree with it or not. But for me, you labeling me with a diagnosis was not going to make me well, to be in wellness, to be in recovery, to know who I am, you know, to take the steps of the journey to figure out who am I in this world? In this world of mental health, you know?

Keris: So basically, *being given* a diagnosis of a mental health condition, that the world calls a quote 'serious mental health condition,' whatever the heck that means. And because of my diagnosis, I was highly encouraged to go into the public system. And then after I don't know what number of involuntary hospitalizations, I was given three groups to contact. One was the DBSA (Depression Bipolar Support Alliance), one was Emotions Anonymous [12 steps], and the other was NAMI (National Alliance on Mental Illness). So, I first went to DBSA and I didn't feel comfortable talking about my experience, because the experiences they were talking about were not ones that I had. So, then I went to Emotions Anonymous, and I couldn't understand it. It seemed like I was blaming myself, but giving myself permission not to blame myself? And then I didn't like the fact that they said the Lord's Prayer at the end. What if I don't believe in that? Okay, so this isn't for me either. Then I went to a NAMI meeting called Share and Care. Oh, my goodness, it's hilarious. The story. So, I went to the NAMI Share and Care Meeting and I opened the door and I thought, 'holy shit, what the hell is this?' I opened the door and it's all of these older white, white-haired, majority women, some men sitting in a room around a table, and I thought, 'is this the right room? Oh, myyyyy, I am in the wrong room.' So, I asked them, 'is this NAMI Share and Care?' And they responded, 'yeah,' and so I said, Okay, well, you know, three strikes, you're out. If this doesn't work, I'm probably going to end up back in the hospital.

So, I sat in the room. And, you know, everybody introduced themselves and I introduced myself. And then they kept asking me, 'so are you a consumer or family member?' And I said, 'of course I'm a family member. Isn't everyone a member of some kind of family?' [They say] 'Oh okay, so who's the consumer in your family?' And I'm like, 'consumer of what? The consumer of the grocery store? The consumer of technology, consumer of what?'

So, I was like, 'what?' Finally, they said, you know, 'who's the "ill" one in your family,' and then I got their lingo and said, 'Oh, that's me.'

You should have seen these old people get up and run. A few people said, 'Oh, no. Oh no, honey, this meeting is not for you and blah, blah, blah.' And I thought, wait, what's happening? And they said, 'wait a minute, how did you get here?' This is two days after being discharged from the hospital. I said, 'I got here in my car,' very literal: I didn't understand they meant who referred you here. They said, 'wait a minute, tell us more.' And I said, 'look: I have no family here. My parents do not live here. I have no support here. And my psychiatrist who referred me here, and to other groups thought I could use more support in my own community. So he referred me here.' I'm telling you, those older ladies and men turned into parents, right quick.

'Somebody get her some coffee. Somebody get her some water. Hey, we got cookies over there. Would you like some cookies?'

And then they just kind of loved me. And when I say loved me, I mean, they were loving to me. Because, you know, I didn't have anybody here, and that really spoke to their hearts.

So that was my first entree in a way, and then I just kind of stuck with them. And they stuck with me. And I learned more about mental health advocacy. From there, I got introduced to the consumer movement by Jim McNulty and Kathryn McNulty, who did the peer-to-peer training for NAMI. Later, I would meet Jacki Mckinney[1], who has a similar diagnosis as myself. . .

Anyways, Jim was very, very involved in the consumer advocacy movement. And he helped me go to one of the Alternatives conferences [a psychiatric-survivor-run conference that started in the early 1970s]. He got funding for me to go and help them with some projects. So, for two or three years, I helped them with projects, through NAMI, at Alternatives, which is kind of interesting [laughs].

Alternatives is, well how to describe . . . the narrative . . . yeah, NAMI? Family? No. Y'all are out. Y'all are always trying to have us held against our will, and medicated. Yeah, so, there's a contentious relationship between the consumer movement and NAMI, in particular, family movement. So, Jim and Kathryn are there as people with lived experience. . . developing these peer programs was one way to ensure that there was a place for people with lived experience within NAMI. And we were doing work actually on increasing cultural competency and getting information at . . . Alternatives where we knew we could meet large groups of people with lived experience.

I am oddly, not oddly, but I'm saying oddly, because most people don't see me this way: I'm an incredibly introverted and shy person. So, to be at an Alternatives conference was almost overwhelming for me, because it was entirely too many people that I didn't know. And if people didn't come up to talk to me, I wouldn't go up and talk to people. Because I'm just shy... I don't know how to do those kind of conversation things. I just suck at it. But because I was there with a purpose, I had to sit at a table, and we had to do group interviews. It's kind of like focus group interviews. . . And Jim, of course, knew everybody, as did Kathryn. So, Jim was very good at introducing me to a number of people.

But the hardest thing for me is once people kind of got it that I was with NAMI, I was sort of never really—and still to this day—not a full part of what I would call the consumer movement. I get a lot of, you know, people attack me a lot and stuff. Which is sort of sad because they haven't taken two and a half seconds to get to know me and know what I believe and kind of know why I had started with and stuck with NAMI, quite frankly.

The assumption is that, I mean, I guess in the Black community, I don't know if we have a term for it, but maybe I was like an 'Auntie Tomasina,' you know Uncle Tom, meaning I was not fully supportive of the consumer movement, its philosophies and its vision and its mission, because I was so involved with NAMI.

Yet, in fact, what people didn't kind of understand about me is: I'm a big Black woman, let's just put it that way. When you see me, that's what you are going to see. There's no two cents about it. I'm a big Black woman with a deep voice. And when I show up in a room, maybe that's why I'm shy, some people will say, 'Oh, you have this commanding presence.' And it's like, 'No, I don't want to command anything. Don't even look at me. [Laughs] I think I found ways to kind of say, 'Okay, I might be this person who walks into a room and yeah, you're gonna kind of take notice she's there. And then when I open my mouth, this sort of deep voice, I had figured out that my gift of advocacy is one of soft-spoken, for the most part . . . listening to others, repeating back, very reflective. And bridge-building. I'm a global Nomad. I was brought up all over the world. I was born in Germany and wherever we went, we had to learn the language; where we lived, we lived in the culture. Only once did we live on base, army base, usually, we lived off base with the community. And so, I had to learn how to navigate all sorts of different types of people and cultures and languages and food, music, and everything.

I think that's a gift that I've been able to bring into what I do, is this ability to sit in sometimes places that are not comfortable, because they're not my culture. But I'm able to hear kind of what's going on there. And then also hear what's going on over there. And then figure out, how do I bring those two things together in ways that we can all get along?

So, it was tough. And it's still tough because people don't understand what I'm doing. They don't understand why I might sit on particular tables. Why do I do so much with the American Psychiatric Association? You know, we can change them on the outside by yelling at them. Yes, yes, yes, that's called protest. Right? That definitely works. But doing inside advocacy also works. I think you need both and I don't think it's an either-or situation. And I'm gifted on the inside. If I'm loud, and I put my fist in the air and start yelling, as a big Black woman, that is not protest, that is aggression in the eye of the person on the opposite end of that action. To them that may be seen as aggression. And then when aggression happens, people become defensive, and they cannot hear a word I'm saying. And I need people to hear what I'm saying.

Vanessa: I had a lived experience of having a single episode of clinical depression, so I was coming from that lens. And because I also had been, prior to doing that, I worked in protection and advocacy . . . And so in that I happen to land in Georgia at the time when our state was going through the Olmstead lawsuit[2]. . . . So, I came in with an advocacy perspective. Anyway, I had been a longtime activist in the Black women's health movement, and so I always came in with that lens. And then when I had my experience with depression, and because I'd also been an activist, had already been a legal advocate, I sort of knew how to navigate that system. So, I had a lot of privilege navigating that system, but that allowed me to say like, oh, I can see how people get really trapped. So that was my entree in and that's why Pat Deegan invited me to be part of the project because I did have a lived experience. . . I came in that research door through Pat Deegan. And so Pat invited me in along with Pemina Yellow Bird. . . Pat was doing the cemetery project[3], Pemina was doing Native people's history, and I was doing African American psychiatric history. And so that was my entree into working with the [Movement]; consumer, survivor, ex-patient isn't the way I really identified myself... I was a student of people who taught me how I had my lived experience, I certainly didn't have the kind of experiences like psychiatric incarceration and that kind of stuff. And so it really was for me, people allowing me into a space and to learn from them. So while I had this one experience, it was not by any way my primary identity. . . . I have siblings [with a survivor experience] so I'm also a family member. So when I came in, I just had multiple hats on.

There is a long, often untold, history of the oppression that is faced by Black survivors. What are some of your experiences as Black folks working within or alongside the Mad Movement? How has the Mad Movement handled racism?

Keris: Well, they haven't. Period, full stop. Why would it be handled in the consumer movement if it hasn't been handled in the US? We are a microcosm of a larger movement. Movements move ahead without Black and brown people, and if we look at the arc of movements, POC and LBGTQ folks have to fight their way to the table and lead our own movements. I've had to sit back and go, why would I expect something different if this is the culture we're all brought up in? . . .

Dr. Ruth Shim wrote this letter that basically called out the American Psychiatric Association for being a racist institution, and said, 'you know what, for that reason, I quit. I'm out.' Do you know last month that they came out with an apology letter? I think I read the first line of the apology, and said, 'yeah, okay. Tick tock, tick tock, it's 2021.' And I also feel the reason that it came out was because Ruth Shim called you all out, and they have been called out before. Many many times before. . .

The picture that I always show of Jacki [McKinney] and I, we're on this little bus that went from where the conference was in DC for Mental Health America. And that was the year my mom fell into a coma, she had a heart attack on my birthday. . . . And we're going to see St. Elizabeth's Hospital, where she [Jacki] was institutionalized. And we get to the hospital grounds, what they're doing is they are breaking ground for the cemetery project. . . . They showed us how the old cemetery was, how they are putting all the things together, and putting the numbers with the names so they can create this beautiful garden, which they did. I was struck by it, because I had never heard about this in the cemetery project, and I don't walk in graves, that's not a Native thing, that's a no-no, I was just able to hear what was happening. You know, they would bury the patients, no name, a number on the grounds. But if you were Black, they put you in the swamp land. If you were Native, they put you in the swamp land. I was like, 'I'll be damned. Not only can we not have a name, but we are also so inhuman, even in death where we can cause you no problem, you are going to put us in the swampy part of the graveyard and segregate us.' That's structural racism.

Vanessa: I remember going to my very first Alternatives when I just was starting the research and people didn't know who I was, maybe [in the year] 2000. And when I come into someone else's place, I need to offer respect, because they've been doing the work that I haven't been doing. But one of the things that came up immediately was people were saying that there had been this report that had been conducted around race and diversity that was done by the National Empowerment Center, and no one ever saw it. So of course, in my workshop I said: 'where's that report? People want the report,' which didn't get me any brownie points with them. But what that told me was that there was a unique story . . . of African American experiences within psychiatric systems that wasn't showing up in the wider predominately white movement. . . and the fact that African American people get incarcerated in greater proportion to our numbers, and yet we weren't represented in the leadership of movement work. . . Now, let me be real clear, this is no different than when you go to national mental health conferences, or psychotherapy conferences. It's the same problem there. So it's not unique to this Movement work. . .

It's like the equivalent of the women's lib, white women's movement, and then Black feminists coming in and going, 'we get what you're talking about, but let's talk about this other thing that we have to deal with that you don't have to deal with: racism.' And how we get labeled as psychotic if we come in and say, 'we just lost 15 people, and we're just overwhelmed with grief.' But we want our experiences to be labeled appropriately, and then to have care and support as we move through it. And so that's how racism and white supremacy plays out in, like, who gets to name the problem, how they end the problem, looking at the differences, and then just the whole layer of this economic shift that racism is creating for Black people, which has an impact on access, and control.

And I remember talking to one of my colleagues here, who was working on some peer stuff, he's a Black dude, and he's like, 'how long do I have to keep thanking people? Thank them for doing their damn job like thank you for helping me and thank you for opening up this place where I could come in and share my experience and share my gifts and help other people,' but also felt like he was always being kind of constrained and being asked to be appreciative for being allowed in a peer door.

Celia: During the years, I got reconnected with Judi Chamberlin, Howie the Harp, Joe Rogers, Dick Gelman, an activist from NYC, and I joined a group called Support Coalition International, it's now Mindfreedom. . . Eventually, I became President of Mindfreedom International, and I'm the only person, BIPOC, on the board.

I think at the time they were struggling to get more people of color. When I got in the movement, it seemed like we weren't dealing with each other's race or culture. We were dealing with what the issues were, what happened to me, also what happened to you, and you were being drugged, and so was I; so, we're going to use that idea to connect us. And the Movement has always been that way. And I've had very good friends who are white who were thinking in those terms, and I was thinking in those terms at the time. Now, we're in a new era, and I guess through the years, there has been an absence of people of color. . .

It basically has been a white, middle-class movement, that doesn't mean that everybody had money, but that they were able to advocate just because of privilege. You know what I mean? Now, I understand that I didn't understand it, then. . . .

I'm going to say some good things. And some things that need to be worked on. I think that what happens with white allies is when they're creating their programs for their own healing, or to promote human rights, they're not always consciously thinking, 'Oh, wait a minute, maybe we should, you know, ask a person of color to come in.' So, they'll create their own program, their own boards that don't have a person of color, and then they'll say, 'Oh, well, we need a person of color' as if having one person of color or two is going to make everything better.

Sometimes they expect Black survivors to feel the way they feel about forced treatment and shock. . . But our history is that we have been through a lot, my ancestors . . . slavery, Jim Crow, Civil Rights, everything. And so, it's a little bit different than their frame of reference.

I mean, they can agree that slavery was awful, the Holocaust is awful, all of it's awful. But we're still in this place where, 'Wait, I have to take care of what I need to take care of' on the board they're on or the programs that they're creating, not thinking that this could be a healing rights kind of issue. You can mentor someone, a Black survivor about some of the issues. Black survivors in return, can mentor them or just talk to them about here's the stuff that I go through. And it's not about guilt, it's about this is what I go through, it has nothing to do with your feelings about it. It's, 'I'm a person that's gone through a, b and c, yes, I've experienced racism on the way and this is how it happened.' Those conversations don't happen that much. The good news is that there have been some survivor alternative groups that are asking people to come in and train on anti-racist perspectives. So that is a really good change.

What are the intersections and disconnects between the Mad Movement and Black liberation movements, including Black Lives Matter?

Vanessa: These are related issues. I was just talking to somebody the other day, who works in Black liberation and Black food justice, about how in the last four or five years people in movement work, Black Lives Matter specifically have been saying, 'our folks are committing suicide lately, people were just being disappeared,' all kinds of stuff, and just massive grief and also being assaulted during their actions. And I kept telling: 'y'all need to be talking to the consumer, survivor, ex-patient movement cuz these folks have really been on the ground right and can train you in skills for people with lived experience. These are the people you need to be talking to, you can't just keep sending them to the same five therapists.' . . . everybody's moving in their own little circle. I think one thing that would probably be more helpful for it to shift is for Black folks within the consumer, survivor, ex-patient movement to bop themselves over to like ally in healing and justice forums, to partner with and offer support services at Black Lives Matter events. What I see is the skills and knowledge are in Black consumers, survivors, ex-patients and I think that most of those Movement folks that I know don't have that skill set. . . but so much of it is people are trying to get their head around moving to a broader political movement, trying to build out their network. So there's been some reasons why [there is a disconnect] but I don't think it's for a lack of caring, I think that Black Lives Matter folks completely understand the need to have mental health, emotional support, healing justice.

And, I think we need to have those conversations in our own community. Because, I don't want my sibling being abused, but also [I don't want] my sibling dying on the street when there could have been something available. . . I want to make sure every Black person has the support they need to move through their distress. And we got plenty of distress, because of racism. So I just think that's an internal conversation, that doesn't mean that we're not good advocates around people's right to informed consent, to fully choose alternative ways of healing. But I think we just don't come together that often. I don't see the psychiatric liberation movement being in some of the places where other Black activists are talking about mental health needs, and they need to be in those rooms.

Celia: It's been very difficult to go into [the Black Lives Matter] movement. I don't know what it is. I mean it's as if I need to know someone who knows someone in Black Lives Matter, you know what I mean? And I know that happens in the Movement, somebody knows you or refers you to this person. That's how it is. But I did meet one person from New York that I'm connected with who works a lot in the Bronx. His name is Hawk Newsome [Co-founder of the Greater New York Black Lives Matter Chapter] and what happened with him, we had a Black woman, an older woman, Deborah Danner, who was diagnosed with schizophrenia. And she had a vision that she would be killed by the police, [and then she was]. . . . So, Hawk came out to, let's say, the 40th, maybe the 49th precinct in the Bronx, and he had a rally for her. And I was blown away with that, because here's a person, not only Black, but has a diagnosis, and she was killed. And you're out here supporting her, maybe not knowing all the issues. I thought that was great. I think all of the movements, especially the psychiatric survivor movement, we have to get off the island, all of us know each other.

So BLM, like any group, they don't know about the experiences of the psychiatric survivor movement. So they may say, 'they [Black people] don't need to be shot and killed, but they may need to . . . go to a psychiatric hospital.' So then they would be forced through psychiatry. . . But Black Lives Matter may not have the frame of reference and just think, 'oh, they're going to get help if they're in the hospital.' Now, what we have to do is say, and this will take some education. . . They may say, 'Well, I could just go into hospital, or I can take these meds or whatever.' And they may need it. And I'm not commenting that they shouldn't take it. But they should know that they have a right not to if it bothers them, you know, not just go along with whatever the doctor and the social worker says, you know what I mean? . . .

In 2014, with Eric Garner from Staten Island, and Michael [Brown] from Ferguson . . . I was just really horrified. I have a son who is 25 . . . and I have male nephews and male cousins. And I said, I don't want this to happen to them. And when I'm like that, I want to create, so I said, 'What can we do?' So, I called a couple of Movement people, white and Black, and I said, 'you know, what are we going to do here, we're the Movement, and we can make the change, we can change the world, we can change lives, and we have to work together.' We came up with the name Surviving Race: The Intersection of Injustice, Disability, and Human Rights[4], and it really has been a Facebook page back then so people could talk about police brutality, police murdering us, people with a mental health diagnosis. And try to stop this from happening.

Keris: Wow, so many things to say about this. Black Lives Matter gave an easier way to articulate it in three words: Black. Lives. Matter. Where it might take me a whole paragraph to say what I'm trying to say. Several years ago, here in LA, Mitrice Richardson, a young African American woman had the police called on her because she was not able to pay her bill at a restaurant. The police were familiar with her as a person living with bipolar disorder. She was clearly not well, and they took her to the police station. The police station was on the border of Ventura and LA, and it's called the Lost Hills area. So, she was taken to that station, and she did not have a wallet, she didn't have a purse, cellphone, she didn't have anything. And they released her in the middle of the night in lost hills.

The Lost Hills, for the most part, it's a pretty uninhabited place. They let her go. And then she went missing. And sure enough, they found her 11 months later, dead. Now there are two questions; did the police harm her, such that when she left, she fell and died? Or was she out there long enough that she succumbed to the elements? But at the end of the day, you don't let a woman out, or a man out, no wallet, in the middle of the flipping night in the middle of nowhere, no car, no money, no nothing, because they are free to go. No contact was made with her family who's in LA. No cab was called, no police said, 'let me drive you home.' Nothing. And you know this woman was Black.

When this happened, the first thing I did was call our NAMI affiliates here. And in LA County, we have a very strong criminal justice committee and their leader works very strongly at the state. And I called him directly and I said, 'what are we going to do? What are y'all going to do? Is NAMI going to rise up and say, "What the hell? Why was this woman let go?" Are you going to demand to find out what was going on?' I said, 'this is a travesty and I haven't heard anything, not a peep from NAMI.'

So, they told me, 'Oh, no, we can't do that. We don't really want to upset the police.' And I said, 'if it was one of your kids, you know, you would do it. You would do it in a heartbeat. But because she's Black, you don't give a shit.' And it's just like we're throwaway people. Throwaway people.

So, I said [to myself] I gotta watch you guys and hold you accountable to everything. So, then I went to NAMI Urban LA—started by Bebe Moore Campbell, which is where National Minority Mental Health Month comes from because of her and her advocacy at the hill in DC to get it passed to be recognized—so I went to NAMI Urban LA and they helped to follow up. So, I think what I'm saying here is that there was no BLM then, but there was a movement to try to figure out why there were all these disparities happening to Black and brown people around criminal justice and criminal justice involvement, inequities in health care, placement of mental health care, and ensuring those services meet the needs of the community.

And all this time Yvonne Smith, Effie Smith[5], who passed away recently, Celia Brown, Jen Padron, were really trying to get the consumer movement to wrap its head around Black and brown people and others in prison because of a mental health condition and stuck there. Consumer movement said, 'oh no, we're not touching it.'

It was years before BLM. So here we are at BLM and they [consumer movement] want to make statements, they want to talk about their privilege, and they want to give things to us because of their privilege and they want to call us and ask, 'do you know any more Black people.' But I can't help you now. Maybe if I have this podcast of Black people talking about what it is we want to see in our Movement and for our people, and if white people want to listen, y'all can listen in, that's your education, but we're doing it for us. We're not doing it to educate you.

What guidance do you have to share for allies doing or ready to do the ongoing work for black liberation in the Mad Movement?

Vanessa: I think that they need to engage in an intensive anti-racism learning project for themselves . . . not just diversity and inclusion crap, but really saying how have we perpetuated white supremacy in our own movement? Where have we not invested in leadership opportunities for folks of color? Where have we grabbed the microphone, when we should have been passing it? I think it's the same questions that the National Association of Social Workers and the APA should be asking. . . How do we create spaces and accept the leadership and celebrate the leadership of people of color? What are the experiences that people of color are having in our Movement, but also within these systems that are different because they're folks of color? How do we create responses that lift everybody, and if you lift folks of color, you're going to lift everybody anyway. . . .

I get invited in to do diversity, inclusion, and belonging [trainings]. . . Teaching tolerance, diversity is the same stuff that hasn't worked for over 25 years . . . we came out of [the] anti-sexual assault [movement] like, people want to call it 'date rape.' That's rape, people. So sometimes we give certain titles to things so we don't offend the perpetrator. So, people feel better about having implicit bias versus being straight up racist. If you're experiencing their behavior, it doesn't feel any different.

Anti-racism is much more focused on getting to the roots of stuff and looking at how white supremacy, specifically, the hoarding of resources and power, the privileging of certain histories and information . . . so it's great if you feel okay about me, but if you keep in place the same systems that at this point are almost working automatically. You almost don't have to do anything, you have to push a button to make it work. If you don't disrupt those systems and it becomes so normal that you don't think that there's a way to stop it versus saying, how does this system get to be this way? How does the way the system is currently set up to disadvantage folks of color? Is it necessary to have this system work this way, in order for people to get quality mental health treatment? Or to run our organization? Who does it privilege when we have these conversations? So this is a fundamentally different set of questions.

Celia: I would tell them to first deal with whatever your biases are, because I have them, we all have to deal with that first. They need to work on their own biases and maybe racism on their own. It's not the job of people of color to educate you. You know, it's too hard. If we educate you, and you say no, that's not something I believe, and that is invalidating the person of color.

Be prepared to ask questions and to listen to the person. It may be a little bit disturbing to you. But listen, and then after you listen, then you can ask another question, but don't assume you know, without speaking to that person, what they've actually gone through the experience of racism.

White allies have to let go of being the person that always makes the decisions, always has people around them that look like them, but that there are other voices that may be completely different. But one thing I think they (white allies) could do is not . . . speak for us all the time. They do it unintentionally. But we need to speak for ourselves, our voices need to be there and they're not always there. . .

[At the beginning of Covid in March 2020], . . .me and my colleague friend Jen developed a Covid Crisis Peer Support network and had these dialogues and trainings with people from Surviving Race. Surviving Race has now grown into a coalition and received a grant. They are funding us to have a retreat in Savannah, Georgia. We are inviting white allies and BIPOC psychiatric survivors and we are going to have a dialogue and we'll have some facilitated questions and we'll write up a report.

A friend of mine, totally against psychiatry, she's doing research on how slavery turned into asylums, psychiatric asylums for colored people, white people, and then prisons. It's fascinating research. And because they used to think that slaves that ran away that there was, you know, something wrong with them.

We're not only talking about that, we're talking about how slavery was oppressive to our people, how they separated families, like they're separating immigrant families now. And that person may have to go miles to see their daughter, you know, the mother, who's a slave to go see their kids, I'm just giving you an example. None of that even comes up, that, 'Oh, that must have been hard for you, hard for your ancestor or your great great grandmother,' you know. So, racism can cause trauma, I think you know this, and it's very hard to heal from it. My mother was in the civil rights movement. And she was around Jim Crow. Sometimes we're just talking about maybe the weather or how I'm doing, how she's doing, and she will remember something that's happened that she had to drink at the colored water fountain. [She'll] bring up these things, and she said to me the other day . . . you know . . . she might need healing. I'm going to call it intergenerational healing, because it's still with her. These things don't go away because the incident is now in the past. It's still within you.

Keris: I certainly think there is some level of starting to do their own education and not rely on people to educate them. Dr. Annelle Primm said, 'You are not everybody's magical Negro.' I was like, 'Oh no she didn't!' . . . she did. I pride myself when somebody asked me, you know, to teach them, but I have to say to myself, I'm not their magical Negro. And I'll recommend a book or an article. So, I think there are ways in which people can learn on their own.

Attend the conferences that may not be about them, because they can learn about the other. The only way to learn about the other is to go sit by and listen to the other, I think not always invite the other to come to your house, but you go to the other person's house.

Think about who is in your circle of acquaintances, friends and colleagues. If they 100% all look like you, I think that's a little problematic. So instead of asking people, can you find x kind of person for me, actually develop authentic friendships and collaborations and working relationships with people who are from different walks of life from you.

If you're putting together a conference making sure every panel and the keynote lineup has diversity in it. And reaching out to different groups to encourage people to apply that might not think about it. There has to be an intention, not a 'check the box' . . . but definitely a level of intentionality, dedication, perseverance, until it is baked into the consumer movement. It's not baked in right now. . . .

Look around your community and look at where the injustices are in your communities. I don't know a community that would be exempt from it. To me, injustice will breed compromised mental health. Why? Because, there's your trauma, there's your emotional wellbeing, it's out the door. I don't think people understood MLK's speech to the American Psychological Association in 1967. They quote it all the time and say we just need to be 'creatively maladjusted.' But I don't think people really understood that he was saying, this is our trauma, and our trauma really is creative maladjustment. We've found ways to make shit work when it shouldn't. And that is because if we become adjusted to this, that would be pathological. And I think that's what Martin Luther King was saying. If you become adjusted to discrimination, that's actually maladjusted. You should be maladjusted to injustice. You should be very maladjusted to injustice, but that's not an illness. And he was trying to tell the psychological association, 'you use this term maladjusted to talk about illness and I'm saying, no, it is a way and state of being for Black Americans, because we have to live in a world in which there is injustice, and we will never, ever become adjusted to that, so we creatively "maladjust" to it.'

> You who are in the field of psychology have given us a great word. It is the word maladjusted. . . It is a good word; certainly, it is good that in dealing with what the word implies you are declaring that destructive maladjustment should be destroyed. You are saying that all must seek the well-adjusted life . . .

> But on the other hand, I am sure that we will recognize that there are some things in our society, some things in our world, to which we should never be adjusted. There are some things concerning which we must always be maladjusted if we are to be people of good will. We must never adjust ourselves to racial discrimination and racial segregation. We must never adjust ourselves to religious bigotry. We must never adjust ourselves to economic conditions that take necessities from the

many to give luxuries to the few. We must never adjust ourselves to the madness of
militarism, and the self-defeating effects of physical violence.

Martin Luther King Jr, 'The Role of the Behavioral Scientist
in the Civil Rights Movement,' Distinguished Address
delivered at the APA Annual Convention, 1967.

Honoring Celia Brown

In dreaming up this piece, I never thought Celia Brown would not be here to read the
final copy of her contribution and work. Deeply loved and admired by so many, I felt
it was important to include messages from her family, dearest friends and colleagues
who she deeply impacted through her activism. This is a reminder to me and so many
to ensure we give people their flowers while they are here, as now for Celia we will
have to give them after she has passed.

A message from Keris Jän Myrick, M.B.A., M.S., Ph.D.c, National and
International Mental Health Advocate and Longtime Colleague

One of the hardest things to do is write about someone who has a major impact
in your life and work in memoriam. What I write, however, was not unknown to
Celia, because during her life, I let her know how much she meant to me and how
she impacted my life (and I know countless others). When I was looking for someone
who looked like me who openly talked about living with a mental health condition,
Ms. Jacki McKinney wasted no time introducing me to Celia Brown. When others in
the mental health consumer/survivor/ex-patient-peer movement wouldn't accept
me as a person who included their family as part of the recovery journey, Celia
supported me and asked me to tell her and others about what family means especially
to those in the Black community.

Celia Brown was not only a remarkable mental health advocate, but also an
inspiring champion for race equity as an African American woman. Her tireless
efforts to promote awareness and fight against systemic racial injustices have had a
profound impact on me and countless others. Celia's ability to navigate and address
the intersectionality of mental health and racial disparities has shed light on the unique
challenges faced by marginalized communities. Her advocacy work has empowered
individuals like me to engage in conversations about race, equity, and mental health.
Celia's unwavering dedication and resilience in advocating for both mental health
and racial equity, especially within the peer movement, make her a true force for
positive change.

A message from Jonathan P. Edwards, Ph.D., Peer Support Workforce
Advocate and Researcher, Colleague and Longtime Friend

When I entered the peer support workforce community nearly two decades ago, Celia
Brown was one of the first pioneers of the consumer/survivor/ex-patient movement

I met; she soon became an ally, a mentor, and a deeply close personal friend. Celia possessed unparalleled wisdom and skill navigating historically oppressive systems while simultaneously 'changing the narrative' within these same hierarchies. She was a tireless advocate, possessed a buoyant spirit, and was intentional about supporting others. Celia inspired her fellow advocates to speak out against inhumane practices, racism, and stigma. She skillfully and inimitably traversed her multiple roles with grace and discretion.

Mere words cannot capture the breadth and depth of support Celia exchanged with her peers, friends, and family. On a very personal note, I always experienced a sense of excitement, hope and rejuvenation talking with Celia. Regardless of what was going on in our lives and throughout the world, we always found something to be grateful for and laugh about. We sought comic relief to buffer the harshness of police violence, political upheaval, and structural racism. Celia and I share a birthday and were born in the same year. I am fortunate to have worked with Celia on planning the New York City Conference for Working Peer Specialists for the past 17 years; convening the Inaugural Surviving Race Dialogues this past summer in Savannah, Georgia; and hosting virtual peer support groups on Saturday afternoons for 14 months during the pandemic. Celia sought to change systems one person at a time and never deemed any cause insurmountable. I will miss her immensely and will always be enriched by her dedication, friendship and support.

A message from The Brown Family

Celia was a pillar of strength to her community, but also to her family. While many of her constituents depended on her to lead, to make power moves, to advocate for the disenfranchised, her home and family is where she recharged. Her partner and son especially understood the value of her work. Her son, Kevin talks about how devoted she was to the needs of her community. Endless hours were spent talking on the phone, helping to find housing for consumers in half-way houses or shelters. Oftentimes, she listened and counseled her peers by offering kind words, redirection and sound alternatives to their problems. She was patient, considerate, nurturing and compassionate about the needs of others. Celia was a multi-tasker who juggled various projects, travelled to speaking engagements, organized conferences, Zoom calls, rallies, while still finding time to tend to her family. Celia was the best person to talk to because she heard every word you said and addressed the concern with truth and reason.

In her youth, when Celia was first diagnosed with mental health issues, it was the assumption that she would have to be taken care of for the rest of her life. She fooled us all. Celia's 360 turnaround from mental health consumer to advocate is a testament that everyone has a choice to pave their own way, and that mental challenges can be managed with the right support. It is our hope that the legacy of Celia's body of work as a mental health advocate and survivor will continue to encourage, motivate and help others to save lives.

The Brown family would like to give special thanks to the authors of the book.

Notes

1 Jacki McKinney was a survivor of incarceration in the psychiatric and criminal justice systems and her advocacy focused on Black women and families. She was the founding member of the National People of Color Consumer/Survivor Network. She was a board member for National Association for Rights Protection and Advocacy (NARPA). She died in 2021.

2 The Olmstead lawsuit was initiated by Lois Curtis and Elaine Wilson who received diagnoses of mental health conditions and developmental disabilities and were admitted to the psychiatric unit in the State-run Georgia Regional Hospital. Following the women's medical treatment there, mental health professionals stated that each was ready to move to a community-based program. However, the women remained confined in the institution, each for several years after the initial treatment was concluded. They filed suit under the Americans with Disabilities Act (ADA) for release from the hospital. On June 22, 1999, the United States Supreme Court held in Olmstead v. L.C. that unjustified segregation of persons with disabilities constitutes discrimination in violation of title II of the Americans with Disabilities Act. The Court held that public entities must provide community-based services to persons with disabilities when (1) treatment professionals determine community placement is appropriate; (2) the impacted persons do not oppose community-based treatment; and (3) community-based services can be reasonably accommodated, considering the resources available to the public entity and the needs of others who are receiving disability services from the entity. Olmstead became one of the most important civil rights decisions for people with disabilities.

3 From the mid-1880s to the 1960s, over 45,000 people passed away while living in a state institution. Usually, their remains are in mass gravesides, unmarked, or have a faded number marker. Due to the unrelenting efforts of mental health activists, some state hospitals have invested in cemetery restoration projects, in an effort to restore cemeteries where individuals are buried and preserve the history of those who have died in state institutions.

4 Founded in 2014 by Celia Brown, Surviving Race: The Intersection of Race, Disability and Human Rights is a coalition comprised of Black, Indigenous, People of Color (BIPOC) who are mental advocates and survivors and speak on police brutality, white privilege, disability, race, LGBTQI2SA, human rights, psychiatry, and anti-psychiatry. Their mission is to create and support local and national antiracist activities to expose and eliminate police killings, police brutality, and mass incarceration generally and specifically as it relates to the mental health system and survivor/other movements.

5 Ethel 'Effie' Smith was the founder of Consumer Action Network (CAN), a peer-run non-profit and spent over two decades working with the Washington DC Department of Behavioral Health to improve mental health services. Effie also focused her advocacy efforts on incarcerated women with trauma histories. She died in 2020.

References

American Psychological Association [APA]. (2021). *APA's apology to Black, Indigenous and people of color for its support of structural racism in psychiatry.* https://www .psychiatry.org/newsroom/apa-apology-for-its-support-of-structural-racism-in -psychiatry

Jackson, V. (2002). In our own voices: African American stories of oppression, survival and recovery in the mental health system. *University of Dayton Medical Journal.* https:// dulwichcentre.com.au/wp-content/uploads/2014/08/In_Our_Own_Voice_African _American_stories_of_oppression_survival_and_recovery_in_mental_health_ systems.pdf

Ken Schlosser, K. (1999). *Issues of Race and Ethnicity in the Mental Health System and the Psychiatric Survivors Movement: A Collective Assessment.* Diversity Project National Empowerment Center.

King, M.L. (1968). 'The Role of the Behavioral Scientist in the Civil Rights movement.' APA Annual Convention, *1967. Journal of Social Issues*[reprint] (*Vol. 24, No. 1, 1968*).

Shim, R. S. (2020, June 30). Structural racism is why I'm leaving organized psychiatry. *STAT.*https://www.statnews.com/2020/07/01/structural-racism-is-why-im -leaving-organized-psychiatry

Stuhler, L. (2011, July 10). *The Inmates of Willard 1870 to 1900 / A Genealogy Resource.* https://inmatesofwillard.com/

Trinkley Ph.D., M., & Hacker, D. (2009). 'Southerland, N. Preservation Assessment of St. Elizabeths East Campus Cemetery, Washington, DC.' *Chicora Research Contribution 514.* Chicora Foundation, Inc. June 15, 2009.

Interviews

K.J. Myrick, personal communication, February 20, 2021

V. Jackson, personal communication, February 23, 2021

C. Brown, personal communication, March 12, 2021

Chapter 38

Mad Resistance/Mad Alternatives

DEMOCRATIZING MENTAL HEALTH CARE[1]

Jeremy Andersen, Ed Altwies, Jonah Bossewitch, Celia Brown, Kermit Cole, Sera Davidow, Sascha Altman DuBrul, Eric Friedland-Kays, Gelini Fontaine, Will Hall, Chris Hansen, Bradley Lewis, Audre Lorde Project, Maryse Mitchell-Brody, Jacks McNamara, Gina Nikkel, Pablo Sadler, Madigan Shive, David Stark, Adaku Utah, Agustina Vidal, and Cheyenna Layne Weber

Summary

Over the last century there have been multiple attempts to reform mental health systems and to develop new models. Most of these innovations, however, have come from clinical experts using top-down approaches. Potential service users, the key stakeholders, are rarely included in the process of imagining, building, and staffing mental health approaches. Mad pride activism works to open this process, taking seriously the rallying cry of "nothing about us without us" and lobbying for more democratic practices in mental health. But this work is slow and difficult because expert stakeholders are reluctant to share their authority or truly embrace a democratic option.

Activists are increasingly responding to this situation through direct action and by taking matters into their own hands. In addition to lobbying the mental health system to build alternatives, many activists are also building them directly. This multi-authored chapter, written by a group of activists, outlines the rationale for direct action around mental health and highlights several direct-action examples. The authors discuss four main alternative approaches: (1) mutual aid and resilience strategies; (2) alternative professional support; (3) hybrid approaches; and (4)

DOI: 10.4324/9781003148456-43

advocacy approaches. This chapter was first published in 2020 and not all of the options discussed are still available. But the chapter remains a classic and gives an excellent sense of how to use direct action to democratize mental health—even when the mainstream itself is reluctant to develop options. None of these activists are asking mental health systems to change, they are simply changing the world of mental health by adding new possibilities.

*

NOTHING ABOUT US WITHOUT US!!
> (Protest poster outside American Psychiatric Association)

If justice is what love looks like in public, then deep democracy is what justice looks like in practice.
> Cornel West (*Hope on a Tightrope*)

Introduction

Contemporary efforts to improve treatment and care in community mental health are heir to a range of historical reform efforts in psychiatry. The very founding images of psychiatry begin with Philip Pinel's libratory reform of unchaining Parisian "insane" (Cohen & Timimi, 2008). Follow-up reforms include William Tuke's efforts to create a moral treatment, Sigmund Freud's efforts to discover and interpret unconscious conflicts, Jacques Lacan's efforts to keep Freud's work true to its potential, community psychiatry's efforts to spread psychiatric treatment to a broader public, Thomas Szasz's efforts to rid psychiatry of philosophical category mistakes, R. D. Laing's efforts to make space for the existential value of psychic suffering, Carl Rogers' efforts to develop person-centered care, family therapy attempts to include the family dynamics of mental difference, Aaron Beck's efforts to bring evidential and cognitive rigor to psychotherapy, Robert Spitzer's efforts to make psychiatry more scientifically operational and consistent, biological psychiatrists' efforts to develop pharmaceutical treatments, and third-wave cognitive therapy's attempts to bring mindfulness practices to psychotherapy. In short, throughout the history of mental health care we see a range of reform efforts designed to benefit the psychically different and those who suffer from psychic pain.

Despite the tremendous diversity of these reforms, they all have at least one thing in common. They were all created and designed by clinical experts through a top-down process. In each case, a clinical expert, or a small band of experts, undertook a critique of current mental health paradigms and institutions and then imagined alternative treatment systems—which offered different and sometimes radically different approaches to psychiatry. The expert then joined with others to spread the new system out into the field. The net result in each case was that new ideas for mental health care came from a small handful of relevant stakeholders. And, more strikingly, the most important stakeholders, the potential service users, were excluded from the process. Even in the most radical of these examples, service users themselves did not articulate the critique or design the improved system. In each of these historical efforts the process moved from expert analysis to expert solution.

We draw a clear lesson from this history. Reforming community mental health's clinical practice must include a larger democratic reform of mental health. No matter how wellmeaning the reform intentions, when a clinical system of knowledge and practice is set up without input from the main stakeholders the system risks being skewed and biased away from stakeholders' needs, preferences, and priorities. In all probability, the system ends up skewed in rough proportion to the relative input and power dynamics of those involved (Bucchi, 2009; Hall, 1997). Future libratory reforms efforts in community mental health must not fall in this top-down trap. Rather, future reforms must be developed through a process of inclusiveness. Key stakeholders must be involved in all levels of the reform—not just empathic listening and shared decision-making at the point of service, but also in considering and researching problems, in designing alternatives, in educating the public, and in providing care. In short, the next wave of libratory reform in mental health care should not be driven by top-down practices; it should be inclusive by design, driven by democracy. The call for progressive libratory reform in mental health should be a call for democracy in mental health.

Democracy-Based Practices: Historical and Theoretical Background

The history of mental health care reform spearheaded by top-down clinicians could be called the "above-ground" history of mental health. We can gain a better understanding of this aboveground history if we put it in context with an "underground" history of mental health. This underground history is the history of the consumer movement, of mad pride, of the recovery movement, and of the disability rights movement. There are many ways to tell these underground histories and some of the important narrative highlights have been worked through in other chapters of this book. For the purposes of this chapter, the key insight for an emerging generation of contemporary mental health activists, what we are calling the "mad resistance," is that the most powerful way to plot that underground history is through the organizing frame of *increasing democracy* (Bossewitch, 2015).

Plotting the underground history of mental health through increasing democracy connects this history with the long revolution of progressive politics. Democratic theorists Ernesto Laclau and Chantal Mouffe explain that the language and goals of democracy have been pivotal "fermenting agents" behind the women's movement, African-American civil rights, gay and lesbian liberation, and environmental activism (Laclau & Mouffe, 1985, p. 155). This same democratic imaginary inspired abolitionists to combat slavery, suffragettes in their struggles for the vote, and anti-imperialists in their resistance against colonial rulers (Smith, 1998, p. 9). Moreover, egalitarian discourses have played an increasing role in collective identification for the last 200 years: "At the beginning of … the French Revolution, the public space of citizenship was the exclusive domain of equality, while in the private sphere no questioning took place of existing social inequalities. However, as de Tocqueville clearly understood, once human beings accept the legitimacy of the principle of equality in one sphere they will attempt to extend it to every other sphere" (Laclau & Mouffe, 1990, p. 128). Once democracy gets started, it tends to spread into ever new domains, including domains such as mental health care that have been traditionally far removed from the discourse of democracy.

It is important to understand that, historically, antidemocratic knowledge formations regarding gender, race, nation status, and sexual preference link directly to the oppressive social structures of sexism, racism, colonialism, and heterosexism. Similarly, with physical and mental difference, antidemocratic practice links to the oppressive structures of *ableism* and *sanism*. The slide from antidemocratic human inquiry into oppressive knowledge formations, such as sexism and sanism, happens despite well-meaning intentions to make inquiry "objective" and "value free." Regardless of rational or empirical "rigor," antidemocratic human inquiry inevitably risks representing the other as inferior and subordinate. In sexist, racist, colonialist, and heterosexist representations, the other is seen as naturally and essentially substandard and lesser. In antidemocratic medical and psychiatric representation, where the physically or mentally different or impaired are excluded because of lack of "credentials" and "expertise," *the other is overly categorized as disordered, dysfunctional, and pathological.* This medical and psychiatric representational bias goes beyond the familiar problem of "stigma." Rather, it creates ableist and sanist structures of exclusion, subordination, and condescension all too similar to oppressive structures of sexism, racism, colonialism, and heterosexism (Linton, 2013; Lewis, 2013; Poole et al., 2012).

As a result, contemporary mad activists take up the call for mental health reform through democratic self representation and direct action. They are struggling to assert their right to substantively engage in the conversation around their own identities and self-care. They want to participate in the production of the knowledge that governs their diagnosis and treatment, and they are questioning the very language and narrative frames used to talk about their mental health and wellness. Their argument, embodied in their stories, represents a shift from the antipsychiatrist, psychiatric survivors, and the consumer movements that preceded them. Many contemporary mad activists have moved away from an oppositional, head-butting critique of the psychiatric–pharmaceutical alliance, and their demands have begun to focus on questions of voice. In the tradition of the disability rights movement, this new generation of the mad resistance has taken up the democratic cry "Nothing about us without us."

James Charlton cataloged the centrality of this phrase to disability rights in his book *Nothing About Us Without Us: Disability Oppression and Empowerment* (Charlton, 1998). Charlton first heard the expression invoked by leaders of the South African disabled people's group in 1993, who claimed to have heard it used earlier at an Eastern European international disability rights conference. Two years later he saw a front-page headline in a Mexico City daily about thousands of landless peasants marching under the banner *Nunca Mas Sin Nosotros* (Never Again Without Us), and adopted "Nothing About Us Without Us" as the rallying cry for the disability movement.

Charlton quotes Ed Roberts, a leader of the international disability rights movement: "if we have learned one thing from the civil rights movement in the U.S., it's that when others speak for you, you lose" (Drieger, 1989, p. 28). On the surface, the proposition "nothing about us without us" may seem like a timid assertion, easy to satisfy. However, it has proven to be one of the most radical demands that mental health activists can make. It has radical implications for the ways in which human conditions are investigated and addressed. It also challenges the binary distinction between objectivity and subjectivity, and calls into question the possibility of objective knowledge devoid of context. This problematic has shaped mental health activism throughout its history, and the emerging wave of mad resistance has begun to confront this impasse directly.

The transformational shift in mad resistance can be construed as a shift from advocating for a particular ontology to advocating for a new democratic epistemology (Harding, 2006; Brown, 2009). More than a discursive face-off disputing the nature of reality, the disagreement focuses on the question of how to approach controversies and establish consensus. For example, many antipsychiatrists and psychiatric survivors in the 1970s argued (and continue to argue) that there is no such thing as mental illness. We argue that the newly emerging wave of mad resistance operates on a different plane. It is more concerned with ensuring that all of the relevant stakeholders have seats at the tables of power, where their voices can be included in the production of psychiatric knowledge. First and foremost is the primacy of their own voices in the understanding of their situation and the cocreation of their stories. Crucially, their insistence on coconstructing their own identities and narratives underlies their platforms, critiques, and actions.

Mental health researchers are starting to use community-based participatory research to partially address this issue (Roberts, 2013). But, more to the point of this chapter, mental health activists are using direct action techni ques to develop on-the-ground alternative approaches to mental health care (Hall, 2016; Stastny & Lehmann, 2007). What these alternatives all have in common is that they are either spearheaded or deeply informed by the key stakeholders in mental health—people with lived experience of mental difference or mental suffering.

Democratic Mental Health Examples: What Are People Doing?

In this section we give some examples of these alternatives. Examples are critical for understanding the contemporary democratic fermentation because, by definition, one cannot plan democracy through top-down rational, ethical, or scientific inquiry—one must see what people want, what they are creating, and what they are advocating. We do just that in this section and we divide our examples into five groups: (1) *individual strategies*, (2) *mutual aid and resilience strategies*, (3) *alternative professional support*, (4) *hybrid approaches*, and (5) *advocacy approaches*. These groupings are loose heuristics, they could be arranged in other ways, and they easily blend into each other. We only use them for an initial orientation into this domain.

For examples of "individual strategies" we refer the reader to www.mindfreedom .org/p-ersonal-stories, http://igotbetter.org/, www.freedom-center.org/section /speakout, and "What Helps Me if I go Mad" in *Alternatives Beyond Psychiatry* (Stastny & Lehmann, 2007, pp. 44–75). Our "mutual aid and resilience strategies" section provides examples of organized self-help. Our "alternative professional support" section provides professional examples deeply informed by democratic principles.

"Hybrid approaches" are emergent examples of individuals with lived experience who are developing alternative approaches to care outside standard credentialing, regulation, and reimbursement structures. And, finally, "advocacy" provides examples of organizations devoted to democratic promotion in mental health through cultural, political, academic, or economic support.

Our goal with these examples is not to give an exhaustive list of all the possible alternatives. "Nothing about us without us" is a rallying cry that is on the streets and in the air, and it is beginning to yield a diverse range of new approaches. We only scratch the surface. But, in the spirit of encouraging others to follow suit, we hope to give a substantial sense of direct action strategies that exemplify and promote democratizing mental health. The examples are in the words of the organizers.

Mutual Aid and Resilience Strategies

The Audre Lorde Project, http://alp.org/

The Audre Lorde Project (ALP) is a Lesbian, Gay, Bisexual, Two Spirit, Trans and Gender Non-Conforming People of Color (LGBTSTGNC POC) community organizing center, focusing on the New York City area. Through mobilization, education and capacity-building, we work for community wellness and progressive social and economic justice. Unlike most mainstream approaches, we see these issues as all connected rather than separate or compartmentalized. Committed to struggling across differences, we seek to responsibly reflect, represent and serve our various communities.

Our 3rd Space Support program is for individuals who struggle with issues around employment, education, health care and immigration status. It is a place to give and receive sustainable support; where creation, invention and innovation will be practiced. We draw from our resilience to support ourselves. Within this 3rd Space we hold on to the idea that LGBTSTGNC POC communities have always found ways to support each other and survive outside of systems. The 3rd Space Support program hopes to encourage and create space for these organic methods of community support and community building.

At the same time, ALP acknowledges that LGBTSTGNC POC community members also engage within systems to find support and get their needs met. Therefore, ALP also engages with these systems to provide advocacy, resources and referrals for community members around the issues, employment, education, health care and immigration status. In the words of Audre Lorde: "When we are silent, we are still afraid. So it is better to speak remembering we were never meant to survive …" At ALP we practice these resiliency strategies knowing we must for our collective survival.

Icarus Project, http://theicarusproject.net/

The Icarus Project (TIP) is a support network and education project by and for people who experience the world in ways that are often diagnosed as mental illness. We advance social justice by fostering mutual aid practices that reconnect healing and collective liberation. We transform ourselves through transforming the world around us. TIP's approach offers an invitation to exploration and identification beyond the sometimes alienating mental health mainstream. Since 2002, TIP has crafted online support, member art, talks, community events, dynamic publications, and a network of allied local groups—all creating space for thousands of people to share their wisdom and learn from each other's stories.

We use the following strategic programs to support our mission:

- We create diverse and accessible **resources** that resonate with the lived experiences of people of color, women, LGBTQI people, and disabled people/people with disabilities, among other marginalized groups. These resources help readers explore the impacts of issues like racism, transphobia, homophobia, sexism, and intergenerational trauma on mental health, and offer community-based strategies for individual and collective healing.
- We foster **community and support** for people who feel isolated by the mental health mainstream. Between our online forum and Facebook presence, we count over 10,000 people sharing virtual support and political education.
- We use **education** to build the capacity of our communities to create change and shift the language and culture of mental health in the United States.

At TIP, we envision a world with more options to navigate mental health issues: options that support self-determination, center people who are most impacted by mental health-based oppression, and, most critically, uplift social transformation as central to individual wellbeing. We do this work in the service of achieving that vision.

Intentional Peer Support, www.intentionalpeersuupport.org

> As peer support in mental health proliferates, we must be mindful of our intention: social change. It is not about developing more effective services, but rather about creating dialogues that have influence on all of our understandings, conversations, and relationships.
>
> Shery Mead, Founder of IPS

Intentional Peer Support (IPS) is a way of thinking about and inviting transformative relationships. Practitioners learn to use relationships to see things from new angles, develop greater awareness of personal and relational patterns, and support and challenge each other in trying new things. IPS is used across the world in community, peer support, and human services settings, and is a tool for community development with broad appeal to people from all walks of life. IPS is different from traditional service relationships because:

- Relationships are viewed as partnerships that invite and inspire both parties to learn and grow, rather than as one person needing to "help" another.
- IPS doesn't start with the assumption of a problem. With IPS, each of us pays attention to how we have learned to make sense of our experiences, then uses the relationship to create new ways of seeing, thinking, and doing.
- IPS promotes a trauma-informed way of relating. Instead of asking "What's wrong?" we learn to ask "What happened?"

- IPS examines our lives in the context of mutually accountable relationships and communities—looking beyond the mere notion of individual responsibility for change.
- IPS is a practice which provides tools for mindfulness and self-reflection in relationships. There are three principles which shift the focus–from helping to co-learning, from the individual to the relationship, and through fear to hope. The four tasks are connection, worldview, mutuality, and moving toward.
- IPS encourages us to increasingly live and move toward what we want instead of focusing on what we need to stop or avoid doing.

Western Mass Recovery Learning Community, www.westernmassrlc.org /

The Western Massachusetts Recovery Learning Community (RLC) is built upon the work of years upon years of advocacy dedicated to the idea that peer supports should be valued monetarily and funded throughout the state. We use the legacy of that dedication to support healing and growth for the community and individuals who have been impacted by psychiatric diagnosis, trauma, extreme states, homelessness, addiction and other life-interrupting challenges. Several themes run throughout our work, including (but not limited to): *Social justice and anti-oppression are key*. We have repeatedly witnessed that—when supports such as what the RLC has to offer become divorced from a broader context of undoing oppression (not just psychiatric oppression but also racism, transphobia, sexism, classism, and so on)—co-optation and replication of the system are the most likely outcomes.

Making meaning is a personal process. We do not believe in any one way of understanding emotional or mental distress, and find that the one-size-fits-all medicalized explanations that are elevated in current society have often been harmful (especially when presented as the only way). Our community creates many spaces and opportunities for people to explore and learn from their own experiences, and (most importantly) take ownership over their own story.

Connection is healing. Ultimately, we believe that connection with other human beings (in all their imperfections) can be healing. Thus, our community is designed to facilitate connection not just with people in paid roles, but with others who are taking part in any number of ways, including:

- Peer-to-peer support and opportunities for genuine human relationships
- Access to alternative Healing Practices like yoga, acupuncture, Reiki, and meditation
- Learning Opportunities including trainings, film screenings, and public events
- Advocacy at an individual and systems level

Alternative Professional Support

Narrative Psychiatry

Despite the dominance of biomedical and technological models in psychiatry, the field also contains robust critical, ethical, and recovery-oriented practitioners that work to correct the field toward the values of autonomy, empowerment, and democracy.

All of this critical professional work shares an understanding that there is more than one way to tell the story of human difference and human suffering.

Narrative psychiatry brings to this critical community the fruits of recent work in narrative theory, narrative medicine, and narrative psychotherapy (Lewis, 2011; Hamkins, 2014; Thomas, 2014). These narrative approaches deepen our understanding of the way human stories are organized by metaphors, plots, narrative identifications, and points of view. When these narrative elements are systematized by clinical communities they become clinical models, such as biological, cognitive, psychoanalytic, family, social, creative, spiritual, etc., that compete or integrate with each other in a bid for dominance of the field. But, from a narrative perspective, they are all possibilities for meaning making. The question is not which story is right, but who gets to decide, and what choices are available for people to decide from?

Narrative psychiatry joins with critical, ethical, and recovery-oriented approaches to help develop real-world options where people are empowered to create the narratives, or combination of narratives, best for them. In this way, narrative psychiatry is in political struggle with the mainstream and at the same time a clinical version of "sly normality" that passes as nothing more than "good psychiatry" (Mills, 2014). As a result, narrative psychiatrists can serve, even in the most dogmatic and antidemocratic clinical settings, as underground railroads to alternatives beyond the mainstream for those people who are unhappy with the dominant options.

Parachute NYC, www1.nyc.gov/site/doh/health/health-topics/crisis-emergency-services-parachute-nyc.page

In 2012, the Fund for Public Health in New York, Inc., on behalf of the New York City Department of Health and Mental Hygiene (DOHMH), was awarded $17.6 M three-year grant to launch Parachute NYC. The project was supported by funding from Centers for Medicare and Medicaid Services, Center for Medicare and Medicaid Innovation. Parachute NYC has made progress toward democratizing mental health services on several levels: staffing the project's range of services (four mobile teams, four respite centers, and a "warm-line" call-in center) with peer specialists and training all staff in Intentional Peer Support (IPS) and therapeutic approaches drawn from Needs Adapted Treatment/Open Dialogue (NAT/OD) practices.

A central tenet of these new practices is that neither the peer specialist nor the service provider is an expert in the traditional sense. Rather than focusing on diagnosis and psychoeducation, the emphasis is on the development of mutual relationships in which professionals support the service user (and their social network, in the case of NAT/OD) in constructing meaning and making choices based on their experiences. Both of these approaches privilege holding multiple and often contradictory "truths," equally valuing the "voice" of everyone involved, and tolerating the uncertainty of any given circumstance so that new and often unforeseen "ways of going on" can emerge (Mead, 2014; Seikkula, 2011).

In addition, both the home-based mobile teams and respites created new, more democratic mental health settings embedded in the community and away from traditional institutional power structures. The introduction of these practices continues to evolve, with the long-term hope of establishing a more egalitarian community of practice involving many stakeholders in NYC's diverse and multicultural mental health service system.

Third Root Community Health Center, http://thirdroot.org/

Third Root is a worker-owned holistic health-care center in Flatbush, Brooklyn. We currently consist of six proud and diverse member-owners and several staff offering acupuncture in both community and private settings, herbal medicine and herbal medicine education, massage, and yoga, as well as numerous workshops and forums that address healing. We were founded in 2008 with the mission of being accessible to our communities; collaborative in our work and healing modalities; and empowering to the people we engage with, communities we belong to, and all the workers at our center. Our services are offered at sliding scale rates and work exchange volunteers support our administrative team. Worker-owners (all of us healers in various modalities) are all paid the same wage, and worker-owners can get services from each other at no cost. In this way we recognize the profound bridges of interdependence between provider and client; work place and place of nourishment; and individual and community.

While we welcome people of all backgrounds to our space, we actively work to center people of color, LGBT and gender non-conforming people, low income people, people with disabilities (identities we share as a collective), and all marginalized people who experience barriers to holistic healthcare. We challenge the notion that holistic healing is only a spa experience to pamper the wealthy, and place our modalities (with multiple roots in global traditions) firmly in the realm of effective, life-sustaining primary care. We see and treat people with a wide range of conditions affecting mind, body, and spirit; and are coconspirators with each patient/client/student in sustainably supporting their health and healing. Because we regard this work as supporting communities within movements for social justice, we call ourselves a healing justice center.

Windhorse, www.windhorseimh.org

The Windhorse model is a contemplative, environmental approach to supporting people in their recovery from extreme mind states. The underlying view that forms the foundation for this approach is that we all possess the same "brilliant sanity," that sanity is a spectrum upon which we all move along throughout our lives and even throughout a given day. Moreover, even in the depths of an extreme mind state, we have moments or "islands" of clarity, when our sanity shines through and we are more connected to our present environment. This view stands in stark contrast to any notion that there are those of us who are "sane" on one side of the line, and those who aren't on the other.

The Windhorse approach emphasizes creating an environment of safety and sanity, supported and enriched by genuine, compassionate relationships. This kind of physical and relational environment is co-created by a team, which can include the client or person at the center of concern, a therapeutic housemate, a principal psychotherapist, a wellness nurse, a team leader who coordinates care, and one or two counselors or peer counselors who—along with the team leader—practice basic attendance together.

Basic attendance is used to describe a grounded, compassionate, human-to-human way of being with someone who is struggling to recover. This kind of attention is supported by one's contemplative practice—particularly mindfulness and compassion practice— which is an essential part of the ongoing training of anyone doing Windhorse work. Paying attention in this way naturally invites the attendee to compassionately be with and gain perspective on his or her inner and outer experience, thereby synchronizing mind to body and to environment. Furthermore, genuinely connecting in this way can offer a much needed bridge to others and to life as a whole. Recovery, then, at Windhorse, is not a matter of people who are "well" helping someone who is "sick," but a journey of mutual learning and mutual recovery.

Hybrid Approaches

Sascha Dubrul: T-Maps, www.mapstotheotherside.net/t-maps/

Transformative Mutual Aid Practices (T-MAPs) is an emerging set of community-developed workshops that provide tools and space for building a personal "map" of resilience practices and cultural resources. T-MAPs was initially inspired by advanced directives and related recovery tools for planning mental health treatment options in times of crisis. Our T-MAPs practice goes beyond the usually defined mental health concerns to articulate larger strategies, life-goals, and social visions that are helpful not just in times of distress but also in times of flourishing. Rather than approaching advanced directives as primarily a mental health practice, we turned it into a group practice of mutual aid, imagination, and prefigurative cultural change. Through a mix of collective brainstorming, creative story-telling, theater games, art/collage making, and breath/mindfulness practices, the group is guided through a process to develop greater personal wellness and collective transformation. We work together to envision, articulate, and build the world we want to live in now.

Each participant collaborates with the group to complete a personalized booklet (or "T-MAP"). These booklets are guides for navigating challenging times, coming back to what we care about, and communicating with the important people in our lives. We ask each other questions like "What is most important to me?" and "What am I like when I am most alive?" as jumping off points for conversation and leaving written trails for ourselves.

Initially developed as an informal mutual aid tool in the Icarus Project community, over the years I (Sascha DuBrul) have come to see the importance of mentorship and structured practice for personal and collective transformation. Today I am pursuing further mental health training and have begun the dance between the worlds of the clinical and the peer. I continue to be inspired by the possibilities of hybrid map making workshops that stay true to the advantages of mutual aid and also add guidance from more formal clinical grounding.

Harriet's Apothecary, www.harrietsapothecary.com/

Harriet's Apothecary is an intergenerational, healing village led by the brilliance and wisdom of Black Cis Women, Queer and Trans healers, artists, health professionals, magicians, activists and ancestors. Our village, inspired by Harriet Tubman and founded by Adaku Utah is committed to co-creating accessible, affordable, liberatory, all-body loving, all-gender honoring, community healing spaces that recognize, inspire, and deepen the healing genius of people who identify as Black, Indigenous and People of color and the allies that love us.

The intention of Harriet's Apothecary is to continue the rich healing legacy of abolitionist, community nurse and herbalist Harriet Tubman. Like our courageous ancestor, we expand access to health and healing resources that support our community, specifically Black, Indigenous and PoC folks, in their healing journeys toward freedom. We recognize that there are significant individual, collective and generational consequences to living in a world that systematically oppresses people of color. We know that the consistent, widespread direct and indirect exposure to violence, colonization, loss, burn-out, stress, microaggressions, imperialism, dis-ease and traumatic social conditions permeates and impacts our personal and interpersonal physical, emotional and spiritual well-beings.

This is why we intentionally choose to gather as a healing team of Black Cis Women, Queer and Trans people because our existence and togetherness is fundamentally a form of resistance against the colonization of our bodies, practices and communities. Harriet's Apothecary is committed to being a part of a long legacy of healers who center healing in social justice work for the sake of liberating our bodies and our communities. Our shared goal is to create dynamic healing spaces that supports Black, Indigenous and PoC folks in connecting with a deeper sense of resilience, self worth and acceptance, transformative healing, and inspiration to liberate injustice in their tissues and within the spaces they occupy.

Will Hall, www.willhall.net

> "I do not ask the wounded person how he feels, I myself become the wounded person."
>
> —Walt Whitman

Psychotherapy, borrowing from medicine and the church, denies mutuality. Separating the broken one from the one who will fix them would seem indispensable, but not only is this unnecessary, it is also frequently harmful. Professionals sent me down a spiral of medication, hospitals, and labels that reversed only when I stopped seeking help outside myself. I relinquished my autonomy to the stigma that something was wrong with me. It wasn't until I discovered the recovery movement and mutual self aid peer groups that I began to get better.

Today my own practice as a counselor works alongside the community support that helped me. Medical theories of the brain and psychological theories of the individual obscure social problems in the community. I learned that what we call "mental illness" is disempowerment and isolation, not individual pathology. To move forward people need empowerment and connection, not treatments. I develop social change programs and systems transformation aimed at the society, not just the individual.

In my counseling work I relate as a person, not an expert, and dispense with professional distance, jargon, or interpretation. Research consistently shows that technique is not what makes change happen: it is the relationship itself. Trust, listening, and reciprocity work best. Focusing on one person is a momentary situation, not a permanent difference between helper and helpee.

How can we be honest about why people suffer and how to help each other? By rethinking therapy. We need to support and facilitate the community's own empowerment and healing process, not replace it with dependence on experts.

Jacks McNamara: Red Roots Healing Arts, www.redrootshealingarts.com

Red Roots Healing Arts is a space where I (Jacks McNamara) can be both a survivor—of trauma, and of the psychiatric system—and a practitioner of trauma-informed healing practices. Through somatic counseling, wellness mentoring, and the creative arts, I offer people a compassionate space to heal, reflect, and transform. My goal is not to help people adjust to a sick society—it is to help all of us connect to meaningful life work, loving communities, and the possibility of liberation. Together, we work through the body and the imagination to develop the insight, practices, and tools necessary to bring our loves [and preferred lifestyles] closer to own definitions of health.

In addition to offering one on one work with clients, both in person and across the world via Skype, I have also developed a number of unusual group offerings, including 2 writing courses—Creative Writing for the Creatively Maladjusted, for people living with divergent mental health, and Writing Ourselves Alive—for queer & trans poets—and a community healing group, called Cultivating Resilience, for survivors and other miracles. Through coming together with other survivors in a carefully facilitated space, I help folks discover that they are not alone, and that through community, somatic practices, journaling, and other exercises, they can begin the journey of coming back home to their bodies and their psyches. It is so powerful to do this work with others who have been through the fire.

My approach is deeply informed by the time I spent training with generative somatics, an organization committed to somatic transformation and social justice. I spent 3 years in their Somatics & Trauma practitioner training, where the vast majority of my fellow students were also practitioner/survivors. Some of these folks have gone on to become licensed therapists, and some, like me, have chosen to practice outside the "mental health/mental illness" paradigm altogether, offering the kind of responsive, hybrid approaches that are not usually possible inside large, frequently oppressive systems.

Advocacy For Democratic Alternatives

Foundation for Excellence in Mental Health, www .mentalhealthexcellence.org/

The Foundation for Excellence in Mental Health Care is an innovative approach for improving global mental healthcare toward a greater recovery focus. Although the

Foundation does not provide direct care it helps create private philanthropic funding for innovative research, education, and programs emphasizing increased service user voice and participation in recovery and trauma-informed care. It was founded in February 2011 to match the passion of private philanthropy with the world's top researchers and programs to bring recovery based care to every community.

Under the direction of our Global Scientific Advisory Board research examples include a 20 year follow up study on the long term effects of anti-psychotics in the treatment of schizophrenia, alternative National guidelines for treating attention and depression problems in children, and adapting the Open Dialogue Model for acute crisis to the United States.

Programs we have helped fund include expanding the Hearing Voices approach in the United States, Intentional Peer Support training to communities, and an International Leadership Academy. Education opportunities include Mad in America Continuing Education courses that equip doctors, counselors, and the general public with research on the risks and uses of neuroleptic drugs as well as a broad array of recovery tools, Families Healing Together (an online course for learning about your loved ones mental health challenges and coping tools), and the Dorothea Dix Think Tank. Our website provides a large library of books, papers, videos and other resources such as the Early Psychosis Intervention Program Directory, the RxISK Guide to Stopping Antidepressants, and a well vetted Provider Directory.

The Foundation operates under the premise that it will take each one of us to change the current standard of care and that we must do it together. We offer the financial structure and the global collaborative expertise to affect the way we view excellence in mental health care.

Mad in America, www.madinamerica.com/

Mad in America (MIA) began in 2012 to provide news of psychiatric research, original journalism articles, and a forum for an international group of writers—people with lived experience, peer specialists, family members, psychiatrists, psychologists, social workers, program managers, journalists, attorneys, and more—to explore issues related to the goal of "remaking psychiatry."

It was swept into existence by the response Robert Whitaker encountered to his books *Mad in America* and *Anatomy of an Epidemic* (Whitaker, 2002, 2010). A generation of people whose lives had been affected found validation in Whitaker's critique of the literature that biological psychiatry claimed as its foundation—people whose voices had been systematically dismissed (literally) by a powerful and pervasive institution. A forum was needed to channel that energy into productive dialogue.

In *Anatomy of an Epidemic*, Whitaker found that the best documented "treatment" outcomes are in Tornio, Finland, where Open Dialogue's central premise is that people whose voices are excluded from the dominant dialogue in a social network become increasingly strident and/or bizarre, and are sooner or later labeled "mentally ill." Tornio corrected this by creating ways and means for people to find understanding together, and in this last 30 years reduced their rate of schizophrenia from record-high to record-low.

Inspired by Open Dialogue, MIA committed to hearing voices in as direct, immediate, and "unmoderated" a way as possible (within guidelines of civility, clarity, and relevance). This proved challenging at times, but MIA is committed to the hope is that over time—as Open Dialogue has demonstrated—sunlight would help us make progress toward finding consensus and navigating differences in the world of mental health care.

Madness Radio, www.madnessradio.net

When I (Will Hall) got out of mental hospitals and treatment facilities nothing on the radio made any sense. So I made my own radio show.

After helping start a community FM station in Northampton Massachusetts I began broadcasting Madness Radio, and 15 years later we've done more than 200 hour-long interviews. Patients speak out about abuse they endured in isolation rooms and restraints; voice hearers explore mental difference in a mentally conformist world; whistleblowers challenge pharmaceutical company corruption; scientists refute neuroscience dogma about the brain; artists talk about madness and creative inspiration; activists explore the relation between social oppression and intergenerational trauma; and dissident psychiatrists question labeling and pill pushing. The show has been heard by tens of thousands in Oregon, Massachusetts, and through the Pacific Network; and we have online listeners around the world.

Any system of oppression controls who speaks, who gets heard, and what kind of "official" stories get told. Dominated by the medical and insurance industries, most mental health media follows a script: brave scientists slowly winning a war against brain disorders with the latest treatment breakthroughs; pioneering researchers ignoring social problems and unlocking human suffering in the biology and genes; and patients deluded by illness finally surrendering to expert doctors and finding salvation through the prescription pad.

Madness Radio writes new scripts from the point of view that matters: people who have been diagnosed ourselves. The human mind's capacity for madness is far more mysterious than diagnostic labels and brain scans. Can we start asking different questions than we've had so far? Can we ask instead, "what does it mean to be called crazy in a crazy world?"

MindFreedom International, www.mindfreedom.org/

MindFreedom International is where democracy gets hands on with the mental health system. We are a nonprofit organization that unites 100 sponsor and affiliate grassroots groups with thousands of individual members to win human rights and alternatives for people labeled with psychiatric disabilities. Inspired by the civil rights and other movements, in about 1970, many psychiatric survivors, dissident mental health professionals, and advocates formed a diverse international effort to change the mental health system. MindFreedom is directly rooted in this international social change movement.

Our goals are to

- Win human rights campaigns in mental health.
- Challenge abuse by the psychiatric drug industry.
- Support the self-determination of psychiatric survivors and mental health consumers.
- Promote safe, humane and effective options in mental health.

As we put in our mission statement, "In a spirit of mutual cooperation, MindFreedom leads a nonviolent revolution of freedom, equality, truth and human rights that unites people affected by the mental health system with movements for justice everywhere."

MindFreedom is one of the very few totally independent groups in the mental health field with no funding from or control by governments, drug companies, religions, corporations, or the mental health system. We bring together the power of mutual support with the power of human rights activism. The majority of MindFreedom's members are people who have experienced human rights violations in the mental health system, or *psychiatric survivors.*

However, *everyone* who supports human rights is invited and encouraged to join and become active leaders. Mental health professionals and workers, advocates and attorneys, family members and the general public are all active as equal members and leaders in the MindFreedom International family. Our sponsor and affiliate groups are among the key leading organizations to change the mental health system.

Conclusion

None of these alternatives means that mainstream or clinically organized mental health systems are "bad" or "wrong" in some totalizing way. Just because top-down approaches risk being biased in favor of mainstream or clinical values does not mean that many service users do not share these very same values. Many service users are very grateful for mainstream approaches and many have grown and healed through them. The democratic alternatives that this chapter develops should be seen as just that—alternatives. They are options for people to choose from who do not fit well with mainstream possibilities.

As this chapter demonstrates, taking democracy and diversity seriously in mental health inevitably results in a range of choices rather than a single approach to care. But the need for diversity in mental health should not surprise us. We would not expect everyone to want the same fashion, same music, same art, same films, same cuisine, same religion, etc., and we should not expect everyone to want the same kinds of mental health services. In addition, none of these options means that people have to choose only one approach any more than people have to eat one kind of food or listen to one kind of music. It is very possible to combine approaches to create a combination unique to the particular person's values and concerns.

Finally, from a bioethics perspective, democracy and diversity of mental health services fits well with values-based practice (VBP). The first principle of VBP gets at the heart of the issue: "All [mental health] decisions stand on two feet, on values as well as on facts, including decisions about diagnosis (the "two feet" principle)" (Fulford, 2004, p. 208; Fulford, Thornton, & Graham, 2006, p. 498). The two feet principle of

VBP means that data and evidence alone cannot determine clinical decisions or choice of care and support models. Even if there is good data for aggressive chemotherapy, for example, that does not mean that everyone wants aggressive chemotherapy. The final decision depends on how potential interventions line up with the person's life choices, life goals, and narrative identity (who the person wants to be). But VBP, like informed consent more broadly, will only work if there are true options available. Otherwise it becomes a shibboleth or a ruse—one is given a choice among a few options, or at best a range of options organized by a similar top-down structure. For choice to be real, options must also be real. And for options to be real, we need a strong democracy in mental health.

Note

1 Originally printed in *Community Mental Health Reader,* edited by Samuel J. Rosenberg and Jessica Rosenberg, and published by Routledge. Reprinted with permission.

References

Bossewitch, J. (2015). *Dangerous gifts: Towards a new wave of mad resistance* (Dissertation). Columbia University Press.

Brown, Mark B. (2009). *Science in democracy: Expertise, institutions, and representation.* Cambridge, MA: MIT Press.

Bucchi, Massimiano. (2009). *Beyond technocracy: Science, politics and citizens* (Adrian Belton, Trans.). Dordrecht: Springer.

Charlton, J. (1998). *Nothing about us without us: Disability, oppression, and empowerment.* Berkeley, CA: University of California Press.

Cohen, C., & Timimi, S. (2008). *Liberatory psychiatry: Philosophy, politics, and mental health.* Cambridge: Cambridge University Press.

Drieger, D. (1989). *The last civil rights movement: Disabled People's International.* New York: Macmillan.

Fulford, K. W. M. (2004). Facts/values: Ten principles of values-based medicine. In J. Radden (Ed.), *The philosophy of psychiatry: A companion* (pp. 205–236). Oxford: Oxford University Press.

Fulford, K. W. M., Thornton, T., & Graham, G. (2006). *Oxford texbook of philosophy and psychiatry.* Oxford: Oxford University Press.

Hall, S. (Ed.). (1997). *Representation: Cultural representation and signifying practices.* London: Sage.

Hall, W. (Ed.). (2016). *Outside mental health: Voices and visions of madness.* Madness Radio.

Hamkins, S. (2014). *The art of narrative psychiatry.* Oxford: Oxford University Press.

Harding, S. (2006). *Science and social inequality: Feminist and postcolonial issues.* Chicago, IL: University of Illinois Press.

Laclau, E., & Mouffe, C. (1985). *Hegemony and socialist strategy: Towards a radical democratic politics.* London: Verso.

Laclau, E. & Mouffe, C. (1990). Post-Marxism without apologies. In E. Laclau (Ed.), *New reflections of the revolutions of our time*. London: Verso.

LeFrançois, B. A., Menzies, R., & Reaume, G. (Eds.). (2013). *Mad matters: A critical reader in Canadian mad studies*. Toronto: Canadian Scholars Press.

Lewis, B. (2011). *Narrative psychiatry: How stories can shape clinical practice*. Baltimore, MD: Johns Hopkins Press.

Lewis, B. (2013). A mad fight: Psychiatry and disability activism. In L. Davis (Ed.), *The disability studies reader* (4th ed.). New York: Routledge.

Linton, S. (2013). Reassigning meaning. In L. Davis (Ed.), *The disability studies reader* (4th ed.). New York: Routledge.

Mead, S. (2014). *Intentional peer support—An alternative approach* (4th ed.). Bristol, VT: Sherry Mead.

Mills, C. (2014). Sly normality: Between quiescence and revolt. In B. Burstow, B. A. LeFrançois, & S. Diamond (Eds.), *Psychiatry disrupted: Theorizing resistance and crafting the (r)evolution*. Montreal: McGill-Queen's University Press.

Poole, J., Jivraj, T., Arslanian, A., Bellows, K., Chiasson, S., Hakimy, H. … Reid, J. (2012). Sanism, "mental health," and social work/education: A review and call to action. *Intersectionalities: A Global Journal of Social Work Analysis, Research, Polity, and Practice, 1*, 20–36.

Roberts, L. (2013). *Community-based participatory research for improved mental healthcare: A manual for clinicians and researchers*. Dordrecht: Springer.

Seikkula, J. (2011). Becoming dialogical: Psychotherapy or a way of life? *The Australian and New Zealand Journal of Family Therapy, 32*(3), 179–193.

Smith, A. M. (1998). *Laclau and Mouffe: The radical democratic imaginary*. London: Routledge.

Stastny, P., & Lehmann, P. (Eds.). (2007). *Alternatives beyond psychiatry*. Berlin: Peter Lehmann.

Thomas, P. (2014). *Psychiatry in context: Experience, meaning, and communities*. Monmouth: PCCS.

West, C. (2008). *Hope on a tightrope: Words and wisdom*. Carslbad, CA: Smiley.

Whitaker, R. (2002). *Mad in America: Bad science, bad medicine, and the enduring mistreatment of the mentally ill*. Cambridge: MA: Perseus.

Whitaker, R. (2010). *Anatomy of an epidemic: Magic bullets, psychiatric drugs, and the astonishing rise of mental illness in America*. New York: Broadway.

Chapter 39

Black Resilience in the Face of Bullshit

WELLNESS AND SAFETY PLAN

Adaku Utah

Summary

Wellness plans within public mental health systems, sometimes called "advance directives" or "safety plans," have been reclaimed and adapted as a crucial strategy among mutual aid groups and radical mental health communities for decades. Yet wellness plans, both within and outside the mental health system, have historically excluded or minimized experiences of multiple and intersecting forms of oppression. Utah and Harriet's Apothecary emphasize that a wellness plan should also deliberately address healing from racism, ableism, classism, white supremacy, transphobia, and patriarchy, honoring that wellness looks dramatically different when foregrounding the "distinct definitions of healing & resilience, various shades of access and a wide spectrum of significant realities, that are often changing." The questions elicited by this manual, such as "What does my Black body need to feel safer?" and "What brings my body joy?" are powerful in and of themselves yet also reveal a vision of healing, safety, and thriving spaces for Black people, Indigenous people, and people of color. As a result, "Black Resilience in the Face of Bullshit" offers a practical guide and reflection questions for developing a wellness plan in times of crisis, to define what help, support, and healing mean to each individual even, or especially, when it may mean utilizing community support to stay out of violent or corrupt systems.

The following pieces have appeared previously online and on social media, in different forms and with the author's original artwork. Please head to www.harrietsapothecary. com or follow the @Harrietsapothecary on Instagram to view the original versions of the plan.

*

DOI: 10.4324/9781003148456-44

BLACK RESILIENCE IN THE FACE OF BULLSHIT WELLNESS & SAFETY PLAN

EVERY PART OF YOU IS SACRED

These reflection questions are grounded in a compassionate understanding of our experiences at the edges and centers of multiple sites of intersecting oppressions and privileges. Regardless of your legacy, present and/or future
YOU ARE LOVED
AND
WORTHY OF CARE!

REMEMBER

We each come from distinct
definitions of healing &
resilience,
various shades of access and a
wide spectrum of significant
realities, that are often changing.

This will impact how you create
and maybe change your wellness
plan over time.

REMEMBER

Safety and wellness planning
can support us in minimizing
the current,
potential and future levels of
harm and increase our capacities
to feel safer and resilient.
As we take action to address,
reduce, and/or prevent violence,
we engage in a radical act of
Black love, vast and mighty
enough to transform us in the
present and carry us into the
future we long for and deserve.

HEALING IS NON-LINEAR

this safety plan is also a non-linear process.
you may take 2 steps forward
and 10 steps back.
and vice versa.
that's totally okay AF

YOU ARE WORTH THE TIME

YOUR PLAN WILL TAKE
Developing a plan takes time.
Feel free to answer in one or
more settings. Preferably, pick
a time(s) and place that will
offer you the least distractions
and the most support.

feel free to add additional
questions that make sense for
your Black body.

WATCH OUT FOR...

oppressive internalized narratives
that might arise as you fill this out like
. "i am not worthy", "other things are more
important than my care", "I am too _ _ _ _ _ _ _ _ _
_ _ _ to do this", "I am not enough", "I'm having
a hard time and I don't think anyone can help
someone like me because I am _ _ _ _ _ _ _ _ _ "
These inherited and very well practiced
narratives often haunt us as we seek liberation
in our vessels.
All part of the strategic design of racism,
sexism, ableism, classism, transphobia
white supremacy and
patriarchy.

REFLECTION QUESTIONS

- What historically and currently impacts my ability to be well and/or resilient in my body? (consider individual, community, familial and/or systemic challenges).

- When I am feeling well (physically, emotionally, spiritually well).
  I am… (describe yourself when you are feeling safer and well).

- What brings my body joy?

- What people, places, and/or practices support my body in feeling safer and/or resilient?

- How often does my Black body need to be engaging with these people, places and/or practices? – daily, monthly, weekly, yearly etc.

IN TIMES OF CRISIS...

- How do I want my body to be supported? What are my short- and long-term needs? Which of these would I prefer to do on my own? Which would I prefer support from others?

- What does my Black body need to feel safer?

- Who do I trust to support me?

- Who do I NOT trust to support me?

- What physical, emotional, and/or spiritual symptoms reveal to me and others that I need support caring for my Black body?

IN TIMES OF CRISIS...

- What are my **preferred** practices, rituals, earth medicines, and/or medications?

- What are my **acceptable** practices, rituals, earth medicines, and/or medications?

- What are my **undesirable** practices, rituals, earth medicines, and/or medications?

- What are signs that my wellness plan needs to change?

- Who do I need to share this plan with?

Chapter 40

Demolition, Abolition, and Inherited Legacies of Madness

Leah Harris

Summary

Using the brutalist architecture and demolition of the psychiatric asylum to expand on the harrowing nature of their existence, Harris chronicles the inherited legacy of pain, violence, and systematic abuse perpetrated by the state. "I am still fighting to get the hospital out of me, out of all of us who live with its legacy," Harris states, revealing how they were torn from their mother's arms at birth and the ways in which they have been guided back to a connection with their mother even after her death.

Harris tracks their own and others' reactions to the demolition of asylums, asking those sympathetic to psychiatric asylums to consider protesting "the treatment of the people trapped inside them with equal fervor." They ask: "What is the point of preserving these places as monuments of remembrance, when the abuses of the past continue to reach into the present?" urging us to remember that the abuses of the asylum are far from over. Harris plays within the nuance of relief at seeing the asylum, the site of immense trauma and oppression, demolished, yet simultaneously feeling despair at "how the asylum just keeps evolving, changing, rebuilding, and calling itself by different names." In the end, Harris encourages hope, asserting that when we say, "tear it down," we are fighting for not only an end to violence but also a future of collective care.

*

I've been internet-stalking the Charles W. Landis Mental Health Complex in Wauwatosa, Wisconsin, for 20 years, watching and waiting for its end. Within the hideous, Brutalist architecture, inside its brown brick walls, my beautiful poet mother was psychiatrically incarcerated 24 times between 1968 and 1993, before she died at age 46 in 1996. While the caseworker's final note in her psychiatric chart claims that her death appeared to be from "natural causes," I don't agree at all. There is nothing natural about a 46-year-old woman dying in her sleep. There is nothing natural about being locked in a psych ward two dozen times over the course of a life. There is nothing natural about the brutal treatment she experienced in the Brutalist building, the slow process of giving up prompted by being repeatedly treated as less than human. There was nothing natural about the heavy-duty doses of psychiatric

DOI: 10.4324/9781003148456-45

drugs she was forced to take for her entire adult life, drugs that are well known to cause all manner of metabolic and other adverse effects, including death. This architectural eyesore of a state psychiatric facility was the site of her slow murder. I want it demolished, dead and gone, disappeared from this earth.

Implosion is one of the most dramatic ways to demolish a building, a marvel of science and detonation. The implosion itself occurs in mere seconds, but it can take painstaking years to plan. It involves a carefully orchestrated placement of explosives at the vertical supports, collapsing a building down to what is known as its "footprint," or the boundaries defined by the perimeter of its structure. Implosions are often attended by hundreds of bystanders, a spectator sport.

Included in the toppling of buildings that have outlived their usefulness to systems and society there is the genre of the psychiatric hospital demolition video. One such video on YouTube (Jabbow, 2008) documents the 1989 demolition of the Edgewood Hospital, part of Pilgrim Psychiatric Center in Deer Park, New York, formerly known as Pilgrim State Hospital, once the largest hospital of any kind in the entire world (New York State Office of Mental Health, n.d.), holding captive over 13,000 souls during the height of the asylum era in the 1950s.

In the minutes prior to the implosion, an electric buzz of chatty anticipation moves through the mingling bystanders gathered behind a tall, protective chain-link fence. A low-pitched, mournful siren sounds for several seconds, signaling the building's imminent destruction, eliciting a smattering of onlookers' cheers. Next, a visible flash of explosives from deep within the bowels of the 13-story building; a thunderous double boom as they detonate, making the frame shake. The entire structure drops downward, as if to its knees. The right tower leans slightly and goes down, followed by the central portion of the hospital and its peaked roof, and then the left tower topples over in an almost reluctant, slow-motion crash. More cheers, whistling, and scattered applause erupt from the crowd. Smoke and debris billow into the air, liberating the ghostly imprints, the densest, most painful memories that have been trapped within the walls, producing an ominous greying of the sky as the spectators slowly disperse.

My mother's 24 psychiatric incarcerations at the Mental Health Complex over the course of decades were a direct result of Milwaukee's criminally dysfunctional mental health system. *Chronic Crisis: A System That Doesn't Heal*, a 2013 series by Meg Kissinger in the *Journal-Sentinel*, revealed that one person was committed there 196 times in six years. One-third of people treated at the emergency room returned within 90 days. Experts who studied the system over the past 20 years said it depended on emergency psychiatric treatment more than any system in the United States, neglecting community-based supports that would have stymied the vicious revolving-door cycle. Kissinger's (2013) description of the *Chronic Crisis* series reads: "Despite scandals, studies and promises of reform, the system is like many of its patients: It never gets better."

At a time when many asylums were permanently closing around the United States, the Milwaukee County Mental Health Complex was being built. It was erected in 1968 to replace the Milwaukee County Asylum, which was in turn built to replace the Milwaukee County Asylum for the Chronic Insane, constructed in 1880. The

Wauwatosa County Grounds is a palimpsest of poorhouses, asylums, institutions, and hospitals.

I went on Google Reviews to see what people had to say about the Mental Health Complex in its final years. One reviewer wrote:

> The people they hire are more interested in terrorizing patients than helping them. The only way they helped me was treating me so badly that I wanted to get better so I could get the hell out of there. Do everything you can to keep your loved ones out of this hell hole.

Another review said, "Worst Psych Ward ever. Not even one star. I give it 0 stars." Yet another former patient said, "Major mistreatment of residents, I have never feared for my life like I did when I was here. I still have nightmares of this place." In a 2013 *Milwaukee Journal-Sentinel* interview on YouTube, a former patient who'd been there many times said of the place, "I feel safer in jail than being at the mental health facility." The testimonies only increased my fierce longing to see the building disappeared.

Demolition using a high-reach arm, also known as a long-reach excavator, is typically used instead of implosion on buildings that are higher than 60 feet. It is done with a base machine such as an excavator, fitted with a long demolition arm with a telescopic boom. Demolition tools such as a crusher, shears, or a hammer are affixed to the end of the arm and allow it to crumble the building from the top down. There are many drone videos on YouTube documenting high-reach-arm demolitions of old asylums, such as the Greystone Park Psychiatric Hospital, a magnificent Kirkbride-style building in Parsippany, New Jersey, famed for incarcerating Woody Guthrie within its walls for five years. A group of preservationists had fought the state on demolition and lost; it was finally torn down in 2015. Someone even went to the trouble of creating a romanticized drone video reversing the demolition, resurrecting the building, with massive stones and bits of debris flying vertically upward through the air to return to their former locations, all overlaid with sad piano music and audio clips of people calling the demolition a "tragedy."

The hideous legacy of the beautiful building lives on, five years after it ceased to exist. A woman who was repeatedly raped by an orderly while incarcerated at Greystone between 1989 and 1990, when she was just 17, filed a lawsuit in 2020 against the New Jersey Department of Human Services. And there are several current lawsuits pending regarding sexual violence and abuse at the new Greystone Park Psychiatric Hospital, built in 2009 to replace the old asylum. I wish that those who protest the "tragic" demolition of these places would protest the treatment of the people trapped inside them with equal fervor. What is the point of preserving these places as monuments of remembrance, when the abuses of the past continue to reach into the present?

In June 2001, five years after my mother's death, I traveled to the Mental Health Complex to retrieve her psychiatric records before they were destroyed for good. Grief and the longing to gather up the lost pieces of her story maneuvered me down the fluorescent-lit corridors of the place my mother slept, ate, cried, fought her captors, and dreamed of escape.

The mental death complex, she used to call it, on the few occasions I ever remember her talking about the place.

As I wound my way to the records room, I became convinced that one of the people in one of the hallways would mistake me for an escaping patient. They'd call a code and an orderly's hands would grab me, and they wouldn't let me out until I could prove that I didn't belong in there. My chest tightened in on itself until my breath stuck shallow and panicky in my throat. The corridors seemed to stretch and elongate, telescoping ahead of me as I moved.

Follow the signs on the wall, I told myself. *Just follow the signs*.

One of the rooms was marked "chapel," and I dared to peek inside. It was empty, except for an uncared-for disarray of orange chairs and a few beams of sunlight speckled with dust streaming in through an abstract stained-glass window. As I blinked into the dusty bands of light, whispery sounds filtered through my ears. *Help. Let me out. Please. God*. The whispered prayers grew louder, crowding in on me. All the air went out of the chapel. I willed my body to move, but my limbs were frozen in place.

Hurry, my mother's voice said, as the voices stilled.

The chapel finally let me out.

My body continued to move toward the medical records room, passing the sign for the courtroom where the judges meted out the involuntary commitments. Once you're declared seriously mentally ill or disabled, they almost never believe your side of the story. Such a short and convenient trip from the courtroom to the locked ward.

Retrieving the records was an anticlimactic, transactional experience. "I told you all you needed were the admission and discharge records, which I already sent to you," the older woman employee said in a bored monotone. "But here is all of it." *I told you. All you needed*. People working in places like this like to tell you what you need, even if you're not a patient. I did not speak of the vastness of my need to know what happened to my mother within these walls.

The woman handed me a heavy white cardboard box filled with the ream of records, including at least 100 pages of caseworker notes that she had refused to send me by mail. I was being charged 50 cents per page, and there were a lot of pages.

"That'll be $194.65," she said. I wrote out the check.

Get out of there, my mother said. Gripping onto the records with both hands, I moved as fast as I could while still passing for sane. Time slowed and collapsed as I headed for the exit. I held the double glass door in my sights, barely allowing myself breath until I pushed it open and emerged unscathed into the sunny parking lot. Once I was safely inside the car, I released my vice-grip on the box of records and placed it gently onto the passenger's seat. The white box looked like an urn carrying the storied remains of my mother. The story of how they saw her, anyway. I'd have to read between the lines for the rest.

My breath surged once again into my lungs. *I made it out*, I whispered to myself, to the box, to her. But the fact of the Mental Health Complex remained, solid and casting its shadow.

I currently live in the state of Virginia, where America's first asylum, the Public Hospital for Persons of Insane and Disordered Minds, later to be renamed Eastern

State Hospital, was erected in 1773. The asylum came into being in large part due to the efforts of Francis Fauquier, Royal Governor of the then-colony of Virginia. In 1766, Fauquier addressed the House of Burgesses with these words:

> It is expedient I should also recommend to your Consideration and Humanity a poor unhappy set of People who are deprived of their senses and wander about the Country, terrifying the Rest of their fellow creatures. A legal Confinement, and proper Provision, ought to be appointed for these miserable Objects, who cannot help themselves. Every civilized Country has an Hospital for these People, where they are confined, maintained and attended by able Physicians, to endeavor to restore to them their lost reason.
>
> (Library of Congress, 1766)

Reading Fauquier's words, I'm struck by how closely they resemble those of former Congressman Tim Murphy, a zealous psychologist who seized, parasite-like, on the horrors of Sandy Hook and subsequent mass shootings in America in 2013, scapegoating mad and disabled people for the violence to advance a punitive and regressive legislative agenda. His legislation would have made it easier to force people into treatment and incarcerate them in inpatient facilities for long periods of time, eroding civil rights standards that were specifically designed to prevent the abuses of the asylum era (Harris, 2016).

The first time I sat in a congressional hearing on Tim Murphy's proposed mental health law at the stately House Rayburn Building, I stared into his thin, grim, owlish face as he railed on about "serious mental illness," fairly salivating about how violent and dangerous we are when untreated; how we lack insight into our condition and must be forced into treatment for our own good. For Murphy and the conservative think tanks and family groups that supported him, we are still Fauquier's "miserable objects," "terrifying our fellow creatures," unable to help ourselves or each other. We advocates fought his brutal, regressive agenda at every turn, with the main advantage in our favor being the inability of Congress to get anything substantive done on mental health.

Every time I heard or saw this man speak, I thought: *He is an abuser.* Sure enough, in 2018, Murphy abruptly resigned from Congress due to an infidelity scandal (DeBonis, 2017), along with simultaneous revelations that he had verbally abused his staff and created a toxic work environment (Fuller, 2017). But I could not linger in *schadenfreude* around his downfall for long, because while it stopped the grinding momentum of his legislation, his agenda to get us back into the asylums and under the thumb of carceral state control continues to live on. In December 2019, President Donald Trump held a "mental health summit" at the White House, in which he called for the rebuilding of institutions and getting "very dangerous people" off the streets. Tim Murphy was in the audience.

Despite the pontifications of politicians and pundits, the asylum has never really gone away. It just continues to change form. Three times destroyed by fire, Eastern State Hospital, America's first asylum, continues to operate, although in the 1930s it was moved to a larger parcel of land a few miles away from its original location.

In 1985, the original Georgian-style colonial-era main building, an imposing red brick structure crowned with a cupola and weathervane, was rebuilt, and it is now a museum at the Colonial Williamsburg tourist attraction, complete with replicas of the prison-like cells (Colonial Williamsburg, 2015).

The lore surrounding Dr. John Galt, Eastern State's Civil War-era superintendent, highlights the whitewashing of the racism that has always undergirded mental health care in America and continues to this day. On Eastern State Hospital's (n.d.) account of its history, Galt is lauded as a proponent of the moral treatment philosophy, "an incontrovertibly brilliant physician" who treated patients "without regard to race." Dr. King Davis (2018), scholar on race and psychiatric care in the United States, has corrected this official historical record of Galt's racial benevolence, noting the doctor's hypothesis that enslaved Africans were "immune from mental illness." Popular accounts of Galt's ghost haunting the Colonial Williamsburg museum accord with the state's official view of the doctor as a "compassionate," long-suffering soul driven to suicide by the impact of the war on his patients at the asylum (Phelps, 2020). There is conveniently no mention of race in any of these spooky tales. Such narratives, both official and supernatural, affect another kind of demolition—the demolition of history.

Unused buildings at Eastern State were not demolished by machines or explosives but abandoned to nature. YouTube abounds with videos posted by people who have snuck onto the grounds, exploring the remaining decaying 20th-century era buildings, which have now been halfway reclaimed by lush green foliage. The explorers give each other tips on how to sneak onto the grounds and evade being caught by security. They point their cameras and send their drones down moldering hallways covered in graffiti, searching for ghosts and turning up the strangest items, such as lifeguard noodles and moldy pink baby dolls with unblinking eyes.

The first time I was confined to a psychiatric ward, I was a newborn. I never would have believed it, if I hadn't requested the records from every place I knew of where my mother had been locked up. But there it is in black and white, undeniable on a mimeographed page: as a six-week-old baby, I was admitted to St. Michael Hospital in Milwaukee along with my mother, her mind and body unraveling from postpartum distress.

"At this time, she was blatantly psychotic. She was unable to care for herself and her baby," the summary reads. My mother, always the rebel, refused to take meds so that she could continue to nurse me. In the anything-but-therapeutic atmosphere of an institution, her mind would not settle down. "She has deteriorated, become more angry, more incoherent, and less cooperative in this period of about 7 weeks." The hospital staff did not force her to stop nursing so they could put her on meds. Instead, the state removed me from her custody and transferred her to the Mental Health Complex.

In 2011, St. Michael Hospital was demolished to make way for a family care clinic. News reports quote an administrator who blamed poor and uninsured people seeking emergency care at the hospital, causing the hospital to lose millions of dollars a year ("Milwaukee's St. Michael Hospital to Shut Down," 2006). Photos of the St. Michael demolition on the internet show a white high-reach excavator that resembled a clawing, skeletal arm ripping off the facade of the multi-story red brick building, leaving dangling shards of concrete like flaps of skin, protruding steel-beam innards in its wake.

"This is going to hurt," read the caption of one of the photos.

St. Michael was torn down via a process known as selective demolition, or strip-out, in which materials from the original building are reused, recycled, and incorporated into the new construction. I imagine the family care clinic absorbing into its facade bits of salvaged, decades- old brick and fill that once comprised the walls that held my mother and me as a tiny baby.

The apartment building on Center Street, the only place my mother and I ever lived together, still exists. Google Maps shows me a narrow, nondescript, two-story beige brick building with a hair extension salon below. We lived in a one-bedroom apartment on the second floor, with windows facing the street. A neon sign advertising a dentist's office in the building next door blinked red and blue and green incessantly through our windows. When I try to remember anything at all about the building, all I can see is that neon sign, blinking.

My mother had tried so hard to make a good home for us there, raising me alone while forced to take zombifying quantities of Haldol. My parents were not married when I was conceived, which amounted to a *shonda*, a shameful scandal, in my immigrant Jewish family. But my mother believed in the *shonda* dream of us as much as my father rejected it, not willing to admit that I was of his flesh until a judge proclaimed it. He had his own mental health issues and couldn't, or didn't, help with child support. And so, a combination of poverty and ableism set my mother up to stumble and fall, until the courts stripped her of parental rights when I was four. She was not alone: it turns out that 50 percent of mothers diagnosed with schizophrenia lose their children. Today, at least 30 states have a designation called "predictive neglect," which allows courts to preemptively terminate a parent's rights for having a mental illness diagnosis that authorities *think* will limit the parent's capacity to raise a child.

My family tried to help us where they could, but they were a product of settler colonial values that broke the bonds of traditional, extended-family networks into nuclear-sized entities. That left my mother and me as an isolated island in a stormy sea. When the state subdivided that family unit of two even further, I was put on a plane and sent to live with my maternal grandmother and her second husband in Allentown, Pennsylvania, far away from the influence of my mother's madness.

Losing custody sent my mother speeding down the streets of Milwaukee in her car; court records say that she took the cops on a chase at over 70 miles an hour until they were able to maneuver in front of her car and make her stop. While waiting for her criminal case to be tried, she was committed to the forensic unit of Winnebago Mental Health Institute, itself built upon the site of Northern State Hospital for the Insane, an asylum built in 1873. Once restored to competency, she was eventually found not guilty "by reason of mental defect."

"She has to learn to live in the real world," a doctor's letter to the judge said.

On one of my childhood visits back to Milwaukee after I was taken away, I went with my grandfather to pick up my mother at discharge from some place or another.

Maybe I was eight, or nine. Was it at the Mental Health Complex or one of the other institutions she'd been locked up in over the years? There my memory is blank, and there is no one alive who would remember. Now I realize that she must have managed to finagle a discharge right as I arrived for my visit. How hard she must have played along with the staff to do that, to not demand anything or get angry, or cry, or do anything that would get her in trouble and add days onto her sentence.

My memories tell me that the hallway where we wait for her on the other side of the locked ward door is colorless and smells faintly of urine. And then she is there, beyond the locked door, with her wild, frizzy hair and her hazel eyes, her red lipstick, smiling and smiling, holding a plastic bag containing her possessions. I bound into her arms. She holds me so tight, and for so long. She smells like cigarettes and institutional soap.

Wrecking-ball, or crane-and-ball demolition, is one of the oldest and most well-known forms of building demolition. In fact, the term has become a kind of shorthand used by the press to describe any kind of demolition, even if it's not the precise method that will be used. The ball itself, cast from forged steel, can weigh anywhere from 1,000 to 13,000 pounds. It's suspended from a crane by a cable, whose operator drops or swings it against the structure, repeatedly landing severe and punishing blows until the building is no more.

I could not find any pictures or videos of a wrecking-ball demolition of an asylum. Perhaps they are simply too big and sprawling, too laden with asbestos and other contaminants, for this method to make sense—especially when newer, more efficient technologies are available.

"You came to us as damaged goods!" my maternal grandmother said to me whenever I cried or yelled too loudly or in any way acted like the traumatized child I was. In the 1980s, it was commonly believed that children did not mourn.

"Damaged goods!" My grandmother screamed at me, over and over, until the words swam in my bloodstream and beat in my pulses until I accepted the fact of my essential, inherited damage. I've often wondered what would prompt someone to say those words to a child. I suspect it was likely motivated by her shame about my mother's madness, what I represented by extension. More than anything, she feared history repeating itself. Which it did, once I began to take a wrecking ball to myself.

The hormonal changes associated with puberty transformed the facade of my body into one I no longer recognized. Self-injury was my initial chosen method of demolition, tiny fuses that I placed in strategic places on the body to distract from the long-buried memories and intolerable sensations. This behavior brought on the doctors, seeking to patch up my cracked foundation with pills. At 14, each day I swallowed doses of Prozac that created further fissures in the world beneath my skin. On psychiatric drugs, the impulse to self-harm morphed into full-on suicidal urges. I became determined to find a way to bring my body/building completely down. Much like the careful planning that goes into a building implosion, I systematically plotted out my own collapse down to the footprint.

"My existence is pointless," I wrote in my suicide note at age 15.

"If you don't get help at Charter, get help somewhere," the for-profit hospital chain's TV and radio commercials pleaded to prospective customers throughout the late 1980s and 1990s. You can still find these old television commercials uploaded to YouTube (VHSofDeath, 1996), mostly by people who have themselves been harmed there. As a suicidal teen, I was stashed away, not in a state-run asylum of old, but in the newer, corporate version: Charter Hospital. White privilege and access to private health insurance insulated me from the public mental health system or the juvenile (in)justice system. My young bodymind was confined within the fluorescent-lit hallways of this modern asylum, with its rose-colored carpeting and pictures of abstract flowers on the walls—like you'd find in a hotel room. What I had no way of knowing then was that the carceral logic of these places had barely changed, just the methods of punishment. The lobotomies, ice baths, and cold packs were exchanged for seclusion rooms and five-point restraints. They don't keep you locked away for life as they did in the old asylum days, but as my friend and advocate Chacku Mathai once shared, quoting Shery Mead, creator of the Intentional Peer Support framework: "I wonder if we are not only supporting each other to get out of the hospital and stay out. Maybe we are also supporting each other to get the hospital out of us."[1]

I am still fighting to get the hospital out of me, out of all of us who live with its legacy.

In 2001, when my adult self was ready to remember what my younger self had submerged, I tried to obtain my records from Charter Hospital. I was a year too late. They sent a letter informing me that the records had all been destroyed. The Charter Behavioral Health empire imploded in 2000, when it filed for Chapter 11 bankruptcy. Its downfall was swift. In 1998, the corporation settled with the DOJ after whistleblowers revealed patterns of Medicare fraud (US Department of Justice, 1998), in which elders were admitted without medical necessity and held for as long as possible against their will. Then, in a 1999 *60 Minutes* expose (Reporters' Committee for Freedom of the Press, 1999), Ed Bradley revealed findings from an undercover whistleblower, that staff working with youth were receiving little to no training. At least one child died from injuries caused by blunt-force restraint techniques (CBSNews.com, 1999).

Psychiatric hospital systems are like a multi-headed hydra: when one topples, another grows in its place. After Charter Behavioral Health went under, 12 of its hospitals were bought for $105 million by Universal Health Services (George, 2000), America's largest for-profit behavioral health hospital chain. UHS was soon profiting from the same shady billing practices as Charter had. By 2017, the corporation was under investigation by three federal agencies for Medicare, Medicaid, and private insurance fraud, holding people against their will for as many days as their insurance would pay (US Attorney's Office, Eastern District of Pennsylvania, 2020). UHS is also notorious for cutting corners to save costs; chronic understaffing has resulted in numerous documented cases of neglect and abuse of patients.

When I read in the *Journal-Sentinel* in 2015 that Milwaukee County could permanently shut down the Mental Health Complex (Boehm, 2015) as part of a plan to transition away from its historic overreliance on institutional care, my cells vibrated with giddiness. I thought about how, if Mama were alive, I'd call her to talk about it and we would be celebrating the possibility of the hospital's long-overdue demise.

My excitement waned when I discovered that the replacement for the County Mental Health Complex would be a brand-new facility run by none other than UHS: Granite Hills, a 120-bed, $33 million hospital, not in Wauwatosa but in West Allis (Anderson, 2021). The County's Behavioral Health Division hoped to grant the contract to a local health system, but UHS was the only bidder. The Fortune 500 corporation had long been wanting to break into the Milwaukee market. As the contract with the County Behavioral Health Division was finalized and signed, UHS was paying the federal government and states' attorneys $127 million to settle allegations of Medicare and Medicaid fraud.

Will this brand-new hospital, slated to open this summer, be yet another snake pit in the making? Will historic and ongoing patterns of harm now be privatized behind a glass-paned, light-filled, state-of-the-art facade? Will I be reading disturbing reports about this place in the near future? I worry and wonder, and I think I know the answer.

When I despair at how the asylum just keeps evolving, changing, rebuilding, and calling itself by different names, I hold dear the words of my own Jewish tradition in the ethical text *Pirkei Avot*: "You are not obligated to complete the work, but neither are you free to desist from it." And I remember the words of abolitionist organizer Mariame Kaba, who refers to "hope as a discipline." In an interview in *We Do This 'Til We Free Us*: *Abolitionist Organizing and Transforming Justice*, Kaba (2021) says:

> I don't take a short-term view. I take the long view, understanding full well that I'm just a tiny, little part of a story that already has a huge antecedent and has something that is going to come after that. I'm definitely not going to be even close to around for seeing the end of it. That also puts me in the right frame of mind: that my little friggin' thing I'm doing is actually pretty insignificant in world history, but if it's significant to one or two people, I feel good about that.

I draw strength and sustenance from the wisdom of elders and contemporary organizers, and from the knowledge that all of us who believe in abolition, inclusive of psychiatric abolition, are coconjuring a believed-in hope for a future we may never live to see, the end of history echoing within newer and shinier institutions. Together we fight for a world where all the sites and structures of carceral control are torn down or abandoned, to make way for the liberation of all her people and good stewardship of the planet. Together we fight for a world where all forms of the asylum are eclipsed and made obsolete by the rise of communities of deep belonging and mutual aid, where we collectively care for and with one another in ways that wall off madness no more.

I do not know if I will ever have the opportunity to be a spectator at the planned demolition of the Charles W. Landis Milwaukee County Mental Health Complex. Even if I am not able to see any part of the take-down of this hideous brown structure in person or on the news, I will bear witness in the realms of my imagination, and I will invite my mother to join me. In my dreams, I imagine us on a Milwaukee spring day, setting down lawn chairs behind the tall construction fence and watching the machines go to work. We observe the destruction, brick by brick, wall by wall, reveling in the noisy commotion.

"Tear it down, baby, tear that shit down," Mama says.

"Demolish the mental death complex. Demolish them all!" I yell, thrusting my middle finger forcefully into the air toward the building. We look at each other and laugh, hurling our mad cackles into the wind and dust and din.

Note

1 Conversation between Chacku Mathai and Shery Mead. (2003). Peer Bridger Dialogue. New York.

References

Anderson, Lauren. (2021, September 16). Granite Hills behavioral health hospital in West Allis preparing to welcome patients this fall. *BizTimes*. https://biztimes.com/granite-hills-behavioral-health-hospital-opens-in-west-allis/

Boehm, Don. (2015, October 21). County could demolish old day hospital at mental health complex. *Milwaukee Journal-Sentinel*. https://archive.jsonline.com/news/milwaukee/county-to-demolish-old-day-hospital-at-mental-health-complex-b99600860z1-335249401.html/

CBSNews.com. (1999, April 21). Unsafe restraint. *60 Minutes*. https://www.cbsnews.com/news/unsafe-restraint/

Colonial Williamsburg. (2015, August 28). *The public hospital of 1773 at Colonial Williamsburg*. [Video]. YouTube. Retrieved January 10, 2022, from https://youtu.be/n9LsZ60FQCA

Davis, King. (2018, May 1). Blacks are immune from mental illness. *Psychiatric News*. https://psychnews.psychiatryonline.org/doi/full/10.1176/appi.pn.2018.5a18

DeBonis, Mike. (2017, October 5). Rep. Tim Murphy resigns from Congress after allegedly asking woman to have abortion. *The Washington Post*. https://www.washingtonpost.com/powerpost/rep-tim-murphy-resigns-from-congress-after-allegedly-asking-woman-to-have-abortion/2017/10/05/7a68a414-aa08-11e7-850e-2bdd1236be5d_story.html

Eastern State Hospital. (n.d.) *The history of Eastern State*. https://esh.dbhds.virginia.gov/History.html

Fuller, Matt. (2017, October 13) Capitol hell: Inside Rep. Tim Murphy's toxic congressional office. *Huffington Post*. https://www.huffpost.com/entry/tim-murphy-toxic-office_n_59e0b4c9e4b0a52aca173676

George, John. (2000, August 7). Analysis: Charter deal too good to pass up. *Philadelphia Business Journal*. https://www.bizjournals.com/philadelphia/stories/2000/08/07/story3.html

Harris, Leah. (2016, November 23). Washington's horrible mental health legislation. *Huffington Post Blog*. https://www.huffpost.com/entry/washingtons-horrible-mental-health-legislation_b_8623226

Jabbow, Gerard. (2008, November 16). *Edgewood demolition pilgrim state hospital.* [Video]. YouTube. Retrieved January 10, 2022, from https://youtu.be/llsGvmAh1HI

Kaba, Mariame. (2021). *We do this 'til we free us: Abolitionist organizing and transforming justice.* Haymarket Books.

Kissinger, Meg. (2013) Chronic crisis: A system that doesn't heal. *Milwaukee Journal-Sentinel.* https://archive.jsonline.com/news/milwaukee/chronic-crisis-a-system -that-doesnt-heal-milwaukee-county-mental-health-system-210480011.html#!/gaps -in-the-system/

Library of Congress. (1766). *The speech of the Honble Francis Fauquier, Esq.; his Majesty's Lieutenant Governour, and commander in chief of the Colony and Dominion of Virginia.* Retrieved January 10, 2022, from http://www.loc.gov/resource/rbpe .1780020c.

Milwaukee Journal-Sentinel. (2013, June 3). *A patient's view of the Milwaukee county mental health complex.* [Video]. YouTube. https://youtu.be/9Uxe0hLe1yU

Milwaukee's St. Michael Hospital to Shut Down. (2006, May 9). *Daily Reporter.* https:// dailyreporter.com/2006/05/09/milwaukees-st-michael-hospital-to-shut-down/

New York State Office of Mental Health. (n.d.). *About pilgrim psychiatric center.* Retrieved January 10, 2022, from https://omh.ny.gov/omhweb/facilities/pgpc/

Phelps, Linda Landreth. (2020, September 28). Haunted Williamsburg. *House and Home Magazine.* http://thehouseandhomemagazine.com/culture/haunted-williamsburg/

Reporters' Committee for Freedom of the Press. (1999, May 3). *Court refuses to restrain '60 Minutes II' broadcast.* https://www.rcfp.org/court-refuses-restrain-60-minutes -ii-broadcast/

US Attorney's Office, Eastern District of Pennsylvania. (2020, July 10). *Universal health services, Inc. to pay $117 million to settle false claims act allegations.* https://www .justice.gov/usao-edpa/pr/universal-health-services-inc-pay-117-million-settle-false -claims-act-allegations

US Department of Justice. (1998, August 19). *Psychiatric hospital settles allegations of Medicaid fraud.* https://www.justice.gov/archive/opa/pr/1998/August/378civ .html

VHSofDeath. (1996). *Worried about your teenager?—Charter PSA.* [Video]. YouTube. https://youtube/XpRp9KR9Whk

A Critical Overview of Mental Health-Related Beliefs, Services and Systems in Uganda and Recent Activist and Legal Challenges[1]

Kabale Benon Kitafuna

Summary

Researchers and journalists such as China Mills and Ethan Waters have brought attention to the export of psychiatry to the Global South and to the complexity around whether Western psychiatric models and treatment undermine indigenous knowledge, create even greater human rights issues, and/or provide access to desirable modern services such as psychotropic medication. As Mills writes in *Decolonizing Global Mental Health*, questions about psychiatry as a colonial export leave us

> in a strange place, where we are led to wonder whether we should call for equality in global access to psychiatry, in global psychiatrization, whether "everyone, everywhere" should have the right to a psychotropic citizenship, and whether mental health can, or should, be global.

The ways in which psychiatry weaves itself within the current systems, legislation, and values of a place will be drastically different around the world. Mental health and human rights activists, especially in the Global South, face an interesting challenge, as they are often criticized for advocating for community programs, peer support, and an end to coercive treatment when some view these "alternative" methods as a "luxury" they cannot afford in places where there may be little or no access to treatment of any kind.

In this chapter, Kabale hones in on the attempts made in Uganda to bring equity, dignity, and basic human rights to those with mental health concerns. He describes the structural manifestations of human rights violations in Uganda due to colonial psychiatry, the rise of the asylum, and the budding formalized role of peer support

DOI: 10.4324/9781003148456-46

workers in an already fraught field. He points to the lag time between human rights legislation and implementation, and the corruption that often fails to capture the full extent of the accountability needed to truly end discrimination and violence, isolation, and exclusion.

*

Witchcraft and Mental Illness in Ugandan Society

Throughout the pre-colonial and colonial periods, Ugandan culture positioned supernatural factors as the primary cause of mental illness. And, unlike high income, Anglophone countries, witchcraft was the subject of criminal sanctions well into the 20th century (Mutungi, 2011), with laws regarding witchcraft still remaining active as of 2021. Under the Ugandan Witchcraft Act of 1964, the court was able to issue "exclusion orders" explicitly banning occupants from a given community for a set length of time, but also penalizing false accusations of witchcraft. While in theory this might have provided some protection to individuals with mental illness, in reality the Act was not explicit enough to curtail discrimination and those with MI were therefore often convicted. Meanwhile, some have argued that the Act simultaneously defined 'witchcraft' in such a way as to also limit potentially possible or therapeutic alternative cultural healing practices (cf. Mulumba et al., 2021).

Outside spheres of (neo-)colonial control, however, traditional healers were and continue to be called on to provide treatment or intervention in some form. In general, traditional healers have viewed those affected by MI as possessed by spirits or demons or suffering from the effects of witchcraft in other ways. Healers may use herbs and spiritual rituals to appease ancestral spirits, to purge the ostensible victim, or remove the effects of witchcraft. In some cases, these practices involve binding, chaining or force, in other cases actively contribute to healing and are perceived by those affected as beneficial (Abbo et al., 2012; Abbo, 2011). Over the past century, practices have also become increasingly syncretic or integrative, and some traditional healers actively integrate more biomedical "Western" practices, and frequently refer families to medical care (Akol et al., 2018; Teuton et al., 2007).

Early Colonial Psychiatry

In the early 20th century, colonial government administrators introduced segregated institutional care in response to perceptions of an increased number of Ugandans with mental illness (cf. Pringle, 2015, 2019b). In the early 1920 s, the District commission in Hoima ordered 'mad men and women' to be removed to a garrisoned prison in a small town in southern Uganda. The primary motivation behind this removal was not treatment but rather the ostensible 'protection' of the public and their property from allegedly destructive "lunatics"; administrators wanted to reassure community members that they would be safe from the "dangerousness" of those affected by mental illness. As the Mulago Mental Hospital Superintendent, Charles Baty, wrote in the early 40s:

Many years ago there were no Mental Hospitals in Africa and mad people just went walking about and sometimes died, and sometimes they killed people and set fire to houses and stole and did damage to other peoples [sic.] property...Sometimes...they were caught and chained up in a little house and kept there until they died or got better' [but altogether these conditions were] very troublesome both for the people who look after mad people and for the mad people themselves, so Uganda like all other African countries came to have a Mental Hospital because lunatics are less troublesome and the country is much safer when lunatics are kept in a place by themselves where they are properly looked after.

(Baty quoted in Pringle, 2019a).

In reality, the prison facility cum asylum in southern Hoima was poorly ventilated and never cleaned. Patients were looked after by prison wardens and staff, generally with no training in mental health or illness, who made no attempts to interact with patients beyond slipping containers of food through the small space created when patients' doors were cracked open during meal times. While these "patients" were nominally separated from prisoners, and categorized as patients rather than prisoners, they were in fact provided only custodial care, and had no right or ability to leave the prison-asylum.

Professionalized Care in the First Half of the 20th Century

Over the following decades, colonial medical practitioners and administrators eventually intervened, determining that the "mentally sick" should be removed from a prison environment and instead treated as "sick" patients in a more hospital-like setting (see Baty quote above; cf. Pringle, 2019a). During the early 1930s, a site on Mulago Hill, 100 m from the main hospital was identified. (Due to perceptions that those experiencing mental illness would disrupt patients and visitors at the main hospital, the psychiatric facility was intentionally located some distance away (Wood, 1968). In 1934, construction of the ward was completed. Between 1936 and 1937, at least forty patients were admitted to the 'old Mulago,' as it eventually came to be known. In contrast to Hoima Prison, at Mulago the patients were looked after by nursing attendants. These attendants did not have formal training but were nevertheless encouraged to learn to engage with mental health patients on the job. Then, in 1938, a mental treatment ordinance passed, paving the way for the introduction of what were framed as 'modern' and 'scientific' psychiatric services. This ordinance later became an act of parliament. In 1940, the first forty patients from Hoima prison were transferred to Old Mulago hospital, adding to the existing cohort of patients and leading to overcrowding. The wards became overwhelmed and difficult to manage, and because they were close to the road, commentators at the time described patients visibly smearing themselves with excreta, undressing, and sometimes throwing excreta at those passing by on the road. Pressure on administrators to address these problems grew.

The National Mental Referral Hospital and Formal
Nursing and Psychiatric Training and Certification

To address the situation then, a 600 square yard piece of land was identified that was located 8 km east of Kampala city on the shores of Lake Victoria (Ndyanabangi et al., 2004). This land would become Uganda's "national referral hospital" designed to admit patients from all over the country. The facility was named Butabika Hospital, a name derived from the Lugandan word *kutabika* (literally "to become mentally disturbed"). In 1954 the first Butabika wards, kitchen and an office block were constructed, and in 1955 the buildings officially opened. Men and women, explicitly required to be physically strong, were recruited to manage inpatients and each ward had a capacity of 50 beds. In 1956, formal training of nursing attendants began in the wards, led by predominantly European ward leaders (Pringle, 2019b). In a short space of time, Butabika hospital became the largest and most efficient mental health institution in sub-Saharan Africa. Butabika's forensic unit, the "broadmore" (now known as *kirinya* ward) opened in 1959.

A nurses training school was opened at Butabika in 1960, initially led by a European nurse tutor – Hope Wood; the first African principal nursing tutor was Vincent B. Wankiri (Pringle, 2019b). While there was initially no registration associated with nursing, by the late 1960 s, psychiatric nursing had become a registered profession and the first registered nurses qualified in 1972. Among psychiatrists, the first Ugandan Medical superintendent, Dr. Steven Bossa, assumed leadership in 1968, later becoming the first African-Ugandan professor of psychiatry. Although an official department of psychiatry (headed by a doctor with specialization in psychiatry) was opened in the early 60 s, the challenges involved in establishing psychiatry as a legitimate medical specialty were substantial. For example, there was a chronic shortage of teaching staff and lack of scholarly training materials and resources (Pringle, 2019b). By 1970, Uganda had barely five psychiatrists. These persistent shortages ultimately led to the decision to train a cadre of psychiatric personnel mid-way between a psychiatric nurse and a psychiatrist, whose primary role was to help supplement services that would otherwise have been provided by psychiatrists. Eventually, these personnel were titled psychiatric clinical officers (PCOs), and formalized as a Diploma Level position (Kigozi et al., 2010; Ndyanabangi et al., 2004). Formal training of PCOs began in 1979 and candidates were typically selected from among already registered psychiatric nurses.

Human Rights and the Law in Uganda Circa 1950–2018

Turning to modern legal history, Uganda's first Mental Health Treatment Act, modelled after the Mental Health Treatment Act of 1959 in the UK, was signed into law in 1964, only a few years after Butabika opened. Replacing all earlier mental health treatment ordinances, the Act has been described by legal scholars as "welfarist or medical model legislation [that] focuses on promoting the role of medical professionals" (Nyombi et al., 2014). Among other things, the Act made it possible for magistrates to sign temporary detention orders (known as "reception orders") and place patients at the hospital under legal surveillance. No criteria were provided for involuntary detention, essentially allowing medical professionals to request or certify involuntary treatment without either procedural safeguards or standards. The Act also created a "Minister's order" for patients who were charged with crimes that were ostensibly due to 'insanity,' leading to a form of legal jeopardy in which the judicial branch was forced to share powers with the executive (i.e. Minister's office). The result was that often Minister's orders aimed to protect individuals from criminal adjudication failed because they were over-ruled or circumvented by judges.

A 2010 review of the Act by the Mental Health and Poverty Project (MHaPP) using a World Health Organization (WHO) tool developed for the evaluation of mental health laws identified numerous violations, concluding that it is "prejudiced and hostile to persons with mental illness" and "fails to promote and protect the rights of persons with mental illness both within the health care context and in the community" (MHaPP, 2010).

While the Act remained in force until a recent overhaul (see below), interim human rights laws and policies helped to somewhat mitigate the violations unaddressed by the 1964 Act. For example, the Uganda Human Rights Commission (https://www.uhrc .ug/) was formed in 1995 as a governmental oversight body mandated to investigate and hear cases of human rights violations or abuses (cf. Hatchard, 1999). Designed to cover human rights violations of all kinds, the Commission's work has nevertheless been limited by both insufficient funds and a political atmosphere in which it is often difficult or impossible to carry out conclusive and timely investigations in mental health institutions or hospitals and as well violations occurring in the community. One legal scholar has gone so far to describe the Commission as a "toothless bulldog" (Matshekga, 2002). Among other complicating factors specific to psychosocial disabilities, police officers often tasked with investigations are often themselves implicated in rights violations and even when not directly involved, lack the knowledge to investigate crimes against individuals with disabilities.

Meanwhile, an initial Ugandan Persons with Disabilities Act was passed by Parliament in 2006 and modified in 2016. A review by the United Nations Office of the High Commissioner for Human Rights nevertheless noted a history of delays in implementation, ambiguities of wording that in effect leave the status quo in place, and failures to include explicit policies to ensure the greater inclusion of persons with disabilities, including provisions for disability-based accommodations or affirmative action (UNOHCHR, 2018). Thus, in spite of some policy advances, we still witness significant stigma and discrimination against persons with mental disabilities (Cooper et al., 2010; Drew et al., 2013; Enonchong, 2017; Mfoafo-M'Carthy et al., 2021). On a regular basis, many Ugandans with mental health challenges are deprived of their right to be treated as valued individuals, and are instead stigmatized and marginalized in their own communities, as well as in treatment facilities where they are commonly subjected to wide ranging forms of human rights violations. Specifically, ongoing violations documented by domestic and international human rights groups include arbitrary use of seclusion without proper regulations and supervision, violation of rights to privacy (removal of clothes while in forced seclusion), overmedication with the primary purposes of controlling the movement of patients, and overcrowding beyond bed capacity (MDAC, 2014a, 2014b; MDAC et al., 2015). Structural rights violations also include unequal funding allocations to mental health care relative to other health section budget lines.

Legal Developments after 2018

In 2019, Parliament passed a new Mental Health Treatment Act, in theory strengthening protections in several key areas. For example, the Act requires the implementation of a new mental health board (the Uganda Mental Health Advisory Board), requires consent for treatment (except under designated circumstances), and [provides some degree of protection for individuals with mental illness in institutional settings. The new Act also provides that a person who ill-treats or tortures an individual with mental illness, knowing that the individual in question is a person with mental illness, can be held criminally liable, with punishments including a fine not exceeding one hundred and eighty currency points, a term of imprisonment not exceeding eighteen months or both. Section 27 of the Act requires the investigation of deaths related to mental illness and provision of all such reports to the Mental Health Advisory Board.

While implementation of at least some of these protections should be straightforward, at the time of writing (fall 2021) there had already been extensive implementation delays since the Act was first signed into law on in December 2019. As of late 2021, the minister of health had not yet begun formal implementation of the Act, nor has moved to implement changes in practice based on initial draft mental health policy guidelines and regulations designed to align with the Act's new policies.

Meanwhile, the Ugandan Human Rights Enforcement Act (HREA) of 2019 ostensibly provides another avenue for the enforcement of human rights. In response to historical limits on judicial independence and power, HREA gives the judiciary substantive leverage in the enforcement of court decisions, bolstering the ability of the courts to protect human rights. In addition, in response to older policy which disallowed individual public officers from being held accountable for violations of human rights, the HREA specifically allows for criminal proceedings against public officers, even if working in an official capacity at the time of the violation. If fully implemented, HREA would therefore help ensure accountability at an individual level while also creating mechanisms for the compensation of the victims of human rights violations. Once again, however, as of late 2021, there appears to have been little headway in implementation, and minimal awareness of the Act among either government leaders or the institutions (including psychiatric wards) where rights are regularly violated. Legislation can only bring about change if it is implemented and enforced.

Efforts to Improve the Status of Persons with Psychosocial Disabilities outside of Government and Law

Activism and Advocacy

In the last decade, mental health activists and peer supporters have made significant strides in advocating for the rights of persons affected by mental illness in Uganda. These efforts have included legal challenges to existing law and policy, initiatives to increase public awareness and challenge discriminatory attitudes and language, and the development of peer support. With respect to legal advocacy, in at least a handful of cases, grassroots activists and public interest law groups have successfully held individual staff or hospitals accountable through litigation of human rights violations in courts of law (see e.g. Kabale, companion article in press). Civil society organizations have taken steps to change legal practices by drafting judicial guidelines relevant to the handling of mental health cases in court; however, as of writing these recommendations have not yet be adopted by the judiciary or acknowledged by the chief justice of Uganda.

National and international human rights policy and advocacy efforts have helped Ugandan activists leverage the legal system in the service of change. For example, in 2013 the United Nations special rapporteur for the Committee on Torture called on member states to impose an absolute ban on forced and/or nonconsensual medical interventions targeting persons with disabilities. And 2012 Ugandan anti-torture laws (Prohibition and Prevention of Torture Act of 2012) holds that electro-convulsive therapy (ECT) when forced on persons with psychosocial disabilities "satisfies both [the] intent and purpose required under article I of the Convention against Torture" notwithstanding medical professionals claims of good intentions.

Turning to mutual aid, the Butabika – East London Link, a project to promote bidirectional exchange between the East London National Health Service (NHS) and Butabika Hospital, sponsored an initial two-year peer worker training and implementation scheme in 2012–2013 (see Baillie et al., 2015; Hall et al., 2017; Ryan et al., 2019). Building on the successes of this initial effort, the joint project established a recovery college on the Butabika Hospital grounds in 2015. The Recovery College was co-designed by former patients trained as peer support workers or recovery trainers alongside hospital staff/professionals in the mental health field. However, as has been true in other countries, recovery trainers have encountered challenges and push-back as they navigate the boundaries between peer support work within the hospital and advocacy work focused on systems change (challenging hospital practices). Tensions have played out both within Butabika Hospital and in the community. On the community side too, peer support workers have sometimes found themselves forced to choose between working within civil society organizations or organizing independent community-based organizations (CBOs) or non-governmental organizations (NGOs) that allow for more direct decision making and advocacy able to more directly challenge existing institutions and institutional practices.

Peer support workers and activists representing different Ugandan organizations have also been involved in the United Nation's Universal Periodic Review (with a focus on human rights issues). The International Disability Alliance and its African arm, the Africa Disability Forum, have also been key in empowering some peer support workers to move into administrative leadership roles and represent Ugandan activist perspectives at continental and international levels, including within the United Nations Convention on the Rights of Persons with Disabilities' Human Rights Council (IDA, 2016).

At the country-level, in 2017, a group of psychosocial disability activists formed the Mental Health Coalition of Uganda, an independent psychosocial disability advocacy organization. The Coalition has helped strengthen independent activist voices and has helped hold hospitals and hospital staff accountable for human rights violations including seclusion and death in mental health institutions, rape, and other forms of torture. While enormous problems and challenges remain, progress across both the independent advocacy sector as well as through the integration of peer support workers and initiatives within existing systems nevertheless represent a significant advance over the landscape in prior decades.

Discussion and Conclusion

The core human rights principle of "dignity" – honor and respect for persons, regardless of identity or disability – was first introduced into legal frameworks through the Universal Declaration of Human Rights of 1948 (UDHR): "all human beings are born free and equal in dignity and rights." The concept of dignity is interlinked with social justice, requiring equal opportunities and privileges in society in a way that explitly [sic] includes members of historically marginalized groups including, in this context, persons living with mental, intellectual or psychosocial disabilities. In "Justice as Fairness," John Rawls (1991) argued that social justice is fundamentally tied to ensuring the protection of equal access to liberties, rights and opportunities universally for all humans, as well as the moral duty to provide care and support for the least advantaged members of society. As is true around the world, Ugandans with mental illness are and have been subject to marked stigma, social exclusion and punitive treatment in institutions and jails. Both cultural Ugandan belief systems and Western colonial frameworks have contributed to discriminatory practices at key historical junctures.

Nevertheless, over the past 2–3 decades, the country has experienced both incremental improvements and more revolutionary advancements, as individuals and activists with psychosocial disabilities have acquired power, increased community awareness of the treatment of individuals with mental illness, and pushed for change. This momentum has been aided by international developments, including the UN CRPD, as well as international disability alliances, and shifts in international law.

Declarations

Conflict of interest The author reports no conflicts of interest relevant to the writing of this manuscript. This paper does not involve human subjects research.

Note

1 Originally printed in: *Community Mental Health Journal*, Vol. 58, pp. 829–834 by Springer Nature. Reprinted with Permission.

References

Abbo, C. (2011). Profiles and outcome of traditional healing practices for severe mental illnesses in two districts of Eastern Uganda. *Global Health Action*, 4(1), 7117–7127.

Abbo, C., Okello, E. S., Musisi, S., Waako, P., & Ekblad, S. (2012). Naturalistic outcome of treatment of psychosis by traditional healers in Jinja and Iganga districts, Eastern Uganda–a 3-and 6 months follow up. *International Journal of Mental Health Systems*, 6(1), 1–11.

Akol, A., Moland, K. M., Babirye, J. N., & Engebretsen, I. M. S. (2018). We are like co-wives: Traditional healers' views on collaborating with the formal child and adolescent mental health system in Uganda. *BMC Health Services Research*, 18(1), 1–9.

Baillie, D., Aligawesa, M., Birabwa-Oketcho, H., Hall, C., Kyaligonza, D., Mpango, R., et al. (2015). Diaspora and peer support working: Benefits of and challenges for the Butabika–East London link. *BJPsych International*, 12(1), 10–13.

Cooper, S., Ssebunnya, J., Kigozi, F., Lund, C., Flisher, A., & MHaPP Research Programme Consortium. (2010). Viewing Uganda's mental health system through a human rights lens. *International Review of Psychiatry*, 22(6), 578–588.

Drew, N., Funk, M., Kim, C., Lund, C., Flisher, A. J., Osei, A., et al. (2013). Mental health law in Africa: Analysis from a human rights perspective. *Journal of Public Mental Health*, 12, 1.

Enonchong, L. S. (2017). Mental disability and the right to personal liberty in Africa. *The International Journal of Human Rights*, 21(9), 1351–1377.

Hall, C., Baillie, D., Basangwa, D., & Atukunda, J. (2017). Brain gain in Uganda: A case study of peer working as an adjunct to statutory mental health care in a low-income country. In Ross G. White, Sumeet Jain David M.R. Orr, & Ursula M. Read. *The Palgrave Handbook of sociocultural perspectives on global mental health* (pp. 633–655). London: Palgrave Macmillan.

Hatchard, J. (1999). A new breed of institution: The development of human rights commissions in commonwealth Africa with particular reference to the Uganda Human Rights Commission. *Comparative and International Law Journal of Southern Africa*, 32(1), 28–53.

International Disability Alliance (IDA). (2016). Compilation of UN human rights recommendations-Uganda. Retrieved January 6, 2022, from https://www.internation aldisabilityalliance.org/resources/compilation-un-human-rights-recommendations -uganda

Kigozi, F., Ssebunnya, J., Kizza, D., Cooper, S., & Ndyanabangi, S. (2010). An overview of Uganda's mental health care system: Results from an assessment using the world health organization's assessment instrument for mental health systems (WHO-AIMS). *International Journal of Mental Health Systems*, 4(1), 1–9.

Matshekga, J. (2002). Toothless bulldogs-the human rights commissions of Uganda and South Africa: A comparative study of their independence. *African Human Rights Law Journal*, 2, 68–81.

Mental Health Disability Advocacy Center (MDAC). (2014a). *Psychiatric hospitals in Uganda: A human rights investigation*. MDAC.

Mental Health Disability Advocacy Center (MDAC). (2014b). *They don't consider me as a person: Mental health and human rights in Ugandan communities*. MDAC.

Mental Health Disability Advocacy Center, Mental Health Uganda & Heartsounds Uganda. (2015). DPO/NGO information to the 4th pre-sessional working group of the United Nations Committee on the Rights of Persons with Disabilities for consideration when compiling the List of issues on the first report of the Republic of Uganda under the convention on the rights of persons with disabilities (CRPD). Retrieved January 6, 2022, from https://tbinternet.ohchr.org/Treaties/CRPD/Shared%20Documents/UGA/INT_CRPD_ICO_UGA_21584_E.doc

Mental Health and Poverty Project (MHaPP). (2010). Policy brief 3: Mental health law reform in Uganda. Retrieved January 6, 2022, from http://www.rodra.co.za/images/countries/uganda/research/Mental%20Health%20Law%20Reform%20-%20Uganda.pdf

Mfoafo-M'Carthy, M., & Grischow, J. (2021). "Hope deferred...": Meeting the challenges of stigma toward Ghanaians diagnosed with mental illness. *Social Work in Mental Health*. https://doi.org/10.1080/15332985.2021.1996504.

Mulumba, M., Ruano, A. L., Perehudoff, K., & Ooms, G. (2021). Decolonizing health governance: A Uganda case study on the influence of political history on community participation. *Health and Human Rights*, 23(1), 259–270.

Mutungi, O. K. (2011). Witchcraft and the criminal law in East Africa. *Valparaiso University Law Review*, 5(3), 524–555.

Ndyanabangi, S., Basangwa, D., Lutakome, J., & Mubiru, C. (2004). Uganda mental health country profile. *International Review of Psychiatry*, 16(1–2), 54–62.

Nyombi, C., Kibandama, A., & Kaddu, R. (2014). A critique of the Uganda mental health treatment act, 1964. *Mental Health Law & Policy Journal*, 3(1), 505–526.

Pringle, Y. (2015). Investigating "mass hysteria" in early postcolonial Uganda: Benjamin H. Kagwa, East African psychiatry, and the Gisu. *Journal of the History of Medicine and Allied Sciences*, 70(1), 105–136.

Pringle, Y. (2019a). A place on Mulago Hill. In *Psychiatry and decolonisation in Uganda. Mental health in historical perspective*. Palgrave Macmillan. https://doi.org/10.1057/978-1-137-60095-0_2.

Pringle, Y. (2019b). The 'Africanisation' of psychiatry. In *Psychiatry and decolonisation in Uganda. Mental health in historical perspective*. Palgrave Macmillan. https://doi.org/10.1057/978-1-137-60095-0_3.

Rawls, J. (1991). Justice as fairness: Political not metaphysical. In *Equality and Liberty* (pp. 145–173). London: Palgrave Macmillan.

Ryan, G. K., Kamuhiirwa, M., Mugisha, J., Baillie, D., Hall, C., Newman, C., et al. (2019). Peer support for frequent users of inpatient mental health care in Uganda: Protocol of a quasi-experimental study. *BMC Psychiatry*, 19(1), 1–12.

Teuton, J., Dowrick, C., & Bentall, R. P. (2007). How healers manage the pluralistic healing context: The perspective of indigenous, religious and allopathic healers in relation to psychosis in Uganda. *Social Science & Medicine*, 65(6), 1260–1273.

United Nations Office of the High Commissioner for Human Rights (OHCHR). (2018). The rights of persons with disabilities in Uganda: An assessment of selected national laws. Retrieved January 6, 2022, from https://uganda.ohchr.org/Content/publications/National%20Disability%20Analysis%20Report.pdf

Wood, J. F. (1968). A half century of growth in Ugandan psychiatry. In Stuart A. Hall (Ed.), *Uganda Atlas of disease distribution* (p. 118). Dept. of Preventive Medicine, Makerere University College, Kampala.

Editor's Reference

Mills, C. (2014). *Decolonizing global mental health: The psychiatrization of the majority world*. London: Routledge.

Original Publisher's Note Springer Nature remains neutral with regard to jurisdictional claims in published maps and institutional affiliations.

Chapter 42

Letter to the Mother of a "Schizophrenic"

WE MUST DO BETTER THAN FORCED TREATMENT

Will Hall

Summary

In this chapter, written as a letter to the mother of a son who is dealing with trauma and extreme states, Will Hall presents the case against forced psychiatric treatment. Hall tells a compassionate story of his encounter with this young man and reflects on his own reactions to him as one who has also been labeled with mental illness. His reflections reveal the dangers of reducing sufferers to patients who must receive treatment even if it violates their own desires. Hall also reveals to us the complex and brilliant mind of the son as he grapples with reality and nonreality. We learn that there can be viable relational alternatives to mainstream medical treatment for schizophrenia—grounded in trust, respect, and humanity—that could better serve this son and countless others. Forced treatment remains a controversial issue in psychiatry among patients, clinicians, and family members. By telling this very human story, Hall shows us what individuals and families could gain if we expanded our thinking about schizophrenia, trauma, and treatment and made space for human connection.

*

A few months ago I met your son. He said he would be waiting for us in the Berkeley park near where he sleeps outside at night, but at the last minute he called and was in San Francisco. He said he was at "the Mrs. Doubtfire house" with a photograph of his best friend, and that the photo showed numbers and codes predicting Robin Williams' suicide. He found the house where Williams made one of his films and was trying to talk to the owner: it was all part of a complex plan, marked mathematically in signs and omens he was collecting.

DOI: 10.4324/9781003148456-47

We drove across the Bay, worried. Were we too late? Would he be arrested and end up in the hospital again, this time for trespassing and harassment, a psychotic man caught bothering someone at a private residence?

When the GPS showed we were getting near the address he gave, I started to see people milling around, a commotion, cars stopped. My first thought was that something had happened. Maybe we weren't in time, maybe he was already in trouble with the police, arrested at the house he seemed obsessed with?

At Steiner and Broadway, we found your son, sitting on the sidewalk—but he wasn't alone. He wasn't the only one interested in the Mrs. Doubtfire house. The sidewalk was strewn with flowers, and dozens of other people were also there. What first seemed crazy, now seemed normal: many people, like your son, were drawn to the private residence where a Robin Williams film was made, to commemorate the actor's suicide with a pilgrimage.

I walked up to your son and greeted him, unsure how this young disheveled man would respond to me. I had been told he was considered "severely mentally ill," the worst of the worse, so beyond reach in his delusions that clinicians were considering using force to bring him to the hospital for treatment. But as soon as we made eye contact I was surprised. There was a clear feeling of affinity and communication. He explained in rapid speech about the numbers and messages on the photo, Robin Williams' middle name, and the sidewalk code. It was all part, he said, of an alphanumeric psyche that communicates to him through signs and coincidences.

It was exhilarating and exhausting keeping up with the math calculations, anagrams, and nimble associations that flowed when he spoke. But he also at times talked normally, planned a walk up the street to a coffeehouse, and explained what had happened about our meeting. I lost the thread at different points in our discussion, but one thing was clear: your son is brilliant. I was not surprised when he told us he got a perfect score on the SAT. "It was easy," he explained when I asked. "Anyone can get a perfect score if they take the practice tests."

We were quickly engrossed in conversation, and when he suddenly wove the author Kurt Vonnegut into the pattern, my eyes widened. Just moments before our meeting I was talking with my colleague, telling my own story of meeting Vonnegut. And now here your son was mentioning the author. I was amazed by the coincidence. As your son's talk became wilder and more complex, referencing the Earth Consciousness Coordinating Office, SEGA Dreamcast, and numerology, and as he did math equations instantly to prove his obscure points, I sensed an uncanny power and clairvoyance in the air. I was in the presence of someone in a different reality, but a reality with its own validity, its own strange truth. A different spiritual view.

Perhaps I am eager to emphasize your son's talents because today he finds himself so fallen. I don't romanticize the suffering that he, or anyone, endures. His unusual thoughts and behavior led to a diagnosis of schizophrenia and seem to be part of deeper emotional distress he is struggling with. I don't romanticize because I've been through psychosis and altered states myself. I've been diagnosed schizophrenic, many years and many life lessons ago, moving on with my life only after I found ways to embrace different realities and still live in this one.

So when we met your son I was completely surprised. The "severely mentally ill man" I was told needed to be forced into treatment was intelligent, creative, sensitive—and also making sense. Like someone distracted by something immensely important, he related to us in bits and pieces as he sat in conversation. Living on the street and pursuing an almost incomprehensible "calorie game" of coincidences on food wrappers isn't much of a life, perhaps. And maybe it's not really a choice—at least not a choice that most of us would make, concerned more with getting by than we are with art, spirit, and creativity. What surprised me was the connection I had with your son. Because I took the time, and perhaps I also have the background and skill, I was quickly able to begin a friendship.

By taking interest in his wild visions, not dismissing them as delusional, and by telling him about my own mystical states, not acting like an expert to control him, we began to make a bond. I spoke with respect and interest in his world, rather than trying to convince him he "needs help." What, after all, could be more insulting than telling someone their life's creative and spiritual obsession is just the sign they need help? That it has no value? By setting aside the professional impulse to control and fix, I quickly discovered, standing on that cold sidewalk and then over hot tea in a cafe, that your son is able to have a conversation, can relate, communicate, even plan his day and discuss his options. Some topics were clearly pained, skipped over for something else, and he was often strangely distracted—but it was after all our first meeting, and I sensed some terrible and unspoken traumas present that were still not ready to be recognized. To me, clearly, he was not "unreachable."

That we had a connection in just a short time made it very hard for me to understand why you or anyone would want to use force—to use violence—to get him into mental health treatment. A traumatic assault, instant mistrust, betrayal, restraint, then a complex web of threat, coercion, and numbing medications to impose compliance, possibly a revolving door of re-hospitalization, more medications, more threats and force and police… Surely creating a relationship, building trust, and interacting with compassion over time is a much better way to show concern and offer help?

When you think you know what is best for someone, it might seem faster to send a patrol car and force them off the streets and into a locked hospital cell. But would that really be safer? For whom? Or would it push someone farther away, undermine the connection needed to find a real way out of crisis?

You've become an outspoken public advocate of new legislation to empower clinicians to intervene drastically in the life of your son and others like him. In pushing for so-called "Laura's Law" the idea is to pressure, through force, compliance with medication and hospital care. Your son, homeless and in an altered state, is today held up as a perfect example of why force is needed. I share your desire to help people in need; that's why I went to meet your son in the first place. And I agree that our broken mental health system needs fixing, including new legislation and new services. I do want your son to get support. I want there to be more resources, more access to services, more connection, more caring, more healing. But I do not see your son, or people like him, as so "unreachable" that they cannot form a relationship with someone genuinely interested. That just wasn't the man I met that day. I don't see him as so less than human that his own voice and perspective should be ignored, rather than understood. I don't see strange beliefs and outsider lifestyle on the street in any way justifying the violence of forced treatment. I don't see him as any different than any other human being, a human who would be terribly damaged by the violence of force, confinement, and assault, regardless of it being perpetrated in the name of "help."

That day I met a man possessed by a mysterious artistic and spiritual quest that others around him can't understand. He is homeless and perhaps very afraid deep down, but he is a person with feelings, vulnerabilities, and emotions. Alongside the rapid-fire associations that I couldn't keep up with, he was also capable of connecting. His pilgrimage to Robin William's Mrs. Doubtfire house wasn't some lone obsessive symptom, the sign of schizophrenia and a broken brain, but understandable when put in context. His ranting was not a meaningless mutter but a creative and encyclopedic stream of enormous intellect. Yes, he seemed to be in touch with some other reality, an altered state that demanded most of his attention. Yes, I would love to see him living indoors, less afraid, more cared for, and more caring for himself. I'd like to see the many homeless people in the Bay Area have the same. But no, this is not a man I would want to force into restraints, injections, and confinement. I would not want anyone to be subjected to such violence—and it is violence, as people who have endured it will tell you. I would not want to destroy my emerging friendship with him with such an attack, because I know it is friendship—long, slow, developing connection and understanding—that can truly heal people who are tumbling in the abyss of madness.

Concerned and wanting to help, wouldn't it be better for us to find the resources to gently befriend your son, to learn more about him, create trust, and meet him in his life and world? Even if this took patience, skill, and effort? Isn't this how we want others to approach us if we seem, in their opinion, to be in need of help? Don't we want our voice respected if we disagree with someone about what is best for us? How can friendship and trust possibly come out of violence?

Again and again, I am told the "severely mentally ill" are impaired and incapable, not quite human. I am told they are like dementia patients wandering in the snow, with no capacity and no cure, not to be listened to or related to. I am told they must be controlled by our interventions regardless of their own preferences, regardless of the trauma that forced treatment can inflict, regardless of the simple duty we have to regard others with care, compassion, and respect, regardless of the guarantees of dignity we afford others in our constitution and legal system. I am told the "high utilizers" and "frequent flyers" burden services because they are different than the rest of us. I am told the human need for patience doesn't apply to these somehow less-than-human people.

And when I finally do meet the people carrying that terrible, stigmatizing label of schizophrenia, what do I find? I find—a human being. A human who responds to the same listening and curiosity that I, or anyone, responds to. I find a human who is above all terrified, absolutely terrified, by some horrible trauma we may not see or understand. A human being who shows all the signs of flight and mistrust that go along with trauma. A person who may seem completely bizarre but who still responds to kindness and interest— and recoils, as we all would, from the rough handling and cold dismissal so often practiced by mental health professionals. Listening and curiosity might take skill and affinity, to be sure, when someone is in an alternate reality. But that just makes it our responsibility to provide that skill and affinity. Do we really want to add more force and more violence to a traumatized person's life, just because we were not interested in finding a different way?

Your son may be frightened, may be in a different reality, may spend most of his time very far away from human connection. But his life, like everyone's, makes sense when you take time to understand it. He deserves hope for change, and he deserves careful, skilled efforts to reach him and to connect—not the quick fix falsely promised by the use of force.

Even under the best of circumstances, mothers and sons sometimes have a hard time communicating. Many young people refuse help—just because the hand that offers it is the hand of a parent they are in conflict with. Perhaps the need for independence is stronger than the need to find refuge in the arms of a parent. Perhaps children flee their parents in spite of themselves, because of some complex reality they are seeking to overcome. So maybe the help that is needed is not just for the sick individual but for repairing a broken relationship. I say this because after my own recovery from what was called "schizophrenia," I became a counselor with families. I see again and again—and the colleagues I work with also see again and again—that by rebuilding relationships, not tearing them down with force, healing can occur. A young person whose promising life and career were interrupted by psychosis can regain hope for that possible future.

A simple look at the research literature over the past 50 years shows that recovery from what is diagnosed schizophrenia is well documented and a real possibility—for everyone. Not a guarantee, but a possibility worth striving for. It is only in the past few decades that we forget this basic clinical truth about the prognosis of schizophrenia and psychosis, and instead predict chronic, long-term illness for everyone. Such a prediction threatens to become a self-fulfilling prophecy, as we lower our expectations, give up hope, and relegate people to a lifetime of being controlled and warehoused in the identity of "severely mentally ill."

I do believe help is needed, help not just for your son, but help for everyone in the family affected by the strange and overwhelming experience of psychosis. But when parents, who are alone and desperate to change their children, resort to pleas for force and coercion, they risk sacrificing the very connection and bond that can be the pathway toward getting better.

I hear the claim that Yes, we should respect the right to refuse help, but when people are suffering so greatly and everything else has been tried, we have no choice but to infringe on freedom. This is false. *We haven't already tried everything we can.* We have not tried everything we can with your son, or with you. There is a huge wellspring of creative possibilities, skills, and resources possible if we just direct our mental health system to try harder and do better for you and your son—and the many people like you. It takes money, vision, and political willpower, but people struggling with mental illness deserve the dignity of true help, not false promises.

We can, and must, do better. We must think outside of the false choice between coercive help or no help. We might start by asking people who have recovered from psychosis—and there are many—what they needed to get better and give them a leading role in shaping our mental health policies. We might start by respecting people's decision to avoid treatment and seek to understand the decision rather than overpower the person making it. When you have been traumatized by those offering help, avoiding treatment might even be a sign of health, not madness.

Maybe some of us, when we are terrified, discover different realities to hide in. And maybe some of us, when we are terrified about people we love, reach for desperate measures—like forced treatment policies and Laura's Law—to help. I believe that people who are afraid, perhaps such as your son and yourself, need caring, kindness, patience, and listening. Trying to force you, or him, to change may only drive us all farther apart.

I believe it is often the most brilliant, sensitive, artistic, and yes sometimes even visionary, telepathic, and prophetic people who get overwhelmed by madness. We need to discover who they are and meet them as we would ourselves want to be met, rather than giving up hope for human connection.

At the cafe where we talked, the waiter was polite, but kept his eye on your son, seeing only a dirty and homeless schizophrenic, not the human being I was getting to know, not the son you love dearly. When we said goodbye, I tried to imagine what it would be like, living rough on the street, facing suspicion or worse from everyone I passed. I imagine it would be lonely, that I might fall asleep at night missing my childhood home, missing my mother.

Chapter 43

With the Launch of Mad in Denmark, a Global Network for Radical Change Grows Stronger[1]

Robert Whitaker

Summary

Robert Whitaker, a prize-winning science journalist, started the Mad in America (madinamerica.com) website in the aftermath of his two groundbreaking books *Mad in America: Bad Science, Bad Medicine, and the Enduring Mistreatment of the Mentally Ill* (2002) and *Anatomy of an Epidemic: Magic Bullets, Psychiatric Drugs, and the Astonishing Rise of Mental Illness in America* (2010). These books carefully consider the scientific evidence around the current "brain disease" model of mental health and illness. They show the many evidence flaws in the model and the need for the model to be replaced by one that emphasizes our common humanity and promotes robust, long-term recovery and wellness.

Mad in America has become a go-to site for the activist community and for anyone concerned about the limitations of today's dominant models in mental health. As the website explains, Mad in America contains:

> news of psychiatric research, original journalism articles, and a forum for an international group of writers—people with lived experience, peer specialists, family members, psychiatrists, psychologists, social workers, program managers, journalists, attorneys, and more—to explore issues related to this goal of "remaking psychiatry."

What is equally important about this work is that it is expanding globally. The network is continually adding affiliates and now having global meetings. For example, a feature on the website, "Decolonizing Psychiatry in Pakistan: A Reckoning with our Colonial Past and a Call for Reconstruction," was first published by Mad in South Asia. This global expansion tells of a larger global resistance to the disease model that is now being promoted around the world.

*

DOI: 10.4324/9781003148456-48

When we started Mad in America more than a decade ago, we never envisioned that our webzine would one day bloom into a global network of Mad sites. Mad in Denmark, which is newly launched, is the 11th affiliate in that network, and three others are expected to launch later this year.

Personally, I have been waiting for a Mad in Denmark for a number of years. Olga Runciman is a long-time board member of Mad in America, and so it makes for a particularly happy moment that she and her Danish colleagues have launched this site.

I can no longer remember when I first met Olga, but we have been fellow travelers now for at least a decade, spending time together at conferences held in countries that now have a "Mad" site. I mention this because our friendship is emblematic of the spirit that unites the growing network of global Mad sites—there is a commonality of purpose and a shared joy at pursuing radical change together.

Here is Mad in America's mission statement:

> Mad in America's mission is to serve as a catalyst for rethinking psychiatric care in the United States (and abroad). We believe that the current drug-based paradigm of care has failed our society, and that scientific research, as well as the lived experience of those who have been diagnosed with a psychiatric disorder, calls for profound change.

Our affiliate sites, while they all have editorial independence, share this mission. The roots of this shared mission go back to 1980, when the American Psychiatric Association (APA) published the third edition of its Diagnostic and Statistical Manual (DSM). That is when the APA adopted a "disease model" for diagnosing and treating psychiatric disorders, and in the ensuing decades, that model of care, with pharmaceutical funding at its back, spread around the globe. People everywhere heard of how major psychiatric disorders were caused by chemical imbalances in the brain, and how the drugs fixed those chemical imbalances and thus were like insulin for diabetes.

However, that was not a story of science. Rather it is better understood as a marketing story, one that served psychiatry's interests as a medical guild and the financial interests of drug companies. And here it is 43 years later, and the public health outcomes with this model of care are clear: the disease model has produced a public health debacle. The global "burden" of psychiatric disorders has notably increased over the past four decades, and there is a growing body of research that tells of how psychiatric drugs worsen long-term outcomes. The diagnoses in the DSM are understood to be "constructs," as opposed to validated diseases, and the chemical imbalance story has collapsed.

The failure of that disease model makes it a ripe time for a paradigm shift in psychiatry. Indeed, the rapid rise in the number of sites in the "Mad" network tells of how disenchantment with the disease model has spread far and wide. There is a grass-roots rebellion in the making.

While there exists a shared purpose among the Mad sites, each reports news and publishes voices specific to its culture, and the landscape for promoting such radical change may vary widely from country to country. The network provides a means for all of us to learn from each other.

For the sites in our Latin American countries—Brazil and Mexico (soon to be joined by Argentina)— this struggle within psychiatry is understood to be part of a larger political struggle, one related to the protection of human rights for oppressed populations. That is a lesson to be learned: in the US, challenges to a medical specialty are mostly seen as specific to that specialty, as opposed to a struggle that is political in kind.

In the UK, there is a strong critical psychiatry movement and a strong user movement, which for years have advocated for a paradigm shift in psychiatry. Mad in the UK helps provide a public platform for those voices for change. At the same time, the struggle for such change in the UK seems tied, in part, to the delivery of services within the National Health Service. Get the NHS to change, and the public's understanding of psychiatric disorder will similarly evolve.

There is a strong user movement in Ireland too. There have been pockets of Mad activism in Ireland for some time, which have brought together professionals and psychiatric survivors, and the activism there has served as a seed for activism in other European countries. Leaders of these activist efforts have come together to publish Mad in Ireland, and like in the UK, that activism has given this affiliate a head start in terms of making a mark in the Irish community.

In the United States, we tend to lump Scandinavian countries together, and see them all through rose-colored lenses. However, there are distinct differences in the psychiatric landscapes in Finland, Sweden, Norway, and Denmark.

Tornio, in the north of Finland gave rise to Open Dialogue therapy, an innovative approach to treating people with psychotic disorders that is now being adopted in countries throughout much of Europe and beyond. When I wrote *Anatomy of an Epidemic*, which was the book that prompted the creation of the Mad in America website, I presented Open Dialogue as the example of an alternative to the disease model that could dramatically improve outcomes for psychotic patients, and it seemed that Finland, as a country, could be a beacon for systemic change. Yet, much of Finnish psychiatry has been hostile to Open Dialogue and its methods. Indeed, it has been Finnish psychiatrists who, in recent years, have published findings designed to restore belief in the long-term merits of antipsychotics. In addition, there isn't much of a "psychiatric survivor" presence in Finland, which, as history has shown, is a vital catalyst for change. As such, Mad in Finland in many ways is introducing to the public ideas that challenge the existing paradigm of care, as opposed to further fueling a discussion that is already common in the country.

In Sweden, psychotherapy has a strong presence, and that does open up a possible challenge to the disease model of care. At the same time, there isn't much of a "psychiatric survivor" presence in Sweden, and, unlike in the UK, there doesn't seem to be much of a "critical psychiatry" movement among professionals in the country. Carina Håkansson was one such voice, and she led the way for the creation of the International Institute for Psychiatric Drug Withdrawal, but that organization is now centered in the UK. As such, Mad in Sweden editors, much like the Mad in Finland editors, are engaged in the earlier stages of a struggle to remake psychiatry, introducing the research, for example, that tells of a need for such change. In much of Sweden, the story of drugs that fix chemical imbalances is still seen as a scientific truth.

Now cross the border to Norway. In that country, there has been a vigorous ongoing effort for radical change for some time. In large part, this is the result of there having been a strong psychiatric survivor movement in Norway dating back to 1968, when the group We Shall Overcome was formed. In 2015, a coalition of user groups successfully lobbied the Norwegian Health Ministry to order its four health districts to provide "medication free" treatment for those who wanted such treatment.

The editorial team at Mad in Norway is composed of both professionals and psychiatric survivors, and its readership, on a per-capita basis, is greater than our readership at Mad in America. Norway, in short, is a country where ideas of a paradigm shift are percolating in the public mind, and one that can serve as an international model for change. Yet even here the battle lines are drawn. Conventional psychiatry in Norway is quite biological, with forced treatment more common than in most European countries.

Denmark has much of the same resources for a successful Mad site as Norway: a strong user movement, the long-time presence of Hearing Voices groups, and ongoing public debates about the merits of psychiatric drugs, a debate fostered in part by Peter Gøtzsche, a co-founder of the Cochrane Collaboration. Olga Runciman is internationally known for her leadership in the Hearing Voices movement, and she served as a consultant on a World Health Organization publication in 2022 that called for a paradigm shift in mental health care. The editorial team also brings together a group that has been active in promoting such change for years, both through the publishing of books and through the delivery of services.

As such, Mad in Denmark can hope to gain a considerable readership quickly, and—if the country pioneers alternatives to conventional care—the site can provide reports that will inspire such change elsewhere.

That is the importance of the network of Mad sites: it provides an international forum for the exchange of information, ideas, and initiatives that can inspire change in multiple countries. As such, the network can have an impact that is far beyond the sum of its individual parts. Ours is, in many ways, a David versus Goliath struggle, and yet, with each new affiliate, the voice for change grows stronger and louder.

Note

1 Originally published online at www.madinamerica.com. Reprinted with permission.

Chapter 44

Defunding Sanity

Raj Mariwala

Summary

Philanthropy as usual has a top-down dynamic that functions within normative capitalistic frameworks. This structural situation raises critical questions for mad studies advocate Raj Mariwala in their role as director of the Mariwala Health Initiative (MHI) in India. MHI is devoted to grant-making and advocacy that also has a deep social justice mission (https://mhi.org.in/). To do this work, MHI has had to ask itself a series of questions. Can philanthropy and social justice go together? Is it possible to fund against epistemic and structural injustice? Can one work against the grain of philanthropy as usual in mental health, which overwhelmingly tends to uphold a narrow biomedical model? Unfortunately, for most mental health philanthropy, the answer has been no. History reveals that, without serious rethinking, philanthropy "not only reinforces and supports a Eurocentric biomedical lens, but also propagates a philanthrocapitalist approach and plays a significant role in supporting ableist, expert-led narratives of mental health."

Despite this difficulty, Mariwala shows how MHI has found ways to work around dominant medicalized approaches, which all too often "uphold societal norms around race, gender, ethnicity, caste, religion, ability, and so on" The Mariwala Health Initiative has done this through queering mental health and through partnering with organizations and programs in India that foreground community-based support, social inclusion, and those informed by user-survivor movements. They have also worked to get a public audience for non-normative perspectives through their ReFrame series.[1] The result is a philanthropy that reverses top-down approaches and is deeply sensitive to the ways that social, economic, and institutional exclusion contributes to psychosocial distress.

*

A few systems—capitalism, pharma-complex, psychiatry—have been interrogated in the manner by which they uphold ableism and sanity and pathologize mental difference, but has philanthropy?

How does one engage in philanthropy and marginalization? The politics of funding has, by its own definition, a top-down dynamic, functioning within traditionally

DOI: 10.4324/9781003148456-49

capitalist frameworks and systems of welfare or charitable "giving." Philanthropy, thus, doesn't destabilize systemic inequity but rather reinforces, in some ways, the current status quo (Giridharadas, 2020). Given this dynamic, is it even possible to "give" in ways that directly support those who are oppressed? What does this mean for *philanthropy in mental health*? Just as there are conversations on how philanthropy may reflect White supremacy or Global North supremacy, it is also critical to reflect on the ways in which philanthropy reflects ableist neurotypicality.

While the overwhelming focus is on the lack of resources provided in mental health, what role does philanthropy play in *upholding* the biomedical in mental health? Amidst calls for increased funding and "investment," has the social justice discourse informed mental health funding, just as we have seen calls for philanthropy's support of movements such as Black Lives Matter? The only visible critique within philanthropy seems to be that the category of "mental health and substance abuse" received less than 1% of development assistance for health during 2000–2015 (Charlson et al., 2017).

Before exploring this, it's important to ask: Can one fund *against* epistemic and structural injustice? Can one fund resistance and dissent? Or do we, in our "giving," reinforce a paternalistic colonization of counternarratives and the appropriation of struggle, of a tokenistic inclusion in the "mainstream"? So how can funding— "giving"— destabilize these systems?

This chapter takes a foray into ways to start such a conversation in mental health, even as we examine ways in which philanthropy in mental health may replicate the dominant narrative. I conduct this examination in my role as director of the Mariwala Health Initiative (MHI), a grant-making and advocacy organization working on mental health domestically in India. We have found that to develop effective strategies in mental health philanthropy we had to understand and work against the grain of philanthropy as usual in mental health. It's also important to state that counternarratives have always existed as a source of resistance, critique, and dissent; so, do they need to be funded within this paradigm?

The History of Money in Madness

"Charity" and "profit-making" have played a significant role in the history of mental health—the source of funding has been either religious, charitable, or philanthropic, by the state or led by a profit motive. In the 13th century, a charity institution called the Bethlem Royal Hospital (or Bedlam) was established to provide treatment or incarceration of those deemed unmanageable by their families or "insane" (Arnold, 2009). Apart from "charity," private entrepreneurs also established for-profit institutions all by the 16th to17th centuries. (Scull, 2016). Seen in many parts of Europe, "asylums" were born of financial investment—whether philanthropic or private—and were not necessarily run by trained doctors or experts but by interested individuals such as priests, physicians, and entrepreneurs (Porter, 2004).

It was this investment or funding that enabled the building of psychiatric and psychological systems of knowledge and treatment via the asylum (Foucault, 1973). The spread of the asylum to many parts of the world such as South Asia and Africa happened via colonialism, and thus began the practice of seclusion of certain types of people (Davar, 2015). Similarly, the role of profit-making entities such as private practice, sanatoriums in spa towns, and psychopharmacology, as well as government budgets and investments toward long-stay institutions, took root for "curable" patients in the 19th century (Scull, 2016). Through centuries, irrespective of the type of investment, financial backing seems to have consistently upheld expert-led exclusion of those marked "abnormal."

The push toward deinstitutionalization and community-based mental health services was partially due to the lack of government funding to keep large institutions running, as well as user-survivor movements in the 21st century (Novella, 2010). However, the focus on the biomedical, on the "disease-" or "diagnosis-" led model, has remained despite the efforts of deinstitutionalization and demedicalization. This may be partly due to the significant influence exerted by entrepreneurship and the profit motive in the mental health field, whether via the pharma-complex, the wellness industry, or artificial intelligence applications.

Nutbeam (2000) says that "this century has seen greater gains in health for the populations of the world than at any other time in history" (p.1). Many gains in health were due to social safety nets and inclusion, as well as medical advances—but mental health has not seen the same attention or progress (Desjarlais, 1997). Partly, this contention is borne out by simply looking at government funding or philanthropy in mental health—which is not at parity with spending on physical health. On average, countries spend less than 2% of their health budgets on mental health. While figures between high-income countries (HIC) and low- and middle-income countries (LMIC) vary greatly, many countries allocate this spending to tertiary care, hospitals, and state-based institutions rather than to community-based mental health primary care (Kesner, 2021).

Comparatively, philanthropy or donations toward mental health account for 0.5% of all philanthropic health spending. While this is not at parity with physical health, it is approximately 30% of total mental-health-sector funding (Iemmi, 2020). Partly, it seems to be widely believed that such funding can be more easily channeled toward civil society and community-based mental health efforts as opposed to funding from states or governments (Kesner, 2021).

Recent efforts to increase philanthropic investment in mental health, especially in LMIC settings, have only intensified with calls from multiple actors, such as the World Health Organization, the World Federation for Mental Health, and private entities such as United for Global Mental Health. In the calls for increased funding, the most commonly used arguments seem to be calling attention to how mental health contributes to the global burden of disease, or how it accounts for lost or reduced productivity due to anxiety and depression. Other fund-raising rationales offered include the dollar-value loss of poor mental health to the world economy and the "return on investment" for putting money into mental health.

Just as colonialism aided the spread of Euro-Western psychiatry, the pattern of development assistance for mental health mirrors this movement. Multilateral organizations, global health initiatives such as the Global Fund to Fight Aids, Tuberculosis, and Malaria, and private foundations from the Global North dominate funding—choosing where, what, and how to fund mental health. South and Southeast

Asia received the largest proportion of funding for mental health in 2013 (Charlson et al., 2017). Apart from reinforcing these status-quo dynamics, philanthropy seems to have taken a decidedly biomedical approach to funding mental health—with the language of treatment, of focus on "conditions" such as depression and anxiety, or of providing "cure" or symptom remission.

While there are limited data on what is funded within the field of mental health—the bulk of mental health funding seems to go toward two broad categories—"mental health treatment" and "substance abuse" (Charlson et al., 2017). Another area that receives considerable funding is mental health research, which mirrors similar dynamics—a focus on substance dependence and depression as well as an overwhelming concentration on the Global North. Additionally, the impetus to center voices of lived experience—articulated as users/survivors of psychiatry—has been limited to very few funders.

Whether in research or in mental health services, it is clear that a Eurocentric, diagnosis-based, English-language-led model of mental health is the lens predominantly used by philanthropy. Even as actors in the Global North may decide to allocate funding toward depression, one may wonder about a decontextualized search or mapping of symptoms to the *Diagnostic and Statistical Manual of Mental Disorders (DSM)* in order to access such funding in LMIC contexts. While much more can be explored in the context of such funding, such as reliance on Eurocentric visions of administering "treatments" in order to achieve symptom reduction, resilience, or recovery—such an exploration is beyond the ambit of this essay. Philanthropy, largely, not only reinforces and supports a Eurocentric biomedical lens but also propagates a philanthrocapitalist approach and plays a significant role in supporting ableist, expert-led narratives in mental health.

Global North and Global South Is a Binary Like Any Other

Does philanthropy that originates in the Global South or is local to an LMIC differ vastly from the pathways and flows of money detailed above? This question is especially important considering the location of the writer—South Asia, and India in particular—as one of the major recipients of philanthropic funds for mental health. Domestic philanthropy is marked with a similar power dynamic—with foundations or individuals funding locations of their preference or communities they personally relate to, rather than issue areas or locations in most need (Vikas Anvesh Foundation, 2021).

If anything, an existing review of the literature around philanthropy in India points out that Indian philanthropy is not intentionally cognizant of social justice, historical oppression, and structural injustice. According to Minj et al. (2021):

> If philanthropy originated as a colonial system in the West, then its practice in India, which is heavily influenced by the West in contemporary times too, retains these colonial principles. When combined with the experience of internal colonialism it produces a layered form of colonial power dynamics.
>
> (p. 12)

Moreover, multiple sources point to philanthrocapitalism as a dominant approach in Indian giving—which has explicitly included philanthropy in mental health. Apart from that, the larger discourse around Indian philanthropy hasn't called into question issues of transparency or, specific to mental health, conflict of interest due to donations from the pharmaceutical industry. Furthermore, the colonial legacies of the psy-disciplines remain strong in the South Asian context—steadfastly upholding the Eurocentric standard of normal as an able-bodied cis-heterosexual male. Thus, the framework of Global North versus Global South is rendered meaningless when we look at the role of philanthropy in upholding the neurotypical and sane ideal. The decolonization of the disease model can happen only from the margins.

The Revolution Needs Funding, Said No One Ever

Before exploring whether philanthropy can play a role in challenging top-down psy-discipline, it's important to ask—can one fund *against* epistemic and structural injustice? Can one fund resistance and dissent? Or do we, in our "giving," reinforce a paternalistic colonization of counternarratives and the appropriation of struggle, of a tokenistic inclusion in the "mainstream"? So how can funding, "giving," destabilize these systems? One thing is clear—funding is based on privilege, privilege that reproduces across generations, that embodies itself precisely by the action of marginalization. So how can funding, "giving," destabilize these systems? What is it to claim an act of philanthropy as an act of defiance, as a redistribution of power and wealth? Is it even possible to *fund* madness? Or must one *defund* sanity?

Counternarratives, or lived realities, have always existed. One cannot fund the creation of knowledge, of new epistemological structures, when they have *always already* been a part of marginalized discourse. It would be vain to think the queers, the cripples, the persons of color, and the crazies need to be funded into being. There has never been an *absence*—there has been erasure. The hegemony of dominant narratives has not stopped counternarratives from resisting, from pushing back, from defiance—it has created the cisgender, able-bodied, able-minded, Savarna ideal; it has imbued that ideal with power. But the margins are not powerless; there is power in resistance. There is power in critique, in the articulation of self, in support systems and social networks.

What are the ways to embed such an understanding of structural oppression in mental health philanthropy? How do we add to the current calls for accountability around race, ethnicity, and gender and include disability? Or, critically, from the writers' locations—caste, without which we cannot hope to begin a conversation on decolonizing mental health.

Operationalizing

A host of these questions are what we use to conceive of and build Mariwala Health Initiative's (MHI) work as a grant-making and advocacy organization working on mental health domestically in India. At the very outset, our focus was defined as accessible and appropriate mental health services and support for marginalized communities. Thus, it was important for us to begin this journey by partnering with organizations and programs that foregrounded community-based mental health support, social inclusion, and autonomy of those who live with mental health conditions. General support services for common life stressors or addressing socioeconomic distress also fell within this ambit. Such work stands on the shoulders of user-survivor movements, and while such labor continues to inform mental health and resists the violence embedded in these systems, it does not adequately address the historical legacy of the psy-disciplines.

Psychiatry colluded with systems of power to exclude, build carceral systems, and propagate a certain idea of "normal" (Dave & Mariwala, 2020). Not only did it have a monopoly on defining the abnormal and thus the normal—it also developed tools for social disciplining of behaviors and people. These histories clearly tell us that the psy-disciplines and their allied institutions reflected social hierarchies more than they did illness. The deployment of the biological and medical frame of reference contributed to the idea of the psy-disciplines as objective and scientific. The dominant top-down narratives in mental health are not only about disease or diagnoses—they are about using the badge of expertise to uphold societal norms around race, gender, ethnicity, caste, religion, ability, and so on.

In an Indian context, mental health as an institution reinforces and reenacts compulsory cis-heteronormativity and able-bodiedness/mindedness, along with caste supremacy, an urban subject, and linguistic hegemony. And following this, user-survivor visibility is largely limited to those who are Savarna, cis-heteronormative, Hindu, and English-speaking with class privilege.

Conversations about LGBTQIA+ mental health for Black, Asian, and minority ethnicity are recent. They all call into question how the most visible mental health services and narratives are also the most privileged ones. For example, why are workplace mental health conversations never about what happens on the factory floor? So, in terms of MHI's approach, the understanding was that, to challenge mainstream conceptions of mental health, counternarratives from the margins are a valid critique of the power systems that may be reproduced within that mainstream. The composition of MHI's leadership and team allowed us to engage with queer-trans mental health from lived experience and build a course called Queer Affirmative Counselling Practice (QACP), which draws on disability studies, user-survivor narratives, mad studies, and queer feminist politics to create ways to modify mental health practice.

Queering Mental Health

This approach necessitates the interrogation of the "normal" and "expert" in multiple ways. While a biomedical approach definitely pathologizes the body and mind, the psychosocial approach, too, can exert methods and modes of normalization—for example, challenging the knowledge systems in psy-disciplines that have pathologized homosexuality or trans lives. The *DSM* and *ICD* only declassified homosexuality in 1973 and 1990, respectively, but these diagnostic manuals continue to carry variations of pathologizations around queer, trans, and intersex identities. Mental health systems continue to collude with social norms to uphold heteronormativity and the gender-body binary. This compulsory heterosexuality is also deeply connected to compulsory able-bodiedness (McRuer, 2006).

The legacy of this violent history continues because mainstream and traditional curricula of the psy-disciplines have not deconstructed the disciplinary expertise that enabled the "othering" of queer-trans folx. A different framework is needed—a queer-trans lens built from and by the margins—to counter the expertise built on "normality." Ranade et al. (2022) say:

> Knowledge in general, and particularly within the psy disciplines, is usually knowledge by and about the dominant. Since the psy disciplines engage, primarily, with the deviant, they do create knowledge about those of us who are on the margins—knowledge created by the dominant about the margins.
>
> (p. 84)

However, challenging pathologization and criminalization also means finding ways to center the historical complicity of the psy-disciplines to be responsive and affirmative to the needs of queer-trans clients (Chakravarty, 2019). Taking an affirmative stance versus the scientific myth of a "neutral" approach is also critical if we are to systemically counter power imbalances and epistemic violence in mental health and advocate beyond mental health to dismantle structural cis-heterosexuality and other forms of systemic discrimination such as ableism/neurotypicality at their roots

Built and taught by LGBTQIA+ mental health practitioners (MHPs) themselves, QACP both covers perspective-building to recognize inequalities and their impact on mental health and provides tools and techniques to address distress and promote the well-being of LGBTQ persons. The idea of QACP is also to engage with the ethics of mental health—what needs to change in frameworks and in clinical or counseling practice—as well as engaging with intersectionality and spectrums of experience to inform ideas of recovery and neurotypicality (Chakravarty, 2019).

Nothing about Us without Us

Any "expert intervention" or mental health practice should necessarily be situated alongside peer groups, networks, and allying communities. All the years that mental health care was nonexistent or hostile toward queer-trans folx has meant decades of care work, activism, and advocacy by trans and queer activists and collectives. So MHI believes in the subversive potential of shared marginalization as a resource and operationalizes this through a course called *Peer Support Practice* (PSP) with LGBTQIA+ communities, queer collectives, and organizations. The PSP module borrows from mental health practice skills to work with support seekers and ethics around power and boundary-setting that exist between support seekers and support givers. Nair (2020) explains why PSP is integral:

> speaks not just about loosening the grip of social institutions over lives, but simultaneously reimagining spaces as those where possibilities for

healing exist in plenty. As peer support in the queer-trans communities
has repeatedly shown, healing and growth is not the monopoly of Psy
disciplines; it never was.

(p. 30)

To work toward depathologization and dismantling sanism and ableism, instead of
focusing on the neoliberal notion of empowerment, perhaps one must find ways to
strategically disempower, or redistribute resources from, mainstream narratives and
power structures. So, accessible mental health support through professionals and
peers must be carried out alongside a range of social, legal, and economic inclusion
measures. Thus, MHI actively partners with and funds LGBTQIA+ collectives and
community-based organizations—who provide not just peer support or professional
mental health support but also legal and medical support. For example, the youth-
led Ya_All collective in Manipur works to enable easy access for queer youth to
information and services in health, education, and sexuality. At its drop-in center,
queer-friendly counselors and MHPs provide free mental health services to queer
youth, for whom the center also serves as an informal space to interact. Other
examples, such as Raahi or Moitrisanjog, are LGBTQ+ collectives that work
extensively with persons in crisis or rural trans folx, along with their allies, on issues
related to mental health stemming from their identity—providing shelter, legal and
medical support, and mental health care.

Structures of Oppression Are Necessarily Linked

Heteronormative imaginings are also necessarily cisgender, able-bodied/minded,
and Savarna. So challenging the resources used to speak that dominant language—to
make space for madness in movements and vice versa—is critical to decolonized,
queer, crip futures. For philanthropy to be accountable to the idea of neurodivergent,
nonableist schemas that query the construction of "normal" or of "natural," it is
necessary to follow Kafer (2013): "If disability is everywhere once we start looking
for it, then why not look for it in other social justice movements?" This tells us that
philanthropy in mental health must engage with structures like caste and islamophobia
to begin the process of decolonizing mental health.

Psychiatry is a social institution that derives power out of such structural forces
and maintains it through conformity to them. This adherence and submission
manifests in labels of abnormality on all those who are not politically productive for
the stability of the status quo, who dissent, who challenge these structural forces, and
who demand a reorganization of power. Perhaps, at this point, it is very telling to
state that we were able to envision and create a program like QACP because queer-
trans folx with caste and allied privileges have been able to access the psy-disciplines
and their "expertise." For those who are marginalized by caste, religion, and certain
disabilities, opportunities to study and practice mental health have been severely
limited. Alongside this gatekeeping, mental health praxis manifests as a spectrum of
violence, negligence to obvious inaccessibility literally and metaphorically, and a lack
of affirmation and of culturally and structurally appropriate support for those who
are marginalized.

Keeping in mind these realities, MHI is working toward the principle that the only path to a holistic, universally accessible mental health ecosystem is through challenging structural inequalities and countering systems of expert knowledge, privilege, and power, all from the margins.

If we are to take disability as a site for collective reimagining (Kafer, 2013), it allows us the freedom to ask much more of mental health. How does one approach recovery narratives if as a Dalit you live in a violently casteist environment? Or a trans person in a heteronormative environment? What is the scope for recovery when the diagnostic system in mental health says you have a gender identity disorder?

Some of the ways in which MHI is attempting to confront the status quo is redistribution of resources by approaching funding as creating an absence in dominant narratives by denying support to this hegemony. An example of this is working with and supporting Samvada, who work on education and livelihood support with youth marginalized by caste, religion, gender and sexuality, and disability in a range of socially critical areas such as mental health and agriculture. For those young persons who are studying mental health, there is an intersectional, structural, and psychosocial understanding of mental health alongside feminist mental health. All the other disciplines taught also have mental health components, in terms of self-care, as well as an understanding that is relevant to their discipline. For example, farming students engage with farmer distress and deaths by suicide. In this manner, MHI hopes to support the fostering of future mental health professionals who work with a sociopolitical view on mental health and rebuild narratives from their lived experience and the margins (Samvada, 2021).

While this process is ongoing, it is also important to support community work in Dalit, Bahujan, and Adivasi communities so that there are spaces for the psychosocial and the building of a grassroots narrative. For too long, we have been talking about very narrow definitions of mental health—that are applicable to only certain kinds of people. Mental health as the process of foregrounding agency, control over life choices; access to education, public transport, public spaces, health care, and workspaces; and freedom from violence, poverty, and food insecurity is an economic, political, cultural, and critical psychosocial process. This is exemplified in the work done by Adivasi leaders such as Deepa Pawar, who founded the Anubhuti Trust, which works with multiple marginalized communities in urban settlements. Even as cultural idioms of distress are centered alongside advocacy work, such projects are building the contextual frameworks of mental health that are informed by their particular sociocultural, economic, and personal circumstances. Anubhuti's work on a campaign for the "right to pee," for example, centers the exclusion and the mental health dimensions of access to sanitation for women, Adivasis, trans persons, and persons with disability.

The intersection of identity in such spaces and politics is an attempt at defunding not just sanity/ability, but also caste supremacy, class, cis-heteronormativity, and urbanization. Similarly, MHI partners like WAYVE and Ohana provide a chance to work with, support, and train grassroots women leaders in fundamental and constitutional rights—rights related to social protection, education, and economic and political participation, as well as mental health—and counseling skills. If we are to imagine the possibility of futurities that are not able-bodied/minded and cis-heterosexual and are decolonized, by necessity those futurities will foreground access to justice and healing.

Defunding and decolonizing the places of compulsory able-bodiedness and able-mindedness, breaking down the social construction of normal and natural is a process by which we are continuously learning from the margins and standing on the shoulders of such activism. Philanthropy must and should be held accountable to deplatform ableist neurotypicality. Currently, with the example of MHI, our approach underlines the need to be informed by and be in solidarity with activist movements such as anticaste movements, disability rights, LGBTQIA+ rights, and labor movements. We cannot sidestep the need to address social, economic, and institutional exclusion that contributes to psychosocial distress—which means widening our ambit beyond affirmative mental health policy and services to demand freedom from violence and food insecurity, and access to the provision of social safety nets, labor rights, and LGBTQIA+ rights and human rights.

Note

1 The Mariwala Health Initiative website can be accessed here: https://mhi.org.in/resources/research/

References

Arnold, C. (2009). *Bedlam: London and its mad*. Pocket Books.

Chakravarty, S. (2019). Queering mental health. *Reframe: Bridging The Care Gap, 2*, 24–26. https://mhi.org.in/media/insight_files/MHI_ReFrame_II_21.06.15_edited.pdf

Charlson, F. J., Dieleman, J., Singh, L., & Whiteford, H. A. (2017). Donor financing of global mental health, 1995–2015: An assessment of trends, channels, and alignment with the disease burden. *PLoS One, 12*(1). https://doi.org/10.1371/journal.pone.0169384

Davar, B. (2015). Disabilities, colonisation and globalisation: How the very possibility of a disability identity was compromised for the "insane" in India. In H. Spandler, J. Anderson, & B. Sapey (Eds.), *Madness, distress and the politics of disablement* (pp. 215–227). Policy Press.

Dave, A., & Mariwala, R. (2020). Clinical legacies and counter-narratives. *Reframe: Beyond Clinical Contexts, 3*, 5–12. https://mhi.org.in/media/insight_files/ReFrame2020_Beyond_Clinical_Contexts.pdf

Desjarlais, R. (1997). *World mental health: Problems and priorities in low-income countries*. Oxford University Press.

Foucault, M. (1973). *Madness and civilization: A history of insanity in the age of reason*. Vintage Books.

Giridharadas, A. (2020). *Winners take all: The elite charade of changing the world*. Penguin Books.

Iemmi, V. (2020). Philanthropy for global mental health 2000–2015. *Global Mental Health*, 7. https://doi.org/10.1017/gmh.2020.2

Kafer, A. (2013). *Feminist, queer, crip*. Indiana University Press.

Kesner, C. (2021). *Funding the future of mental health* (p. 11). United for Global Mental Health, NM Impact, Arabella Advisors. Retrieved September 25, 2021, from https://unitedgmh.org/sites/default/files/2021-07/Philanthropic%20Finance%20Report.pdf

McRuer, R. (2006). *Crip theory cultural signs of queerness and disability*. New York University Press.

Minj, N., Hembrom, R., & Nag, C. (2021). *The current landscape of philanthropy for Adivasi and tribal women at the grassroots* (pp. 3–17). Centre for Social Impact and Philanthropy.

Nair, P. (2020). I get you. *ReFrame: Beyond Clinical Contexts, 3*, 28–30.

Novella, E. J. (2010). Mental health care and the politics of inclusion: A social systems account of psychiatric deinstitutionalization. *Theoretical Medicine and Bioethics, 31*(6), 411–427. https://doi.org/10.1007/s11017-010-9155-8

Nutbeam, D. (2000). Health promotion effectiveness—The questions to be answered. In D. Boddy (Ed.), *A report for the European commission by the international union for health promotion and education. The evidence of health promotion effectiveness: Shaping public health in a new Europe* (2nd ed., pp. 1–11). European Commission.

Porter, R. (2004). *Madmen: A social history of madhouses, mad doctors and lunatics*. Tempus.

Ranade, K., Chakravarty, S., Nair, P., & Shringarpure, G. (2022). *Queer affirmative counselling practice: A resource book for mental health practitioners in India*. Mariwala Health Initiative.

Samvada. (2021, August 7). *Baduku community college*. Retrieved October 3, 2021, from http://samvadabaduku.org/

Scull, A. (2016). *Madness in civilization: A cultural history of insanity from the Bible to Freud, from the madhouse to modern medicine*. Princeton University Press.

Vikas Anvesh Foundation. (2021). *Big philanthropy in India: Perils and opportunities*. Azim Premji Foundation.

Chapter 45

Making the Case for Multiplicity

A HOLISTIC FRAMEWORK FOR MADNESS AND TRANSFORMATION

Jazmine Russell

Summary

In this chapter, Russell details her "first episode of psychosis" and the crisis of meaning that followed as she navigated healing outside hospital walls. Stubbornly unwilling to reduce her experience and those of her clients to a singular narrative, Russell uses her own story as a primary case study to explore five frameworks for understanding mental health crises and finding meaning in pain. She dives into the critically intertwined factors of complex trauma, autoimmunity, ancestral wounding, spiritual experiences, and structural oppression. These lenses offer not only vital information around root causes of mental health concerns but also unique pathways for hope, possibility, and healing.

Russell argues that, while we may want a simple concise answer to why we experience mental and emotional pain or extreme states, "the minute someone gives you a diagnosis, a label for your most intimate inner experiences, using a language that is not your own, you lose the right to define yourself and the freedom to define your own reality." Reclaiming that right requires a willingness to face uncertainty and multiplicity. This chapter seeks to redefine "holistic" as more than a word or modality centering mind-body interactions, but rather a way of approaching healing that defines crisis as a learning opportunity ripe with possibility.

*

Going mad is the beginning of a process. It is not supposed to be the end result.
—Jeanette Winterson, *Why Be Happy When You Could Be Normal?* (2011, p. 170)

DOI: 10.4324/9781003148456-50

On one particular afternoon in October, I slowed my standard New York City walking pace and sat on the narrow path overlooking the subway cars on the Williamsburg bridge, feet dangling in between the bars. Looking up at the sky, I succumbed to the kind of life-weariness that most trauma survivors know well. I screamed out to the universe, "Get this out of me, please!'" There was nothing but an empty void in my stomach, emotional and physical pain radiating throughout my whole body. I wanted it all gone. I spent most of my life attempting to outrun madness. Beyond moments of forced emotional processing in the therapy office, I ran forward in life as fast as I could, looking back only to track the distance that madness had gained on me. This was the day it outpaced me.

Shortly after, I spent three months going in and out of altered states, also known as a "first episode of psychosis."[1] "Psychosis" felt like someone pulling all the seams out of my carefully stitched together body until I spilled out all over the floor. I merged with the world until I was nothing. I became undeniably permeable, my thin skin unable to hold me in anymore. I had no identity, just overwhelm and paranoia. I experienced psychic pain in obscure parts of my body. I watched the past, present, and future meld into one. I felt what everyone around me seemed to feel and had no idea what was mine and what was not.

Surprisingly, "psychosis" also felt like a great purge. At times, I could almost visibly watch the darkness being expelled from my body, as if I was throwing up pain in the form of screams, visions, wounding, old identity, old patterns, and memories. All of it was freed and eliminated from my being. While some moments were harrowing and I prayed for death, others were blissful and liberating.

There is a trajectory that follows once you've admitted to seeing, hearing, and believing things that other people don't see, hear, or believe. I understood this deeply, not just from books or movies, but because while I navigated this crisis, I was also working within the public mental health system. It was my job to conduct psychosocial assessments, confer with psychiatrists, school psychologists, and other specialists, and offer home-based crisis support. I knew what happened when a person gets diagnosed with a "serious mental illness" because I watched it happen to many of my clients. Medication and hospitalization hang in the air as inevitable, imminent events. People stop asking you what you need or want and start telling you. You become a "high risk" patient, even if you feel your only risk is in trusting near strangers with name tags with your intimate feelings, thoughts, and experiences they cannot seem to hold and do not truly understand. Your every feeling or thought is considered a symptom of a disease, your brain rendered faulty. I couldn't help but think this system seemed so contradictory to healing.

Still, I took the subway home from work past Woodhull Hospital every day and considered checking myself in. I tried to hide what was happening for a long time, until I finally quit my job, unable to stitch the fabric of my own reality together. I decided against telling any doctor or clinician what was happening to me – not because I thought that it was right to deny myself help or I wasn't terrified by the serious nature of what was happening to me. I kept this crisis to myself for one simple reason: the minute someone gives you a diagnosis, a label for your most intimate inner experiences, using a language that is not your own, you lose the right to define yourself and the freedom to define your own reality.

Somehow I managed to assemble a small scrappy team of unofficial peer supporters and healers. I was adamant that I wanted to stay out of the hospital and off medication, choices afforded to me by my privilege – my whiteness, careful strategy, and supportive community – and choices that are often unavailable to most of my clients and those entangled in the public mental health system. I knew there was far more to my story than a broken brain, or mere "psychosis." I had a raw gut sense that this experience could be incredibly transformative if I chose to dive into it, rather than resist or run from it. I wanted to be my own case study for a different, more humane way of understanding and healing from altered states. I wanted to explore and answer questions I had about my own experiences such as: What factors contribute to experiences that get labeled as "psychosis"? What does this experience mean to me existentially, spiritually? How can I move through it safely and become more myself on the other side? Is there a wisdom to altered states?

A Crisis of Meaning

It is not unusual to seek answers to quell the wild uncertainty that crisis brings. We want to know what to do, how to fix it, and who has the correct information to apply to the situation. More so than easy answers, I have consistently found that meaningful questions have the capacity to heal – specifically questions that open up possibilities beyond the theoretical containers we've been given in life. Now, in private practice as a holistic counselor, some of the most frequent questions I get from my clients are: "Am I suffering from a mental illness or is it [my brain chemistry, hormones, my autoimmune disease, etc.]? Is this a spiritual/existential experience or is there something really wrong with me? Am I crazy or am I just living in a world that wasn't built for me?"

In the midst of crisis and emotional pain, some variation of the question "Is it me or is it…?" inevitably emerges, opening up a range of possibilities for exploration. What does it really mean to have a "mental illness"? What does it mean for someone's sense of self and worldview if we decide that an experience can be attributed to *just* a chemical imbalance, *just* a spiritual experience, or *just* society? As I see it, the kinds of experiences that can get labeled as mental illness are not *just* anything. They are layered, complex, and nuanced.

"Is it me, or is it…?" is not just a question seeking to answer why or to elucidate causality. This is a question with many further inquiries embedded within, such as: Is this experience normal? Can I trust my experiences? Is it something within me (internal) or outside of me (external)? Do other people experience this? Am I inherently wrong/broken/sick/crazy/dysfunctional? Should I feel ashamed or proud?

How we – as healers, clinicians, researchers, activists, or supporters – choose to navigate these questions has a dramatic impact on how someone moves forward in their process, which avenues of support they seek, and perhaps most importantly, how they come to see themselves and the world around them. In other words, these moments can be considered a crisis of meaning, where we have the opportunity to offer options, choices, and frameworks that can help shape the person's life narrative.

In helping others navigate these questions, and facing my own crisis of meaning, several realizations have informed how I think about madness. First, multiplicity is key. While we may want to define our experiences in terms of cause and effect, there are usually multiple, interconnected roots of mental health concerns. Second, there may be elements of our mental and emotional experiences we would rather heal or move beyond, and elements we may want to harness that feel generative or are simply part of who we are. Living in this both/and makes our experiences richer. Lastly, I believe crisis to be a generative force. The emotional pain and/or extreme states we experience are not the problems in and of themselves, but rather the messengers. They carry crucial information, signaling us toward deep transformation.

To get to the roots of what our body-minds are trying to show us, I've found curiosity to be vital. This curiosity has led me to understand "psychosis" as a response to the critically intertwined factors of complex trauma, autoimmunity, historical and ancestral wounding, spiritual experiences, and structural oppression. Each of these frameworks, described in depth in the following sections, has deepened my understanding of mental health and provided unique pathways for healing. As human beings, we are infinitely dynamic, and the strategies or lenses we use to help us understand our pain and our healing must be too.

Trauma: What Haunts Us Can Heal Us

Through metaphor and symbols, altered states force us to reconcile with seemingly insurmountable traumatic circumstances. At the height of my "psychosis," I became fixated on the idea that the blood running through my veins wasn't my own. I believed it was my father's blood, that it was dirty, and that being his daughter was a curse. I wanted desperately to tear myself open and drain myself of any connection to him. At my core, I was grappling with the identity of being a daughter that had been sexually abused by her father.

I believe there is no *right* way to respond to horrifying violence and abuse. So many of the experiences we label as mental illness are people attempting to make sense of extreme pain. Extreme experiences beget extreme states. I maintained this belief, despite telling the story of my trauma to a man with a prescription pad, who concluded that I suffered numerous mental disorders – specifically catatonic schizophrenia, bipolar mania, and depression – and offered me Abilify, an antipsychotic, to heal the wounds (although, he did add "situational" in front of the depression diagnosis, noting that *perhaps* my life circumstances were contributing). I was 17 years old, encountering psychiatry for the first time. This was five years before my first run-in with psychosis. Even as a teenager, I knew deeply that my body, my mind, and my spirit were trying to cope with flashback memories of 13 years of sexual abuse and the (then-recent) suicide of my best friend. I'd spend the next five years in dissociation, developing stomach ulcers, re-enacting and running from trauma, and trying to survive estrangement from my family, most of whom silently disowned me once I revealed the truth about my father's actions.

It is a fairly modern framework to view mental and emotional pain as strictly pathological, as a chemical imbalance, or a brain defect. It feels reductive, transactional, and offensive to any body-mind that has had to endure both overt and invisible wounding to be further invalidated as nothing more than an "imbalance." It struck me, even then, that my body was desperately trying to show me the pain it was in. While I wanted that pain to end, what I wanted even more was to understand it deeply. Somehow I sensed that I *needed* to feel it all, not cut it off at the waist – or rather, the skull.

Psychotherapist Thomas Moore (1992) describes this process of honoring our deep pain and trauma as "soul work," stating "if we avoid the compensatory move into support and positive thinking, we can instead learn to honor the symptom and let it guide us in close care of the soul" (p. 116). If honoring deep pain was a form of caring for the soul, "psychosis" was the ultimate soul work. Altered states brought every unexamined inch of my trauma to the surface, purging it from my body. What makes altered states so terrifying is that the emotional pain can take over without your consent, whether you feel ready to face it or not. With nowhere left to run or hide, I was forced to face the impact that years of complex trauma had on my body, my worldview, my core beliefs, and my psyche. The altered states were the vehicle for my trauma to be revealed, and like a skillful healer or ancient medicine, the pain worked its way through me. I spent most of my life feeling suspicious of my pain, betrayed by it, believing that I should somehow be able to expel or avoid it. "Psychosis" taught me to trust my pain. It wasn't coming up to haunt me, it was coming up to heal me.

Activists, survivors, clinicians, and scholars have long countered the dominant narrative that "psychotic breaks" are purely pathological in nature, and/or that the content of delusions and hallucinations are meaningless. Research shows that those who experience trauma, whether as children or adults, are more likely to be diagnosed with a psychotic disorder (Hammersley et al., 2003; Sheffield et al., 2013). The greater the adversity, the more likely they are to experience symptoms of psychosis (Read et al., 2005). Interestingly, childhood sexual abuse seems to be most correlated to experiences of hallucinations (Read et al., 2003). We could simply consider the correlation between trauma and "psychosis" an unfortunate coincidence, but I have often wondered if there may be more to it. What if altered states serve some utility in healing trauma, in the right context and with the right support? What if "auditory or visual hallucinations or delusions" don't signal a deficit, but rather, serve as a way for our bodies to reveal psychic content that is deeply buried and richly meaningful?

I find that uncovering the content of our altered states can be similar to interpreting dreams. When we focus too hard on any one aspect, things seem elusive, perplexing, and trivial. Yet when we consider themes, archetypes, and patterns, we can garner vital information about our hopes, fears, and inner demons. Altered states take us back to our original means of communication, language before words, meaning made of symbols and metaphors. In my experience, this ancient language is incredibly conducive to healing.

It's also important to recognize that altered states and extreme experiences labeled as "psychosis" can be traumatizing and sometimes life-threatening for many reasons. With police often serving as first responders to crises, many people in extreme states wind up incarcerated or face brutal violence at the hands of individuals and institutions (Watson et al., 2008). In the US, there are virtually no spaces in the public mental health system to be supported, validated, and cared for in the midst of altered states while maintaining a semblance of autonomy. It is still common practice for hospitals and inpatient centers to use force and coercion, and to deter patients from discussing the content of their altered states at all. Given the strong correlation between trauma and "psychosis," I wonder what even a small dose of trauma-responsive crisis care could do for those in extreme states. When we come to understand that there are often complex reasons why people experience altered states, we can find ways to create safety and support.

Biology: It's Not All in Your Head, but It's Not All in Your Brain Either

Experiencing altered states, as terrifying as they were, quite literally saved my life. During the very first hallucination at the onset of my "psychosis," I looked down at my stomach to see three holes punctured through my gut by three demonic figures. My roommates weren't home; they'd find me in the shower later that evening, yelling incantations trying to banish my demons – to no avail. At the time, I believed these shadowy forces were trying to harm me, but later I'd find their message to be an eerily accurate one.

I was chronically ill at the time without knowing it and on the path to an early death. I experienced extreme physical pain, sleeplessness, panic, and malnutrition, and moreover, was dissociating from all of my symptoms. I had spent years suffering stomach pain, ulcers, hormonal imbalances, allergic reactions, and systemic inflammation that wreaked havoc on my body. Amid an enormously drawn out and maddening series of medical evaluations that yielded no explanation for my chronic pain, one friend of mine suggested that perhaps I had an autoimmune disorder and should get tested for celiac disease, a condition he also had. The test came back positive. It turned out that the demons, not the doctors, were correct in showing me that my gut was indeed too permeable (hence the common phrase "leaky gut").

Although the Western medical system has a strong track record of addressing acute crises such as broken bones and infections, it is not so adept at treating or preventing chronic illness. In the case of autoimmunity and chronic inflammation, there is much still yet to be understood about causation, but many doctors point to a complex combination of environmental toxins, poor diet, extreme stress, allergies, genetic pre-disposability, and lifestyle. The rate at which people are being diagnosed with autoimmune diseases is rising so dramatically with each generation that it's hard to believe increased testing or awareness could be the sole explanation (Lerner, Jeremias, & Matthias, 2015).

While we have a growing awareness of autoimmunity and chronic illness, it's less commonly understood that those diagnosed with autoimmune disorders are also likely to be diagnosed with psychiatric conditions at higher rates than the general population (Jeppesen & Benros, 2019). Links between autoimmunity, especially celiac disease, and psychotic disorders have been found, showing higher levels of inflammation and genetic associations between them (Jungerius et al., 2008). Individuals with a history of celiac disease, for example, may have three times the risk of developing schizophrenia (Greenblatt & Delane, 2018). Unsurprisingly, one of the possible explanations underpinning the association between autoimmunity and psychiatric diagnoses is childhood trauma. Those with higher scores on the Adverse Childhood Experiences Scale (ACES) and those diagnosed with PTSD are more likely to develop and be hospitalized with an autoimmune disease (Dube et al., 2009; O'Donovan et al, 2015). While far more research at this intersection is needed, there does appear to be a correlation between autoimmunity and mental health concerns, often mediated by trauma.

Head of the psychiatry department at Cambridge University, Dr. Edward Bullmore, has built his career on studying the immune system's role in mental health. In his book, *The Inflamed Mind: A Radical New Approach to Depression* (2018), he describes the vast intersections of mental health and immune dysfunction. Bullmore calls for an end to the era of Cartesian dualism, as well as the overtly reductionist chemical imbalance theory that dominates understandings of mental health, asserting that our immune system significantly influences both mental and biological health – which are inseparable. In other words, just because mental health concerns often have roots in our biology doesn't mean it's all in the brain, nor that our lived experiences can't play a role. Bullmore and many others make a compelling case that one pathway for mental health concerns to develop or worsen is through chronic inflammation in the body, a condition that can also develop or worsen through exposure to trauma and extreme stress (Bullmore, 2018).

My own practice has surfaced heaps of anecdotal evidence at this intersection. I see clients diagnosed every day with chronic health conditions such as pediatric acute-onset neuropsychiatric syndrome (PANS), marked by an OCD diagnosis brought on by an acute strep infection that has long-term consequences; chronic inflammation brought on by mold exposure that worsens anxiety and OCD; multiple food allergies; Lupus; celiac; endometriosis, rheumatoid arthritis; and more. Each of these conditions has long-term mental health consequences. I have rarely seen a client present solely with mental/emotional concerns without some kind of moderate to severe physical health concern that seems to worsen, if not instigate, brain fog, depression, anxiety, hallucinations, and other symptoms. Yet public discourse offers very little to those who desire more complex explanations for these co-occurrences. Many of us are shuffled from specialist to specialist, told our physical symptoms are a psychosomatic result of being mentally ill, or that we are mentally ill because of our poor physical health. It is extremely rare for a mental health concern to be acknowledged as associated with a physical health concern outside of the chemical imbalance theory; when it is, we usually explain away emotional and mental distress as simply a byproduct of being physically ill, rather than a complex interaction within the body-mind as a whole system.

It is far too simplistic to say that mental health concerns are *caused* by biological phenomena and also too reductive to imply that a chronic illness simply makes one depressed or mentally unwell as a side effect of knowing you're ill. We need the capacity to hold infinite possibilities that lie in between these extremes, and the understanding that mental and physical health *influence each other simultaneously*. As research demonstrating the link between inflammation and autoimmunity to mental health concerns advances, I'm wary of the labels like "autoimmune-induced psychosis" or "gluten-psychosis" (Lionetti et al., 2015). These new diagnoses are deemed distinct from typical definitions of psychosis and fail to capture the very complex ways that biology, trauma, life experience, and so much more weaves together to co-create our experience of health and illness. As the functional medicine principle states, "One symptom, many causes. One cause, many symptoms" (Hyman, 2019). In other words, there are multiple roots to our pain, and multiple ways our pain can manifest, mentally, emotionally, spiritually, and physically.

Even beyond "psychosis" or autoimmunity, our experiences of health and illness are also deeply related to the everyday stressors that our bodies encounter. Most of us spend such little time on sleep, rest, exercise, nutrition, creativity, connection with people, and basic fundamental aspects of life. Many of us cannot afford to, as these basic needs have become commodified and sold to us as luxuries within a society that places increasing demands on our time and energy. Tending to the basics is one of the best forms of preventative medicine we have, and many who live with mental health diagnoses will tell you that letting our basic needs slip is one of the first signs that something is off. It seems silly to remind ourselves that tending to basic care of our bodies has extraordinary effects, yet decades of nutritional and exercise-based interventions for mental health have shown positive results in decreasing and helping to prevent depression and anxiety, partially by way of reducing inflammation in the body (Norwitz & Naidoo, 2021; Naidoo, 2021; Marx et al., 2017; Purnomo et al., 2017). It is a radical act to tend to our basic needs. Simultaneously, we must also look to the societal factors that make it challenging, if not nearly impossible, to meet our basic biological needs, and the band-aids that our system, especially psychiatry, attempts to place on deeply structural issues.

Ancestral Wounding: Manifestations of Historical Trauma

Just as certain genetic information is passed down through generations, so too are our emotional legacies, whether we're aware of the living narratives behind them, or not. My grandfather was from the Philippines but grew up in Hawaii. I was told for most of my life that his parents were "farmers," but that narrative quickly dissipated when he told me they left their home on a broken promise of good pay, housing, food, and education from American sugar cane companies. "They separated us: Filipinos over there, Chinese and Japanese over here. Our homes were made from sticks. I couldn't get a job so I joined the Army. My English was bad. I spoke Pidgin English. I was so *stupid*," he would say, shaking his head.

I used to think *Pidgin English* (what I heard as *Pigeon* English) was a self-effacing term my grandfather made up in the heat of his shame. Later on, scouring Wikipedia, I found that "Hawaiian Pidgin" was a real term to describe a mix of Hawaiian, English, Japanese, Cantonese, and Portuguese, a language used to combat the hierarchical caste system set up by plantation owners to prevent organized resistance among laborers ("Hawaiian Pidgin," 2022). My grandfather never used the words "racism" or "oppression" to describe his experiences, though he described countless instances of them to me; nor would he so much as utter a word of anger toward the people who enslaved our family. Instead, all he would say is "I'm stupid. Don't be ignorant like me."

My grandfather was prone to bursts of rage, my mother to depression and dissociation, and both of them had a rather authoritarian parenting style. My grandfather's promise to his kids was that he would never beat them the way his stepfather beat him. Instead, he used words, threats, and emotional bombs. His greatest wish was that we all became educated – "unlike me," he would add. In this environment, falling short of expectations was not an option for me. By the time I experienced my "first episode of psychosis," I had already graduated magna cum laude from NYU on a scholarship with an honors thesis under my belt. This achievement didn't put so much as a dent in my deep-seated impostor syndrome, shame, and self-doubt. Like my mother and my grandfather, I believed I was unworthy of any opportunity that came my way and that I needed to prove myself in any situation. Academia certainly didn't help this cause, only fanning the flames of perfectionism, burnout, and exhaustion.

Once revealed to me, my grandfather's history taught me that some of us – especially those who are marginalized, really anyone who is not white, cisgender, male, able-bodied, neurotypical, and heterosexual – are *made* to feel like impostors living in a society that is built upon our exploitation. With greater connection to my ancestral story, I could see that my feelings of shame, doubt, self-hate, and impostordom weren't individual defects or personal failings. As Resmaa Menakem says in *My Grandmother's Hands: Racialized Trauma and the Pathway to Mending Our Hearts and Bodies* (2017), "what we call out as individual personality flaws, dysfunctional family dynamics, or twisted cultural norms are sometimes manifestations of historical trauma" (p. 37). In truth, the wounds that plagued me were far older than me: the pain of not belonging, of being raised in a mixed race family hiding within and striving for whiteness, the threat of being seen as an impostor and unworthy within capitalism and white supremacy culture. Ancestral pain carries a particular weight, a sense that my story is not just my own, that something is trying to be healed through me.

I've learned that ancestral wounds are often so insidious and invisible that they repeat until they are recognized. Often the vehicle for this transfer of pain is internalized shame. When we name its origin – in my family's case, the pineapple and sugarcane companies, protagonists of white supremacy and colonialism that ignited much of my ancestors' suffering – as key players in a complex game, we are less likely to turn against ourselves and our families. Shame that can be named can also be healed.

Researchers have defined historical trauma as a wound that is shared among a community or group of people and passed down through multiple generations. Intergenerational trauma is similarly a wound or trauma passed down through multiple generations within families but does not necessarily imply shared group or communal trauma (Sotero, 2006). Psychologists have identified that historical and intergenerational trauma is transferred via three main channels: (a) family dynamics, narratives, and norms; (b) biologically via epigenetics and DNA expression; and (c) corrupt systems, societal norms, abusive institutions, and systemic oppression (Menakem, 2017).

It can be relatively easy to identify the ways in which family patterns are passed down through narratives (e.g., "we are a family of survivors") or similar emotional or behavioral patterns (e.g. "I'm just as anxious as my mother was"). We are also more aware than ever of the impact systemic abuse and violence has on the lives of communities and families, such as police brutality, redlining, and mass incarceration of Black people in America. Yet, what's fascinating to me is that we may also be physically primed to experience changes in our physiology depending on the trauma our ancestors experienced. Dr. Rachel Yehuda, a researcher in epigenetics at Mount Sinai, has explored the changes in physiology passed down from parent to child and found that children of Holocaust survivors, for example, are born with low levels of cortisol like their parents, leaving them three times more likely to suffer PTSD and three to four times more likely to experience anxiety and depression having never experienced the original trauma themselves (Yehuda, Halligan, & Grossman, 2001). A similar result was seen in pregnant mothers who developed PTSD after the 9/11 World Trade Center attacks (Yehuda et al., 2005). These findings give significantly greater depth to our understanding of the way trauma lives deep within our bodies, as warning signals from the blood and bone of those who came before us. We can then know that we are not alone in our pain and that when we heal, we are healing on behalf of our whole family line.

Mystical Experiences: The Potential for Generativity

I know I'm not alone in considering my "psychosis" a spiritual initiation of sorts. While certainly not everyone experiences a mystical element to altered states, in my case it was hard to deny. Time seemed to skip and bend, allowing me to pick up threads. "Psychosis" left me raw, vulnerable to a pervasive sense of expansiveness. I could feel energy moving around me and pick up information that lingered in an empty room. The existential or mystical quality of altered states carried a wide valence, at times far too heavy or too light to bear.

During one powerful "episode," I found my reality morphing. I looked down to find my skin was painted green. At the foot of my bed, small figures emerged, their skin also green with adornments on their heads. "You're here," they said, "we knew you'd be coming!" They were celebrating something much bigger than I. It was a ceremony. I felt them carry my body into a coffin and close the lid. Frightened, I wondered if they thought I was dead, if they would leave me there to rot. Instead, they cast the coffin into a river and let me float downstream. At the end, a similar group of beings took me out, opened the lid, and celebrated. "We've been waiting for you!" they said. The fear finally dissipated from my body. I didn't die, but a part of me did, and I emerged from the coffin feeling very much alive.

I came to interpret this experience as a rite of passage. I could celebrate all that I let die within me to make room for a new way of being. In a society with few initiations and markers of transition, and so little regard for expansive ritual, altered states gave me an unconventional way to experience this death and rebirth.

Spiritual and religious experiences are incredibly common among "psychosis" experiencers (Menezes & Moreira-Alameida, 2010). Qualitative analyses of post-traumatic growth following psychosis reveal that these experiences can lead to people feeling a renewed appreciation of life, making positive life changes, and having more compassion for themselves and others (Jordan, Malla, & Iyer, 2019). Some people report having awakened gifts, wisdom, or a renewed sense of peace. Psychologists who support the notion that altered states have the capacity to bring about generative growth and change call them "spiritually transformative experiences" (Rominger, 2013). Regardless of whether these states are experienced as harrowing or uplifting, they are nevertheless valuable for their capacity to dissolve "the outlines of the confining selfhood" (Phillips, Lukoff, & Stone, 2009). When in these states, the layers of who we think we are in relation to the world, society, the void, the mystery all crumble. By remaining open to such an experience, even impossibly painful ones, we can begin to unravel the breadcrumb messages left behind in metaphor and symbols – or, as Thomas Moore (1992) describes it, "the necessary changes requested" by disruptive feelings and extreme states (p. 6).

Throughout the three-month duration of my altered states, despite moments of wanting to end it all, I couldn't shake the feeling that these states were not only deeply meaningful, but also necessary. The changes they instigated in my life were absolutely vital to my survival and my healing. I moved out of the city to live in a forest where I could find more ease and energetic spaciousness. I quit my job in the mental health system and dedicated my work to organizing with other survivors. I finally learned how to nourish my body, and gained empathic and emotional skills I couldn't have otherwise. These "necessary changes requested" by altered states don't negate the pain and terror. The gifts of "psychosis" are not silver linings. If anything, these generative qualities are the result of the willingness to honor the experience in its totality.

Structural Oppression: From Gatekeeping to Mad Organizing

When I was working for home-based crisis intervention, one of my client's teachers called me in for a meeting. My client was 13, and her older brother, whom she missed desperately, had been psychiatrically hospitalized for years. Her mom worked several jobs to care for all four kids alone. My client was isolated and in the midst of her own breaking point. Her teachers sat me down and said, "You need to talk to her. She won't do work. She's in tears and being dramatic. We found something in her notebook saying she wants to die." They ultimately concluded, as I later learned many school officials do, that this was a ploy to get out of schoolwork. I begged to differ.

When my client and I spoke, it was clear to me that she didn't want to die, and that she wasn't going to act on her feelings; she simply didn't want to be living the life she was living anymore, as is the case for many of us who experience suicidal ideation. My supervisor instructed me to have my client's mom take her to the psychiatric emergency room. I protested, asking if there was any other support we, as a crisis team, could offer. After all, aren't we supposed to be providing the kind of wrap-around support that prevents hospitalization, using it only – if ever – as a last resort? My supervisor's decision was final.

I saw my client the next day. She looked worse than before. With tears in her eyes, she explained that the doctor concluded she had major depressive disorder, and since she wasn't at "high risk," she should try to take her medication, smile, and be happy. He told her that sometimes "fake it 'til you make it" was the best strategy. I asked, "What do you think?" She said, "I think that sounds impossible."

This was the first of many moments in which rage took hold in me – not toward burned out doctors, social workers, colleagues, or school officials, but toward the system that manipulated us all to be gatekeepers and enforcers of a dangerous "medicate and separate" logic. In this logic, the goal is to return to the "status quo," without recognizing that many of us who get labeled with diagnoses are suffering precisely because of the society we live within. For the first time, I found myself complicit in a system that systematically fails and abuses people, refuses them the support they truly need, offering only band-aids – all while proliferating a narrative of "biomedical disease" that erases the many roots of our suffering.

As for my own suffering, if unhealed interpersonal and ancestral trauma, an undiagnosed autoimmune disease, and a spiritual crisis weren't enough to create the perfect storm, watching people suffer in a system that often creates more harm than good, and knowing I was an arm of that system, pushed me over the edge. I quit my job, not just to heal myself, but also to find the people who were already working to combat the madness of the mental health system. I found a home first with the New York City Icarus Project doing events and organizing work for the "mad underground" (DuBrul, 2017). I then became a peer-specialist on an Open Dialogue team, a therapeutic approach to "first episode psychosis" that seeks to understand how the whole family and community context contributes to mental health challenges, bringing together multiple practitioners and offering in-home crisis support. I was, ironically enough, working for the same umbrella organization as before, but in a radically different program.

Around that time, I also met a psychiatrist, Dr. Peter Stastny, who was equally passionate about uplifting alternative models to the biomedical paradigm. We discovered our shared interest in creating trainings that are co-developed by those with lived experience and those with clinical training. Together, alongside a group of inspiring leaders, we started The Institute for the Development of Human Arts (IDHA) as a training institute for professionals, activists, and survivors. In the years since, IDHA has also grown into a powerful hub for movement building, community organizing, and mad activism, drawing in members from around the world.

In building IDHA, I connected with people who had been doing this work for decades. We intentionally created space for complexity, multiplicity, and nuance in our shared vision, which allowed me to bring all pieces of my story to the table. I reconciled spiritual emergence with ancestral pain, systemic oppression with trauma and generativity. Most importantly, I didn't have to choose a narrative or try to fit every part of my experience neatly together as if they were puzzle pieces completing a picture. Eliminating the need for a nice, neat, and composed story was perhaps the biggest relief of all.

Principles of Holistic Thinking

Regarding that central, inciting question: "Is it me or is it…?" I realize that "perhaps all of the above" is likely not as satisfying as receiving one singular answer in the form of a particular diagnosis or label. One of the things that makes psychiatry so attractive is the way that it conjures certainty and limits, which inevitably narrows possibility. Psychiatry operates on a very specific set of largely unquestioned assumptions. During a crisis, one of the last things we want to feel or explore is uncertainty. And yet, diving into the complexity of our stories is the very thing that could heal us.

Each of these ways I've come to frame my own experience offer a wildly different set of assumptions, pathways for healing, and further unanswered questions. I can never know if, had I not experienced childhood trauma, or developed an autoimmune disease, I would have still experienced altered states. To me, this part isn't important. What matters is the life-giving qualities each of these avenues have provided me.

Today, I practice outside of the mental health system, utilizing holistic principles, and co-creating opportunities for meaning-making. The term "holistic," at this moment in time, is often associated with or limited to herbal and nutritional remedies, commercialized spirituality, and the Goop brand. However, I use the term as a nod to the grounding principles of holistic medicine, which offer fundamental insight that mental health and psychiatry could draw on for future directions. According to the Academy of Integrative Health and Medicine, these principles are as follows:

- Holistic physicians embrace a variety of safe, effective options in diagnosis and treatment, including: (a) education for lifestyle changes and self-care; (b) complementary alternatives; and (c) conventional drugs and surgery.
- Searching for the underlying causes of disease is preferable to treating symptoms alone.
- Holistic physicians expend as much effort in establishing what kind of patient has a disease as they do in establishing what kind of disease a patient has.
- Prevention is preferable to treatment and is usually more cost-effective. The most cost-effective approach evokes the patient's own innate healing capabilities.
- Illness is viewed as a manifestation of a dysfunction of the whole person, not as an isolated event.
- A major determinant of healing outcomes is the quality of the relationship established between physician and patient, in which patient autonomy is encouraged.
- The ideal physician-patient relationship considers the needs, desires, awareness, and insight of the patient as well as those of the physician.
- Physicians significantly influence patients by their example.
- Illness, pain, and the dying process can be learning opportunities for patients and physicians.

- Holistic physicians encourage patients to evoke the healing power of love, hope, humor, and enthusiasm, and to release the toxic consequences of hostility, shame, greed, depression, and prolonged fear, anger, and grief.
- Unconditional love is life's most powerful medicine. Physicians strive to adopt an attitude of unconditional love for patients, themselves, and other practitioners.
- Optimal health is much more than the absence of sickness. It is the conscious pursuit of the highest qualities of the physical, environmental, mental, emotional, spiritual, and social aspects of the human experience. (Academy of Integrative Health & Medicine, n.d.)

These principles emphasize root causes, centering the person, the quality of the supportive relationship, crisis as a learning opportunity, and defining health as far more than the absence of sickness. The fields of psychiatry and psychology would benefit greatly from re-evaluating their own operating principles and underlying assumptions. Until they do, those of us dedicated to the work of transformative mental health will continue to uplift "the practice of personal and collective healing rooted in systemic change, experiential knowledge, and holistic care" (Institute for the Development of Human Arts, n.d.). We will continue to build networks of support predominantly from the outside, building bridges with those in the system who choose to be part of these changes, and keeping our vision for transformation alive.

I believe it will take collective action to realize this vision, but I also believe it begins at home, with how we orient ourselves toward our own healing. Are we willing to be with ourselves in the vast range of our human emotions? Are we willing to let ourselves repeatedly break open, expanding our capacity to feel and honor the totality of our experiences? Are we willing to refuse our own fragmentation, so when we are met with another's suffering, we don't recoil or instantly attempt to fix, control, or change them?

I engage in a transformative practice every Sunday night when I lay down to do a variation of Holotropic Breathwork, a meditative practice that involves deep belly breathing, evocative music, and somatic awareness. I carve out this time for myself to engage in the mystery of my body and emotions – to dive in and honor the complexity. I choose this practice specifically for its ability to gently induce altered states, akin to a deep meditation or dream state, and its emphasis on embodiment and emotional release.

In a way, I am still that younger version of myself, looking up at the sky on the Williamsburg Bridge, screaming "Get this all out of me!" But this time, I trust in the process, I trust my pain, and I trust my body. As I breathe, I feel all the frameworks merging. I feel my ancestors around me, showing me the path forward. I feel my heart opening, my stomach releasing trauma-holding patterns, and my inner child taking a deep sigh. I feel a connection to a divine spirit, while my nervous system re-learns how to experience safety. I feel a commitment to a collective power, and I feel what it's like to be situated deeply in my own energy.

This practice often reminds me that healing is an innate ability; it is what our bodies know how to do best when we can get out of our own way and trust the process. I've found that healing does not come from constructing a strict narrative around our wounds, analyzing or assessing our patterns, or fighting with our demons. Rather, it's a homecoming: a willingness to trust in the wisdom of our bodies, our emotions, and our capacity to transform.

Note

1 I use the term psychosis in this chapter, often in quotation marks, as a shorthand for experiences marked by altered and extreme states of consciousness. I seek to challenge the idea that psychosis is a disease or disorder, reclaiming the term to honor the vast range of experiences that it may signify.

References

Academy of Integrative Health & Medicine (n.d.). *Principles of holistic medicine*. American Holistic Health Association. Retrieved June 20, 2022, from https://ahha.org/selfhelp-articles/principles-of-holistic-medicine/

Bullmore, E. (2018). *The inflamed mind: A radical new approach to depression*. Picador.

Dube, S. R., Fairweather, D., Pearson, W. S., Felitti, V. J., Anda, R. F., & Croft, J. B. (2009). Cumulative childhood stress and autoimmune diseases in adults. *Psychosomatic Medicine*, *71*(2), 243.

DuBrul, S. A (2017, June 13). The next generation of the mad movement in NYC looks like this. *Mad In America*. https://www.madinamerica.com/2017/06/the-next-generation-of-the-mad-movement-in-nyc-looks-like-this/

Greenblatt J. & Delane D. (2018, May 16). Beyond the gut: The relationship between gluten, psychosis, & schizophrenia. *Integrative Medicine for Mental Health*. https://www.immh.org/article-source/2018/5/16/s7msy4lerz1s1vl2zqn7wc62b3oz6y

Hammersley, P., Dias, A., Todd, G., Bowen-Jones, K., Reilly, B., & Bentall, R. (2003). Childhood trauma and hallucinations in bipolar affective disorder: Preliminary investigation. *British Journal of Psychiatry*, *182*(6), 543–547. doi:10.1192/bjp.182.6.543

Hawaiian Pidgin. (2022, June 25). *Wikipedia*. https://en.wikipedia.org/wiki/Hawaiian_Pidgin

Hyman, M. (2019, December). *One condition, many causes: One cause, many conditions* [Video]. Institute for Functional Medicine. https://video.ifm.org/one-condition-many-causes-one

Institute for the Development of Human Arts. (n.d.). *Transformative mental health*. Retrieved June 29, 2022, from https://www.idha-nyc.org/about-idha

Jeppesen, R., & Benros, M. E. (2019). Autoimmune diseases and psychotic disorders. *Frontiers in Psychiatry*, *10*, 131.

Jordan, G., Malla, A., & Iyer, S. N. (2019). "It's brought me a lot closer to who I am": A mixed methods study of posttraumatic growth and positive change following a first episode of psychosis. *Frontiers in Psychiatry*, *10*, 480.

Jungerius, B. J., Bakker, S. C., Monsuur, A. J., Sinke, R. J., Kahn, R. S., & Wijmenga, C. (2008). Is MYO9B the missing link between schizophrenia and celiac disease?. *American Journal of Medical Genetics Part B: Neuropsychiatric Genetics*, *147*(3), 351–355.

Lerner, A., Jeremias, P., & Matthias, T. (2015). The world incidence and prevalence of autoimmune diseases is increasing. *International Journal of Celiac Disease, 3*(4), 151–5.

Lionetti, E., Leonardi, S., Franzonello, C., Mancardi, M., Ruggieri, M., & Catassi, C. (2015). Gluten psychosis: Confirmation of a new clinical entity. *Nutrients, 7*(7), 5532–5539.

Marx, W., Moseley, G., Berk, M., & Jacka, F. (2017). Nutritional psychiatry: The present state of the evidence. *Proceedings of the Nutrition Society, 76*(4), 427–436.

Menakem, R. (2017). *My grandmother's hands: Racialized trauma and the pathway to mending our hearts and bodies.* Central Recovery Press.

Menezes, A., & Moreira-Almeida, A. (2010). Religion, spirituality, and psychosis. *Current Psychiatry Reports, 12*(3), 174–179.

Moore, T. (1992). *Care of the soul: A guide for cultivating depth and sacredness in everyday life.* Harper Perennial.

Naidoo, U. (2021). Eat to Beat Stress. *American Journal of Lifestyle Medicine, 15*(1), 39–42.

Norwitz, N. G., & Naidoo, U. (2021). Nutrition as metabolic treatment for anxiety. *Frontiers in Psychiatry, 105.*

O'Donovan, A., Cohen, B. E., Seal, K. H., Bertenthal, D., Margaretten, M., Nishimi, K., & Neylan, T. C. (2015). Elevated risk for autoimmune disorders in Iraq and Afghanistan veterans with posttraumatic stress disorder. *Biological Psychiatry, 77*(4), 365–374.

Phillips III, R. E., Lukoff, D., & Stone, M. K. (2009). Integrating the spirit within psychosis: Alternative conceptualizations of psychotic disorders. *The Journal of Transpersonal Psychology, 41*(1).

Purnomo, K. I., Doewes, M., Giri, M. K. W., Setiawan, K. H., & Wibowo, I. P. A. (2017, March). Exercise prevents mental illness. In Ade Gafar Abdullah, Asep Bayu Dani Nandiyanto, & Ari Arifin Danuwijaya (Eds.), *IOP conference series: Materials science and engineering* (Vol. 180, No. 1, p. 012167). IOP Publishing.

Read, J., Agar, K., Argyle, N., & Aderhold, V. (2003). Sexual and physical abuse during childhood and adulthood as predictors of hallucinations, delusions and thought disorder. *Psychology and Psychotherapy: Theory, Research and Practice, 76*(1), 1–22.

Read, J., van Os, J., Morrison, A. P., & Ross, C. A. (2005). Childhood trauma, psychosis and schizophrenia: A literature review with theoretical and clinical implications. *Acta Psychiatrica Scandinavica, 112*(5), 330–350.

Rominger, R. (2013). Integration of spiritually transformative experiences: Models, methods, and research. *Journal of Near-Death Studies, 31*(3), 135–150.

Sheffield, J. M., Williams, L. E., Blackford, J. U., & Heckers, S. (2013). Childhood sexual abuse increases risk of auditory hallucinations in psychotic disorders. *Comprehensive Psychiatry, 54*(7), 1098–1104. doi:10.1016/j.comppsych.2013.05.013.

Sotero, M. (2006). A conceptual model of historical trauma: Implications for public health practice and research. *Journal of Health Disparities Research and Practice, 1*(1), 93–108.

Yehuda, R., Engel, S. M., Brand, S. R., Seckl, J., Marcus, S. M., & Berkowitz, G. S. (2005). Transgenerational effects of posttraumatic stress disorder in babies of mothers exposed to the world trade center attacks during pregnancy. *The Journal of Clinical Endocrinology & Metabolism, 90*(7), 4115–4118.

Yehuda, R., Halligan, S. L., & Grossman, R. (2001). Childhood trauma and risk for PTSD: Relationship to intergenerational effects of trauma, parental PTSD, and cortisol excretion. *Development and Psychopathology, 13*(3), 733–753.

Watson, A. C., Morabito, M. S., Draine, J., & Ottati, V. (2008). Improving police response to persons with mental illness: A multi-level conceptualization of CIT. *International Journal of Law and Psychiatry, 31*(4), 359–368.

Winterson, J. (2011). *Why be happy when you could be normal?* Grove Press.

List of Contributors

1. "Icarus Wings," "National Association for the Eradication of Mental Illness," and "Taking Care of the Basics"

The Icarus Project (TIP), active from 2002–2020, was a mutual-aid group of people affected by experiences that are commonly labeled as psychiatric conditions. TIP envisions a new culture and language that resonates with participants' actual experiences of "mental illness" rather than trying to fit into a conventional framework. They believe these experiences are mad gifts needing cultivation and care, rather than diseases or disorders. By joining together as individuals and as a community, the intertwined threads of madness, creativity, and collaboration inspired hope and transformation in an oppressive and damaged world. Participation in TIP helps overcome alienation and tap into the true potential that lies between brilliance and madness. TIP archive project has collected material from when the project was active: https://icarusprojectarchive.org/.

2. Mad Studies and Mad-Positive Music

Mark Anthony Castrodale, PhD, engages in education and spatial justice research. His work centers on critical pedagogy, critical disability studies, mad studies, and mobile research methodologies. He has been published in *Disability & Society*, *Journal of Qualitative Inquiry*, *Disability Studies Quarterly*, *Canadian Journal for the Study of Adult Education*, and *Manifestos for the Future of Critical Disability Studies*.

3. Woody Guthrie's Brain

Issa Ibrahim finds meaning and purpose as an artist, musician, writer, filmmaker, activist, 30-year artist-in-residence at Creedmoor Psychiatric Center's Living Museum, and now as a member of Fountain House Gallery. Author of the memoir *The Hospital Always Wins*, published in 2016, Issa has been featured on German Public Television, an HBO documentary, and an Edward R. Murrow and Third Coast award-winning NPR audio story.

4. The Invisible Line of Madness

Sabrina Chap is a Brooklyn-based songwriter, performer, and writer. Her three critically acclaimed albums have centered her as a creative force in the neo-burlesque/variety revival. Chap is also the editor of the Lambda-nominated anthology, *Live Through This: On Creativity and Self Destruction* (Seven Stories Press). Other activist work includes *Cliterature*, *Letters to the Revolution* and *Audio Protest*. She lectures internationally on madness, creativity, and gender. Her website is www.sabrinachap.com.

5. Cry Havoc: The Madness of Returning Home from War

Stephan Wolfert, MFA, is a military veteran who left a career in the Army and became an award-winning playwright and actor after receiving his MFA in 2000. He is the founder of DE-CRUIT, which uses Shakespeare with veterans to mitigate the effects of trauma and is currently an MSW candidate at Simmons University.

6. Betty and Veronica

Emily Allan and Leah Hennessey are playwrights and performers from NYC. Their work explores "slash fiction," a genre of fan fiction that focuses on homoerotic pairings of canonically straight characters. This genre was developed primarily by women writers and uses the power of the erotic imagination to undermine patriarchal traditions of authorship and ownership. Allan and Hennessey first began working together in a larger collective as co-creators of the web series Zhe Zhe, a camp satire of the New York City performance scene. Their two-person show Slash, called "fast and campy, and as clever as anything the New York stage has seen in some time" (Vogue) was deemed the "ultimate fanfiction play (Syfy)." Slash ran for four months at MX Gallery, one night at Joe's Pub at The Public Theater, and one night (under the direction of John Cameron Mitchell) at Ars Nova in 2019. Their last play Star Odyssey, a commissioned piece by MoMA PS1, explored themes of imperialism, inter-species empathy, and biowarfare. Most recently, they collaborated on the film Byron and Shelley: Illuminati Detectives, developed during their 2019 residency at CERN in Geneva for the Biennale de l'image en mouvement 2021 at the Centre d'Art Contemporain Genève.

7. The Uses of Depression: The Way Around is Through

David Budbill was an American poet and playwright. During his prolific career he authored eight books of poems, seven plays, two novels, a collection of short stories, two picture books for children, dozens of essays, and the libretto for an opera. He also served as an occasional commentator on National Public Radio's All Things Considered. Life in rural Vermont provided much of the inspiration for his work, be it cutting wood, putting a vegetable garden to bed, a bird's song, or the struggles of working folks.

8. Inbetweenland

Jacks McNamara is a neurodivergent, genderqueer writer, artist, activist, podcaster, educator, and healer in Santa Fe, NM. Author of the poetry collection *Inbetweenland* and co-author of *Navigating the Space Between Brilliance and Madness*, Jacks leads The Big Queer Poetry Class and hosts the podcast So Many Wings. They are the co-founder of The Icarus Project, and their life and work are the subject of the poetic documentary *Crooked Beauty*. Plus, their artwork adorns the cover of the reader!

9. Sometimes/I Slip

Lyo Demi (L. D.) Green is a queer and non-binary poet, essayist, screenwriter, graphic novelist, and community college professor who has been published in Salon, The Body is Not an Apology, Foglifter, and elsewhere. They co-edited *We've Been Too Patient: Voices from Radical Mental Health* with Kelechi Ubozoh, published by North Atlantic Books and distributed by Penguin Random House, and they authored *Phoenix Song*, published by Nomadic Press and now distributed by Black Lawrence Press. Their queer and trans rom-com fantasy screenplay and graphic novel *Journey to the Enchanted Inkwell* was a finalist in the Script2Comic Contest and Screencraft Virtual Pitch Contest in 2023.

10. The Mystery of Madness through Art and Mad Studies

Ekaterina Netchitailova is a doctor of philosophy, a university lecturer, and a lover of cats, fine wine, dancing, theatre, and human eccentricity. She is also a novelist who explores the phenomenon of "madness" in her books. Ekaterina's personal struggles have made her appreciate the manifestations of weirdness that exist everywhere. Born in the Soviet Union (Moscow), she grew up in both Russia and Donbas. Despite a surname—Netchitailova—that translates from Russian into English as "unreadable," her great passions in life are reading and writing.

11. Mad Art Makes Sense

Lorna Collins, FHEA, FRSPH, is an artist, filmmaker, writer, journalist, and arts educator. She is the author of *Making Sense: Art Practice and Transformative Therapeutics* (Bloomsbury) and a series of children's fiction, beginning with *Squawk: A Book of Bird Adventures* (Pegasus). She is co-editor of *Deleuze and The Schizoanalysis of Visual Art* (Bloomsbury). She has written articles about mental health, the NHS, creativity, and art in *The Independent, The Guardian, and The British Medical Journal.* Lorna's TEDx Talk is called "How Creativity Revived Me."

12. Are You Conrad?

Sofia Szamosi is an artist and zinester from New York City. Her first graphic novel, *UNRETOUCHABLE* (Lerner / Graphic Universe), tackles social media and image manipulation. She is currently working on her second book, a graphic memoir about her adolescence in the troubled teen industry.

13. Theoretical Considerations in Mad Studies

Erica Hua Fletcher, PhD, is a qualitative researcher at Veterans Affairs Greater Los Angeles Mental Illness Research, Education and Clinical Center. Her work examines the impact of mental health social movements on US public mental health systems. Her scholarship spans the health humanities, social medicine, mad studies, and social work. She writes about community health and healing, peer support, care work, and the education of healthcare providers. She is currently collaborating on a project to adapt the Hearing Voices approach for Veteran voice-hearers.

14. Obsession in Our Time

Lennard J. Davis is distinguished professor of liberal arts and sciences at the University of Illinois at Chicago where he has affiliations in the departments of English, Disability and Human Development, and Medical Education. He is the author or editor of over 25 books and numerous additional articles, essays, and op-ed pieces. His most recent work is *Poornography: How Those with Money Depict Those Without* (Duke UP 2024).

15. A (Head) Case for Mad Humanities: *Sula*'s Shadrack and Black Madness

Hayley C. Stefan, PhD, (she/her) is a lecturer in the Montserrat Program and Department of English at the College of the Holy Cross in Worcester, Massachusetts. Her work focuses on the relationship between disability and race in American contemporary, children's and young adult literature and media, and across the digital humanities. You can read her recent work in *American Literature*, *Research on Diversity in Youth Literature*, and *Screen Bodies*, and learn more about her pedagogy and research on her website: www.hayleystefan.org.

16. How to Go Mad without Losing Your Mind: Notes toward a Mad Methodology: From "How to Go Mad without Losing Your Mind: Madness and Black Radical Creativity"

La Marr Jurelle Bruce is an interdisciplinary humanities scholar, philosopher, fever dreamer, and associate professor of American Studies at the University of Maryland, College Park. His writings on black, mad, and queer expressive cultures appear in *African American Review*, *American Quarterly*, *The Black Scholar*, *GLQ*, *Social Text*, *TDR*, and elsewhere. Bruce's debut book, *How to Go Mad without Losing Your Mind: Madness and Black Radical Creativity* (2021) earned the MLA Prize for a First Book and the Nicolás Guillén Outstanding Book Award. Now he's in the thick of a project on—and experiment in—convergences of love and madness.

17. Commercialized Science and Epistemic Injustice: Exposing and Resisting Neoliberal Global Mental Health Discourse

Justin M. Karter, PhD, is a practicing psychologist and academic in affiliation with the Center for Psychological Humanities and Ethics at Boston College. He has led the research news team for the social justice-oriented mental health webzine *Mad in America* since 2015. He works at the intersections of critical psychology, philosophy of psychology, and critical disability studies.

Lisa Cosgrove, PhD, is a clinical psychologist, professor, and faculty fellow at the Applied Ethics Center at the University of Massachusetts, Boston. Her research addresses the ethical and medical-legal issues that arise in organized psychiatry because of academic-industry relationships. Lisa was a research fellow at the Edmond J. Safra Center for Ethics, Harvard University (Lab on Institutional Corruption), co-chair of the task force on Depression Outcome Measures, Agency for Healthcare Research and Quality, and is the co-founder, with Julie Hannah, of the Centre for Mental Health, Human Rights and Social Justice. Lisa also served as a consultant to the United Nations Special Rapporteur on the Right to Health. She is co-author, with Robert Whitaker, *of Psychiatry under the Influence: Institutional Corruption, Social Injury, and Prescriptions for Reform*.

Farahdeba Herrawi, MA, is a PhD candidate at the University of Massachusetts Boston, in the Counseling and School Psychology Department. She holds a master of arts in Mental Health Counseling and Behavioral Medicine from the Boston University School of Medicine. Her research and clinical interests are focused on immigrant and refugee health and human rights, as well as rights-based approaches to mental healthcare.

18. "Structural Competency" meets Mad Studies: Reckoning with Madness and Mental Diversity beyond the Social Determinants of Mental Health

Nev Jones is an activist scholar, interdisciplinary mental health services researcher, and assistant professor in the School of Social Work at the University of Pittsburgh. Deeply grounded in personal and family experience of what has been socially constructed as "schizophrenia," her work seeks to fundamentally shift the way we think about and respond to experiences falling under the "psychosis" umbrella.

19. The Neoliberal Project: Mental Health and Marginality in India

Zaphya Jena, MA, from the Indian Institute of Technology Gandhinagar, is an independent researcher, and has previously worked with organizations such as Population Council in New Delhi, Aksha Centre for Equity and Wellbeing, and Mariwala Health Initiative in Mumbai. Her work has focused on youth mental and reproductive health, social justice, and development in the Global South.

20. Child as Metaphor: Colonialism, Psy-Goverance, and Epistemicide

China Mills (she/her) is head of research at Healing Justice Ldn, where she also leads the Deaths by Welfare project—investigating how welfare policies harm people and what can be learned from the strategies of disabled people and bereaved families in fighting for justice. Before leaving academia, she was a senior lecturer at City, University of London where she researched and taught global mental health with a focus on state and corporate production of harm, distress, and deaths by suicide. China is author of the book *Decolonizing Global Mental Health: The Psychiatrization of the Majority World* (published in 2014 by Routledge).

Brenda A. LeFrançois is a university research professor at Memorial University of Newfoundland in Canada. Their scholarship focuses on the psychiatrization of young people and on anti-sanist, anti-colonial, and anti-racist praxis. They are a co-editor (along with Geoffrey Reaume and Robert Menzies) of the edited volume *Mad Matters*, which is currently being developed into its second edition (along with a new co-editor, Idil Abdillahi).

21. Beyond Disordered Brains and Mother Blame: Critical Issues in Autism and Mothering

Patty Douglas is the inaugural Chair in Student Success and Wellness and associate professor of disability studies in the Faculty of Education at Queen's University. Her research focuses on transforming deficit approaches to disability and difference in education using critical and creative approaches including disability studies, critical autism studies, mad mothering, decolonial studies, intersectionality theory, and arts-based methodologies. Douglas leads the Re•Storying Autism in Education project, a multimedia storytelling project that reimagines autism, disability, and educational practice in ways that affirm difference. Douglas is a former special education teacher and mother of two sons, one of whom attracted the label of autism. She is a white settler deeply committed to decolonizing research and identifies as neurodivergent and invisibly disabled. Her book *Unmothering Autism: Ethical Disruptions and Affirming Care* is in production with UBC Press.

Estée Klar holds a PhD in critical disability studies from York University. Her dissertation, *Neurodiversity in Relation: An Artistic Intraethnography* is a collaborative work with Adam Wolfond, now a published writer and the first non-speaking classically autistic MA student in Canada. Klar is also a facilitator and an artist and co-founder with Wolfond of *dis assembly*, a lab for neurodiverse artistic experimentation involving processes that explore conditions and techniques for human and more-than-human relation and support located at Artscape Youngplace in Toronto. She collaborates with others around the world in these projects. Klar is also the founder/director of the former Autism Acceptance Project (2006–10) and its subsequent artistic-activist events, and the original blogger at The Joy of Autism (2004–2008), which over the years has resonated throughout the autistic community. She is an artist and filmmaker and her can be seen at www.esteerelation.com and dis-assembling.com.

22. Enacting Activism: Depathologizing Trauma in Military Veterans through Theatre

Alisha Ali, PhD, is an associate professor in the Department of Applied Psychology at New York University. She heads the Advocacy and Community-based Trauma Studies (ACTS) lab which investigates empowerment-based and arts-based interventions for the effects of various forms of trauma, oppression, and violence.

Luke Bokenfohr, MEd, is a practicing registered clinical counselor specializing in individual and group trauma therapy. He is a former HM Forces' Royal Marines Commando and combat veteran of both Iraq and Afghanistan. He currently works as a front-line, operational police officer within the Mental Health Unit of the Vancouver Police Department.

23. Mental Illness Is Still a Myth

Dr. Thomas Szasz was professor of psychiatry at SUNY Upstate Medical University in Syracuse. He wrote 35 books, including "Myth of Mental Illness" with hundreds of written pieces and presentations. In this work, he was always lucid, witty, and provocative. Dr. Szasz was a deep critic of psychiatry and has been seen by many as humanist, libertarian, and "the biggest of the antipsychiatry intellectuals."

24. The Emergence of the UK Critical Psychiatry Network: Reflections and Themes

Pat Bracken, MA MD MRCPsych PhD, is an independent consultant psychiatrist. He has sought to promote the importance of "critical reflection" in mental health work. He was co-editor of the book *Rethinking the Trauma of War* with Dr Celia Petty, published in 1998. His own book *Trauma: Culture, Meaning and Philosophy* was published in 2002. With Prof Phil Thomas, he published the book *Postpsychiatry: A New Direction for Mental Health* in 2005.

Duncan Double is a retired consultant psychiatrist. He was a founding member of the Critical Psychiatry Network. He was the editor of *Critical Psychiatry: The Limits of Madness* (2006) and blogs on relational psychiatry at http://criticalpsychiatry.blogspot.com.

Suman Fernando, MD (Cantab.) FRCPsychiatry, is professor emeritus of social sciences in the School of Social Sciences, London Metropolitan University, United Kingdom. He was formerly consultant psychiatrist in the British National Health Service until he retired early to focus on academic work. His recent books include *Global Psychologies; Mental Health and the Global South,* co-edited with Roy Moodley (2018), *Institutional Racism in Psychiatry and Clinical Psychology; Race Matters in Mental Health* (2017), and *Mental Health Worldwide; Culture, Globalisation and Development* (2014). He is currently working on a new fourth edition of his book *Mental Health Race and Culture,* first published in 1991.

Joanna Moncrieff is professor of critical and social psychiatry at University College London and works as a consultant psychiatrist in the NHS in London. She researches the over-use and misrepresentation of psychiatric drugs and the history, politics, and philosophy of psychiatry more generally. She is co-founder of the Critical Psychiatry Network. Her books include *A Straight Talking Introduction to Psychiatric Drugs Second edition* (PCCS Books), *The Bitterest Pills: The Troubling Story of Antipsychotic Drugs* (2013), and *The Myth of the Chemical Cure* (2009) (Palgrave Macmillan). Her website is https://joannamoncrieff.com/, Twitter handle @joannamoncrieff.

Philip Thomas worked as a consultant psychiatrist in the NHS for over 20 years before leaving clinical practice in 2004 to write. He was professor of philosophy, diversity, and mental health at the University of Central Lancashire from 2006 to 2009 and is probably best known for his work with Pat Bracken on postpsychiatry. He has written or co-authored four books and over 20 chapters in books. Until recently he was chair of Sharing Voices Bradford, a community development project working with the City's diverse communities in mental health.

Sami Timimi is a consultant child and adolescent psychiatrist and a visiting professor of child psychiatry and mental health improvement at the University of Lincoln, UK. He writes from a critical psychiatry perspective on topics relating to mental health and childhood and has published many articles, chapters, and books. His latest book, published in 2021 is *Insane Medicine: How the Mental Health Industry Creates Damaging Treatment Traps and How You Can Escape Them.*

25. Crisis Response as a Human Rights Flashpoint: Critical Elements of Community Support for Individuals Experiencing Significant Emotional Distress

Peter Stastny was born in Vienna, Austria, where he graduated from medical school in 1976. For nearly 30 years, he was on the faculty at the Albert Einstein College of Medicine in the Bronx and has conducted several publicly funded research projects in the area of vocationalrehabilitation, social support, and self-help. Currently, Peter is working on the development of alternative services that supplement or replace traditional psychiatric intervention and offer autonomous paths toward recovery and full integration. Recently, he has spearheaded Parachute New York, a federally funded project to provide crisis alternatives in New York City. These activities have engendered a close collaboration with the user-survivor movement, as manifested by joint research projects, publications, service demonstrations, and community work. Peter has also worked as an expert witness on numerous legal actions against psychiatric hospitals and practitioners for issues relating to involuntary commitment and alleged harm sustained by the defendants. He is a founding member of the International Network Toward Alternatives and Rights-based Supports (INTAR), the Institute for the Development of the Human Arts (IDHA) and Reimagining Psychiatry Network. Peter has also directed a number of documentary films related to mental health and the Shoah. In the clinical realm, Peter worked as a psychiatrist for state-operated inpatient and outpatient services, as well as for the NYU and Pratt Institute student counseling centers. He is in private practice in Chelsea, New York.

Anne M. Lovell trained in anthropology (PhD, Columbia university) and is currently senior research scientist emerita at the French national health institute (Inserm). Her over 40 years of research in France, Italy, the US, and Senegal have focused on mental health, public health, and health democracy, often with health activist and psychiatric survivor groups. Her other research areas include addiction, the anthropology of disaster and care philosophies. *Her latest book, Reimagining Psychiatric Epidemiology in a Global Frame: Towards a Conceptual and Social History* (co-edited with Gerald M. Oppenheimer) was published by Rochester University Press in 2022.

Julie Hannah is a lecturer in the School of Law, director of the International Centre on Human Rights and Drug Policy based at the Human Rights Centre, and co-founder of the Centre for Mental Health, Human Rights, and Social Justice, a global research consortium. Her research focuses on the intersections between medicalization, criminalization, and human rights. She has a particular interest in international drug control policy, mental health, and the human rights aspects of the pursuit of social justice. From 2015–2020, Julie was the senior advisor to the United Nations Special Rapporteur on the Right to Health. Since 2012, Julie has supervised a range of projects in the Human Rights Centre Clinic, which has involved the production of research for UN human rights mechanisms, national and global networks of people who use drugs, and a range of social justice focused civil society actors. Julie previously spent a decade working in refugee protection and resettlement in the United States and Southeast Asia. She has an LLM (distinction) in international human rights and humanitarian law from Essex University and BA in Foreign Affairs from the University of Virginia.

Daniel Magalhães Goulart is an assistant professor at the Department of Theory and Foundations of the Faculty of Education of the University of Brasilia. He graduated as a psychologist from the University of São Paulo and completed his PhD at the Faculty of Education of the University of Brasilia, Brazil. His latest books are: Subjetividade, sujeito e vida: diálogos com Fernando González Rey [*Subjectivity, Subject and Life: Dialogues with Fernando González Rey*]; *Theory of Subjectivity* *from a Cultural-Historical Standpoint: González Rey's Legacy* (Ed., Springer, 2021), and *Subjectivity and Critical Mental Health: Lessons from Brazil* (Routledge, 2019)

Alberto Vásquez Encalada is co-director at the Center for Inclusive Policy (CIP) and works at the intersection of disability, mental health, and human rights. He is a Peruvian lawyer with an LLM in international and comparative disability law and policy from the National University of Ireland, Galway. He has worked as a research coordinator at the Office of the UN Special Rapporteur on the rights of persons with disabilities and as a consultant to various UN agencies. In Peru, he has been actively involved in drafting, advocating, and monitoring laws and policies relating to persons with disabilities and mental health, working at the Ombudsperson Office and the Peruvian Congress. He is also president of Sociedad and Discapacidad—SODIS and a board member of the Redesfera Latinoamericana por las Culturas Locas, la Diversidad Psicosocial, la Justicia, el Buen Vivir y el Derecho al Delirio.

Seana O'Callaghan received her master's diploma in international public health (DIPH) from the University of Medicine in Berlin, Charitè. She has worked as the CEO of a mental health foundation, business owner, mental health research project manager, research assistant, non-profit grant writer, chief cook, and bottle washer. Her research focus is the dialectic between evidence-based practice and alternative medicine in community-based psychiatry and international health.

Dainius Pūras is professor of child psychiatry and public mental health at Vilnius University, Lithuania. He is also a consultant child and adolescent psychiatrist at the Child Development Center of Vilnius University Hospital. Among the positions he held, Dainius Pūras was President of the Lithuanian Psychiatric Association, Dean of the Medical Faculty of Vilnius University, and Director of the Human Rights Monitoring Institute. During the years 2007–2011, Dainius Pūras was a member of the UN Committee on the Rights of the Child. During the years 2014–2020, he served as a UN Special Rapporteur on the right to physical and mental health.

26. Sanism: Histories, Applications, and Studies So Far

Stephanie LeBlanc-Omstead, PhD, OT Reg (Ont), is a maddened occupational therapist, university lecturer, carer, researcher, and scholar. Informed by mad studies and her own experiential knowledge, her research critically examines the practice of "service user involvement" in health professional education programs. Her writing, learning, teaching, and practice have focused on the interruption of epistemic injustice and sanism in the health professions, as well as on the importance of engaging with experiential knowledges and establishing anti-sanist praxis in these spaces.

Jennifer (Jen) Poole (she/her) is a first-generation white settler from England living in Toronto, Canada. She is a maddened community peer supporter. She is also an associate professor in the School of Social Work at Toronto Metropolitan University (formerly Ryerson) where her teaching, learning, and research is focused on sanism, madness, grief, and interrupting colonialism in education.

27. On Being Insane in Sane Places: Breaking into the Cult of the Mental Health Industry

Noel Hunter, PsyD, is a clinical psychologist and the director of MindClear Integrative Psychotherapy in NYC. Her work focuses on complex trauma, the oppressive nature of the mental health system, and advocating for change. She is also the author of the book *Trauma and Madness in Mental Health Services*.

28. Therapy as a Tool in Dismantling Oppression

Gitika Talwar, PhD, (she/her/we/us) is a community clinical psychologist who served the student community at the University of Washington, Seattle. As an international student from India, she earned her PhD from the University of Maryland Baltimore County. A trauma-informed, liberation-focused psychologist, she remains committed to the decolonization of mental health practices and centering the needs of communities frequently silenced in mainstream mental health practices. From 2022 to 2024, she served on the American Psychological Association's Presidential Taskforce on Decolonial and Liberation Psychology.

29. Decolonizing Psychotherapy by Owning Our Madness

Debbie-Ann Chambers, PhD, is a counselling psychologist and certified poetry therapy practitioner. She serves as the head of unit of the University Counselling Service at The University of the West Indies (Mona) in Jamaica. Debbie-Ann provides trauma-informed, culturally informed, and creative therapies in a quest to address the post-colonial wounds/legacy burdens of her community.

30. Creating a Cultural Foundation to Contextualize and Integrate Spiritual Emergence

Katrina Michelle is a psychotherapist who completed her PhD research on the phenomenology of emergent states of consciousness and our resistance to them. Her interest is in evolving mainstream systems to create a cultural context for embracing the fullness of the human experience and its generative potential.

31. The Establishment and the Mystic: Musings on Relationships between Psychoanalysis and Human Development

Marilyn Charles, PhD, ABPP, is a psychologist and psychoanalyst at the Austen Riggs Center, Chair of the Association for the Psychoanalysis of Culture and Society (APCS), and Scholar of the British Psychoanalytic Council. Affiliations include the Chicago Center for Psychoanalysis; Boston Graduate School of Psychoanalysis; Universidad de Monterrey; and Harvard Medical School. Books include *Patterns*;

Constructing Realities; *Learning from Experience*; *Working with Trauma*; *Psychoanalysis and Literature; Introduction to Contemporary Psychoanalysis; Fragments of Trauma and the Social Production of Suffering* (with Michael O'Loughlin); *Women and Psychosis* and *Women and The Psychosocial Construction of Madness* (with Marie Brown); and *The Importance of Play in Early Childhood Education* (with Jill Bellinson).

32. Rethinking Psychiatry with Mad Studies

Bradley Lewis, MD, PhD, is a psychiatrist and psychotherapist with interdisciplinary training in the arts, humanities, and continental philosophy. He is associate professor at New York University's Gallatin School of Individualized Study and has affiliations with the Department of Social and Cultural Analysis and the Disability Studies Program. He is on the editorial board of the *Journal of Medical Humanities*. His books include *Moving Beyond Prozac, DSM, and the New Psychiatry: The Birth of Postpsychiatry* and *Narrative Psychiatry: How Stories Can Shape Clinical Encounters*, and *Experiencing Epiphanies in Literature, Cinema, and Everyday Life* (forthcoming).

33. The Ex-Patients' Movement: Where We've Been and Where We're Going

Judi Chamberlin was a pioneer in the psychiatric survivors' movement, spending four decades as an activist leader. After several voluntary hospitalizations for depression as a young woman, Chamberlin was involuntarily committed in 1971. Her experiences in the mental health system galvanized her to take action on patients' rights, and she helped found the Mental Patients' Liberation Front in Cambridge, Mass. Her book, *On Our Own: Patient Controlled Alternatives to the Mental Health System* (1978), is considered a key text in the intellectual development of the movement. In recognition of her advocacy, she was awarded the Distinguished Service Award by the President's Committee on Employment of People with Disabilities in 1992, the David J. Vail National Advocacy Award, and the 1995 Pike Prize, which honors those who have given outstanding service to people with disabilities.

34. The Icarus Project: A Counter Narrative for Psychic Diversity

Sascha Altman DuBrul, MSW, was a co-founder of The Icarus Project (https:// icarusprojectarchive.org/) and is now a lead trainer with the Institute for the Development of Human Arts (www.idha-nyc.org/). For more than two decades, DuBrul has been laying the foundations for a Transformative Mental Health movement which understands human suffering and mental difference as a catalyst for generative change, rather than pathology. He is an Internal Family Systems practitioner and can be reached at: https://www.saschadubrul.com.

35. Ending Coercion

Alberto Vásquez Encalada (see Chapter 25).

36. Language Games Used to Construct Autism as Pathology

Nick Chown is a book indexer who undertakes autism research alongside autistic colleagues in the Independent Autism Research Group. He co-edited *Neurodiversity Studies: A New Critical Paradigm* (2020), reviews for autism and disability journals, and has written numerous academic articles. He is a member of a small international group of scholars who founded Autistic Scholars International in November 2023.

37. The Black Wisdom Collective

Kelechi Ubozoh is a Nigerian-American writer, mental health advocate, coach, and facilitator with over a decade of experience working in the California mental health system in the areas of research and advocacy, community engagement, suicide prevention, youth development and peer support. Her story of surviving a suicide attempt is featured in *The S Word* documentary, *O, The Oprah Magazine* and *CBS This Morning with Gayle King*. Her book with LD Green, *We've Been Too Patient: Voices from Radical Mental Health*, elevates marginalized voices of lived experience who have endured psychiatric mistreatment is featured in curriculum at Boston University and New York University. Learn more at kelechiubozoh.com.

38. Mad Resistance/Mad Alternatives: Democratizing Mental Health Care

Jeremy Andersen is a senior clinician and education manager at Windhorse Integrative Mental Health in Northampton, Massachussets. Before joining Windhorse, Jeremy worked as a psychotherapist in urban and rural community mental health clinics, as a counselor for a therapeutic afterschool program, and as a direct care worker for people with developmental disabilities. He has served in leadership positions at the Berkeley and Pioneer Valley Shambhala Centers and is an authorized meditation instructor in the Shambhala Buddhist tradition. Jeremy has a BA in transpersonal psychology from Burlington College, an MA in integral counseling psychology from the California Institute of Integral Studies, and a CAGS in professional counseling from Union Institute and University.

Ed Altwies, PsyD, was the program manager for the Queens Parachute NYC mobile team and a clinician on the Brooklyn early episode team. He participated in hundreds of Open Dialogue-style network meetings with more than 35 families from a diverse range of cultural backgrounds. He was also a consultant to the NYC Department of Health where he was a co-trainer to three of the Parachute training cohorts. Prior to working with Parachute NYC, Ed completed two years of training at the Institute for Dialogic Practice. He is currently in private practice in NYC and staff clinician at Kings County Hospital.

Jonah Bossewitch, PhD, is a technologist, writer, and educator who lives in Connecticut with his partner and young son. A native New Yorker, Jonah grew up in the city and studied communications at Columbia University. His doctoral dissertation, *Dangerous Gifts: Towards a New Wave of Psychiatric Resistance*, examined significant shifts in the politics of psychiatric resistance and mental health activism. He is an advocate for mental health and cares deeply about free speech, the environment, and social justice. He has over 20 years of experience as a professional software architect, engineering leader, and free software contributor. He earned a master's in communication and education at Teachers College (2007) and graduated from Princeton University (1997) with a BA cum laude in philosophy and certificates in computer science and cognitive studies. He blogs intermittently at https://alchemicalmusings.org.

Celia Brown was a longtime leader in the mad pride movement. She presented nationally and internationally on topics such as self-help, peer counseling, human rights, trauma, and cultural competency. She was president of the board of MindFreedom International, and she promoted choice, alternatives, and human rights in mental health. Celia was instrumental in developing the first peer specialist civil title in the country, and she was a founding member of the National People of Color/Consumer Survivor Network. She was the Regional Advocacy Specialist at the NYC field office of the NYS Office of Mental Health and a co-founder of the International Network Towards Alternatives and Recovery. She graduated from the Center to Study Recovery in Social Contexts, Nathan Klein Institute.

Kermit Cole, MFT, was the founding editor of the *Mad in America* webzine. He began working in residential settings with people in psychotic states in 2002 while participating in research on schizophrenia at Harvard—inspired, in part, by Bob Whitaker's "Mad in America." This experience, along with learning the value of working with families (from direct experience as well as the inspiration of Open Dialogue) led Kermit to become licensed as a marriage and family therapist. He and his partner run the Santa Fe Relational Therapy Center, where they work with couples and families seeking alternative ways of working with madness.

Sera Davidow is an activist, advocate, filmmaker, author, and mother of two. She has spent most of the last two decades as a part of the leadership team for the Wildflower Alliance (formerly known as Western Massachusetts Recovery Learning Community or RLC) where she has sought to change the dominant narratives about suicide, self-injury, and what constitutes a "crisis," as well as what "help" should look like when someone is struggling. Sera is also a founding member of the Hearing Voices USA Board of Directors and a frequent contributor to *Mad in America*. You can learn more about her life and work in the 2017 *Sun Magazine* article, "An Open Mind" (thesunmagazine.org/issues/496/an-open-mind).

Sascha Altman DuBrul (see Chapter 34).

Eric Friedland-Kays is a senior clinician and administrator at Windhorse Integrative Mental Health, in Northampton, MA, where he has worked since 2000. He earned a master's degree from the School for International Training and has been a psychotherapist for many years trained in intensive psychotherapy, psychosynthesis, and contemplative traditions. He has also been a meditator deeply connected with Vipassana meditation, in the tradition of S. N. Goenka, since the early 1990s. He lives in Western Massachusetts with his wife, seven-year-old daughter, and two Cornish Rex cats.

Will Hall (see Chapter 42).

Chris Hansen is a co-director of Intentional Peer Support and has been co-teaching and developing Intentional Peer Support internationally with Shery Mead and now Lisa Archibald for the past 17 years. Chris has spent 25 years involved in local, national, and international peer support and advocacy initiatives from a lived experience perspective. Chris was a member of the New Zealand delegation to the United Nations for the development of the Convention for the Rights of Persons with Disabilities, has served on the board of the World Network of Users and Survivors of Psychiatry, and has played a key role in the development of a number of peer-run crisis respites and alternatives.

Bradley Lewis (see Chapter 32).

Audre Lorde Project (ALP) is a Lesbian, Gay, Bisexual, Two Spirit, Trans and Gender Non-Conforming People of Color center for community organizing, focusing on the New York City area. Through mobilization, education, and capacity building, we work for community wellness and progressive social and economic justice. Committed to struggling across differences, we seek to responsibly reflect, represent, and serve our various communities. Initiated as an organizing effort by a coalition of LGBTSTGNC People of Color, ALP was first brought together by Advocates for Gay Men of Color (a multi-racial network of gay men of color HIV policy advocates) in 1994. The vision for ALP grew out of the expressed need for innovative and unified community strategies to address the multiple issues impacting LGBTSTGNC People of Color communities.

Maryse Mitchell-Brody (they/them) is a white, Jewish, and trans facilitator, fundraiser, and radical social worker. They are director of development at the Third Wave Fund—dedicated to youth-led, intersectional gender justice activism. Maryse has been active in movements for healing justice, sex worker organizing, racial justice, economic justice, and LGBTQI+ liberation for over 25 years. In 2018, Maryse co-organized the Sex Worker Giving Circle (SWGC), the first sex worker-led fund housed at a US foundation and joined Third Wave's staff in 2019 to continue that work. Today, they focus on fundraising for Third Wave's Spotlight Funds: the SWGC, the Accountable Futures Fund, and the Disability Frontlines Fund. Raised in NYC, Maryse now lives on Mahican land in the Northern Catskills region of New

York with their partner and dog, along with their many non-human neighbors in the beech-maple forest.

Jacks McNamara (see Chapter 8).

Gina Nikkel was the president and CEO of the Foundation for Excellence in Mental Health Care, a community foundation that matches the passion of private philanthropy with researchers and programs to bring recovery practices to every community. She is associate clinical professor of psychiatry at Oregon Health and Sciences University, and she served as executive director of the Association of Oregon Community Mental Health Programs for 11 years before taking the helm of EXCELLENCE. She has worked extensively in mental health and addiction policy, leadership and management, health care financing, and political advocacy. As a community mental health therapist, adolescent program director, and clinical supervisor, she brings experience in all aspects of community mental health. Gina's public service includes two terms as a Tillamook County commissioner and vice president of the Association of Oregon Counties. She has a BA in theater and dance, an MS in counseling from Portland State University, and a PhD in education, focusing on social public policy and leadership, from the University of Oregon.

Madigan Shive, also known as Bonfire Madigan, is an American songwriter, performing artist, community organizer, and musician. She is contributing author to the anthology *Live through This: On Creativity and Self-Destruction*. www.bonfiremadigan.com

David Stark is a peer educator and a peer counselor at Windhorse Integrative Mental Health in Northampton, Massachusetts. An account of his time as a Windhorse client was published by Springer in 2000 as "Sanity Recovered" in *Housecalls: Psychosocial Interventions in the Home*. He is currently a graduate student in the community mental health and clinical mental health counseling program at Southern New Hampshire University.

Adaku Utah hails from Nigeria and is an award-winning liberation educator and organizer, healer, and performance ritual artist committed to healing and liberation within oppressed communities. For over ten years, her work has centered on movements for radical social change, with a focus on gender, sexuality, race, youth, and healing justice. She is the founder and director of Harriet's Apothecary, a healing village led by Black Cis Women and Queer and Trans folks committed to living out Harriet Tubman's legacy of liberation in our tissues and our lineage. She is also the founder of BeatBox Botanicals, a local sliding-scale, love-centered, and community-inspired plant medicine and healing practice. Adaku has taught, organized, created sacred healing spaces, and performed both nationally and internationally as a Social Change Initiatives Coordinator, rape crisis counselor, youth organizer, intuitive healer, advocate against gender-based violence, dancer, liberation trainer, sex education teacher, herbalist, sexual violence organizing educator, and board member for several organizations including Yale University, Chicago Foundation for Women, the Illinois Caucus for Adolescent Health, Black Lives Matter, Students Active for Ending Rape (SAFER), Lincoln Center, Brooklyn Museum, Sadie Nash Leadership

Project, and more. Her greatest desire is to embody the sacredness and wholeness of love and support herself, humanity, and our larger ecosystem in garnering and using our tools of love, healing, and liberation to fashion just and sustainable realities.

39. Black Resilience in the Face of Bullshit: Wellness and Safety Plan

Adaku Utah (see Chapter 38)

40. Demolition, Abolition, and the Legacy of Madness

Leah Harris, writer and advocate with over 20 years of experience training and facilitating in trauma-responsive and social justice approaches in mental health, writes of their intimate journey to remember their mother, who faced repeated violence and oppression within psychiatric asylums.

41. A Critical Overview of Mental Health-Related Beliefs, Services and Systems in Uganda and Recent Activist and Legal Challenges

Kabale Benon Kitafuna is a human rights defender, mental health care activist, and executive director of the Mental Health Recovery Initiative.

42. Letter to the Mother of a "Schizophrenic": We Must Do Better Than Forced Treatment

Will Hall, MA, is a schizophrenia diagnosis survivor and therapist trained in Open Dialogue and Jungian psychology. Host of Madness Radio and author of the *Harm Reduction Guide to Coming Off Psychiatric Drugs* and *Outside Mental Health: Voices and Visions of Madness*, Will's disability advocacy has won several awards, including the Judi Chamberlin award. He appears in the documentaries *Crazywise* and *Healing Voices*, and is co-founder of the Hearing Voices Network USA, co-founder of Freedom Center, and past co-coordinator of The Icarus Project.

43. With the Launch of Mad in Denmark, a Global Network for Radical Change Grows Stronger

Robert Whitaker is the author of five books, three of which tell of the history of psychiatry. In 2010, his *Anatomy of an Epidemic: Magic Bullets, Psychiatric Drugs, and the Astonishing Rise of Mental Illness* won the US Investigative Reporters and Editors book award for best investigative journalism. Prior to writing books, he worked as a science reporter at the *Albany Times Union* newspaper in New York for a number of years. He is the founder of madinamerica.com, a website that features research news and blogs by an international group of writers interested in "rethinking psychiatry."

44. Defunding Sanity

Raj Mariwala is director, Mariwala Health Initiative, an advocacy, capacity building, and grant-making organization in India that focuses on mental health and marginalization. Using the standpoint of lived experience of mental illness and learning/developmental disabilities, their interest areas and activism lie at the intersection of feminist, queer-trans, and mad studies. Raj is also a practicing canine and feline behaviorist.

45. Making the Case for Multiplicity: A Holistic Framework for Madness and Transformation

Jazmine Russell is a holistic counselor, mental health educator, and scholar at the intersection of mad studies, critical psychology, and neuroscience. She is the host of "Depth Work: A Holistic Mental Health Podcast" and co-founder of the Institute for the Development of Human Arts, a training institute that brings together people with lived experience and professional knowledge to educate and build community around transformative mental health practices.

Index

For Product Safety Concerns and Information please contact our EU representative GPSR@taylorandfrancis.com Taylor & Francis Verlag GmbH, Kaufingerstraße 24, 80331 München, Germany